Inflammatory Diseases of the Central Nervous System

4125

This book is to be returned on or before the last date stamped

09. JUN 1 ?.

4132

Inflammatory Diseases of the Central Nervous System

Professor Trevor Kilpatrick MB BS PhD FRACP
Professor of Neurology and Director
Centre for Neuroscience
The University of Melbourne
Parkville, Victoria, Australia

Professor Richard M. Ransohoff MD
Director
Neuroinflammation Research Center
Department of Neuroscience
Lerner Research Institute
Cleveland Clinic
Cleveland, Ohio, USA

Professor Steven Wesselingh MBBS PhD FRACP
Dean
Faculty of Medicine, Nursing and Health Sciences
Monash University
Clayton, Victoria, Australia

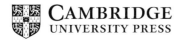

CAMBRIDGE
UNIVERSITY PRESS

CAMBRIDGE UNIVERSITY PRESS
Cambridge, New York, Melbourne, Madrid, Cape Town,
Singapore, São Paulo, Delhi, Dubai, Tokyo

Cambridge University Press
The Edinburgh Building, Cambridge CB2 8RU, UK

Published in the United States of America by
Cambridge University Press, New York

www.cambridge.org

Information on this title: www.cambridge.org/
9780521888745

First published 2010

Printed in the United Kingdom at the University Press,
Cambridge

*A catalog record for this publication is available from the
British Library*

ISBN 978-0-521-88874-5 Hardback

Contents

List of Contributors   *page* vii
Preface   ix

Section 1: Interactions between the immune and nervous systems

1   **Effectors and determinants of the innate and adaptive immune responses**   1
Edgar Meinl & Hartmut Wekerle

2   **Microglia: protective and pathogenic mediators**   15
Bevyn Jarrott & Karina Apricò

3   **The role of dendritic cells in neuro-inflammation**   27
Heather Donaghy, Edwina J. Wright & Anthony L. Cunningham

4   **Negotiating the brain barriers: access of immune cells and pathogens into the CNS**   35
Britta Engelhardt

Section 2: Autoimmunity

5   **Immune effector heterogeneity in multiple sclerosis and related CNS inflammatory demyelinating disorders**   47
Shanu F. Roemer & Claudia F. Lucchinetti

6   **Multiple sclerosis: neuro-immune cross-talk in acute and progressive stages of the disease**   75
Martin Kerschensteiner & Reinhard Hohlfeld

7   **CD8+ T cell-mediated autoimmune diseases of the CNS**   87
Lisa Walter & Matthew L. Albert

8   **Acute disseminated encephalomyelitis: determinants and manifestations**   97
Eppie M. Yiu & Andrew J. Kornberg

9   **Primary angiitis of the CNS and its mimics**   109
Tina Chadha, George F. Duna & Leonard H. Calabrese

Section 3: Microbiological and traumatic challenges to the CNS

10   **Acute viral encephalitis: role of the immune system in viral clearance from the CNS and in the generation of pathology**   125
David N. Irani & Natalie Prow

11   **Chronic HIV infection of the CNS: role of the immune system in virological control and the generation of pathology**   137
Carolyn F. Orr & Bruce J. Brew

12   **Brain inflammation during bacterial meningitis**   161
Trine H. Mogensen & Lars Østergaard

13   **Parasitic infections of the brain: malaria and beyond**   173
Stephen J. Rogerson & Danny A. Milner Jr

14   **Role of the inflammatory process in traumatic brain damage**   185
Cristina Morganti-Kossmann, Laveniya Satgunaseelan, Nicole Bye, Phuong Nguyen & Thomas Kossmann

Section 4: Therapy

15   **HIV-associated neurocognitive disorders: clinical features and therapeutic challenges**   201
Nicoline Schiess & Justin C. McArthur

16 **Role of immunomodulation in management of infections of the CNS** 221
Miles H. Beaman

17 **Neuro-inflammation: an emerging therapeutic target in neurological disease** 245
Joseph M. Antony & Christopher Power

Index 261

The colour plates are to be found between pages 86 and 87

Contributors

Matthew L. Albert MD PhD
The Laboratory of Dendritic Cell Immunobiology, Institut Pasteur, Paris France

Joseph M. Antony PhD
Developmental & Stem Cell Biology Program, Hospital for Sick Children, Toronto, Ontario, Canada

Karina Apricò BSc PhD
Department of Human Physiology & Anatomy, School of Human Biosciences, La Trobe University, Melbourne, Victoria, Australia

Miles H. Beaman MBBS FRACP FRCPA
Department of Microbiology, Western Diagnostic Pathology, Perth, WA, Australia; Department of Medicine, University of Notre Dame, Freemantle, WA, Australia

Bruce J. Brew MBBS MD FRACP
Department of Neurology, St Vincent's Hospital, Darlinghurst, NSW, Australia

Nicole Bye BSc
National Trauma Research Institute, The Alfred Hospital/Monash University, Melbourne, Victoria, Australia

Leonard H. Calabrese DO
Rheumatic & Immunologic Disease, Cleveland Clinic, Cleveland, OH, USA

Tina Chadha MD
Department of Immunology, Allergy & Rheumatology, Baylor College of Medicine, Houston, TX, USA

Anthony L. Cunningham MD
Centre for Virus Research, Westmead Millennium Institute, Sydney, NSW, Australia

Heather Donaghy PhD
Centre for Virus Research, Westmead Millennium Institute, Sydney, NSW, Australia

George F. Duna MD
Department of Immunology, Allergy & Rheumatology, Baylor College of Medicine, Houston, TX, USA

Britta Engelhardt PhD
Theodor Kocher Institute, University of Bern, Bern, Switzerland

Reinhard Hohlfeld MD
Institute of Clinical Neuroimmunology, Ludwig Maximilians University, Munich, Germany; Department of Neuroimmunology, Max Planck Institute of Neurobiology, Martinsried, Germany

David N. Irani MD
Department of Neurology, University of Michigan Medical School, Ann Arbor, MI, USA

Bevyn Jarrott PhD BPharm
Florey Neuroscience Institutes, University of Melbourne, Melbourne, Victoria, Australia

Martin Kerschensteiner MD
Institute for Clinical Neuroimmunology, Ludwig Maximilians University, Munich, Germany

Andrew J. Kornberg FRACP
Department of Neurology, The Royal Children's Hospital, Melbourne, Victoria, Australia

Thomas Kossmann MD
Epworth Healthcare, Melbourne, Victoria, Australia

Claudia F. Lucchinetti MD
Department of Neurology, Mayo Clinic, Rochester, MN, USA

Justin C. McArthur MBBS MPH
Department of Neurology, Johns Hopkins
University School of Medicine, Baltimore,
MD, USA

Edgar Meinl MD
Institute of Clinical Neuroimmunology, Ludwig
Maximilians University, Munich, Germany;
Department of Neuroimmunology, Max Planck
Institute of Neurobiology, Martinsried, Germany

Danny A. Milner Jr MD
Department of Pathology, Brigham & Women's
Hospital, Boston, MA, USA

Trine H. Mogensen MD PhD
Department of Infectious Diseases, Aarhus
University Hospital, Skejby, Aarhus, Denmark

Cristina Morganti-Kossmann PhD
National Trauma Research Institute, The Alfred
Hospital/Monash University, Melbourne,
Victoria, Australia

Phuong Nguyen
National Trauma Research Institute, The Alfred
Hospital/Monash University, Melbourne,
Victoria, Australia

Carolyn F. Orr MBBS PhD FRACP
Department of Neurology, St Vincent's Hospital,
Darlinghurst, NSW, Australia

Lars Østergaard MD PhD DMSc
Department of Infectious Diseases, Aarhus
University Hospital, Skejby, Aarhus, Denmark

Christopher Power MD FRCPC
Department of Medicine (Neurology), University
of Alberta, Edmonton, Alberta, Canada

Natalie Prow
Department of Molecular Microbiology &
Immunology, Johns Hopkins Bloomberg
School of Public Health, Baltimore,
MD, USA

Shanu F. Roemer MD
Department of Neurology, Mayo Clinic,
Rochester, MN, USA

Stephen J. Rogerson PhD MRCP FRACP
Department of Medicine, University of
Melbourne, Parkville, Victoria, Australia

Laveniya Satgunaseelan
National Trauma Research Institute,
The Alfred Hospital/Monash University,
Melbourne, Victoria, Australia

Nicoline Schiess MD
Department of Neurology, Johns Hopkins
University School of Medicine, Baltimore,
MD, USA

Lisa Walter PhD
Department of Pharmacology, University
of Cologne, Cologne, Germany

Hartmut Wekerle MD
Department of Neuroimmunology,
Max Planck Institute of Neurobiology,
Munich, Germany

Edwina J. Wright
Infectious Diseases Unit, Alfred Hospital,
Melbourne, Victoria, Australia

Eppie M. Yiu MBBS
Department of Neurology, Royal Children's
Hospital, Melbourne, Victoria, Australia

Preface

When Richard Ransohoff, Steve Wesselingh and I first met to consider editing a book dedicated to inflammatory diseases of the brain, we were all enthused by the important messages it could convey and the niche it could assume. We wanted to convey the sense of excitement that is operative in this field and how new knowledge in basic immunology and its unique nuances within the brain have seeded novel perspectives concerning the pathogenesis and treatment of both autoimmune and infectious diseases of this exquisitely complex organ. For too long, undergraduates have been taught inaccurate dogma concerning the nexus between the immune and nervous systems. This book aims to dispel that dogma and to provide an articulate account of our current understanding of the complex interactions that are operative between immune and neural cells, both in the healthy state and in the context of disease, where not only the nature but also the magnitude of the inflammatory response can be a key determinant of whether it is reparative or pathogenic.

The organization of the book is designed to be both user friendly and easy to negotiate for the practicing clinician. The contents are divided into a section dedicated to basic immunology, with special attention given to features specific and relevant to neuroinflammation; a section focusing on autoimmune diseases; a section that concentrates on microbiological and traumatic challenges to the central nervous system; and finally, a section dedicated to therapy, providing both generic principles and valuable insights relevant to specific infections, including HIV, as well as to the management of autoimmune disease, in particular multiple sclerosis. The book should be a valuable reference for both undergraduates and clinicians but also for basic scientists who wish to establish a broad knowledge base in order to provide a context to their specific research focus.

It has been a privilege to work with Richard Ransohoff and Steve Wesselingh on this book. They are truly leaders in the field of inflammatory diseases of the brain and their complementary interests, one directed to basic immunology and its application to autoimmune disease and the other to infectious diseases, have helped to provide this book with its unique perspective. They have worked tirelessly to bring this project to its fruition. The contributing authors have also provided us with an outstanding set of chapters and I thank them for their dedication to the cause and patience as the book has gone through its various iterations.

I would also like to thank key people at Cambridge University Press for their patience and enthusiasm for this work. In particular, I would like to thank Nicholas Dunton and Dawn Preston who have overseen the project. Special thanks also to Carmel McFarlane, my PA, who has maintained her dedication to the cause throughout, and who has applied herself to the significant task of collating the work with a combination of good humour and skill. My thanks also to Agnes Wong for her considerable role in proofreading the manuscripts.

Effectors and determinants of the innate and adaptive immune responses

Edgar Meinl and Hartmut Wekerle

Introduction

Multicellular organisms must protect themselves against a plethora of exogenous enemies surrounding them. In the case of microbes, the body relies on several, scaled strategies. Firstly, there are external membranes, such as the skin and mucous membranes, that ward off most potential intruders. The physical barriers are highly efficient, but not perfect; at any time, a few potential pathogens can leak through and invade the tissues. These invaders are dealt with by an intricate system of internal defense, the immune system, which identifies the foreign pathogen and mounts a response with the ultimate aim to neutralize and eliminate it.

There are principally two classes of immune responses, one, the innate immune response, is based on response elements preformed within the body, and thus is immediately available upon contact with a microbial target. The other response type, adaptive immunity, develops following the first contact with the pathogen. It produces specific effector cells and humoral antibodies, which are exclusively programmed to exterminate infectious agents, and it provides an immunological memory (Table 1.1).

Importantly, however, innate and adaptive immune reactions are not strictly separated, but tightly interconnected (Medzhitov, 2001). Thus, in the course of early innate immune reactions, the presentation of antigens to cells of the adaptive immune system is enhanced, while, conversely, ongoing adaptive reactions can trigger or enhance innate reactivity.

The general rules of immune response are of proven validity for most of the body's organs and tissues. They also govern protection of the central nervous system (CNS), although in a modified version that takes into account the particular requirements of these very special tissues. This chapter will discuss how innate and adaptive immune responses function in the CNS to maintain health and to modulate different diseases.

Innate immunity

Innate immune reactivity is the oldest version of immunity. It acts throughout phylogeny, in insects as in mammals, even in plants. Like its adaptive counterpart, the innate immune system must be able to distinguish between foreign structures, which are to be discarded, and the various components of the "self", which must be tolerated. Recognition of infectious non-self is mediated by a limited number of germline-encoded *pattern-recognition receptors* (PRRs), that recognize structural motifs typical for microbial agents, and which trigger rapid inflammatory responses (Medzhitov and Janeway, 1997). Some PRRs can also recognize endogenous "danger signals" (Wagner, 2006), such as mitochondrial components leaking out of a destroyed cell. These receptors alert the immune system to cell damage, independent of microbial infection. Activation of innate immune pathways occurs in the brain classically in infectious diseases of the CNS, but also under "sterile" conditions (Wyss-Coray and Mucke, 2002). Brain injury, neurodegeneration, ischemia, autoimmunity and neoplasia can all give rise to innate immune responses within the CNS tissues. The consequences of innate immune activation in non-infectious CNS diseases are ambiguous. Dependent on the context, the reactions can either mediate damage to neurons or, in contrast, protect them from exogenous insult.

Pattern recognition receptors: TLR, NLR, RLR, and others

Throughout evolution, some structures have remained unchanged while others were either lost or profoundly modified. The PRRs make use of structural motifs that are present in primitive organisms (e.g. bacteria), but which are not expressed in vertebrates. To initiate immune responses, PRRs recognize pathogen-associated molecular patterns (PAMPs). The PRRs are present in

Inflammatory Diseases of the Central Nervous System, ed. T. Kilpatrick, R. M. Ransohoff and S. Wesselingh. Published by Cambridge University Press. © Cambridge University Press 2010

Table 1.1 Innate and adaptive immunity

Property	Innate immune system	Adaptive immune system
Receptors	PRR fixed in genome	Gene segments, rearrangement, diversity
Responding cells	Immune cells, tissue resident cells (microglia, astrocytes, neurons?)	B cells, T cells
Recognized targets	Conserved molecular patterns	Details of molecular structure: proteins, peptides, carbohydrates
Self/Non-self discrimination	Endogenous PRR ligands as danger signals	Autoreactive T cells and B cells are a component of the normal immune repertoire
Memory	Memory of the species	Individual memory

Modified from: Janeway and Medzhitov, *Ann Rev Immunol* 2002, **20**: 197–216.
PRR: Pattern recognition receptor.

three different compartments: soluble in body fluids, immobilized on cell membranes, and internally within the cell, that is within the cytoplasm. The PRRs belong to different families, namely *toll-like receptors* (TLRs), RIG-like receptors (e.g. RIG-I, MDA5), NOD-like receptors (e.g. NOD-1, NALP-3), C-type lectins (e.g. DC-SIGN), scavenger receptors (e.g. CD36), complement factors (C1q, C3), collectins (mannose-binding lectin) and pentraxins (e.g. CRP) (Lee and Kim, 2007).

The TLRs are the best-characterized signal generating receptors among the PRRs. The *Toll* gene was discovered in *Drosophila* as a gene involved in antimicrobial immunity, but subsequent studies also identified related genes in vertebrates (Hoffmann *et al.*, 1999). Currently we know of 13 mammalian TLR paralogues. The TLRs 1, 2, 4, 5, and 6 are located mainly on the cell surface and recognize primarily bacterial components, while TLRs 3, 7, 8, and 9 are located *within* the cell and mainly recognize viral products (Lee and Kim, 2007). The ligands for TLRs 10, 12 and 13 remain unidentified. The TLR family members are not equally distributed across species; for example, TLR10 is expressed in humans but not in mice; TLR8 is not functional in mice; and TLRs 11, 12, and 13 are expressed in mice but not humans (Baccalà *et al.*, 2007). Multiple negative regulatory mechanisms have also evolved to attenuate TLR signaling to maintain immunological balance (Liew *et al.*, 2005).

Two other families of innate receptors, namely NOD-like receptors (NLRs) and RIG-I-like receptors (RLRs), cooperate with TLRs. The NLRs detect bacteria, whereas the RLRs detect viruses. The NLRs and RLRs trigger responses similar to TLRs (Creagh and O'Neill, 2006; Meylan *et al.*, 2006).

Recognition of self by PRR

Importantly, certain TLRs are activated by *endogenous* ligands, components of the body's own tissues. The TLR4, for example, binds numerous ligands, which include fibrinogen, fibronectin, heparin sulfate, hyaluronan, and heat shock proteins (HSPs) (Kielian, 2006). It should be noted, however, that some initial descriptions of endogenous TLR4 ligands could have been obscured by LPS contamination of the "endogenous" antigen preparations (Bausinger *et al.*, 2002). Independent of this, there is now overwhelming evidence that TLRs can also be activated by endogenous ligands. In addition, endogenous RNA and DNA are recognized by the endosomal nucleic acid recognizing TLRs; additionally, evidence for TLR-independent recognition pathways of endogenous nucleic acids has been obtained (Wagner, 2006). Binding of endogenous nucleotides to TLRs (such as TLR7 and 9) seems to be involved in triggering systemic autoimmunity (Marshak-Rothstein, 2006).

There are additional PRRs specific for host endogenous components; for example, scavenger receptors A and CD36 can recognize apoptotic cells and initiate their phagocytosis (Lee and Kim, 2007). In addition, NALP3, a component of a molecular complex called the inflammasome, is critical for recognizing endogenous danger signals such as extracellular ATP and uric acid crystals (Fritz *et al.*, 2006).

Mutations in NALP3 have been found to be responsible for three rare human autoinflammatory disorders: Muckle–Wells syndrome, familial cold autoinflammatory syndrome, and chronic infantile neurological cutaneous and articular syndrome. Interestingly, these diseases respond well to treatment with IL-1 receptor antagonist, redirecting attention to IL-1 as a critical mediator of inflammation (Agostini et al., 2004).

An additional link between PRR engagement and autoimmunity has emerged in a mouse model of spontaneous systemic lupus erythematosus (SLE). In lupus-prone MRL/l mice, functional deficiency of TLR9 enhanced the development of disease, indicating that TLR9 might be involved in the maintenance of tolerance (Ehlers and Ravetch, 2007).

CNS resident cells and innate immune reactivity

Innate immunity is firmly established within the CNS. Several PRRs are constitutively expressed in CNS cells, others require induction. In particular, CD14 and TLR2 have been detected in circumventricular organs, in the choroid plexus and the leptomeninges, all representing CNS areas that lack a complete blood–brain barrier (BBB) and which are particularly exposed to invading pathogens (Rivest, 2003). Inflamed CNS tissues increase production of functional PRRs. Active multiple sclerosis (MS) lesions display high levels of TLR3 and TLR4 in their local microglial cells (Bsibsi et al. 2002).

In general, resident myeloid cells, namely the microglia, are the main players in innate immune responses within the CNS (Aloisi, 2001). However, evidence is emerging that, in addition, astrocytes, the most abundant glial cell population of the CNS, substantially contribute to local innate immune response against a variety of insults (Farina et al., 2007).

Low basal levels of TLR4 expression have been identified in microglia in vivo (Bsibsi et al., 2002). Accordingly, systemic administration of the TLR4 ligand, LPS, leads to rapid up-regulation of TLR2 in microglia and generates an innate inflammatory response that is readily detected and more prominent in BBB-free areas of the CNS but also extends into the brain parenchyma (Farina et al., 2007). Basal levels of TLR3 are noted in the healthy brain, detectable on astrocytes in the hippocampus and striatum (Park et al., 2006). Indeed, several recent in vitro studies have confirmed TLR3 as the predominant TLR expressed by astrocytes. Two reports analyzed the complete human TLR repertoire in human fetal astrocytes by quantitative polymerase chain reaction and pointed to TLR3 as the only TLR with consistent expression in the resting condition (Farina et al., 2005; Jack et al., 2005). The TLR3 was also up-regulated following treatment with inflammatory cytokines such as IL-1β, IFN-β and IFN-γ (Farina et al., 2005).

The central role of astrocytes in regulating neuro-inflammation was recently demonstrated in vivo (Brambilla et al., 2005; van Loo et al., 2006a). Transgenic mice were generated in which NF-kB, an important transcription factor controlling innate immune responses, was selectively inactivated in astrocytes (Brambilla et al., 2005). While these mice displayed normal spinal cord architecture, their functional recovery after injury was dramatically improved. These observations correlated with a drop in leukocyte recruitment into the lesioned area due to the reduced NF-kB-dependent expression of CXCL10 and CCL2 (Brambilla et al., 2005). Similarly, blockade of the NF-kB pathway in neuroectodermal cells of the CNS (including neurons, astrocytes and oligodendrocytes) led to a consistent decrease in pro-inflammatory gene expression during experimental autoimmune encephalomyelitis (EAE) (van Loo et al., 2006b). In summary, the NF-kB pathway in astrocytes is a key regulator of inflammation in the CNS and its inhibition has beneficial effects on tissue regeneration.

In addition to glial cells, neurons can also participate in innate immune reactions. While the production of IFN-γ by neurons was observed some time ago (Neumann et al., 1997a), recent evidence shows that neurons also produce type I interferons (reviewed in Paul et al., 2007). There is also recent evidence that also establishes the expression of TLR3 (Lafon et al., 2006) and TLR8 (Ma et al., 2006) by neurons.

Innate immune activation in the periphery can promote CNS autoimmunity

Several lines of evidence link infections in peripheral tissues and microbial structures to autoimmune processes in the CNS. In a model of spontaneous EAE in transgenic mice, EAE developed more readily in mice housed in a non-sterile facility than in those maintained in a sterile, specific pathogen-free environment (Goverman et al., 1993). Multiple TLR agonists act as potent adjuvants in the induction of autoimmunity (Hansen et al., 2006). The TLR2 agonist PGN is capable of inducing clinical disease in a MOG model of EAE when emulsified in incomplete Freund's adjuvant (IFA), whereas MOG in IFA alone is incapable of inducing disease (Visser et al., 2005). In addition, CpG plus LPS can promote MBP-induced EAE in

Lewis rats (Wolf *et al.*, 2007). Activation of antigen presenting cells (APCs) via innate immune receptors can break self-tolerance and trigger the development of autoimmunity even in a genetically resistant strain (Waldner *et al.*, 2004). These studies indicate that innate immune activation in the periphery promotes autoimmune exacerbations in the CNS.

When considering potential links between microbial infections and autoimmunity, it is also necessary to take account of the so-called hygiene hypothesis, in which some infections are posited to keep the immune system balanced, thereby inducing immunoregulation and preventing allergy and autoimmunity (Kamradt *et al.*, 2005).

Activation of the innate immune system within the CNS modulates brain pathology

The expression of TLRs is up-regulated in the CNS during diseases such as EAE (Zekki *et al.*, 2002). It is intriguing that under sterile conditions, innate immune activation within the CNS can modulate disease activity. Indeed, as a consistent feature of different CNS diseases, microglia and astrocyte activation and enhanced expression of TLRs are observed (Kielian, 2006; Farina *et al.*, 2007; Nguyen *et al.*, 2002). This begs the question as to the repertoire of TLR ligands in sterile CNS diseases. On the one hand, it is possible that pathogen-derived TLR ligands could be imported into the CNS by invading immune cells. Indeed, phagocytes containing a disease-promoting TLR/NOD ligand have been observed in the brain during demyelinating disease in primates (Visser *et al.*, 2006). On the other hand, there are also endogenous TLR ligands (see above), that might engage the up-regulated TLRs within the CNS.

In vivo evidence favoring an active role for TLR in sterile CNS diseases has been obtained in several models. Stereotactic axotomy in the entorhinal cortex results in substantial induction of pro-inflammatory cytokines and chemokines. This reaction is markedly reduced in TLR2-deficient mice, (Babcock *et al.*, 2006). Further, encephalitogenic T cells are less efficient in inducing EAE when transferred into TLR9-deficient hosts, suggesting that endogenous host-derived cells aggravate autoimmune inflammation, presumably via an endogenous danger signal (Prinz *et al.*, 2006).

Mice homozygous for a null-mutation of TLR4 develop increased amyloid Abeta deposits. These changes were documented by thioflavine-S staining of fibrillar Abeta aggregates and by demonstration of buffer-soluble and -insoluble Abeta (Tahara *et al.*, 2006). Together, these observations suggest a role of this pattern receptor in modulating the formation of pathogenic deposits in the brain in Alzheimer's disease. Activation of TLR4 expressed by microglia could induce both oligodendrocyte and neuronal injury (Lehnardt *et al.*, 2002, 2003), but may also promote remyelination (Glezer *et al.*, 2006).

In summary, compelling evidence has now accumulated to indicate that the innate immune system shapes CNS autoimmunity, neurodegeneration, and traumatic tissue injury. On the other hand, the biological consequences can be tissue damage or tissue repair.

Adaptive immune reactivity

Adaptive immune reactivity appears late in phylogeny. Jawed fish are the "oldest" vertebrates to use antigen-specific lymphocytes in the fight against microbial infection. Adaptive immune reactivity ideally complements innate immunity. Both response systems share important features: they protect the body against foreign, potentially menacing organisms, but at the same time largely respect the body's own tissues, displaying immunological self-tolerance. However, protection provided by adaptive immunity is more radical; the distinction between foreign and self that is built up is more clear-cut; and, importantly, adaptive immune responses establish immunological memory. One initial contact with a certain bacterium, for example, conditions the adaptive immune system to mount a faster and stronger response following subsequent encounters. Adaptive and innate immune responses use very different cellular and molecular strategies, but it is important to know that they do not operate separately, independent of each other. Both systems are tightly interconnected to orchestrate concerted actions against particular targets.

Adaptive immunity uses stunningly simple and efficacious principles: clonal diversity of immune cells and immune surveillance of the body's tissues. Clonal diversity implies that the immune system forms a large number of individual lymphocyte clones, each one characterized by a membrane receptor that recognizes one distinct antigen. These lymphocytes patrol through the tissues in permanent search of their antigen; they exert immune surveillance. The actual immune response, however, unfolds in the secondary lymph organs, lymph nodes and spleen. It culminates in the generation of effector mechanisms that are aimed at removing or neutralizing the foreign agent, the antigen, in question.

The adaptive immune response employs three main cellular components. The T lymphocytes are the principal patrollers, migrating through the body and gathering information. During an immune response, they mature either to effector cells that directly attack the antigen, or to regulatory cells that enhance or reduce the activity of the ongoing response. The B lymphocytes, in contrast, are less involved in immune surveillance, but instead they produce humoral antibodies that can bind to antigenic structures and tag them for destruction by macrophages and the complement system.

The third principal player in the immune response is the dendritic cell (DC), a cell type only discovered in the 1970s. The DCs play a pivotal role interconnecting innate and adaptive immune responses. They have the unique ability to sequester protein, to process it, and to ultimately display particular peptide fragments to specific T lymphocytes. The T lymphocytes, in contrast to B lymphocytes, have surface receptors that recognize only *processed* antigen, i.e. antigenic peptide fragments bound to proteins of the major histocompatibility complex (MHC). In addition to serving as the classical APCs to T lymphocytes, DCs are extremely sensitive to stimuli provided by innate immune responses. Thus, DCs display on their membrane PRRs at high density, and following stimuli, they become activated, a process that further intensifies processing of antigen and its presentation to local T lymphocytes.

Does adaptive immunity protect the CNS? Do the main rules of adaptive immune responses apply to the brain and spinal cord? At first glance, this concern may appear moot, but it is not. It should be kept in mind that, until recently, the CNS was deemed exempt from adaptive immune reactivity. After all, the CNS is secluded from circulating immune cells by a tight endothelial BBB, and, in addition, structures critically required for immune responses are missing in the healthy CNS (Wekerle et al., 1986). Indeed, the normal CNS keeps immune reactivity to a minimum. It provides a milieu hostile to immune cells and their function. Normal CNS tissue fails to produce important MHC products, cell adhesion molecules, chemokines and cytokines that are required for successful immune responses. Under a number of pathological conditions, however, the BBB becomes more permeable, and CNS cells can be induced to de novo express molecules

relevant to the adaptive immune response: the CNS tissue milieu turns from immune-hostile to immune-friendly (Wekerle, 2006).

Immune cells in the CNS – T cells

Inflammatory cells invading the CNS were initially described by pathologists, notably in the context of CNS infections and tumors, but also in neurodegenerative disease. Inflammatory infiltrates are particularly notable in active lesions of MS, a CNS disorder, which is not caused by any known specific infectious agent, and which, for several reasons, is thought to be the consequence of an autoimmune attack (Lassmann and Wekerle, 2006).

These observations raise questions of clinical as well as biological importance. What are the conditions that lure inflammatory cells into the normally secluded CNS tissue? How do these cells interact with local CNS components both in health and disease? And, more generally, if there is any immune surveillance of the CNS, how is it organized? Pertinent answers emerge from studies of experimental autoimmune encephalomyelitis (EAE), an animal model of CNS autoimmunity.

T cell migration through the BBB

The endothelial cells lining the microvessels within the CNS are distinct from the endothelia of other organs. They are specialized to form a vascular lining impermeable to most blood macromolecules and cells. The BBB endothelia are interconnected by complex arrays of tight junctions. The few blood-borne molecules required by CNS cells pass through the endothelia by active transport systems (Abbott et al., 2006). Among circulating blood cells, only a few activated lymphocytes and some macrophages seem to be able to pass through the BBB. In health, the BBB inner surface lacks most of the structures required by circulating leukocytes to attach and to navigate through the vessel wall (Engelhardt and Ransohoff, 2005).

The BBB endothelia are, however, readily activated and rendered receptive for leukocytes following several modifications, either initiated systemically, or within the CNS tissue (Ransohoff et al., 2003). In vitro studies have shown that inflammatory stimuli like bacterial lipopolysaccharide (LPS), or cytokines induce BBB endothelia to form cell adhesion molecules or chemokine mediators required for lymphocyte transmigration (Wong and Dorovni-Zis, 2000; Shukaliak and Dorovni-Zis, 2000). In vivo application of these stimuli enhances leukocyte traffic into the CNS in a similar way (Piccio *et al.*, 2002). Importantly, however, leukocyte immigration into the CNS is not only triggered consequent to inflammation, but also in the context of neurodegenerative disease (Ransohoff and Tani, 1998). Loss of neuronal function leads to the production of cytokines that seem to recapitulate much of the events that enhance leukocyte infiltration in microbial infection and autoimmunity (Raivich *et al.*, 2003).

Obviously, interactions between recirculating immune cells and (activated) immune cells are of paramount clinical importance. Such interactions are beneficial in infectious diseases or tumor formation, where the pathogenic process could be limited by incoming immune cells. In these situations, immune cell immigration should be supported therapeutically. In contrast, in cases of anti-CNS autoimmunity (as in MS), invading immune cells are pathogenic. The results of recent trials of anti-integrin α4 antibody natalizumab therapy in MS illustrate this point. These antibodies are reputed to mask a cell adhesion molecule involved in guiding activated T cells through the BBB, and they reduce the number of new relapses and of radiologically demonstrable CNS lesions impressively (Miller *et al.*, 2003). Unfortunately, a small number of patients developed progressive multifocal leukoencephalopathy caused by reactivated JC virus, either dormant in the CNS or transmitted from the periphery (Ropper, 2006). Reactivation might have been caused by compromised anti-microbial immune surveillance, a detrimental side effect of antibody treatment, or alternatively by release of JC virus-containing cells from the bone marrow (Ransohoff, 2007).

Antigen presentation and immune reactivity within the CNS

Previously, we mentioned that, under *normal* conditions, neurons and glial cells within the CNS milieu fail to produce and expose MHC determinants, cell adhesion molecules and soluble mediators necessary for productive immune reactivity. However, we also stressed that CNS cells are by no means unable to produce such molecules. The CNS cells can be induced in varying degrees to produce "immune" genes, and the inducing signals can be provided in the course of processes as diverse as virus infection, tumor growth or, quite surprisingly, neuronal degeneration.

There is a hierarchy of potential APCs within the CNS milieu. Clearly, the most efficient APCs are derived from bone marrow-derived progenitors: resident microglia, as well as macrophages infiltrating from circulating blood. Other glial cells, namely astrocytes and oligodendrocytes, or neurons, may be able to present antigens in the effector stage of immune responses (Wekerle, 1994), and thus can be recognized as targets by effector lymphocytes; their capacity to trigger de-novo immune reactions seems, however, to be confined to discrete circumstances. Under inflammatory conditions, microglia are readily induced to express both MHC class I and class II and to present antigens to T cells. Cytokine-stimulated astrocytes are far less competent in presenting antigens than microglia (Aloisi *et al.*, 2001). Inducibility of MHC class I in neurons is very strictly regulated and full-blown expression of MHC class I on the neuronal cell surface was only observed after treatment of electrically paralyzed neurons with interferon-gamma (Neumann *et al.*, 1995, 1997b).

Autochthonous CNS cells are inducible, facultative APCs, but does the CNS harbor any *professional* APCs, that is DCs? This long-standing debate has, apparently, been answered in the affirmative. Professional APCs are capable of delivering additional co-stimulatory signals to T cells that serve to stimulate the full activation program of naive T cells. Tissue-resident professional APCs are not detected in the normal CNS parenchyma. However, macrophages are activated and substantially increase in number during autoimmune inflammation (Lassmann *et al.*, 1993). Dendritic cells are recruited into the CNS and mainly accumulate in the perivascular area of overt inflammatory foci during EAE (Serafini *et al.*, 2000) and cerebral toxoplasmosis (Fischer *et al.*, 2000). These CNS-associated DCs are credited to play a central role in the pathogenesis of neurological immune diseases; their perivascular location means that they are the first cell type encountered by T cells passing through the microvascular BBB. Presentation of local autoantigen could serve as a guidance signal directing the autoimmune T cells into their target destination (Greter *et al.*, 2005).

Beyond this signaling, DCs, as classical professional APCs, have the ability to recruit naive T cells. Within the CNS, DCs would be the only APCs able to take up and present local autoantigens and thus to activate T cells of specificities other than the original effector cells. Dendritic cells isolated from the brains of mice affected with inflammation contain CNS material and activate a complement of T cells reactive to an extended range of myelin autoantigens (McMahon *et al.*, 2005). Furthermore, recent observations indicate that intracerebral DCs drive naive myelin-specific T cells into the Th17 lineage, the lineage enriched for pathogenic effector T cells (Bailey *et al.*, 2007).

Is there a communication between the CNS and the peripheral immune system? While there is no doubt that inflammatory cells, at least under favorable conditions, are able to cross the BBB and to enter CNS tissue, there is, however, much less evidence of migration in the opposite direction, from within the CNS to the periphery. While emigration of T (and B) cells has never been observed, there are at least circumstantial indications that the extrusion of CNS antigenic material occurs, either by leakage of subcellular material or via carriage within phagocytes. After intracerebral injection, protein markers were seen in local lymphatic organs, mostly the deep cervical lymph nodes (Bradbury and Cole, 1980; Cserr *et al.*, 1992). Moreover, cervical lymph nodes seem to be involved in the EAE response targeted to particular areas of the cerebral cortex (Phillips *et al.*, 1997). More recent studies followed the migration of DC-like cells from the CNS to surrounding lymphoid organs (Hatterer *et al.*, 2006). Indeed, myelin autoantigen is also demonstrable in human cervical lymph nodes from patients with MS (Fabriek *et al.*, 2005) and in primates with EAE (De Vos *et al.*, 2002).

B cells in the CNS

If the healthy CNS fails to provide a favorable milieu for T cells, the same is true with regard to B cells. However, as with T cells, there are pathological conditions that favor the entrance of B cells into the CNS, and their persistence in this location.

In normal CNS tissue, some B lymphocytes can be found, but they are rare (Anthony *et al.*, 2003). B cells are, however, commonly found in inflammatory lesions, such as in MS plaques (Meinl *et al.*, 2006). Intriguingly, there seems to be a certain propensity for B cell lymphomas to expand in brain and spinal cords. Primary lymphomas arising within the CNS are mostly of B cell, and only exceptionally of T cell, origin (Iwamoto and DeAngelis, 2006).

The best-known consequence of B cell activity within the CNS is the appearance of B cell products, immunoglobulin distributed as oligoclonal bands, in the cerebrospinal fluid of patients with MS, or microbial infections. At least some of these immunoglobulins are actively produced within the CNS tissue, or the enshrouding leptomeningeal membranes. In the case of (viral) infections, these antibodies may be specific for the infectious agent. In MS, however, it has been difficult to assign specificity to these antibodies. There is evidence that some of the antibodies bind with low affinity to myelin proteins, but direct evidence of a positive role in the pathogenesis of MS is still elusive. Nevertheless, studies of the primary structure of CSF immunoglobulins indicate a positive, T cell-driven process controlling their production, with evidence of somatic mutation and immunoglobulin class switches.

The intricacies of B cell biology within the CNS are still to be unravelled. For example, it is uncertain whether B cells crossing the BBB respond to either specific signals emanating from the CNS cells proper, or from locally responding T cells, or, whether they merely migrate with invasive T lymphocytes as passive fellow travelers. Most of our present knowledge is derived from experimental models such as EAE. Although most variants of EAE are primarily T cell-mediated autoimmune diseases, there are significant B cell contributions. The B cells act in several stages of the disease. In the emerging autoimmune response, B cells can pick up soluble autoantigen, process it and present it to specific T cells. Then, via the specific repertoire of cytokines that B cells produce, they can help to shape the particular T cell phenotype required to attack the CNS target tissue. Finally, in the effector phase, B cells can act via their autoantibody products, which can bind to CNS membrane structures, and with the help of complement and/or macrophages, can initiate tissue destruction (Schnell *et al.*, 1997).

The CNS milieu for B cells

We have previously emphasized that, in general, the CNS tissue provides a microenvironment adverse to immune cell survival and local immune responsiveness. This statement was mainly directed to T cells and their cooperating cell partners. Interestingly, B cells may find the CNS milieu more hospitable, as suggested by recent investigations (Uccelli *et al.*, 2006). Astrocytes are able to produce and release B cell activating factor (BAF), an essential soluble mediator supporting survival and reactivity of B lymphocytes (Krumbholz *et al.*, 2005). This may explain why some B cells persist over extended periods of time within the CNS.

There is good evidence of structures involved in B cell migration into or within the CNS. It also appears that the CNS parenchyma, either resting or activated, can supply soluble signals that could guide recirculating

B cells through the BBB. For example, the chemokine CXCL12 is detected in both the microvascular wall and in adjacent astrocytes (Krumbholz *et al.*, 2006). In contrast, another B cell chemokine, CXCL13, appeared mainly restricted to inflammatory infiltrates. The level of CXCL13 expression was correlated to the number of infiltrating B cells (Krumbholz *et al.*, 2006).

Studies of an in vitro model of the BBB suggest that the motility of human B cells is similar to that of T cells, and that the two major lymphocyte sets display similar profiles of adhesion molecules and chemokine receptors (Alter *et al.*, 2003), but that they use distinct combinations of proteases to open tissue barriers (Bar-Or *et al.*, 2003).

B cell-containing lymphoid tissues ("ectopic lymphoid tissues")

Transient immune responses take place within the preformed, specialized secondary lymphoid organs, lymph nodes, spleen, gut and bronchus-associated lymphatic tissues. In chronic responses, such as in chronic infection and autoimmune responses, lymphatic tissue can be formed de novo in the vicinity of the actual disease process/target tissue. In rheumatoid arthritis, for example, large lymphatic infiltrations forming germinal centers are typically noted in the inflamed synovial pannus. In Sjögren's syndrome, similar infiltrates change the structure of the lacrimal and salivary glands, and in Hashimoto's thyroiditis they dominate the thyroid (Hjelmström, 2001).

The newly formed lymphoid tissue associated with target organs could contribute to the course and character of the ongoing autoimmune response. Autoantigen produced in the vicinity may enter these lymphoid areas, and there foster the ongoing cellular response. Presentation of these determinants can be expected to activate and recruit pathogenic T cells, and, in addition, give rise to the production of humoral autoantibodies (Aloisi and Pujol-Borrell, 2006).

Germinal center-like formations are common in the avian CNS, where they have been repeatedly described in the pineal gland (Cogburn and Glick, 1981). They have not been noted in healthy mammalian CNS tissue, but occur in a subgroup of patients with MS. In 1979, Prineas described thin-walled microvessels reminiscent of lymphatic vasculature embedded in germinal center-like lymphocyte aggregates. These tissues were located in perivascular areas (Prineas, 1979). An important, and baffling, but not entirely unpredictable, observation was the description of follicle-like organized tissue in the CNS of certain MS cases (Serafini *et al.*, 2004), and these may associate with cortical pathology (Magliozzi *et al.*, 2007). Immunocytochemistry revealed a composition of B cells, T cells, plasma cells and most intriguingly, follicle dendritic cells, the signature cells of differentiated germinal centers (Serafini *et al.*, 2004). These follicle-like structures were noted predominantly within the leptomeningeal membranes, in perivascular areas, and Virchow–Robin spaces, but not within the parenchyma proper (Magliozzi *et al.*, 2007).

Formation of fully differentiated lymphoid tissue involves members of the TNF family of genes. The cytokine, lymphotoxin-alpha (LT-α), LIGHT and other mediators induce the formation of a milieu that promotes the establishment of ordered lymphatic tissues, among them prominently, germinal centers (Ware, 2005). In a chronic-relapsing model of mouse EAE, neutralization of LT-β by a recombinant antagonist protein curbed ongoing disease and at the same time prevented formation of leptomeningeal lymphoid aggregates indicating a central role for LT-β in this activity (Columba-Cabezas *et al.*, 2006). Other cytokines, such as IL-7, also contribute (Meier *et al.*, 2007).

Intrathecal production of immunoglobulins

One hallmark of CNS inflammation, either induced by microbes or autoimmunity, is the formation of oligoclonal immunoglobulin bands in the cerebrospinal fluid (CSF). These immunoglobulins are distinct in their electric charge. As antibody products of a limited number of plasma cells resident within the confines of the CNS they can be readily separated electrophoretically. In contrast, serum immunoglobulins, which are produced by millions of diverse plasmablasts and plasma cells that are present in the peripheral immune repertoire, overlap to form a continuum.

Oligoclonal CSF immunoglobulins in CNS infections commonly include bands that bind structures of the relevant infectious agents such as measles virus in subacute sclerosing panencephalitis (SSPE) (Mehta *et al.*, 1982) and *Borrelia burgdorferi* in neuroborreliosis (Murray *et al.*, 1986). Antigen specificity of infection-associated Ig bands readily indicates their association with an anti-microbial B cell response.

Less clear, however, is the nature and origin of CSF bands in MS. Intensive studies over the past decade were not able to clearly assign antigen specificity to these antibodies. The claim that the oligoclonal bands in MS are specific for *Chlamydia pneumoniae* (Sriram *et al.*, 1999) was not confirmed in other studies (Derfuss *et al.*, 2001). Binding of oligoclonal bands to EBV, a common human virus of the herpes group, was reported (Cepok *et al.*, 2005), but is not yet confirmed in other studies. These shortcomings led to the contention that CSF immunoglobulins have no role in the actual autoimmune disease process. They might rather represent non-specific antibodies generated in the CNS due to bystander processes. Specific antibodies would be absorbed within the target tissue, with non-specific antibodies leaking out into the CSF.

While oligoclonal bands occur in the CSF of both MS patients and patients with an encephalitis with a known infectious agent, one important difference between the intrathecal Ig production of MS patients and other inflammatory neurological disease (OIND) patients has been known for many years: whereas MS patients typically display an intrathecal immune response against many different common pathogens such as measles virus, rubella virus, and varicella-zoster virus, as well as *Chlamydia pneumoniae* and HHV-6, OIND patients do not (reviewed in Anthony *et al.*, 2003). This polyspecific anti-pathogen Ig does not correspond to the major OCB in the CSF and is considered a bystander reaction (Measles–Rubella–Zoster reaction), which can be detected in about 90% of MS patients. The reason for this polyspecific Ig response in MS is unclear; it probably does not simply reflect a consequence of long-lasting disease, since it is typically present at the beginning of MS and is even used as a diagnostic criterion in some clinics. The polyspecific intrathecal Ig response in MS might indicate an environment that promotes enhanced B cell activity long before the clinical disease starts, and could also reflect the individual's history of infections (Anthony *et al.*, 2003).

Immunoglobulins in the brain tissue of MS patients

Early studies eluted antibodies from MS plaque material and identified their oligoclonal distribution (Mehta *et al.*, 1981; Glynn *et al.*, 1982). The identification of antigen specificity of immunoglobulins dissociated from CNS lesions remains a challenge to the present day. While one study initially found binding to native MOG in 50% of samples from MS-derived autopsy material, but not in non-MS control samples

(O'Connor *et al.*, 2005), the same group using more elaborate technology restricted this specificity to a few cases of acute disseminated encephalomyelitis (ADEM), but did not find antibodies to MOG in the serum in classic MS (O'Connor *et al.*, 2007).

In one particular pattern of MS plaques, immunoglobulin bound to myelin debris along with activated complement is the structural hallmark suggesting an active participation of autoantibodies in the pathogenic process (Luchinetti *et al.*, 2000). Furthermore, one group suggested that at least some of these bound antibodies are specific for MOG autoantigen (Genain *et al.*, 1999), a claim, which, however, waits to be formally confirmed by independent studies.

Analysis of Ig rearrangement in the CNS

Frustrating as the search for the target autoantigen may have been, the study of the molecular nature of Ig transcripts in CSF provided important insights into the pathogenesis of MS.

In order to appreciate these data, it should be kept in mind that antigen-driven B cell responses are the result of a complex interaction between helper T cells, mainly of CD4$^+$ lineages, and specific B cells. Both lymphocyte sets recognize the same antigen, through distinct epitopes via distinct mechanisms. Activated T cells ultimately drive B cells to sharpen their antigen specificity via somatic mutation of their immunoglobulin hypervariable regions (complementarity determining regions) and trigger the molecular switch from "primitive" IgM to "effector" isotypes (IgG, IgE, or IgA) (Ahmed and Gray, 1996).

Qin *et al.* used PCR amplification to study CSF-derived B cells and established a hierarchy of sequences that suggested somatic mutation of expanding B cell clones, data that have been supported by other groups. This likely represents a T helper cell-driven B cell response (Qin *et al.*, 1998; Owens *et al.*, 1998; Baranzini *et al.*, 1999; Colombo *et al.*, 2000). More recently, investigators have turned to the study of single B cells, mostly isolated by cytofluorometric cell sorting from CSF (Ritchie *et al.*, 2004), an approach that ultimately allows cloning and expression of paired immunoglobulin, i.e. H and L chains from the same individual B cell (Haubold *et al.*, 2004). Expression of CNS-associated immunoglobulins as recombinant Fab or Fv fragments have been used lately to search for relevant target autoantigens. One study identified polyreactive myelin binding immunoglobulins (Lambracht-Washington *et al.*, 2007), while another pointed to enzymes of the glycolytic pathway as targets that are expressed in neural compartments (Kolln *et al.*, 2006).

B cell models?

There is a deficiency of valid models to study the role of B cells in CNS immune reactivity. In EAE, classical experiments by Linington and colleagues explored the function of anti-myelin autoantibodies by co-transferring relevant MAbs along with encephalitogenic effector T cells (Schluesener *et al.*, 1987; Linington *et al.*, 1988). In these paradigms, the T cells attack the brain white matter and thereby open the BBB to permeation of co-transferred MAbs. This strategy was helpful for studying the role of B cell-derived autoantibodies in the effector phase of an autoimmune attack, such as the interaction of membrane-bound MAbs with complement factors (Piddlesden *et al.*, 1993).

However, the role of B cells in CNS autoimmunity is more complex. The B cells can act as APCs, concentrating and presenting myelin autoantigen to T cells. They also secrete cytokines that influence the character of immune responses. One approach to gain insight into these complexities is the use of transgenic mice with a B cell repertoire dominated by B cells specific for myelin autoantigens; for example, MOG. Litzenburger *et al.* replaced the immunoglobulin J region by the rearranged gene encoding the H chain of the original anti-MOG MAb 8–18C5 and found that about 30% of all mature B cells produced immunoglobulin binding to MOG (Litzenburger *et al.*, 1998). In double-transgenic mice, these B cells actively cooperate with CD4[+] T cells expressing MOG-specific T cell receptors to bring about a spontaneous autoimmune disease involving the optic nerves and spinal cord as primary targets (Bettelli *et al.*, 2006; Krishnamoorthy *et al.*, 2006).

Conclusion

Although innate and adaptive immunity are mechanistically distinct, they reflect components of an integrated response to either exogenous or endogenous danger signals. Much dogma concerning the nature of the CNS immune response and how it interacts with immune activation in the periphery has broken down in recent years. However, the exact nature of these interactions and, in addition, how T and B cells cooperate to induce CNS autoimmunity remain ill-defined. It will be especially important to understand the principles governing these interactions if we are to develop selective strategies that can inhibit CNS autoimmunity but which do not compromise anti-microbial immune surveillance, a major challenge for future research.

References

Abbott NJ *et al.* Astrocyte–endothelial interactions at the blood–brain barrier. *Nature Rev Immunol* 2006; 7: 41–53.

Agostini L *et al.* NALP3 forms an IL-b-processing inflammasome with increased activity in Muckle–Wells autoinflammatory disorder. *Immunity* 2004; 20: 319–25.

Ahmed R, Gray D. Immunological memory and protective immunity: Understanding their relation. *Science* 1996; 272: 54–60.

Aloisi F. Immune function of microglia. *Glia* 2001; 36: 165–79.

Aloisi F, Pujol-Borrell R. Lymphoid neogenesis in chronic inflammatory diseases. *Nature Rev Immunol* 2006; 6: 205–17.

Aloisi F, *et al.* Regulation of T cell responses by CNS antigen presenting cells: Different roles for microglia and astrocytes. *Immunol Today* 2000; 21: 141–7.

Alter A *et al.* Determinants of human B cell migration across brain endothelial cells. *J Immunol* 2003; 170: 4497–505.

Anthony IC, *et al.* B lymphocytes in the normal brain: Contrasts with HIV-associated lymphoid infiltrates and lymphomas. *Brain* 2003; 126: 1058–67.

Babcock AA, *et al.* Toll-like receptor 2 signaling in response to brain injury: An innate bridge to neuroinflammation. *J Neurosci* 2006; 26: 12826–37.

Baccalà R, *et al.* TLR-dependent and TLR-independent pathways of type I interferon induction in systemic autoimmunity. *Nature Med* 2007; 13: 543–51.

Bailey SL, *et al.* CNS myeloid DCs presenting endogenous myelin peptides 'preferentially' polarize CD4[+] TH-17 cells in relapsing EAE. *Nature Immunol* 2007; 8: 172–80.

Baranzini SE, *et al.* B cell repertoire diversity and clonal expansion in multiple sclerosis brain lesions. *J Immunol* 1999; 163: 5133–44.

Bar-Or A, *et al.* Analyses of all matrix metalloproteinase members in leukocytes emphasize monocytes as major inflammatory mediators in multiple sclerosis. *Brain* 2003; 126: 2738–49.

Bausinger H, *et al.* Endotoxin-free heat-shock protein 70 fails to induce APC activation. *Eur J Immunol* 2002; 32: 3708–13.

Bettelli E, *et al.* Myelin oligodendrocyte glycoprotein-specific T and B cells cooperate to induce a Devic-like disease in mice. *J Clin Invest* 2006; 116: 2393–402.

Bradbury MWB, Cole DF. The role of lymphatic system in drainage of cerebrospinal fluid and aqueous humor. *J Physiol* 1980; 299: 353–65.

Brambilla R, *et al.* Inhibition of astroglial nuclear factor kB reduces inflammation and improves functional recovery after spinal cord injury. *J Exp Med* 2005; 202: 145–56.

Bsibsi M, *et al.* Broad expression of Toll-like receptors in the human central nervous system. *J Neuropathol Exp Neurol* 2002; 61: 1013–21.

Cepok S, *et al.* Identification of Epstein–Barr virus proteins as putative targets of the immune response in multiple sclerosis. *J Clin Invest* 2005; 115: 1352–60.

Cogburn LA, Glick B. Lymphopoiesis in the chicken pineal gland. *Am J Anat* 1981; 162: 131–42.

Colombo M, *et al.* Accumulation of clonally related B lymphocytes in the cerebrospinal fluid of multiple sclerosis patients. *J Immunol* 2000; 164: 2782–9.

Columba-Cabezas S, *et al.* Suppression of established experimental autoimmune encephalomyelitis and formation of meningeal lymphoid follicles by lymphotoxin b receptor-Ig fusion protein. *J Neuroimmunol* 2006; 179: 76–86.

Creagh EM, O'Neill LAJ. TLRs, NLRs and RLRs: a trinity of pathogen sensors that co-operate in innate immunity. *Trends Immunol* 2006; 27: 352–7.

Cserr HF, *et al.* Drainage of brain extracellular fluid into blood and deep cervical lymph and its immunological significance. *Brain Pathol* 1992; 2: 269–76.

Derfuss T, *et al.* Intrathecal antibody production against *Chlamydia pneumoniae* in multiple sclerosis is part of a polyspecific immune response. *Brain* 2001; 124: 1325–35.

De Vos AF, *et al.* Transfer of central nervous system autoantigens and presentation in secondary lymphoid organs. *J Immunol* 2002; 169: 5415–23.

Ehlers M, Ravetch JV. Opposing effects of Toll-like receptor stimulation induce autoimmunity or tolerance. *Trends Immunol* 2007; 28: 74–9.

Engelhardt B, Ransohoff RM. The ins and outs of T-lymphocyte trafficking to the CNS: Anatomical sites and molecular mechanisms. *Trends Immunol* 2005; 26: 485–95.

Fabriek BO, *et al.* In vivo detection of myelin proteins in cervical lymph nodes of MS patients using ultrasound-guided fine-needle aspiration cytology. *J Neuroimmunol* 2005; 161: 190–4.

Farina C, *et al.* Preferential expression and function of Toll-like receptor 3 in human astrocytes. *J Neuroimmunol* 2005; 159: 12–19.

Farina C, *et al.* Astrocytes are active players in cerebral innate immunity. *Trends Immunol* 2007; 28: 138–45.

Fischer H-G, *et al.* Phenotype and functions of brain dendritic cells emerging during chronic infection of mice with *Toxoplasma gondii*. *J Immunol* 2000; 164: 4826–34.

Fritz JH, *et al.* NOD-like proteins in immunity, inflammation and disease. *Nature Immunol* 2006; 7: 1250–7.

Genain CP, *et al.* Identification of autoantibodies associated with myelin damage in multiple sclerosis. *Nature Med* 1999; 5: 170–5.

Glezer I, *et al.* Innate immunity triggers oligodendrocyte progenitor reactivity and confines damages to brain injuries. *FASEB J* 2006; 20: 750–2.

Glynn P, *et al.* Analysis of immunoglobulin G in multiple sclerosis brain: Quantitative and isoelectric focusing studies. *Clin Exp Immunol* 1982; 48: 102–10.

Goverman J, *et al.* Transgenic mice that express a myelin basic protein-specific T cell receptor develop spontaneous autoimmunity. *Cell* 1993; 72: 551–60.

Greter M, et al. Dendritic cells permit immune invasion of the CNS in an animal model of multiple sclerosis. *Nature Med* 2005; **11**: 328–34.

Hansen BS, et al. Multiple toll-like receptor agonists act as potent adjuvants in the induction of autoimmunity. *J Neuroimmunol* 2006; **172**: 94–103.

Hatterer E, et al. How to drain without lymphatics? Dendritic cells migrate from the cerebrospinal fluid to the B-cell follicles of cervical lymph nodes. *Blood* 2006; **107**: 806–12.

Haubold K, et al. B-lymphocyte and plasma cell clonal expansion in monosymptomatic optic neuritis cerebrospinal fluid. *Ann Neurol* 2004; **56**: 97–107.

Hjelmström P. Lymphoid neogenesis: De novo formation of lymphoid tissue in chronic inflammation through expression of homing chemokines. *J Leukocyte Biol* 2001; **69**: 331–9.

Hoffmann JA, et al. Phylogenetic perspectives in innate immunity. *Science* 1999; **284**: 1313–8.

Iwamoto FM, DeAngelis LM. An update on primary central nervous system lymphoma. *Hematol–Oncol Clin N Am* 2006; **20**: 1267.

Jack CS, et al. TLR signaling tailors innate immune responses in human microglia and astrocytes. *J Immunol* 2005; **175**: 4320–30.

Kamradt T, et al. Induction, exacerbation and inhibition of allergic and autoimmune diseases by infection. *Trends Immunol* 2005; **26**: 260–7.

Kielian T. Toll-like receptors in central nervous system glial inflammation and homeostasis. *J Neurosci Res* 2006; **83**: 711–30.

Kolln J, et al. Triosephosphate isomerase- and glyceraldehyde-3-phosphate dehydrogenase-reactive autoantibodies in the cerebrospinal fluid of patients with multiple sclerosis. *J Immunol* 2006; **177**: 5652–8.

Krishnamoorthy G, et al. Spontaneous opticospinal encephalomyelitis in a double-transgenic mouse model of autoimmune T cell/B cell cooperation. *J Clin Invest* 2006; **116**: 2385–92.

Krumbholz M, et al. BAF is produced by astrocytes and upregulated in multiple sclerosis lesions and primary central nervous system lymphoma. *J Exp Med* 2005; **201**: 195–200.

Krumbholz M, et al. Chemokines in multiple sclerosis: CXCL12 and CXCL13 up-regulation is differentially linked to CNS immune cell recruitment. *Brain* 2006; **129**: 200–11.

Lafon M, et al. The innate immune facet of brain – Human neurons express TLR-3 and sense viral dsRNA. *J Mol Neurosci* 2006; **29**: 185–94.

Lambracht-Washington D, et al. Antigen specificity of clonally expanded and receptor edited cerebrospinal fluid B cells from patients with relapsing remitting MS. *J Neuroimmunol* 2007; **186**: 164–76.

Lassmann H, Wekerle H. The pathology of multiple sclerosis. In: Compston A, Confavreux C, Lassmann H, McDonald I, Miller D, Noseworthy J, et al., editors. *McAlpine's Multiple Sclerosis*. Churchill Livingstone Elsevier, 2006: 557–600.

Lassmann H, et al. Bone-marrow derived elements and resident microglia in brain inflammation. *Glia* 1993; **7**: 19–24.

Lee MS, Kim YJ. Signaling pathways downstream of pattern-recognition receptors and their cross talk. *Annu Rev Biochem* 2007; **76**: 447–80.

Lehnardt S, et al. The toll-like receptor TLR4 is necessary for lipopolysaccharide-induced oligodendrocyte injury in the CNS. *J Neurosci* 2002; **22**: 2478–86.

Lehnardt S, et al. Activation of innate immunity in the CNS triggers neurodegeneration through a Toll-like receptor 4-dependent pathway. *Proc Natl Acad Sci USA* 2003; **100**: 8514–9.

Liew FY, et al. Negative regulation of Toll-like receptor-mediated immune responses. *Nature Rev Immunol* 2005; **5**: 446–58.

Linington C, et al. Augmentation of demyelination in rat acute allergic encephalomyelitis by circulating mouse monoclonal antibodies directed against a myelin/oligodendrocyte glycoprotein. *Am J Pathol* 1988; **130**: 443–54.

Litzenburger T, et al. B lymphocytes producing demyelinating autoantibodies: Development and function in gene-targeted transgenic mice. *J Exp Med* 1998; **188**: 169–80.

Lucchinetti CF, et al. Heterogeneity of multiple sclerosis lesions: Implications for the pathogenesis of multiple sclerosis. *Ann Neurol* 2000; **47**: 707–17.

Ma YH, et al. Toll-like receptor 8 functions as a negative regulator of neurite outgrowth and inducer of neuronal apoptosis. *J Cell Biol* 2006; **175**: 209–15.

Magliozzi R, et al. Meningeal B-cell follicles in secondary progressive multiple sclerosis associate with early onset of disease and severe cortical pathology. *Brain* 2007; **130**: 1089–104.

Marshak-Rothstein A. Toll-like receptors in systemic autoimmune disease. *Nature Rev Immunol* 2006; **6**: 823–35.

McMahon EJ, et al. Epitope spreading initiates in the CNS in two mouse models of multiple sclerosis. *Nature Med* 2005; **11**: 335–9.

Medzhitov R. Toll-like receptors and innate immunity. *Nature Rev Immunol* 2001; **1**: 135–45.

Medzhitov R, Janeway CA. Innate immunity: The virtues of a nonclonal system of recognition. *Cell* 1997; **91**: 295–8.

Mehta PD, et al. Bound antibody in multiple sclerosis brains. *J Neurol Sci* 1981; **49**: 91–8.

Mehta PD, et al. Oligoclonal IgG bands with and without measles antibody activity in sera of patients with subacute sclerosing panencephalitis. *J Immunol* 1982; **129**: 1983–5.

Meier D, et al. Ectopic lymphoid-organ development occurs through interleukin 7-mediated enhanced survival of lymphoid-tissue-inducer cells. *Immunity* 2007; **26**: 643–54.

Meinl E, et al. B lineage cells in the inflammatory CNS environment: Migration, maintenance, local antibody production and therapeutic modulation. *Ann Neurol* 2006; **59**: 880–92.

Meylan E, *et al*. Intracellular pattern recognition receptors in the host response. *Nature* 2006; **442**: 39–44.

Miller DH, *et al*. A controlled trial of Natalizumab for relapsing multiple sclerosis. *N Engl J Med* 2003; **348**: 15–23.

Murray N, *et al*. Specificity of CSF antibodies against components of *Borrelia burgdorferi* in patients with meningopolyneuritis Garin–Bujadoux–Bannwarth. *J Neurol* 1986; **233**: 224–7.

Neumann H, *et al*. Induction of MHC class I genes in neurons. *Science* 1995; **269**: 549–52.

Neumann H, *et al*. Interferon-g gene expression in sensory neurons: Evidence for autocrine gene regulation. *J Exp Med* 1997a; **186**: 2023–31.

Neumann H, *et al*. MHC class I gene expression in single neurons of the central nervous system: Differential regulation by interferon-g and tumor necrosis factor-a. *J Exp Med* 1997b; **185**: 305–16.

Nguyen MD, *et al*. Innate immunity: The missing link in neuroprotection and neurodegeneration? *Nature Rev Neurosci* 2002; **3**: 216–27.

O'Connor KC, *et al*. Antibodies from inflamed central nervous system tissue recognize myelin oligodendrocyte glycoprotein. *J Immunol* 2005; **175**: 1974–82.

O'Connor KC, *et al*. Self-antigen tetramers discriminate between myelin autoantibodies to native or denatured protein. *Nature Med* 2007; **13**: 211–7.

Owens GP, *et al*. Restricted use of V_H4 germline segments in an acute multiple sclerosis brain. *Ann Neurol* 1998; **43**: 236–43.

Park C, *et al*. TLR3-mediated signal induces pro-inflammatory cytokine and chemokine gene expression in astrocytes: Differential signaling mechanisms of TLR3-induced IP-10 and IL-8 gene expression. *Glia* 2006; **53**: 248–56.

Paul S, *et al*. Type I interferon response in the central nervous system. *Biochimie* 2007; **89**: 770–8.

Phillips MJ, *et al*. Role of cervical lymph nodes in autoimmune encephalomyelitis in the Lewis rat. *J Pathol* 1997; **182**: 457–64.

Piccio L, *et al*. Molecular mechanisms involved in lymphocyte recruitment in inflamed brain microvessels: Critical roles for P-selectin glycoprotein ligand-1 and heterotrimeric G(i)-linked receptors. *J Immunol* 2002; **168**: 1940–9.

Piddlesden S, *et al*. The demyelinating potential of antibodies to myelin oligodendrocyte glycoprotein is related to their ability to fix complement. *Am J Pathol* 1993; **143**: 555–64.

Prineas JW. Multiple sclerosis: Presence of lymphatic capillaries and lymphoid tissue in the brain and spinal cord. *Science* 1979; **203**: 1123–5.

Prinz M, *et al*. Innate immunity mediated by TLR9 modulates pathogenicity in an animal model of multiple sclerosis. *J Clin Invest* 2006; **116**: 456–64.

Qin Y, *et al*. Clonal expansion and somatic hypermutation of V_H genes of B cells from cerebrospinal fluid in multiple sclerosis. *J Clin Invest* 1998; **102**: 1045–50.

Raivich G, *et al*. Lymphocyte infiltration in the injured brain: Role of pro-inflammatory cytokines. *J Neurosci Res* 2003; **72**: 726–33.

Ransohoff RM. Microgliosis: The questions shape the answers. *Nat Neurosci* 2007; **10**: 1507–9.

Ransohoff RM, Tani M. Do chemokines mediate leukocyte recruitment in post-traumatic CNS inflammation? *Trends Neurosci* 1998; **21**: 154–9.

Ransohoff RM, *et al*. Three or more routes for leukocyte migration into the central nervous system. *Nature Rev Immunol* 2003; **3**: 569–81.

Ritchie AM, *et al*. Comparative analysis of the CD19$^+$ and CD138$^+$ cell antibody repertoires in the cerebrospinal fluid of patients with multiple sclerosis. *J Immunol* 2004; **173**: 649–56.

Rivest S. Molecular insights on the cerebral innate immune system. *Brain Behav Immun* 2003; **17**: 13–9.

Ropper AH. Selective treatment of multiple sclerosis. *N Engl J Med* 2006; **354**: 965–7.

Schluesener HJ, *et al*. A monoclonal antibody against a myelin oligodendrocyte glycoprotein induces relapses and demyelination in central nervous system autoimmune disease. *J Immunol* 1987; **139**: 4016–21.

Schnell L, *et al*. Lymphocyte recruitment following spinal cord injury in mice is altered by prior viral exposure. *Eur J Neurosci* 1997; **9**: 1000–7.

Serafini B, *et al*. Intracerebral recruitment and maturation of dendritic cells in the onset and progression of experimental autoimmune encephalomyelitis. *Am J Pathol* 2000; **157**: 1991–2002.

Serafini B, *et al*. Detection of ectopic B-cell follicles with germinal centers in the meninges of patients with secondary progressive multiple sclerosis. *Brain Pathol* 2004; **14**: 164–74.

Shukaliak JA, Dorovni-Zis K. CCL4 (MIP-1b)Expression of the b-chemokines RANTES and MIP-1b by human brain microvessel endothelial cells in primary culture. *J Neuropathol Exp Neurol* 2000; **59**: 339–52.

Sriram S, *et al*. *Chlamydia pneumoniae* infection of the central nervous system in multiple sclerosis. *Ann Neurol* 1999; **46**: 6–14.

Tahara K, *et al*. Role of toll-like receptor signaling in Ab uptake and clearance. *Brain* 2006; **129**: 3006–19.

Uccelli A, *et al*. Unveiling the enigma of the CNS as a B-cell fostering environment. *Trends Immunol* 2006; **26**: 254–9.

van Loo G, *et al*. Inhibition of transcription factor NF-kappaB in the central nervous system ameliorates autoimmune encephalomyelitis in mice. *Nat Immunol* 2006a; 7: 954–61.

van Loo G, *et al*. Inhibition of transcription factor NF-kB in the central nervous system ameliorates autoimmune encephalomyelitis in mice. *Nature Immunol* 2006b; 7: 954–61.

Visser L, *et al*. Pro-inflammatory bacterial peptidoglycan as a cofactor

13

for the development of central nervous system autoimmune disease. *J Immunol* 2005; **174**: 808–16.

Visser L, *et al.* Phagocytes containing a disease-promoting Toll-like receptor/NOD ligand are present in the brain during demyelinating disease in primates. *Am J Pathol* 2006; **169**: 1671–85.

Wagner H. Endogenous TLR ligands and autoimmunity. *Adv Immunol* 2006; **91**: 159–73.

Waldner H, *et al.* Activation of antigen-presenting cells by microbial products breaks self tolerance and induces autoimmune disease. *J Clin Invest* 2004; **113**: 990–7.

Ware CF. Network communications: Lymphotoxins, LIGHT and TNF. *Annu Rev Immunol* 2005; **23**: 787–819.

Wekerle H. Antigen presentation by CNS glia. In: Kettenmann H, Ransom B, (Eds). *Neuroglial Cells.* Oxford, UK: Oxford University Press, 1994.

Wekerle H. Breaking ignorance: The case of the brain. In: Radbruch A, Lipsky PE, (Eds). *Current Concepts in Autoimmunity and Chronic Inflammation.* Berlin: Springer, 2006: 25–50.

Wekerle H, *et al.* Cellular immune reactivity within the CNS. *Trends Neurosci* 1986; **9**: 271–7.

Wolf NA, *et al.* Synergistic interaction between Toll-like receptor agonists is required for induction of experimental autoimmune encephalomyelitis in Lewis rats. *J Neuroimmunol* 2007; **185**: 115–22.

Wong D, Dorovini-Zis K. Upregulation of intercellular adhesion molecule-1 (ICAM-1) expression in primary culture of human brain microvessel endothelial cells by cytokines and lipopolysaccharide. *J Neuroimmunol* 1992; **39**: 11–22.

Wyss-Coray T, Mucke L. Inflammation in neurodegenerative disease – A double-edged sword. *Neuron* 2002; **35**: 419–32.

Zekki H, *et al.* The clinical course of experimental autoimmune encephalomyelitis is associated with a profound and sustained transcriptional activation of the genes encoding toll-like receptor 2 and CD14 in the mouse CNS. *Brain Pathol* 2002; **12**: 308–19.

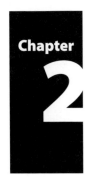

Microglia: protective and pathogenic mediators

Bevyn Jarrott and Karina Apricò

Introduction

Microglia are widely distributed throughout the brain, where they actively sense and respond rapidly to both normal and abnormal neuronal activity through a multitude of receptors and ion channels. Microglia are highly plastic, and undergo significant morphological and biochemical changes when activated in response to either injury or pathogens. These cells can synthesize a cornucopia of different cytokines, chemokines, trophic factors, extracellular matrix components, and transmitters that can exert either a protective or a damaging effect on the adjacent neuronal cells depending upon the extent of injury or duration of exposure to the pathogen.

Background and historical perspective

Microglia are present in all regions of the central nervous system and constitute 5–20% of the glial population and populate the brain as discrete cells that lack physical contact with each other, unlike astrocytes which form a syncytium (Kreutzberg, 1996). Some regions, such as the substantia nigra and the hippocampus, have a greater density of microglia than the cortex and this could have pathological consequences (Lawson *et al.*, 1990). In white matter, the processes of microglia tend to run parallel to axons, whilst in gray matter they have a ramified shape; in both locations, their processes allow the microglia to "sense" a defined region of brain (extending approx 30–50 μm) for alterations in the microenvironment. In view of the distribution pattern of microglia and the well-established observation that microglia become activated at a very early stage to even minor pathological changes in injured or diseased neurons, these cells have been thought of as the brain's resident macrophages (Raivich *et al.*, 1999; Streit *et al.*, 1999). However, it should be noted that there are also macrophages residing in the perivascular spaces of the brain between neural parenchyma and vascular endothelial cells which are bone marrow-derived and which serve as antigen-presenting cells (APCs). These macrophages are phenotypically distinct from microglia and have immunological properties of peripheral accessory cells (Streit, 2002). The perivascular macrophages are thought to come into contact with and process CNS antigens that may seep from the brain parenchyma into the perivascular space. They can then present the CNS antigens to T lymphocytes. On the other hand, microglia in the cerebral parenchyma do not usually encounter T lymphocytes, and so do not act so readily as APCs (Streit, 2002).

The classical view is that injured or diseased neurons emit a signal, such as a transmitter or cytokine, that interacts with receptors on microglia that cause the microglia to become activated and pass from the resting, ramified shape to an intermediate hyper-ramified state, then to a reactive, activated state, before finally becoming amoebid phagocytes that remove dead cells (Streit *et al.*, 1999) and facilitate repair processes, such as angiogenesis and neurogenesis. Activated microglia release inflammatory mediators and also proliferate and migrate in the damaged microenvironment. The phagocytic microglia do not revert to the resting, ramified state and eventually undergo cell death. By analogy with peripheral macrophages, which have been found to have diverse functions including pro-inflammatory apoptotic, phagocytic and anti-inflammatory effects (Duffield, 2003), microglia may similarly represent a heterogenous group of cells within the brain.

Current view of microglia

Origin

Microglia are thought to be derived from blood monocytes that enter the CNS during embryonic development,

Inflammatory Diseases of the Central Nervous System, ed. T. Kilpatrick, R. M. Ransohoff and S. Wesselingh. Published by Cambridge University Press. © Cambridge University Press 2010

where they differentiate into parenchymal cells that express many of the cell surface antigens of blood macrophages (Kim and de Vellis, 2005).

Recently, with the application of molecular biology techniques, it has been possible to breed transgenic mice whose microglia have been labeled with enhanced green fluorescent protein (EGFP), using a plasmid carrying EGFP cDNA under the control of the promoter for ionized calcium-binding adaptor molecule (Iba-1), which is expressed selectively in microglia (Hirasawa et al., 2005). Using these mice, it is possible to visualize microglia in living brain tissue. The authors found that microglial progenitors originate from the yolk sac and are carried to the brain from hematopoietic organs via the bloodstream. They enter the brain parenchyma via the meninges in the prenatal period, although a smaller population enters postnatally at P5–10, which is restricted to particular areas such as the cingulum and the supraventricular corpus callosum, known as the "fountain of microglia" (Hirasawa et al., 2005). Thus, in these transgenic mice, the bone marrow cells are able to pass through the blood–brain barrier (BBB). On the other hand, recent experiments in adult mice using a parabiotic technique employing pairs of syngeneic animals expressing EGFP in all hematopoietic cells except erythroid cells demonstrated that there was no evidence of brain microglia progenitor recruitment from the circulation, despite marked microgliosis after denervation or induction of a CNS neurodegenerative disease (Ajami et al., 2007). These authors concluded that in adult mice, "microglia are maintained and function independently of bone marrow-derived progenitors throughout adult life".

Physiological function

A transgenic strain of mice in which the EGFP reporter gene placed into the *Cx3cr1* locus encoding the chemokine receptor CX3CR1 (fractalkine receptor) has resulted in a major breakthrough in our understanding of microglial function under physiological conditions. Nimmerjahn et al. (2005) used transcranial two-photon microscopy to image the fluorescent microglia for up to 200 μm below the surface of the cortex of these transgenic mice under anesthesia. While the distribution of the fluorescent microglia was homogeneous, with a territorial organization of cell-to-cell distances of 50–60 μm with fixed somata, as determined by observation over several hours, their ramified processes were, unexpectedly, remarkably motile, undergoing random cycles of formation, extension and withdrawal on a time scale of minutes (Figure 2.1). The processes extended and retracted with velocities of approximately 1.5 μm/min, and they displayed bulbous tips with an average lifetime of 4 min. It appeared that the microglial processes were sampling and assessing the microenvironment around neuronal cell bodies, dendrites, astrocytes, and blood vessels. Time-lapse recordings suggested that the brain parenchyma is completely sampled by microglia once every few hours (Nimmerjahn et al., 2005). On the other hand, fluorescently tagged astrocytes showed no comparable movement of their processes, nor did neuronal dendrites. Similar observations were made independently using the same transgenic EGFP mice by Davalos et al. (2005) who found, in addition, that the microglial processes responded within a minute to a laser-induced mechanical injury by extending to the damaged site. After 30 min, all the processes of nearby microglia had reached the damaged site and fused together to corral this region. The authors found that this chemotactic response could be mimicked by the local injection of ATP from a glass capillary inserted into the cortex, and that the ATP appeared to work through the stimulation of P2Y receptors on microglia (Haynes et al., 2006). The papers of Nimmerjahn et al. (2005) and Davalos et al. (2005) thus have changed the traditional dogma that microglia are "resting" or "quiescent", and instead have highlighted the physical motility of microglial processes which, in addition to their known role of responding to CNS injury, may include a "house-keeping" role of phagocytosing secreted proteins and/or membrane debris under normal physiological states.

Another key aspect of microglial biology is their ability to proliferate, particularly after CNS injury, and recent research has focused on the endogenous mitogens that could trigger this response. Unfortunately, the two-photon in-vivo imaging technique of Nimmerjahn et al. (2005) did not show proliferation of microglial somata, probably because of the time limit for maintaining general anesthesia. However, 5-bromo-2'-deoxyuridine (BrdU) incorporation assays using a specific monoclonal antibody have enabled microglial proliferation to be studied both in vitro and in vivo after CNS injury. A recent study (Flanary and Streit, 2006) using cultured rat primary microglia showed that incubation with recombinant rat granulocyte macrophage-colony stimulating factor (GM-CSF)

(a)

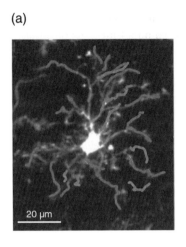

20 μm

(b)

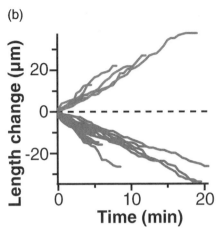

Figure 2.1 A. Transcranial time-lapse recording of a single microglial cell expressing EGFP in the mouse cortex *in situ*. Processes marked in green represent their formation while processes marked in red represent retraction of processes over a 20-min period. B. Plot of length changes amongst the processes depicted in the upper panel as a function of time. (Modified from Nimmerjahn *et al.* (2005). Reprinted with permission from AAAS.)

produced a sustained increase in the proliferation rate from day 2 to day 12, but interestingly, addition of vitamin E (α-tocopherol) produced at least five times the number of dividing microglial cells as GM-CSF over the same time period, and this was accompanied by a decrease in telomere length in the presence of a decrease in telomerase activity. This action of α-tocopherol appeared to be independent of its antioxidative property and could be due to its interaction with key kinases such as protein kinase C, phosphatidylinositol 3-kinases and other cyclin-dependent kinases (Flanary and Streit, 2006).

Microglia also play an important role in CNS development by actively promoting the death of post-mitotic neurons. This has been shown in the case of developing cerebellar Purkinje cells by the elegant experiments of Marin-Teva *et al.* (2004). They showed, using cerebellar slices obtained from postnatal day 3 mice, that microglia promoted the apoptosis of Purkinje cells through the production of superoxide anions similar to the well-established respiratory burst of phagocytes that eliminated microbes in the periphery. Thus, microglia could be responsible for executing the surplus Purkinje neurons and then scavenging the dead cells. Also during fetal development but not later, microglia express thrombospondin, an extracellular matrix protein that regulates synaptogenesis (Chamak *et al.*, 1995).

Pathophysiological function(s)

There is now convincing evidence that microglia play a key role in initiating neurodegeneration in many neurological disorders such as Parkinson's and Alzheimer's diseases, neuropathic pain, stroke, motor neuron disease, multiple sclerosis, and even psychiatric disorders

such as depression and HIV-associated dementia (Marchetti *et al.*, 2005). This is based on animal models of these disorders, as well as post-mortem examination of human tissue and sophisticated positron emission tomography (PET) of the brains of patients with these disorders using ^{11}C-PK11195 (*N*-butan-2-yl-1-(2-chlorophenyl)-*N*-methylisoquinoline-3-carboxamide) (see Banati, 2003). This latter technique enables accurate spatial localization of activated microglia within the CNS which aids in temporal studies of disease progression, as well as the interrogation of secondary neurodegenerative or adaptive responses remote from the primary site of disease (Banati, 2003). However, microglia can also have a beneficial role in these pathophysiological states by releasing neurotrophins and growth factors to initiate the repair of neurons, glia, or blood vessels. Thus microglia are said to function as "double edge swords" or "friend and foe" (Kempermann and Neumann, 2003). This topic has been reviewed extensively in recent years (see Kim and de Vellis, 2005; Minghetti *et al.*, 2005; Sargsyan *et al.*, 2005). This chapter therefore focuses on the known pathogenic and protective mediators released from microglia to expedite these functions, as well as providing an emphasis on experimental drugs that could modulate both types of mediators.

Activation of microglia

As microglia constitute the innate immunity within the brain, it is not surprising that they are the first cells to respond to CNS injury. This occurs within minutes (see above), and can occur in response to a variety of insults, including mechanical damage, ischemia, invasion by microbes, or the influx of toxic chemicals. When the motile processes of microglia encounter either a pathogen or neurotoxic molecules (either endogenous or exogenous chemicals), they undergo dramatic and rapid molecular and phenotypic changes that are collectively referred to as the "activated state". Morphologically, this comprises change from a ramified to an amoeboid shape, followed by proliferation and migration (Streit *et al.*, 1999). It has even been proposed (Nakajima and Kohsaka, 2004) that microglia can sense low oxygen tension and become activated even before neural death has occurred. Recently, Lu *et al.* (2006), studying primary cultures of rat microglia, found that hypoxia up-regulated Hypoxia-Inducible-Factor-1α (HIF-1α) within 4 h in the cytosol, which then translocated to the nucleus where it increased iNOS expression and NO production (see below). However, it is unlikely that this is the sole sensing mechanism, as changes in expression of ion channels and exposure/stimulation by several biochemical agents have been found to activate microglia.

Changes in ion channels

Patch clamp studies of microglia both in vitro and in vivo have shown that microglia express Cl^-, K^+, Na^+, H^+, Ca^{2+} and non-selective cationic channels (Eder, 2005), but these are not permanently expressed and can be dramatically changed by pro- and anti-inflammatory stimuli. Of particular interest are the $K_v1.3$ potassium channel and the $Na_v1.6$ sodium channel. The $K_v1.3$ potassium channel becomes selectively expressed in activated microglia and plays a key role in killing adjacent neurons via release of superoxide anion and, significantly, killing can be prevented by the application of a $K_v1.3$ channel blocker, agitoxin-2 (Fordyce *et al.*, 2005). The $Na_v1.6$ channel is the predominant sodium channel expressed in microglia and there is approximately a fivefold increase in its expression during microglial activation within the spinal cord of mice during experimental autoimmune encephalomyelitis (EAE), as well as in human post-mortem MS spinal cord sections (Craner *et al.*, 2005). These investigators also showed that chronic treatment of mice with EAE with the sodium channel blocker, phenytoin, ameliorated the inflammatory cell infiltrate within the spinal cord.

Biochemical activators of microglia

l-Glutamate

Microglia are well endowed with neurotransmitter receptors that are coupled directly to ion channels or via GTP binding proteins, and which therefore could rapidly "sense" a major change in concentrations of neurotransmitters in their vicinity. In particular, excessive release of the major excitatory transmitter, glutamate is well established as an initial response to brain injury triggering neuronal death (glutamate excitotoxicity). It is significant that glutamate receptors such as the ionotropic AMPA (α-amino-3-hydroxy-5-methyl-4-isoxazole-propionic acid) and kainate subclass and metabotropic glutamate receptors (mGlu2 and 3) are expressed by microglia (Noda *et al.*, 2000; Taylor *et al.*, 2005). These subclasses of glutamate receptors are capable of responding to a wide concentration range of glutamate in the extracellular environment. It is possible that the influx of Ca^{2+} through these receptors serves to activate Ca^{2+}-dependent protein kinases in microglia.

ATP

Not only is ATP a major excitatory neurotransmitter in the brain, it is also released when mitochondria are damaged early after CNS injury. Microglia express ATP receptors, both of the ionotropic P2X family and the G-protein coupled P2Y family, and this allows microglia to sense different concentrations of ATP and thereby activate different transcription processes. For example, the release of tumor necrosis factor-alpha (TNF-α) from microglia requires only low concentrations of ATP, whereas the release of interleukin-6 requires higher concentrations (Inoue, 2006). Stimulation of $P2X_7$ ionotropic receptors by millimolar concentrations of ATP can also induce the formation of cytolytic pores in microglia resulting in: (a) prolonged entry of extracellular Ca^{2+}, K^+ and Na^+ through this ion channel, as well as the release of IL-1β; (b) activation of diacylglycerol lipase; and (c) synthesis and release of the endogenous cannabinoid, 2-arachidonoylglycerol which can function as a protective mediator (see below) (Witting *et al.*, 2004; Inoue, 2006).

Thrombin

Thrombin is a serine protease that is best known as a key factor in the blood coagulation cascade after it is formed from its precursor, prothrombin, which normally circulates in blood at micromolar concentrations. However, prothrombin has also been found to be expressed in the brain, including the cell bodies of dopaminergic neurons in the substantia nigra (Weinstein *et al.*, 1995). Prothrombin appears to be neuroprotective at low concentrations (<50 nM), but at higher concentrations, which, for example, occur after cerebrovascular injury, prothrombin is rapidly converted to thrombin, which then causes toxic responses to neurons and astrocytes and contributes to the breakdown of the blood–brain barrier (Gingrich and Traynelis, 2000). Thrombin also acts via G-protein coupled proteinase-activated receptors (PARs 1 and 4) on microglia (Noorbakhsh *et al.*, 2003; Suo *et al.*, 2003) to increase the synthesis of pro-inflammatory cytokines and to increase the expression of iNOS, which then leads to increased NO formation followed by increased peroxynitrite levels and neurotoxicity (see below). Katsuki *et al.* (2006), using rat midbrain slice cultures, have shown that application of thrombin causes a progressive loss in the number of dopaminergic neurons, in addition to activating microglia and increasing expression of iNOS, which was dependent on mitogen-activated protein kinases (MAPKs) such as extracellular signal-related kinase (ERK), p38 MAPK and c-Jun N-terminal kinase (JNK). Furthermore, these authors demonstrated that depletion of resident microglia in the slices with liposomes containing the cytotoxic drug clodronate markedly attenuated the number of activated microglia, as well as reducing dopaminergic cell death, indicating that activated microglia were essential for thrombin-induced dopaminergic neuronal cell death. In-vivo studies in rats have confirmed that the neurotoxic actions of thrombin involve microglial activation (Choi *et al.*, 2003). These authors injected thrombin into the rat substantia nigra and showed by tyrosine hydroxylase immunohistochemistry that there was a significant loss of dopaminergic neurons in this area, as well as a parallel activation of microglia. Similar to the in-vitro studies of Katsuki *et al.* (2006), Choi *et al.* (2003) found that ERK and p38 MAPK were activated in microglia in the substantia nigra as early as 30 min after thrombin injection. Overall, these results suggest that perturbations of the blood–brain barrier could lead to extravasation of thrombin into the brain, where it could be an endogenous agent that triggers the neuropathological loss of dopaminergic neuronal cell bodies in Parkinson's disease via activation of microglia.

Complement

With the change in shape of the microglial cell membrane, there is a well-characterized up-regulation of a variety of cell-surface molecules including complement receptor 3 (also known as cluster determinant

CD11b). The monoclonal antibody OX-42 is widely used as an immunohistochemical marker of complement receptor 3 on microglia (Robinson *et al.*, 1986), as is a radioiodinated peptide ligand, ^{125}I-CGP42112, enabling the visualization and quantitation of activated microglia (Roulston *et al.*, 2004).

Others

The development of microarray analysis has provided a wealth of information on changes in expression of genes, both up and down, at lesion sites in the spinal cord, as well as in rostral and caudal adjoining areas after a variety of mild, moderate and severe injuries (see, for example, Byrnes *et al.*, 2006). These gene changes are extensive and complex, and a discussion of these changes is outside the scope of this chapter. What is well established is that upon activation, microglia produce and release a variety of biochemicals that can be classified as pathogenic or protective mediators acting upon adjacent neurons, astrocytes and/or cerebral blood vessels. This is discussed in the following sections.

Pathogenic mediators

ROS from NOX

Reactive oxygen species (ROS) have an unpaired electron in the outer orbital of oxygen atoms that makes them highly reactive and chemically unstable. They react with cellular membranes, proteins, and nucleic acids to cause damage that can lead to cell death. The NADPH oxidase (NOX) is a major source of ROS and is present in microglia as a multi-unit complex (Wilkinson and Landreth, 2006). When microglia are activated by ATP, as well as some chemokines and cytokines (Babior, 2004), a cytosolic complex is phosphorylated and translocates to the plasma membrane where it assembles with two membrane subunits (gp91^{phox} and p22^{phox}) of NOX, which then initiates electron flow and generates superoxide anion (O_2^-) from molecular oxygen. The superoxide anion can then kill pathogens. The superoxide anion is normally converted to hydrogen peroxide by the enzyme superoxide dismutase, but can also react with nitric oxide to form the highly damaging substance, peroxynitrite (ONOO$^-$), which is more toxic to neurons than superoxide anion. It is of interest that inhibitors of NOX, such as diphenylene iodonium or apocynin, prevent microglial proliferation in primary cultures of rat glia. On the other hand, continuous generation of hydrogen peroxide in cultures using either exogenous xanthine and xanthine oxidase or glucose and glucose oxidase was able to double their rate of proliferation, thus establishing the role of hydrogen peroxide generated from NOX as a mitogenic signal for these cells (Mander *et al.*, 2006). The formation of peroxynitrite by activated microglia is responsible for the death of premyelinating oligodendrocytes in co-cultures (Li *et al.*, 2005). These authors also demonstrated that blocking the formation of peroxynitrite with a peroxynitrite decomposition catalyst or a superoxide dismutase mimetic protected the premyelinating oligodendrocytes from activated microglial-induced death.

The question then arises as to why peroxynitrite does not kill microglia. Hirrlinger *et al.* (2000) found that microglia have a prominent glutathione system due to high levels of glutathione reductase and glutathione peroxidase activities, and proposed that this reducing agent protected microglia from the ROS produced in either an autocrine or paracrine fashion.

NO from iNOS

Inducible nitric oxide synthase (iNOS, NOS II) is not expressed in the CNS under normal conditions, but is induced in microglia by pro-inflammatory cytokines such as TNF-α and interferon-γ, by bacterial cell wall components such as lipopolysaccharide (LPS) from Gram-negative bacteria that act on toll-like receptor 4, and by lipoteichoic acid from Gram-positive bacteria that acts on toll-like receptor 2 (Arai *et al.*, 2003; Kinsner *et al.*, 2006). In-vivo studies in mice showed that injection of interferon-γ plus either LPS or TNF-α into the lateral ventricle acted synergistically to enhance iNOS expression compared to interferon-γ alone (Kong *et al.*, 2000). Once induced, iNOS produces high, sustained concentrations of nitric oxide that rapidly diffuse into nearby neurons that causes the release of L-glutamate leading to glutamate excitotoxicity. More importantly, NO will react with the superoxide anion (see above) to form the neurotoxic agent peroxynitrite. In-vitro studies of co-cultures of rat primary cortical neurons and microglia by Mander and Brown (2005) demonstrated that neither the induction of iNOS nor the activation of NADPH oxidase alone in the co-cultures resulted in a significant increase in neuronal death, whereas the induction of both enzymes resulted in substantial neuronal death. As this neuronal death was then blocked by the addition of an iNOS inhibitor plus an NADPH oxidase inhibitor, this demonstrated that it was the formation

of peroxynitrite that was the toxic mediator and neither NO nor the superoxide anion. In fact, NO alone can exert neuroprotective actions, as rat strains such as the Brown Norway strain are resistant to EAE and produce increased levels of NO from their macrophages compared to the susceptible Lewis strain (Staykova *et al.*, 2005).

Pro-inflammatory cytokines

Microglia are one of the primary sources of cytokines in the CNS that play a role in inflammatory responses in a variety of neurological disease states, as well as in response to neurotoxic insults (Stoll and Jander, 1999; Raivich *et al.*, 1999; Sriram *et al.*, 2006). Chemokines, which are chemotactic cytokines that elicit leukocyte migration into the brain after ischemic damage, also signal to microglia to undergo chemotaxis (Ubogu *et al.*, 2006).

Tumor necrosis factor alpha (TNF-α)

This is a prominent pro-inflammatory cytokine that is now established to play a key role in neurodegenerative disorders. Stimulation of mGlu2 receptors on microglia causes activation and substantial release of TNF-α (Taylor *et al.*, 2005). The TNF-α is secreted as a 17-kDa polypeptide through enzymatic cleavage from 26-kDa transmembrane TNF by a disintegrin and metalloproteinase, TNF-α converting enzyme (Hallenbeck, 2002). The TNF-α is a pleiotropic cytokine that induces either cell proliferation or cell death depending upon effector cell pathways in the TNF-responsive cells (Kamata *et al.*, 2005). The TNF-α interacts with two distinct receptors, TNFR1 (p55) and TNFR2 (p75), which act as homotrimers, each of which activates different intracellular signal transduction pathways resulting in different biological effects. The TNFR1 has cytoplasmic domains that in most cells induce apoptosis through either a death domain or downstream activation of nuclear factor kappa B (NF-κB). On the other hand, TNFR2 transduces growth and cellular activation signals but can also potentiate TNFR1-mediated cell death and NF-κB induction. In addition, TNF-α stimulates extensive microglial glutamate release in an autocrine manner by up-regulating the enzyme, glutaminase, and facilitating release of glutamate through a connexin 32 hemichannel gap junction (Takeuchi *et al.*, 2006). Furthermore, TNF-α also inhibits uptake of glutamate by a glutamate transporter on astrocytes, namely GLAST (glutamate-aspartate transporter) and GLT-1 (glutamate transporter-1) (Persson *et al.*, 2005). These combined actions could promote glutamate excitotoxicity on adjacent neurons. The TNF-α also stimulates the expression of iNOS in astrocytes and induces activation of adhesion molecule expression on vascular endothelium that then facilitates the passage of leukocytes from the circulation into the ischemic brain (Gregersen *et al.*, 2000).

Interleukin-1 (IL-1)

There are three members of the IL-1 family – IL-1α and Il-1β, which act as agonists, and IL-1 type 1 receptor antagonist (IL-1ra) (Allan *et al.*, 2005). The IL-1α and IL-1β, while having high sequence homology, are the products of different genes which are first synthesized as precursor species, namely pro-IL-1α that is biologically active and then cleaved by calpain to form IL-1α, and pro-IL-1β which is biologically inactive and requires cleavage by caspase-1 to form IL-1β. The third ligand, IL-1ra, is a naturally occurring competitive receptor antagonist that is produced in the same cells that express Il-1β (Allan *et al.*, 2005). All members of the IL-1 family are constitutively expressed in the CNS in very low or undetectable concentrations, but expression of the genes that encode IL-1α and IL-1β is induced by a variety of pro-inflammatory stimuli such as LPS, TNF-α and cellular injury. On the other hand, glucocorticoids and annexin-1 inhibit the transcription of genes encoding IL-1. The IL-1α and IL-1β exert their actions by binding to a specific plasma membrane receptor, the IL-1 type-1 receptor, which then associates with an IL-1 receptor accessory protein, leading to intracellular signal transduction (Allan and Rothwell, 2001). These intracellular signaling pathways culminate in the activation of NF-κB, p38 MAPK, and JNK enzymes. Microglial cells are the main source of IL-1β in the brain, and LPS induces the synthesis and release of IL-1β in its pro-form (Pinteaux *et al.*, 2002).

Chemokines

Previously known as interferon-inducible protein IP10, CXCL10 is strongly expressed in many neurodegenerative diseases by astrocytes, microglia, and neurons as well as on damaged neurons after experimental lesions. The specific receptor of CXCL10 is CXCR3 and is expressed on microglia (Rappert *et al.*, 2004). The CXCR3 receptor controls the migration of microglia to lesioned neurons both in vitro and in vivo, where it is responsible for neuronal reorganization.

Protective mediators

Cytokines

Interleukin-4 (IL-4)

This cytokine is known to suppress superoxide anion production in microglia activated by TNF-α or interferon-γ (Chao *et al.*, 1995) as well as blocking microglia-mediated brain injury (Chao *et al.*, 1993). Recently, Zhao *et al.* (2006) applied IL-4 to co-cultures of primary activated microglia and motoneurons and found that IL-4 protected against motoneuron injury by reducing NO production and suppressing microglial superoxide anion production in the presence of lipopolysaccharide, possibly through an up-regulation of insulin-like growth factor 1 levels and a down-regulation of TNF-α. One potential source of this protective mediator is Th2 lymphocytes, although in-vivo studies are needed to determine whether IL-4 does, indeed, achieve neuroprotective effects by blocking the neurotoxic effects of microglia (Zhao *et al.*, 2006).

Chemokines

Formerly known as fractalkine, CX3CL1 is one of only two chemokines that are constitutively expressed in neurons in the CNS both as a soluble and a membrane-anchored form that is cleaved by a metalloproteinase while its receptor, CX3CR1, is expressed exclusively by microglia (in mice), suggesting that it acts as a molecular messenger in neuron–microglia communication (Ré and Przedborski, 2006). When CX3CL1 is incubated in microglial cultures in the presence of BrdU, it causes a threefold increase in microglial proliferation compared to control cells, which indicates it plays a role in the proliferative response of microglia to injury (Hatori *et al.*, 2002). Elegant experiments by Cardona *et al.* (2006) using three clinically relevant mouse models of neurodegenerative diseases (LPS-induced neuroinflammation, the MPTP model of Parkinsonism, and SOD1^{G93A} amyotrophic lateral sclerosis), in which the *Cx3cr1* gene was replaced with a cDNA encoding green fluorescent protein, revealed that the receptor knockout mice were more susceptible to these neurotoxic insults, as judged both by the extent of microglial activation and by behavioral indices, than wild-type mice. Cardona *et al.* (2006) suggested that CX3CL1 acts in healthy mouse brains as an endogenous neuroprotectant to suppress the microglial neurotoxic phenotype.

Neurotrophins

It is well established that neurotrophins are involved in multiple phases of neuronal development including growth, differentiation and survival, as well as the proliferation of oligodendrocyte precursors. The availability of selective antisera against neurotrophins such as brain-derived neurotrophic factor (BDNF), nerve growth factor (NGF), neurotrophin-3 (NT-3), and neurotrophin-4/5 (NT-4/5) as well their receptors, and their cognate tyrosine kinase receptors (the tropomyosin receptor kinase (Trk) family comprising TrkA, TrkB and TrkC) has made it possible to determine the role of these neurotrophins in the proliferation and function of microglia (Elkabes et al., 1996; Friedman et al., 1998; Dougherty et al., 2000). These studies show that microglia normally express neurotrophins in a heterogeneous manner, suggesting that different subpopulations of microglia subserve different functions, with NT-3, in particular, promoting microglial proliferation and phagocytosis (Elkabes et al., 1996). Of particular significance is the finding that incubation of lipopolysaccharide with cultured microglia differentially altered neurotrophin receptor expression, which results in a marked expression of TrkC receptor but a down-regulation of TrkA receptors (Elkabes et al., 1998). At the same time, LPS also differentially altered neurotrophin expression, with mRNA encoding NT-3 and NGF being elevated four- to fivefold, respectively, within 6 h, whereas NT-4/5 and BDNF mRNA were unaltered. Decreased neurotrophin expression by microglia may be a consequence of aging or of direct insults such as viral infections, for example, HIV (Vilhardt, 2005).

Others

Endocannabinoids

The molecules 2-arachidonoylglycerol and anandamide function as endogenous agonists for the two major classes of cannabinoid receptors (CB_1 and CB_2) in the brain. These endocannabinoids are released after brain injury and inflammation, and attenuate neuronal injury by binding to CB_1 receptors on nerve terminals to inhibit the release of excitatory transmitters such as glutamate. They also act on CB receptors expressed on activated microglia via a novel intracellular negative feedback loop to prevent the release of pro-inflammatory cytokines that would otherwise damage neurons (Eljaschewitsch et al., 2006).

Drugs and toxins acting on microglia

Minocycline is a semi-synthetic tetracycline antibiotic that also has prominent anti-inflammatory actions both in the brain and periphery (Amin et al., 1996). It has been reported that the anti-inflammatory action of minocycline is due not to inhibition of iNOS enzyme activity but to a reduction in iNOS protein levels due to increased degradation of iNOS mRNA in both macrophages and microglia. Studies in primary cultures of rat microglia have shown that exposure to hypoxia (8 h) followed by reoxygenation (24 h) causes a marked increase in NO production (6.3-fold) as well as increased iNOS protein that was mediated through a p38 MAPK pathway, and this was significantly reduced in the presence of minocycline (1 and 10 μM) (Suk, 2004). More recent biochemical studies using the quantitative real-time reverse transcriptase polymerase chain reaction have shown that minocycline treatment reduces the up-regulation of caspase-3 mRNA in rat spinal cord after contusive injury as well as reducing the number of activated microglia seen in tissue sections by immunohistochemistry (Festoff et al., 2006). Minocycline is also an antioxidant with free radical scavenging potency similar to edaravone (Kraus et al., 2005).

However, it should be noted that minocycline could also theoretically affect the expression of protective mediators such as neurotrophins and growth factors. Long-term studies are required to determine whether this might be an important mechanism of action influencing the therapeutic efficacy of minocycline and of similar agents.

Edaravone is a free radical scavenger/antioxidant that is used widely in Japan to treat acute stroke (Edaravone Acute Infarction Study Group, 2003). In primary cultures of mouse microglia stimulated with LPS and IFNγ, edaravone significantly decreased the production of NO by these activated microglia, as well as inhibited the expression of iNOS mRNA in a concentration-dependent manner (Banno et al., 2005). However, edaravone did not inhibit the production of the pro-inflammatory cytokines, IL-1β, IL-6 and TNF-α at the protein or mRNA level after activation of microglia by LPS. In cocultures of primary neurons and microglia, addition of LPS and IFNγ resulted in neuronal death that was characterized by fragmented neurites and shrunken cell bodies and addition of edaravone significantly increased neuronal survival rates.

Opiates

A recent pharmacological study of morphine on cultured rat primary microglia found that a realistic concentration (1 µM) induced morphological changes, namely, from a bipolar, rod-like shape to an amoeboid shape with membrane ruffling at the edge of the cells as early as 10 min after exposure (Takayama and Ueda, 2005). Pretreatment with the selective opiate receptor antagonist, naloxone, at 1 µM had no effect on membrane ruffling, but blocked the effect of morphine when added 30 min later. Morphine enhanced BDNF mRNA expression in a concentration-dependent manner (0.3–1 µM) as early as 1 h after exposure, an effect that was maintained for at least 12 h, and this action was also blocked by naloxone. Interestingly, chemotaxis of microglia studied in a Boyden chamber was stimulated by morphine and closely related to membrane ruffling and was also blocked by naloxone. In-vivo studies in which rats were given morphine daily for 5 days by intrathecal injection resulted not only in the development of tolerance and hyperalgesia to the analgesic effects of morphine, but also in the release of pro-inflammatory cytokines and chemokines, particularly CX3CL1. Interestingly, the co-administration of a neutralizing antibody to the receptor CX3CR1 with morphine potentiated acute morphine analgesia and attenuated the development of tolerance and hyperalgesia (Johnston *et al.*, 2004).

Acrolein

High concentrations of the polyamines spermine and spermidine have been identified within the CNS, but they do not function as neurotransmitters and, instead, are thought to be involved in cell growth, proliferation and differentiation (Tabor and Tabor, 1984). Recently, it has been observed that submicromolar concentrations of spermine and spermidine induce death of cultured microglial cells by apoptotic pathways in the presence of 10% fetal calf serum but not in serum-free medium (Takano *et al.*, 2003). This group has now found that aminoguanidine, an inhibitor of plasma amine oxidase, suppressed the spermine-induced microglial cell death in the presence of fetal calf serum in a concentration-dependent manner, and that the reaction product of spermine and plasma amine oxidase, acrolein, was the causative agent (Takano *et al.*, 2005). Thus, regulation of this activity could play a role in terminating the activation of microglia in pathological states after the microglia have finished phagocytosing cell debris.

Conclusion

The application of molecular biological and in-vivo imaging techniques has given new insight into the role of brain microglia in normal and pathological states. While the rapid activation and proliferation of microglia at the site of injury in the CNS has a beneficial effect in minimizing neuronal damage, it is probable that chronic microglial activation causes neuronal injury through the release of a multitude of endogenous cytotoxic mediators. Several experimental drugs have been found to suppress microglial activation and appear to be neuroprotective in the short term, but more research needs to be done to show functional restoration of neural connections. With advances in genomic and proteomic analysis at the single cell level, it should soon be possible to understand the molecular control of the microglial phenotype, to enable rational pharmacological strategies to promote beneficial microglial activity in a wide range of neurodegenerative disorders.

References

Ajami B et al. Local self-renewal can sustain CNS microglia maintenance and function throughout adult life. *Nat Neurosci* 2007; **10**: 1538–43.

Allan SM, Rothwell NJ. Cytokines and acute neurodegeneration. *Nat Rev Neurosci* 2001; **2**: 734–44.

Allan SM, et al. Interleukin-1 and neuronal injury. *Nat Rev Immunol* 2005; **5**: 629–40.

Amin AR, et al. A novel mechanism of action of tetracyclines: Effects on nitric oxide synthase. *Proc Natl Acad Sci USA* 1996; **93**: 14014–19.

Arai H, et al. Neurotoxic effects of lipopolysaccharide on nigral dopaminergic neurons are mediated by microglial activation, interleukin-1β and expression of caspase-11 in mice. *J Biol Chem* 2003; **279**: 51647–53.

Babior BM. NADPH oxidase. *Curr Opin Immunol* 2004; **16**: 42–7.

Banati RB. Neuropathological imaging: In vivo detection of glial activation as a measure of disease and adaptive change in the brain. *Brit Med Bull* 2003; **65**: 121–31.

Banno M, et al. The radical scavenger edaravone prevents oxidative neurotoxicity induced by peroxynitrite and activated microglia. *Neuropharmacology* 2005; **48**: 283–90.

Byrnes KR, et al. Expression of two temporally distinct microglia-related gene clusters after spinal cord injury. *Glia* 2006; **53**: 420–33.

Cardona AE, et al. Control of microglial neurotoxicity by the fractalkine receptor. *Nature Neurosci* 2006; **9**: 917–24.

Chamak B, et al. Immunohistochemical detection of thrombospondin in microglia in the developing rat brain. *Neuroscience* 1995; **69**: 177–87.

Chao CC, et al. Neuroprotective role of IL-4 against activated microglia. *J Immunol* 1993; **151**: 1473–81.

Chao CC, et al. Modulation of human microglial cell superoxide production by cytokines. *J Leukoc Biol* 1995; **58**: 65–70.

Choi SH, et al. Thrombin-induced microglial activation produces degeneration of nigral dopaminergic neurons in vivo. *J Neurosci* 2003; **23**: 5877–86.

Craner MJ, et al. Sodium channels contribute to microglia/macrophage activation and function in EAE and MS. *Glia* 2005; **49**: 220–9.

Davalos D, et al. ATP mediates rapid microglial response to local brain injury in vivo. *Nat Neurosci* 2005; **8**: 752–8.

Dougherty KD, et al. Brain-derived neurotrophic factor in astrocytes, oligodendrocytes and microglia/macrophages after spinal cord injury. *Neurobiol Dis* 2000; **7**: 574–85.

Duffield JS. The inflammatory macrophage: A story of Jekyll and Hyde. *Clin Sci* 2003; **104**: 27–38.

Edaravone Acute Infarction Study Group. Effect of a novel free radical scavenger, edaravone (MCI-186), on acute brain infarction. Randomized, placebo-controlled, double-blind study at multi-centers. *Cerebrovasc Dis* 2003; **15**: 222–9.

Eder C. Regulation of microglial behavior by ion channel activity. *J Neurosci Res* 2005; **81**: 314–21.

Eljaschewitsch E, et al. The endocannabinoid anandamide protects neurons during CNS inflammation by induction of MKP-1 in microglial cells. *Neuron* 2006; **49**: 67–79.

Elkabes S, et al. Brain microglia/macrophages express neurotrophins that selectively regulate microglial proliferation and function. *J Neurosci* 1 1996; **6**: 2508–21.

Elkabes S, et al. Lipopolysaccharide differentially regulates microglial Trk receptor and neurotrophin expression. *J Neurosci Res* 1998; **54**: 117–22.

Festoff BW, et al. Minocycline neuroprotects, reduces microgliosis, and inhibits caspase protease expression early after spinal cord injury. *J Neurochem* 2006; **97**: 1314–26.

Flanary BE, Streit WJ. Alpha-tocopherol (vitamin E) induces rapid, nonsustained proliferation in cultured rat microglia. *Glia* 2006; **53**: 669–74.

Fordyce CB, et al. Microglia Kv1.3 channels contribute to their ability to kill neurons. *J Neurosci* 2005; **25**: 7139–49.

Friedman WJ, et al. Distribution of the neurotrophins, brain-derived neurotrophic factor, neurotrophin-3, and neurotrophin-4/5 in the postnatal rat brain: an immunocytochemical study. *Neuroscience* 1998; **84**: 101–14.

Gingrich MB, Traynelis SF. Serine proteases and brain damage: Is there a link? *Trends Neurosci* 2000; **23**: 399–407.

Gregersen R, et al. Microglia and macrophages are the major source of tumor necrosis factor in permanent middle cerebral artery occlusion in mice. *J Cerebr Blood Flow Metab* 2000; **20**: 53–65.

Hallenbeck JM. The many faces of tumor necrosis factor in stroke. *Nature Med* 2002; **8**: 1363–8.

Hatori K, et al. Fractalkine and fractalkine receptors in human neurons and glial cells. *J Neurosci Res* 2002; **69**: 418–26.

Haynes SE, et al. The P2Y12 receptor regulates microglial activation by extracellular nucleotides. *Nat Neurosci* 2006; **9**: 1512–19.

Hirasawa T, et al. Visualization of microglia in living tissues using Iba1-EGFP transgenic mice. *J Neurosci Res* 2005; **81**: 357–62.

Hirrlinger J, et al. Microglial cells in culture express a prominent glutathione system for the defense against reactive oxygen species. *Dev Neurosci* 2000; **22**: 384–92.

Inoue K. The function of microglia through purinergic receptors: Neuropathic pain and cytokine release. *Pharmacol Ther* 2006; **109**: 210–26.

Johnston IN, et al. A role for pro-inflammatory cytokines and fractalkine in analgesia, tolerance, and subsequent pain facilitation induced by chronic intrathecal morphine. *J Neurosci* 2004; **24**: 9353–65.

Kamata H, *et al.* Reactive oxygen species promote TNF-α-induced death and sustained JNK activation by inhibiting MAP kinase phosphatases. *Cell* 2005; **120**: 649–61.

Katsuki H, *et al.* Nitric oxide-producing microglia mediate thrombin-induced degeneration of dopaminergic neurons in rat midbrain slice culture. *J Neurochem* 2006; **97**: 1232–42.

Kempermann G, Neumann H. Microglia: The enemy within? *Science* 2003; **302**: 1689–90.

Kim SU, de Vellis J. Microglia in health and disease. *J Neurosci Res* 2005; **81**: 302–13.

Kinsner A, *et al.* Highly purified lipoteichoic acid induced pro-inflammatory signaling in primary culture of rat microglia through toll-like receptor 2: Selective potentiation of nitric oxide production by muramyl dipeptide. *J Neurochem* 2006; **99**: 596–607.

Kong GY, *et al.* Inducible nitric oxide synthase expression elicited in the mouse brain by inflammatory mediators circulating in the cerebrospinal fluid. *Brain Res* 2000; **878**: 105–18.

Kraus RL, *et al.* Antioxidant properties of minocycline: Neuroprotection in an oxidative stress assay and direct radical-scavenging activity. *J Neurochem* 2005; **94**: 819–27.

Kreutzberg GW. Microglia: A sensor for pathological events in the CNS. *Trends Neurosci* 1996; **19**: 312–18.

Lawson LJ, *et al.* Heterogeneity in the distribution and morphology of microglia in the normal adult mouse brain. *Neuroscience* 1990; **39**: 151–70.

Li J, *et al.* Peroxynitrite generated by inducible nitric oxide synthase and NADPH oxidase mediates microglial toxicity to oligodendrocytes. *Proc Natl Acad Sci USA* 2005; **102**: 9936–41.

Lu DY, *et al.* Hypoxia-induced iNOS expression in microglia is regulated by the PI3-kinase/Akt/mTOR signaling pathway and activation of hypoxia inducible factor-1α. *Biochem Pharmacol* 2006; **72**: 992–1000.

Mander P, Brown GC. Activation of microglial NADPH oxidase is synergistic with glial iNOS expression in inducing neuronal death: A dual-key mechanism of inflammatory neurodegeneration. *J Neuroinflam* 2005; **2**: 20–34.

Mander P, *et al.* Microglia proliferation is regulated by hydrogen peroxide from NADPH oxidase. *J Immunol* 2006; **176**: 1046–52.

Marchetti B, *et al.* Glia–neuron crosstalk in neuroinflammation, neurodegeneration and neuroprotection. *Brain Res Brain Res Rev* 2005; **48**: 129–408.

Marin-Teva JL, *et al.* Microglia promote the death of developing Purkinje cells. *Neuron* 2004; **41**: 535–47.

Minghetti L, *et al.* Microglial activation in chronic neurodegenerative diseases: Roles of apoptotic neurons and chronic stimulation. *Brain Res Brain Res Rev* 2005; **48**: 251–6.

Nakajima K, Kohsaka S. Microglia: neuroprotective and neurotrophic cells in the central nervous system. *Curr Drug Targets Cardiovasc Hematol Disord* 2004; **4**: 65–84.

Nimmerjahn A, *et al.* Resting microglial cells are highly dynamic surveillants of brain parenchyma in vivo. *Science* 2005; **308**: 1314–18.

Noda M, *et al.* AMPA-kainate subtypes of glutamate receptor in rat cerebral microglia. *J Neurosci* 2000; **20**: 251–8.

Noorbakhsh F, *et al.* Proteinase-activated receptors in the nervous system. *Nat Rev Neurosci* 2003; **4**: 981–90.

Persson M, *et al.* Lipopolysaccharide increases microglial GLT-1 expression and glutamate uptake capacity in vitro by a mechanism dependent on TNF-α. *Glia* 2005; **51**: 111–20.

Pinteaux E, *et al.* Expression of interleukin-1 receptors and their role in interleukin-1 actions in murine microglial cells. *J Neurochem* 2002; **83**: 754–63.

Raivich G, *et al.* Neuroglial activation repertoire in the injured brain: Graded response, molecular mechanisms and cues to physiological function. *Brain Res Rev* 1999; **30**: 77–105.

Rappert A, *et al.* CXCR3-dependent microglial recruitment is essential for dendrite loss after brain lesion. *J Neurosci* 2004; **24**: 8500–9.

Ré DB, Przedborski S. Fractalkine: moving from chemotaxis to neuroprotection. *Nature Neurosci* 2006; **9**: 859–61.

Robinson AP, *et al.*, Macrophage heterogeneity in the rat as delineated by two monoclonal antibodies MRC OX-41 and MRC OX-42, the latter recognizing complement receptor type 3. *Immunology* 1986; **57**: 239–47.

Roulston CL, *et al.* Non-angiotensin II [^{125}I]-CGP42112 binding is a sensitive marker of neuronal injury in brainstem following unilateral nodose ganglionectomy: Comparison with markers for activated microglia. *Neuroscience* 2004; **127**: 753–67.

Sargsyan SA, *et al.* Microglia as potential contributors to motor neuron injury in amyotrophic lateral sclerosis. *Glia* 2005; **51**: 241–53.

Sriram K, *et al.* Deficiency of TNF receptors suppresses microglial activation and alters the susceptibility of brain regions to MPTP-induced neurotoxicity: role of TNF-α. *FASEB J* 2006; **20**: 670–82.

Staykova MA, *et al.* Nitric oxide contributes to resistance of the Brown Norway rat to experimental autoimmune encephalomyelitis. *Am J Pathol* 2005; **166**: 147–57.

Stoll G, Jander S. The role of microglia and macrophages in the pathophysiology of the CNS. *Prog Neurobiol* 1999; **58**: 233–47.

Streit WJ. Microglia as neuroprotective, immunocompetent cells of the CNS. *Glia* 2002; **40**: 133–9.

Streit WJ, *et al.* Reactive microgliosis. *Prog Neurobiol* 1999; **57**: 563–81.

Suk K. Minocycline suppresses hypoxic activation of rodent microglia in culture. *Neurosci Lett* 2004; **366**: 167–71.

Suo Z, *et al.* Persistent protease-activated receptor 4 signaling mediates thrombin-induced

25

microglial activation. *J Biol Chem* 2003; **278**: 3177–83.

Tabor CW, Tabor H. Polyamines. *Annu Rev Biochem* 1984; **53**: 749–90.

Takano K, *et al.* Microglial cell death induced by a low concentration of polyamines. *Neuroscience* 2003; **120**: 961–7.

Takano K, *et al.* Oxidative metabolites are involved in polyamine-induced microglial cell death. *Neuroscience* 2005; **134**: 1123–31.

Takayama N, Ueda H. Morphine-induced chemotaxis and brain-derived neurotrophic factor expression in microglia. *J Neurosci* 2005; **25**: 430–5.

Takeuchi H, *et al.* Tumor necrosis factor-α induces neurotoxicity via glutamate release from hemichannels of activated microglia in an autocrine manner. *J Biol Chem* 2006; **281**: 21362–8.

Taylor DL, *et al.* Stimulaton of microglial metabotropic glutamate receptor mGlu2 triggers tumor necrosis factor α-induced neurotoxicity in concert with microglial-derived fas ligand. *J Neurosci* 2005; **25**: 2952–64.

Ubogu EE, *et al.* The expression and function of chemokines involved in CNS inflammation. *Trends Pharmacol Sci* 2006; **27**: 48–54.

Vilhardt F. Microglia: Phagocyte and glia cell. *Int J Biochem Cell Biol* 2005; **37**: 17–21.

Weinstein JR, *et al.* Cellular localization of thrombin receptor mRNA in rat brain: Expression by mesencephalic dopaminergic neurons and codistribution with prothrombin mRNA. *J Neurosci* 1995; **15**: 2506–19.

Wilkinson BL, Landreth GE. The microglial NADPH oxidase complex as a source of oxidative stress in Alzheimer's disease. *J Neuroinflamm* 2006; **3**: 30–42.

Witting A, *et al.* P2X$_7$ receptors control 2-arachidonoylglycerol production by microglial cells. *Proc Natl Acad Sci USA* 2004; **101**: 3214–19.

Zhao W, *et al.* Protective effects of an anti-inflammatory cytokine, interleukin-4, on motorneuron toxicity induced by activated microglia. *J Neurochem* 2006; **99**: 1176–87.

Chapter 3

The role of dendritic cells in neuro-inflammation

Heather Donaghy, Edwina J. Wright and Anthony L. Cunningham

Introduction

The brain has long been described as an immune-privileged site due partly to the lack of dendritic cells (DCs) in the central nervous system (CNS). Recent research, however, indicates that DCs infiltrate the CNS both in the steady state and in inflammatory disease.

An understanding of the presence and the role of DCs in the healthy and diseased CNS is an evolving field of research. As the cellular constituents of the inflamed CNS can only be studied by intermittent sampling of the cerebrospinal fluid (CSF), biopsies, or at post-mortem, animal models provide the cornerstone of this evolving understanding. Dendritic cells were first widely recognized to play a role in CNS inflammatory disorders when Serafini et al. demonstrated that DC recruitment into and subsequent maturation within the CNS of mice was pivotal to the development and progression of experimental autoimmune encephalomyelitis (EAE; Serafini et al., 2000), an animal model of multiple sclerosis. Since then, DCs have been shown to be present within the CNS in several neuro-inflammatory disorders, including multiple sclerosis (MS)(Plumb et al., 2003), Guillain–Barré syndrome (GBS) (Press et al., 2005) and also in CNS infections including toxoplasmosis (Fischer et al., 2000), cryptococcosis, leishmaniasis (Abreu-Silva et al., 2003) and bacterial meningitis (Pashenkov et al., 2002b).

In this chapter we provide an outline of different DC subsets within humans and animals and describe the DCs found within the CNS both constitutively and in CNS inflammatory disorders and the role that they play in neuro-inflammation.

Dendritic cells

Dendritic cells are a heterogeneous population of antigen-presenting cells located throughout the blood, tissues and lymphoid organs (Donaghy et al., 2006;

Shortman and Liu, 2002). There are a number of functionally and phenotypically distinct populations in both mice and humans, resulting in a complex system of DCs. This complexity arises from different lineage origins (Rissoan et al., 1999; Robinson et al., 1999), states of differentiation and anatomical location. Dendritic cells are involved in the generation of both innate and adaptive immune responses through the up-regulation of co-stimulatory molecule expression and the release of cytokines (such as IL12, IL10 and IFNα). Unlike other antigen-presenting cells such as tissue macrophages and B cells, which are not usually able to initiate primary immune responses, DCs stimulate naive T lymphocyte clonal expansion. In the peripheral tissues, immature DCs function as sentinels, sampling the environment for pathogens. Upon encounter with pathogens, DCs undergo a maturation process during which they lose their endocytic capacity, process antigens and present them on the cell surface in association with MHC class I or II. This is associated with migration from the periphery to the lymph node and up-regulation of the co-stimulatory molecules CD40, CD80, CD86 and CD83. Together with MHC–antigen complexes and cytokines produced by DCs, these interactions stimulate naive T lymphocyte proliferation.

Dendritic cells are derived from CD34+ stem cells via at least two pathways of generation: myeloid (mDC) and lymphoid. In humans, myeloid DCs are further subdivided into Langerhans cells (LC) in squamous epithelium; interstitial DCs, which include dermal or lamina propria submucosal DCs; and interdigitating DCs in the T cell areas of the lymph nodes and in the blood (CD11c+ CD123–). Human Langerhans cells express CD1a, langerin and e-cadherin, whilst interstitial DCs are CD1a+ DCSIGN+ MR+ (Turville et al., 2002). In addition, DCs can be generated from blood monocytes or bone marrow precursors by stimulation

Inflammatory Diseases of the Central Nervous System, ed. T. Kilpatrick, R. M. Ransohoff and S. Wesselingh. Published by Cambridge University Press. © Cambridge University Press 2010

in vitro with IL-4 and GM-CSF (known as monocyte-derived DCs or MDDCs) or from bone-marrow precursors (Caux *et al.*, 1992; Romani *et al.*, 1994). Monocyte-derived DCs are commonly used in vitro as model DCs because of their accessibility. They most closely resemble interstitial DCs. In contrast, DCs of lymphoid lineage, commonly called plasmacytoid DCs (pDCs), have a more restricted distribution, being found predominantly in the blood (BDCA4+ CD123+) and lymphoid tissues (Grouard *et al.*, 1997; Siegal *et al.*, 1999).

In mice, five different DC subsets are found constitutively in lymphoid organs (Shortman and Liu, 2002). These five populations fall into two main groups based on their migratory capacity. The migratory DCs are tissue-resident DCs such as Langerhans cells and interstitial DCs, which are present in the periphery, mature upon encounter with pathogens and migrate to the lymph nodes to present antigen to T lymphocytes. These DCs are CD8– CD4– CD11c+ CD11b+ and in the lymph nodes they have a mature phenotype (Villadangos and Schnorrer, 2007). Langerhans cells also express CD205 and langerin. Understandably, more migratory DCs are observed in draining lymph nodes of inflamed rather than normal skin. In addition to the migratory DCs are three populations of lymph node-resident DCs. These are CD4+, CD8+ or double negative. The constitutive DCs do not migrate into the lymph from the periphery: rather, they have a role in uptake and processing of antigens within the lymph node. These lymph node-resident DCs have a more immature phenotype than the migratory DCs, which are generally of a mature phenotype once they have arrived in the lymph node.

Another, more recently identified population of DCs is the inflammatory DC that differentiates from monocytes as a consequence of infection or inflammation. An example of this is a DC population that appears in mice following infection with *Listeria monocytogenes* and that produces tumor necrosis factor and inducible nitric oxide synthetase (Serbina *et al.*, 2003).

Animal models for studying the role of DCs in the CNS

Constitutive and peripherally recruited CNS DCs

For many years the brain has been described as immune-privileged because of its lack of a formal lymphatic system and also because of low expression of MHC class II. More recently, the presence of DCs in the brain has been described, initially by Matyszak and Perry, but now by several groups. In healthy animal brains, DCs are present in the meninges, dura mater, choroid plexus, and pituitary gland, but are not present within the brain parenchyma (Hanly and Petito, 1998; Matyszak and Perry, 1996; McMenamin, 1999; Sato and Inoue, 2000; Serafini *et al.*, 2000; Serot *et al.*, 1997; Witmer-Pack *et al.*, 1995). It is unknown whether DCs are constitutively present within healthy animals' CSF.

The presence of constitutive DCs in the brain implies that there is a formalized migratory pathway for DCs to reach their draining lymph nodes. Dendritic cell migration from the CNS has been demonstrated by Carson *et al.* (1999), who injected fluorescently labelled DCs into the spinal theca. They showed a restricted migration of DCs into the CNS parenchyma: the DCs were found in the meninges, the subarachnoid spaces and along the white matter tracts and were rarely found in gray matter. The authors also showed that the DCs migrated to the T-dependent regions of the mouses' cervical lymph nodes (Carson *et al.*, 1999), whilst others have demonstrated migration of DCs to B cell follicles (Hatterer *et al.*, 2006).

DCs in CNS inflammatory disorders

Dendritic cells are found in several inflammatory disorders of the CNS. In animals with experimental CNS inflammatory disease, including experimental autoimmune encephalomyelitis (EAE), cerebral toxoplasmosis, and heat-killed bacillus Calmette–Guérin (BCG)-induced delayed-type hypersensitivity lesions, the location of DCs is typically found within inflammatory cellular infiltrates that are close to the perivascular cuffs and the contiguous parenchymal lesions (Fischer *et al.*, 2000; Fischer and Reichmann, 2001; Matyszak and Perry, 1996; Serafini *et al.*, 2000). Experimental autoimmune encephalomyelitis is a T cell-mediated autoimmune inflammatory disease of the brain and spinal cord in mice and serves as the chief experimental model for MS. Dendritic cells of both myeloid and plasmacytoid origin are found in the CNS of mice with EAE (Bailey *et al.*, 2007; Table 3.1). In relapsing EAE, a more diffuse parenchymal spinal cord infiltrate of DCs is observed (Serafini *et al.*, 2000). Interestingly, in early EAE, Serafini *et al.* noted that DCs appeared to be infiltrating the spinal cord directly from the meninges, suggesting that constitutive CNS DCs are important in the early stages of EAE (Serafini *et al.*, 2000).

Table 3.1 Summary of dendritic cells in the CNS during disease

Disease	DC subset	Tissue	Reference
Humans			
Bacterial meningitis, lyme meningoencephalitis	Myeloid and plasmacytoid	CSF	(Pashenkov *et al.*, 2002b)
Multiple sclerosis, optic neuritis, neuroborreliosis	Myeloid and plasmacytoid	CSF	(Pashenkov *et al.*, 2002a)
Multiple sclerosis	Mature mDC	Demyelination plaques and perivascular inflammatory infiltrates (autopsy)	(Plumb *et al.*, 2003)
Amyotrophic lateral sclerosis	Mature mDC	Ventral horn and corticospinal tracts (autopsy)	(Henkel *et al.*, 2004)
HIV	mDC	Choroid plexus (autopsy)	(Hanly and Petito, 1998)
Guillain–Barré	Immature myeloid and plasmacytoid	CSF	(Press *et al.*, 2005)
Mouse			
EAE, toxoplasmic encephalitis	CD11b+ CD11c+	Perivascular cuffs and contiguous parenchymal lesions	(Fischer and Reichmann, 2001)
Toxoplasma gondii	CD11c+ 33D1+ F4/80+ CD86+	Brain mononuclear inflammatory infiltrate	(Fischer *et al.*, 2000)
Prion infection	CD205+	Cerebral cortex, subcortical white matter, medulla oblongata, thalamus	(Rosicarelli *et al.*, 2005)
Relapsing EAE	CD205+ CD86+	Parenchymal spinal cord infiltrate	(Serafini *et al.*, 2000)
Rat			
Acute EAE, heat-killed bacillus Calmette–Guérin-induced delayed hypersensitivity lesions	OX62+	Perivascular cuffs, CNS parenchyma	(Matyszak and Perry, 1996)

Following prion infection in mice, DCs were detected in the cerebral cortex, subcortical white matter, thalamus, and the medulla oblongata (Rosicarelli *et al.*, 2005). The phenotype of infiltrating DCs suggested migration from the blood in a cortical ischemia model (Reichmann *et al.*, 2002). The DC numbers in the brain were increased by up to 100-fold following cerebral infection with *Toxoplasmosis gondii*, and these cells persisted in an activated state for months (Fischer *et al.*, 2000).

Dendritic cell localization in the human brain and spinal cord

Study of the functions of DCs in human neuro-inflammatory disorders is naturally much more difficult than in animal models of such diseases, and is generally limited to biopsy and autopsy specimens taken at a single time-point or to CSF which can supply serial specimens. In the normal human CNS, the presence of constitutive DCs largely mirrors that of animals in that they are present within the choroid plexus (Hanly and Petito, 1998; Serot *et al.*, 1997, 2000), the meninges (Greter *et al.*, 2005), the dura and cerebral blood vessels (Greter *et al.*, 2005), but are absent from healthy brain parenchyma and spinal cord (Henkel *et al.*, 2004; Plumb *et al.*, 2003).

There are now a large amount of data showing the presence of increased numbers of DCs in the CNS during inflammatory conditions, such as infection or injury (McMahon *et al.*, 2006; Plumb *et al.*, 2003) and also in MS. The chief histopathological findings in MS comprise perivascular CD4 and CD8 cells, mononuclear cell infiltrates and primary demyelination of axonal tracts. In autopsy specimens from patients with MS, mature DCs have been detected in demyelinative plaques and perivascular inflammatory infiltrates (Plumb *et al.*, 2003).

Myeloid and plasmacytoid DCs have been detected in small numbers in the CSF of individuals with non-inflammatory neurological disease, accounting for approximately 1% of CSF mononuclear cells. Elevated numbers of mDCs in the CSF have been observed in several inflammatory conditions including MS, optic neuritis and neuroborreliosis (Pashenkov *et al.*, 2001), bacterial meningitis (Pashenkov *et al.*, 2002b), and Guillain-Barré syndrome (Press *et al.*, 2005). Dendritic cells have also been found within ectopic B-cell follicles in post-mortem tissue sections of the cortical meninges of patients with MS (Serafini *et al.*, 2004).

Dendritic cells have also been found in the ventral horn and the corticospinal tracts of patients with amyotrophic lateral sclerosis (ALS), correlating with elevated levels of the chemokine MCP1 in the CSF (Henkel *et al.*, 2004), The presence of mRNA specific for DCs in the brain was correlated with more rapid disease progression of ALS (Henkel *et al.*, 2004).

In HIV-infected asymptomatic individuals, as well as those with AIDS, there is direct infection of both stromal macrophages and DCs in the choroid plexus in the cerebral ventricles. Indeed, HIV-infected DCs in the brain seem to be confined to the choroid plexus (Hanly and Petito, 1998). The choroid plexus is thought to be one of the sites where HIV enters the brain from the blood, as evidenced by viral sequence clustering analysis (Chen *et al.*, 2000). In addition, DCs in the CSF express the HIV co-receptor CCR5 on their surface (Pashenkov *et al.*, 2001), indicating their susceptibility to the predominant R5 strains of HIV.

The lineage differentiation of dendritic cells in the brain

There is little doubt that inflammation is associated with increased DC numbers in the CNS. However, it is not clear from where these cells originate. There are several possibilities which include infiltration of circulating blood DCs across the blood brain barrier and generation of CNS DCs from intra-cerebral progenitors or differentiation from resident microglia/macrophages.

Support for the infiltration of DCs from blood precursors is provided by observations that mDC levels in the blood are reduced during inflammatory disease and, in parallel, the levels of mDCs in the CSF are elevated (Pashenkov *et al.*, 2001). In addition, when mice received full body irradiation, which would affect peripheral DCs

but not central DC precursors, no DCs were found in an experimentally induced inflammatory lesion (Newman *et al.*, 2005). Furthermore, chemokines such as SDF-1 in the CSF of patients with neural infection were able to induce the migration of in vitro-derived DCs, suggesting that DCs in the CSF could be recruited from the blood (Pashenkov *et al.*, 2002b). Expression of the adhesion molecules L-selectin (CD62L) and P-selectin (CD62P) on endothelial cells of arachnoid vessels and choroid stroma also suggests direct recruitment of leukocytes from the blood to the CSF (Kivisakk *et al.*, 2003). The P-selectin is required for optimal homing of DCs to the thymus through microvessels (Bonasio *et al.*, 2006), suggesting that DCs enter tissues via the same adhesion cascade as other lymphocytes.

It is also possible, however, that a dendritic cell precursor is present in the healthy animal brain. In one recent study, GM-CSF was added to a primary culture of murine cerebral cells and resulted in the development of dendritic-like cells. The phenotype of these cells suggested a myeloid origin (Fischer and Bielinsky, 1999). Subsequent in-vitro work by the same authors used mouse brain cultures infected with *Toxoplasma gondii* bradyzoites to demonstrate subsequent proliferation of dendriform cells. The phenotype of these cells resembled immature, myeloid-derived DCs (CD11C+ 33D1+ F4/80+ CD8ά– DEC-205–/+) (Fischer *et al.*, 2000). These authors postulated that, in the setting of infection within the brain, this novel brain dendritic cell could be derived from either (1) migration into the infected brain from the periphery as reported by Serafini *et al.* (2000), or (2) migration of meningeal DCs into the brain, or (3) the brain's resident microglial cells. However, they argued against a microglial origin because, unlike microglia, the brain dendritic cells possess the DC-restricted markers CD11c+ and 33D1 and they produced large amounts of IL-12 and low levels of IL-10 ex vivo, which is a different pattern of cytokine production to that reported for microglia and brain macrophages as reported by others (Fischer and Reichmann, 2001). Rather, they postulated that these brain dendritic cells arise from intracerebral myeloid progenitors that are stimulated by the presence of intracerebral infection. This could be analogous to the differentiation of monocytes into DCs, as reported in areas of peripheral tissue inflammation (reviewed in Shortman and Naik, 2007). Another study found that both DCs infiltrating from the blood, and activation of resident microglia, can contribute to an increase in DC numbers within the brain during inflammation (Reichmann *et al.*, 2002).

Migration of myeloid DCs into the brain could be mediated by their expression of CCR5 (Pashenkov *et al.*, 2002a) and in response to FMS-like tyrosine kinase ligand (FLT3L) secreted by microglial cells. The FLT3L is a hematopoetic growth factor that induces proliferation of DCs and increases blood DC levels in both mice and humans (Pulendran *et al.*, 2000). In the CNS, FLT3L also plays a role in neuronal survival. Curtin *et al.* (2006) found in a rat model that when FLT3L was expressed by an intracranial tumor, there was improved survival and they postulated that this could have been secondary to an observed increased migration of pDCs into the brain parenchyma.

Role of DCs in induction and remission of CNS inflammation

Following the initial observations that DCs are present within the murine CNS in autoimmune and infectious inflammatory disorders, a number of studies subsequently focused on the functional roles of DCs in these disorders and the molecular mechanisms by which these roles are exerted. Recently, Greter *et al.* utilized a transgenic mouse without secondary lymphoid tissue whose only functional APCs were DCs. Using this model, they showed that vessel-associated CD11c+ DCs were capable of presenting antigen in vivo to T cells primed against myelin, following which clinical signs of EAE developed (Greter *et al.*, 2005). Their model suggests that the presence of DCs in the CNS could play a vital *initial* role in the pathogenesis of CNS inflammation by detecting antigens and presenting them to cognate T cells that are migrating in and through CNS blood vessels (Greter *et al.*, 2005). As a corollary, Zozulya *et al.* studied how DCs migrate into the CNS from the periphery, as opposed to being present constitutively in vessel walls. They found that DC migration through brain microvessel endothelium is regulated by MIP-1α (CCL3) and that DCs both secrete and are dependent upon matrix metalloproteinases for their transmigration (Zozulya *et al.*, 2007).

In the EAE model, once within the brain parenchyma, myeloid DCs appear to play a key role in polarizing CD4+ helper cells towards the IL-17-producing CD4+ effector T cell subset (T_H-17 cells) wherein IL-17 promotes chronic CNS inflammation (Bailey *et al.*, 2007). However, following this initial polarization towards a T_H-17 response, CD11c+ DCs may go on to support CD4+ CD25+ T regulatory cell-mediated immunosuppression. Thus, DCs act at this stage to suppress inflammation and to induce remission in EAE (Deshpande *et al.*, 2007).

In the setting of chronic infection, DCs have been shown to be vital in viral clearance: using the model of chronic infection in mice with lymphocytic choriomeningitis virus (LMCV), Lauterbach *et al.* (2006) showed that without recruitment of DCs into the brain, cytotoxic T lymphocytes do not produce tumor necrosis factor alpha (TNF-α), nor do memory T cells expand, both of which are required for LMCV clearance from the brain.

Thus DCs are involved in the complex regulation of autoimmune and infectious inflammation, inducing and then suppressing it via interaction with different T cell subsets. Despite the ability of DCs to either induce or suppress inflammation, the exact role of these DCs in regulating CNS inflammation remains unclear. Elevated DC numbers in the brain appeared to promote clinical severity of EAE (Greter *et al.*, 2005), and DC mRNA levels correlated with rapid disease progression of ALS (Henkel *et al.*, 2004). In contrast, DCs within the human choroid plexus of dementia patients at post-mortem had an immature phenotype and were IL10+, which may favor an immunosuppressive role (Serot *et al.*, 2000). Initial investigations by Suter *et al.* (2000) suggested that the infiltration of DCs into the CNS was associated with the clinical severity of EAE. However, more recently it was shown by the same group that the infiltrating DCs have a unique phenotype, being unable to stimulate naive T lymphocytes. The authors therefore suggest that DC infiltration may limit rather than induce autoimmunity in the CNS (Suter *et al.*, 2003).

Dendritic cells that express CCR7 (a lymph node homing chemokine receptor) have been found in the inflamed CNS (Kivisakk *et al.*, 2004). Such DCs containing microbial or autoantigens can exit the CNS and migrate directly into cervical lymph nodes via lymphatics, or via blood through arachnoid villi (Cserr *et al.*, 1992; Karman *et al.*, 2004). Dendritic cells emigrating from the brain were sufficient to activate T lymphocytes in the lymph nodes and to enable them to migrate back to the tissue of DC origin (Karman *et al.*, 2004). Dendritic cells arising from CD11b+ cell differentiation in the brain produce IL12 and are able to stimulate naive T lymphocyte proliferation (Fischer and Reichmann, 2001). Thus, this event could also occur directly in the CNS, rather than in the lymph node (McMahon *et al.*, 2005).

Conclusion

The origins and functions of DCs in the CNS remain controversial in animals let alone humans, which are much more difficult to study. Given the diversity of murine DC subsets, some with no apparent human correlates, one should generally be cautious in extrapolating from murine models to human disease. Furthermore, different laboratories often report different roles for DCs in infectious and neuro-inflammatory disorders. Do they initiate or respond to inflammation and does this differ according to the disease? Whether T lymphocyte stimulation occurs in the brain parenchyma or in lymph nodes after DC migration is also controversial. Thus, the biology of mDCs and pDCs in neuro-inflammation is a field deserving of much more intensive study in the future in order to clarify these questions.

References

Abreu-Silva AL, *et al.* Central nervous system involvement in experimental infection with *Leishmania* (*Leishmania*) *amazonensis*. *Am J Trop Med Hyg* 2003; **68**: 661–5.

Bailey SL, *et al.* CNS myeloid DCs presenting endogenous myelin peptides 'preferentially' polarize CD4+ T(H)-17 cells in relapsing EAE. *Nature Immunol* 2007; **8**: 172–80.

Bonasio R, *et al.* Clonal deletion of thymocytes by circulating dendritic cells homing to the thymus. *Nature Immunol* 2006; **7**: 1092–100.

Carson MJ, *et al.* Disproportionate recruitment of CD8+ T cells into the central nervous system by professional antigen-presenting cells. *Am J Pathol* 1999; **154**: 481–94.

Caux C, *et al.* GM-CSF and TNFα cooperate in the generation of dendritic Langerhans cells. *Nature* 1992; **360**: 258.

Chen H, *et al.* Comparisons of HIV-1 viral sequences in brain, choroid plexus and spleen: Potential role of choroid plexus in the pathogenesis of HIV encephalitis. *J Neurovirol* 2000; **6**: 498–506.

Cserr HF, *et al.* Drainage of brain extracellular fluid into blood and deep cervical lymph and its immunological significance. *Brain Pathol* 1992; **2**: 269–76.

Curtin JF, *et al.* Fms-like tyrosine kinase 3 ligand recruits plasmacytoid dendritic cells to the brain. *J Immunol* 2006; **176**: 3566–77.

Deshpande P, *et al.* Cutting edge: CNS CD11c+ cells from mice with encephalomyelitis polarize Th17 cells and support CD25+CD4+ T cell-mediated immunosuppression, suggesting dual roles in the disease process. *J Immunol* 2007; **178**: 6695–9.

Donaghy H, *et al.* HIV interactions with dendritic cells: Has our focus been too narrow? *J Leukoc Biol* 2006; **80**: 1001–12.

Fischer HG, Bielinsky AK. Antigen presentation function of brain-derived dendriform cells depends on astrocyte help. *Int Immunol* 1999; **11**: 1265–74.

Fischer HG, Reichmann G. Brain dendritic cells and macrophages/microglia in central nervous system inflammation. *J Immunol* 2001; **166**: 2717–26.

Fischer HG, *et al.* Phenotype and functions of brain dendritic cells emerging during chronic infection of mice with *Toxoplasma gondii*. *J Immunol* 2000; **164**: 4826–34.

Greter M, *et al.* Dendritic cells permit immune invasion of the CNS in an animal model of multiple sclerosis. *Nature Med* 2005; **11**: 328–34.

Grouard G, *et al.* The enigmatic plasmacytoid T cells develop into dendritic cells with interleukin (IL)-3 and CD40-ligand. *J Exp Med* 1997; **185**: 1101.

Hanly A, Petito CK. HLA-DR-positive dendritic cells of the normal human choroid plexus: A potential reservoir of HIV in the central nervous system. *Hum Pathol* 1998; **29**: 88–93.

Hatterer E, *et al.* How to drain without lymphatics? Dendritic cells migrate from the cerebrospinal fluid to the B-cell follicles of cervical lymph nodes. *Blood* 2006; **107**: 806–12.

Henkel JS, *et al.* Presence of dendritic cells, MCP-1, and activated microglia/macrophages in amyotrophic lateral sclerosis spinal cord tissue. *Ann Neurol* 2004; **55**: 221–35.

Karman J, *et al.* Initiation of immune responses in brain is promoted by local dendritic cells. *J Immunol* 2004; **173**: 2353–61.

Kivisakk P, *et al.* Human cerebrospinal fluid central memory CD4+ T cells: Evidence for trafficking through choroid plexus and meninges via P-selectin. *Proc Natl Acad Sci USA* 2003; **100**: 8389–94.

Kivisakk P, *et al.* Expression of CCR7 in multiple sclerosis: Implications for CNS immunity. *Ann Neurol* 2004; **55**: 627–38.

Lauterbach H, *et al.* Adoptive immunotherapy induces CNS dendritic cell recruitment and antigen presentation during clearance of a persistent viral infection. *J Exp Med* 2006; **203**: 1963–75.

Matyszak MK, Perry VH. The potential role of dendritic cells in immune-mediated inflammatory diseases in the central nervous system. *Neuroscience* 1996; **74**: 599–608.

McMahon EJ, *et al.* Epitope spreading initiates in the CNS in two mouse models of multiple sclerosis. *Nature Med* 2005; **11**: 335–9.

McMahon EJ, *et al.* CNS dendritic cells: Critical participants in CNS inflammation? *Neurochem Int Mol Mech Neuroinflam* 2006; **49**: 195–203.

McMenamin PG. Distribution and phenotype of dendritic cells and resident tissue macrophages in the dura mater, leptomeninges, and choroid plexus of the rat brain as demonstrated in wholemount preparations. *J Comp Neurol* 1999; **405**: 553–62.

Newman TA, *et al.* Blood-derived dendritic cells in an acute brain injury. *J Neuroimmunol* 2005; **166**: 167–72.

Pashenkov M, *et al.* Two subsets of dendritic cells are present in human cerebrospinal fluid. *Brain* 2001; **124**: 480–92.

Pashenkov M, *et al.* Elevated expression of CCR5 by myeloid (CD11c+) blood dendritic cells in multiple sclerosis and acute optic neuritis. *Clin Exp Immunol* 2002a; **127**: 519–26.

Pashenkov M, *et al.* Recruitment of dendritic cells to the cerebrospinal fluid in bacterial neuroinfections. *J Neuroimmunol* 2002b; **122**: 106–16.

Plumb J, *et al.* CD83-positive dendritic cells are present in occasional perivascular cuffs in multiple sclerosis lesions. *Mult Scler* 2003; **9**: 142–7.

Press R, *et al.* Dendritic cells in the cerebrospinal fluid and peripheral nerves in Guillain–Barre syndrome and chronic inflammatory demyelinating polyradiculoneuropathy. *J Neuroimmunol* 2005; **159**: 165–76.

Pulendran B, *et al*. Flt3-ligand and granulocyte colony-stimulating factor mobilize distinct human dendritic cell subsets in vivo. *J Immunol* 2000; **165**: 566–72.

Reichmann G, *et al*. Dendritic cells and dendritic-like microglia in focal cortical ischemia of the mouse brain. *J Neuroimmunol* 2002; **129**: 125–32.

Rissoan MC, *et al*. Reciprocal control of T helper cell and dendritic cell differentiation. *Science* 1999; **283**: 1183–6.

Robinson SP, *et al*. Human peripheral blood contains two distinct lineages of dendritic cells. *Eur J Immunol* 1999; **29**: 2769–78.

Romani N, *et al*. Proliferating dendritic cell progenitors in human blood. *J Exp Med* 1994; **180**: 83–93.

Rosicarelli B, *et al*. Migration of dendritic cells into the brain in a mouse model of prion disease. *J Neuroimmunol* 2005; **165**: 114–20.

Sato T, Inoue K. Dendritic cells in the rat pituitary gland evaluated by the use of monoclonal antibodies and electron microscopy. *Arch Histol Cytol* 2000; **63**: 291–303.

Serafini B, *et al*. Intracerebral recruitment and maturation of dendritic cells in the onset and progression of experimental autoimmune encephalomyelitis. *Am J Pathol* 2000; **157**: 1991–2002.

Serafini B, *et al*. Detection of ectopic B-cell follicles with germinal centers in the meninges of patients with secondary progressive multiple sclerosis. *Brain Pathol* 2004; **14**: 164–74.

Serbina NV, *et al*. TNF/iNOS-producing dendritic cells mediate innate immune defense against bacterial infection. *Immunity* 2003; **19**: 59–70.

Serot JM, *et al*. Ultrastructural and immunohistological evidence for dendritic-like cells within human choroid plexus epithelium. *Neuroreport* 1997; **8**: 1995–8.

Serot JM, *et al*. Monocyte-derived IL-10-secreting dendritic cells in choroid plexus epithelium. *J Neuroimmunol* 2000; **105**: 115–19.

Shortman K, Liu YJ. Mouse and human dendritic cell subtypes. *Nature Rev Immunol* 2002; **2**: 151–61.

Shortman K, Naik SH. Steady-state and inflammatory dendritic-cell development. *Nature Rev Immunol* 2007; **7**: 19–30.

Siegal FP, *et al*. The nature of the principal type 1 interferon-producing cells in human blood. *Science* 1999; **284**: 1835–7.

Suter T, *et al*. Dendritic cells and differential usage of the MHC class II transactivator promoters in the central nervous system in experimental autoimmune encephalitis. *Eur J Immunol* 2000; **30**: 794–802.

Suter T, *et al*. The brain as an immune privileged site: Dendritic cells of the central nervous system inhibit T cell activation. *Eur J Immunol* 2003; **33**: 2998–3006.

Turville SG, *et al*. Diversity of receptors binding HIV on dendritic cell subsets. *Nat Immunol* 2002; **3**: 975–83.

Villadangos JA, Schnorrer P. Intrinsic and cooperative antigen-presenting functions of dendritic-cell subsets in vivo. *Nature Rev Immunol* 2007; **7**: 543–55.

Witmer-Pack MD, *et al*. Tissue distribution of the DEC-205 protein that is detected by the monoclonal antibody NLDC-145: II. Expression in situ in lymphoid and nonlymphoid tissues. *Cell Immunol* 1995; **163**: 157–62.

Zozulya AL, *et al*. Dendritic cell transmigration through brain microvessel endothelium is regulated by MIP-1{alpha} chemokine and matrix metalloproteinases. *J Immunol* 2007; **178**: 520–9.

Chapter

4

Negotiating the brain barriers: access of immune cells and pathogens into the CNS

Britta Engelhardt

Introduction

Before entering the central nervous system (CNS), immune cells or pathogens have to penetrate one of the brain barriers, namely the endothelial blood–brain barrier (BBB), the epithelial blood–cerebrospinal fluid barrier, or the tanycytic barrier around the circumventricular organs. Due to the low number of immune cells entering the CNS under physiological conditions, it was originally assumed that brain barriers inhibit immune cell entry into the CNS. It is now well accepted that immune cells do gain access to the CNS and that immune responses can be mounted inside this tissue, suggesting a rather active role of brain barriers in establishing tight controls to regulate the trafficking of immune cells into the CNS. Whereas studies mostly performed in experimental autoimmune encephalomyelitis (EAE), an animal model for multiple sclerosis (MS), have provided a large body of information on the molecular mechanisms involved in immune cell entry into the CNS, comparatively little is known about the molecular mechanisms involved in leukocyte entry into the CNS under other pathological conditions. Similarly, although it has become evident that pathogens successfully exploit the molecular cell trafficking mechanisms established in the host, our understanding of how they bind and cross the brain barriers at a molecular level is incomplete. This chapter will summarize the current knowledge of the active role of the brain barriers in immune cell and pathogen entry into the CNS.

The brain barriers faced by immune cells and pathogens entering the brain

When considering entry sites for immune cells or pathogens from the periphery into the CNS, the endothelial BBB has been regarded as the most obvious place and has therefore been investigated by most researchers. The "classical" endothelial BBB consists of a complex cellular system of highly specialized endothelial cells, a large number of pericytes embedded in the endothelial basement membrane, perivascular macrophages, and a second basement membrane produced by astrocytes, which cover the abluminal aspect of the brain microvessels with their end-feet (Figure 4.1; Sixt *et al.*, 2001). Although the endothelial cells form the BBB (i.e. the diffusion barrier, proper), they, in isolation, are insufficient to account for the unique barrier properties of CNS microvessels. Rather, it is their interactions with extracellular matrix and cross-talk with adjacent cells that are prerequisites for barrier function (Abbott *et al.*, 2006; Engelhardt, 2003). These interactions, in turn, influence endothelial cell morphology, biochemistry, and function that collectively make BBB endothelial cells unique and distinguishable from any other endothelial cell in the body. Transcellular passage of molecules across the BBB is inhibited by an extremely low pinocytotic activity. The lack of fenestrae and an elaborate network of complex tight junctions (TJ) between the endothelial cells restrict the paracellular diffusion of hydrophilic molecules. On the other hand, in order to meet the high metabolic needs of the CNS tissue, specific transport systems selectively expressed in the capillary brain endothelial cell membranes mediate the directed transport of nutrients into the CNS or of toxic metabolites out of the CNS (Pardridge, 2007). The complex TJs between the brain microvascular endothelial cells are primarily responsible for the barrier function, and unlike simple TJs of endothelial cells elswhere in the body, provide a high electrical resistance (about 2000 $\Omega \times cm^2$) (Crone and Olesen, 1982). The molecular composition of BBB tight junctions has been investigated and found to differ from that of peripheral endothelial cells by the presence of the integral membrane proteins occludin,

Inflammatory Diseases of the Central Nervous System, ed. T. Kilpatrick, R. M. Ransohoff and S. Wesselingh. Published by Cambridge University Press. © Cambridge University Press 2010.

claudins -1,-3, -5, and -12 (Cattelino *et al.*, 2003). Furthermore, the Ig supergene family members junctional adhesion molecule (JAM)-A (Martin-Padura *et al.*, 1998) and endothelial cell-selective adhesion molecule (ESAM)-1 are localized in BBB TJs (Nasdala *et al.*, 2002). Via interaction with the cytoplasmic peripheral membrane proteins of the membrane-associated guanylate kinase (MAGUK) family, such as zonula occludens ZO-1, -2 and -3 (reviewed in Wolburg and Lippoldt, 2002), these integral membrane proteins interact with the actin cytoskeleton, thus providing the molecular link for TJ association with the cytoskeleton. In addition, adherens junctions, which are strongly associated with the cytoskeleton (e.g. via cadherin/catenin interactions), seem to be intermingled with tight junctions at the BBB (Schulze and Firth, 1993). Last but not least, the Ig supergene family member platelet–endothelial cell adhesion molecule (PECAM)-1 (Graesser *et al.*, 2002) is localized to the cell-to-cell contacts of BBB endothelium outside of the structurally organized tight and adherens junctions.

The term "blood–brain barrier" was originally coined to describe the lack of passive diffusion of molecules across the capillary bed within the CNS (reviewed in Engelhardt, 2003). However, strictly speaking, leukocyte extravasation does not take place at the level of the capillary BBB, but rather at the level of post-capillary venules. As some of the unique characteristics of the CNS capillary endothelial cells extend to the endothelial cells of the post-capillary vascular segment, that is the presence of two basal membranes (Sixt *et al.*, 2001), complex tight junctions (Wolburg *et al.*, 2003) and coverage with astrocytic end-feet, thereby equally restricting free diffusion of polar molecules across post-capillary venules, it seemed appropriate to extend the use of the term "blood–brain barrier" to this unique CNS microvascular compartment, when discussing leukocyte migration into the CNS.

Also, although generally referred to as one homogeneous entity, there is emerging evidence that within the brain there might be regional differences in the characteristics of the BBB. Molecular and cellular differences for the meningeal and parenchymal microvascular beds have been described (Allt and Lawrenson, 1997; Rascher and Wolburg, 1997); meningeal microvessels lack astrocytic ensheathment, are more leaky in comparison with parenchymal blood vessels, and are more reactive to pro-inflammmatory cytokines.

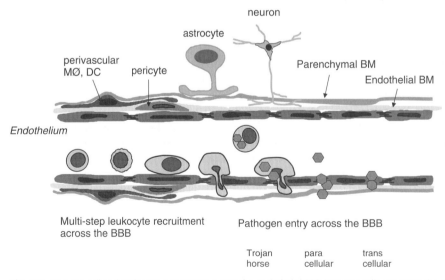

Fig. 4.1 Immune cell and pathogen penetration across the endothelial BBB. Immune cells penetrate the endothelial BBB by a multi-step recruitment cascade involving the molecular mechanisms outlined in the text. Tethering and rolling is followed by chemokine mediated activation of secondary leukocyte adhesion molecules, which mediate the firm adhesion of the leukocyte to the endothelium and finally its diapedesis across the BBB probably via a transcellular route. Pathogens (pink hexagon) can penetrate the BBB via a Trojan horse mechanism inside immune cells or traverse as free pathogens using a paracellular route through the BBB tight junction or a transcellular route through the endothelial cell. BBB = blood brain barrier BM = basement membrane, MØ = macrophage DC = dendritic cell.

In contrast to the classical BBB, until very recently, the epithelial blood–cerebrospinal fluid (CSF) barrier localized at the level of the choroid plexus epithelium has not been considered as an entry site for immune cells or pathogens into the CNS (Engelhardt *et al.*, 2001). The choroid plexus extends from the ventricular surface into the lumen of the ventricles. Its major known function is the secretion of cerebrospinal fluid. It is a structure organized in a villous surface that includes an extensive microvascular network enclosed by a single layer of cuboidal epithelium (Dziegielewska *et al.*, 2001). The microvessels within the choroid plexus parenchyma differ from those of the brain parenchyma, because they allow free movement of molecules via fenestrations and intercellular gaps (reviewed in Betz *et al.*, 1989). Instead, the barrier between the blood compartment and the CSF is located at the level of the choroid plexus epithelial cells, which form tight junctions inhibiting paracellular diffusion of water soluble molecules (Wolburg *et al.*, 2001). These tight junctions are the morphological correlate of the blood–CSF barrier and are characterized by a unique molecular composition of transmembrane proteins with occludin, claudin-1 and claudin-2 and claudin-11 (Wolburg *et al.*, 2001). The latter has been shown to induce morphologically distinct tight junctions appearing as parallel-arrays in freeze fracture microscopy.

Besides the choroid plexus, there are additional structures in the CNS of mammals lacking an endothelial BBB. These areas fulfill neurohumoral and neurosecretory functions, in that the neurons monitor hormonal stimuli and other substances within the blood or secrete neuroendocrines into the blood, and are commonly referred to as the circumventricular organs (CVOs; reviewed in Johnson and Gross, 1993; Leonhardt, 1980b). The CVOs are localized at strategic points close to the midline of the brain within the ependymal walls lining the third and fourth ventricles. Because they lack an endothelial BBB, they lie within the blood milieu and thus form a blood–CSF barrier. Similar to the choroid plexus, a complex network of tight junctions connecting specialized ependymal cells (tanycytes) seals off the remainder of the CNS from the CVOs (Bouchaud and Bosler, 1986; Leonhardt, 1980a). Although, the CVOs have often been referred to as "windows of the brain" with regard to soluble mediators, entry of immune cells into the brain via the CVOs across the tanycytic barriers has not been considered by many to date (Schulz and Engelhardt, 2005).

Molecular mechanism involved in immune cell migration across brain barriers

Introduction

It has been well established that immune cells recirculate through the body via the blood stream and extravasate into the tissue at the level of post-capillary venules. The specificity of the recruitment of circulating leukocytes across the vascular wall into different tissues is mediated by the sequential interaction of different adhesion and signaling molecules on leukocytes and endothelial cells lining the vessel wall (Butcher *et al.*, 1999; Luster *et al.*, 2005). The multi-step interaction starts with an initial transient contact of the circulating leukocyte with the vascular endothelium, mediated by adhesion molecules of the selectin family (E-, P- and L-selectin) and their respective carbohydrate ligands (i.e. P-selectin glycoprotein ligand (PSGL)-1), or by $\alpha4$-integrins. After the initial tether, the leukocyte rolls along the vascular wall with greatly reduced velocity. The rolling leukocyte can then bind chemotactic factors from the family of chemokines presented on the endothelial surface. Chemokines bind to serpentine receptors on the leukocyte surface, delivering a G-protein-mediated inside-out signal to transmembrane adhesion molecules of the integrin family present on the leukocyte surface increasing their avidity through conformational changes and clustering. Only integrins with increased avidity are able to mediate the firm adhesion of the leukocytes to the vascular endothelium by binding to their endothelial ligands of the immunoglobulin (Ig) superfamily. This ultimately leads to diapedesis of the leukocyte. Successful recruitment of circulating leukocytes into the tissue thus depends on productive leukocyte–endothelial interactions during each of these sequential steps. As endothelial cells participate actively in the regulation of leukocyte entry into various tissues, it can be concluded that the specialization of the BBB endothelium extends to CNS-specific trafficking signals for immune cells.

The endothelial blood–brain barrier

As mentioned above, the endothelial blood–brain barrier (BBB) has been considered the obvious place of entry of circulating immune cells into the CNS.

Therefore, most investigations have focused on defining the molecular mechanisms involved in lymphocyte recruitment across the endothelial BBB. Our current knowledge about the molecular mechanisms involved in the migration of inflammatory cells into the CNS is mainly derived from studies performed in the animal model EAE, an inflammatory demyelinating disease of the CNS, which because of its clinical and histopathological characteristics has been considered a prototypic model for inflammatory demyelinating diseases of the human CNS, in particular MS (Martin and McFarland, 1995). It is mediated by activated auto-antigenspecific CD4$^+$ T cells. The target autoantigens of the CD4$^+$ T cells are structural proteins of the CNS myelin such as myelin basic protein (MBP), proteolipid protein (PLP) or myelin oligodendrocyte glycoprotein (MOG). The autoaggressive CD4$^+$ T lymphocytes are activated outside the CNS, can then migrate into the CNS and initiate the cellular events leading to edema, inflammation and demyelination within the white matter. There is evidence provided by in-vivo studies that immunocompetent cells such as T lymphocytes can enter the healthy CNS, irrespective of their antigen-specificity (Hickey et al., 1991). However, the BBB still controls lymphocyte traffic into the CNS, because barrier properties remain intact, and only activated, but not resting, T lymphocytes migrate through cerebral vessels in vivo (Wekerle et al., 1986). Even during inflammation, when the endothelial BBB becomes leaky, lymphocyte recruitment into the CNS seems to be tightly controlled, as T cells detected in the CNS parenchyma are phenotypically distinct from T cell populations detected in other inflamed organs (Engelhardt et al., 1995, 1998b; Zeine and Owens, 1992).

After immune-specific interactions between lymphocytes and cerebral endothelium were excluded as the major determininant of the recruitment of T cells across the BBB (Risau et al., 1990; Sedgwick et al., 1990), adhesion molecules became obvious candidates as the mediators of this process. Yednock and colleagues were the first to demonstrate that T cell recruitment across the BBB critically depends on the adhesion molecule VLA-4 (α4β1-integrin) on the T cell surface (Yednock et al., 1992). This seminal study showed that antibodies blocking α4-integrins inhibit EAE by blocking T cell interaction with the BBB. Numerous follow-up studies confirmed and extended the predominant involvement of α4-integrin interaction with its ligand vascular cell adhesion molecule (VCAM)-1 on the BBB in inflammatory

cell recruitment into the CNS in different EAE models in a number of species (Engelhardt et al., 1998a; Kent et al., 1995; Steffen et al., 1994). Recently, intra-vital microscopy studies have provided direct evidence for α4-integrin-mediated inflammatory cell interaction with the CNS microvasculature in vivo. In inflamed pial venules of mice suffering from EAE, α4-integrins mediate rolling and G-protein-dependent arrest of endogenous leukocytes (Kerfoot and Kubes, 2002). Recruitment of encephalitogenic T cell blasts across the spinal cord white matter microvasculature was shown to depend on α4-integrin-mediated initial capture and G-protein-dependent arrest (Vajkoczy et al., 2001). Taken together, these data demonstrate that α4-integrins play a predominant role in leukocyte recruitment across the BBB, as they mediate both the initial low-affinity interaction of circulating leukocytes with the CNS microvasculature and the subsequent G-protein-dependent arrest requiring high-affinity binding of α4-integrins.

The predominant role of α4-integrins in mediating the initial leukcoyte contact with the BBB during EAE has raised the question about the involvement of selectins and selectin ligands in this process. In inflamed pial vessels, CD8$^+$ T cells from MS patients preferentially rolled via P-selectin glycoprotein ligand (PSGL-1), whereas CD4$^+$ T cells rolled via α4-integrin (Battistini et al., 2003). The contributions of both α4-integrin and PSGL-1 in leukocyte rolling in inflamed superficial brain vessels was confirmed by additional studies by means of intra-vital microscopy (Kerfoot and Kubes, 2002; Piccio et al., 2005). Taken together, these observations are in apparent contrast to previous EAE studies performed by us, where we found that blocking antibodies directed against E- and P-selectin did not influence the development of EAE in the SJL mouse (Engelhardt et al., 1997). Supporting these observations, we and others have demonstrated that although encephalitogenic T cells express functional PSGL-1, neither anti-PSGL-1 antibodies nor the lack of PSGL-1 in PSGL-1-deficient mice inhibit the recruitment of inflammatory cells across the BBB or the development of clinical EAE (Engelhardt et al., 2005; Osmers et al., 2005). Furthermore, blocking another PSGL-1 ligand, L-selectin (Brocke et al., 1999) or lack of L-selectin (Grewal et al., 2001) does not interfere with inflammatory cell recruitment across the BBB during EAE, although L-selectin-deficient C57bl/6 mice fail to develop clinical EAE due to impaired effector cell function.

Thus, although intra-vital video microscopy studies have demonstrated the involvement of selectins and selectin ligands in immune cell interaction with the BBB, other studies have failed to demonstrate an impact of these molecules on EAE pathogenesis. One possible explanation for these apparently discrepant observations could be that different molecular mechanisms are involved in leukocyte recruitment across the BBB in different areas of the CNS. Selectins and selectin ligands could mediate leukocyte interaction with meningeal microvessels, as demonstrated by intra-vital video microscopy or in-vivo homing studies (Carrithers et al., 2000; Carvalho-Tavares et al., 2000; Kerfoot and Kubes, 2002; Piccio et al., 2002). In contrast, inflammatory cell recruitment across the BBB in the CNS parenchyma could mainly rely on α4-integrins mediating both the initial low-affinity interaction of circulating leukocytes with the CNS microvasculature and the subsequent G-protein-dependent arrest requiring high-affinity binding of α4-integrins.

This notion is supported by the observation that targeting leukocyte trafficking across the BBB by blocking α4-integrins with the humanized antibody natalizumab has proven extremely beneficial for the treatment of MS (Polman et al., 2006; Rudick et al., 2006). Unfortunately, an unexpected although small risk for developing progressive multifocal leukoencephalopathy (PML) (Yousry et al., 2006), an often fatal disease caused by JC virus activation or infection of glial cells, has been found to be associated with this treatment. Therefore, future thorough evaluation of MS patients under long-term treatment with natalizumab is required and will allow for a better assessment of its therapeutic mechanisms and its benefits in blocking leukocyte trafficking to the CNS versus its potential increased risk for CNS infections.

The chemokines involved in G-protein-dependent T cell recruitment across the BBB remain to be characterized (reviewed in Engelhardt and Ransohoff, 2005; Ubogu et al., 2006). Chemokines produced by BBB endothelium during EAE include the lymphoid "homeostatic" chemokines CCL19 and CCL21 (Alt et al., 2002; Columba-Cabezas et al., 2003). In vitro these chemokines trigger adhesion of encephalitogenic CCR7-positive T lymphocytes to inflamed brain vessels in Stamper–Woodruff assays; however, their impact in T cell recruitment across the BBB in vivo remains to be investigated. Numerous inflammatory chemokines are produced in the inflamed brain by parenchymal cells such as astrocytes, both in EAE and in MS, and have been demonstrated to be involved in EAE pathogenesis (reviewed by Ubogu et al., 2006). Whether these chemokines are involved in leukocyte migration across the BBB, however, depends on establishing that these chemokines can be translocated from the CNS across the BBB endothelium to be available on the luminal side (Dzenko et al., 2001).

Despite its predominant involvement in T cell interaction with the BBB, in-vitro studies demonstrated that α4-integrin-mediated binding to VCAM-1 is not involved in T cell diapedesis across brain endothelial cells (Laschinger and Engelhardt, 2000). Thus, molecules other than α4-integrin and its ligands mediate this step. At least in vitro, T cell diapedesis across the BBB is mediated by LFA-1/ICAM-1 and ICAM-2 interactions, as blocking antibodies against LFA-1 and ICAM-1 consistently inhibit T cell/brain endothelial interactions (Adamson et al., 1999; Reiss et al., 1998), and studies using ICAM-1-deficient or ICAM-1/ICAM-2-deficient endothelium showed that ICAM-1, and to a lesser degree ICAM-2, is essential for T cell migration across brain endothelium in vitro (Greenwood et al., 2003; Lyck et al., 2003). Furthermore, re-expression of different ICAM-1 mutants in the double-deficient ICAM-1$^{-/-}$/ICAM-2$^{-/-}$ or in the ICAM-1$^{-/-}$ endothelial cell lines enabled the distinction between ICAM-1-mediated T cell adhesion from ICAM-1-mediated T cell diapedesis. The extracellular domain of ICAM-1 suffices to support T cell adhesion, while the presence of the cytoplasmic tail is essential for triggering the activation of endothelial Rho GTPase, which is required for T cell diapedesis in vitro (Adamson et al., 1999; Lyck et al., 2003).

In contrast to the in vitro findings, the contributions of LFA-1/ICAM-1, Mac-1/ICAM-1 and LFA-1/ICAM-2 in inflammatory cell recruitment across the BBB in vivo remain uncertain. Antibody-inhibition studies in a variety of EAE models produced contradictory results, ranging from inhibiting EAE to increasing its severity (Archelos et al., 1993; Cannella et al., 1993; Welsh et al., 1993; Willenborg et al., 1993). These confusing results could be due to the ability of some reagents to alter LFA-1/ICAM-1 interactions within immunological synapses and thus lymphocyte activation (reviewed in Carlos and Harlan, 1994). Using a true ICAM-1^{null} mouse, it has been shown very recently that ICAM-1 is required on multiple cell types for the development of EAE (Bullard et al., 2007). As LFA-1 on encephalitogenic T cells is involved in their diapedesis across the BBB in the spinal cord white matter in vivo (Laschinger *et al.*, 2002), it remains to be demonstrated how endothelial ICAM-1 or ICAM-2 or both contribute to leukocyte diapedesis across the BBB in vivo. The ICAM-1, but not cytokine-unresponsive ICAM-2, is found to be dramatically up-regulated on inflamed vessels in MS lesions (Bo *et al.*, 1996; Sobel *et al.*, 1990) and in EAE (Steffen *et al.*, 1994), and essentially all infiltrating hematogenous leukocytes in MS and EAE lesions are LFA-1[+] (Bo *et al.*, 1996; Engelhardt *et al.*, 1998a; Steffen *et al.*, 1994).

Beyond the involvement of endothelial ICAM-1 and ICAM-2, the cellular pathway involved in leukocyte diapedesis across the BBB is still poorly defined. Based on numerous studies demonstrating that antibodies directed against adhesion molecules localized in endothelial cell–cell contacts block leukocyte diapedesis in vitro and in vivo, the prevalent view is that diapedesis of leukocytes takes place at the endothelial junctions with the leukocyte squeezing through between adjacent endothelial cells (summarized in Johnson-Léger and Imhof, 2003). This type of passage is often envisaged by a zipper-like model, whereby the traversing leukocyte transiently replaces the homophilic interactions of transmembrane proteins present on neighboring endothelial cells (e.g. PECAM-1) via interaction with similar proteins expressed on the leukocyte surface.

In this context, the junctional adhesion molecules (JAMs), which are localized in endothelial and epithelial tight junctions, have attracted significant attention regarding their potential role in mediating paracellular diapedesis of leukocytes (reviewed by Ebnet *et al.*, 2004; Johnson-Léger and Imhof, 2003; Muller, 2003). The JAM family consists of three members called JAM-A, JAM-B and JAM-C, which are immunoglobulin (Ig) superfamily molecules with two extracellular Ig domains and a short cytoplasmic tail ending with a PDZ binding motif (Ebnet *et al.*, 2004). The JAM-A is present in BBB tight junctions and was shown to be involved in neutrophil recruitment during cytokine-induced meningitis in vivo (Del Maschio *et al.*, 1999). However, a second study, blocking JAM-A activity in vivo with the very same reagents failed to prevent leukocyte influx during bacterial-induced meningitis (Lechner *et al.*, 2000). Abnormal endothelial tight junctions and changes in the expression profile of JAM-A have been observed in active MS lesions (Padden *et al.*, 2007; Plumb *et al.*, 2002), further

supporting a role for BBB tight junctions in leukocyte recruitment across the BBB in MS. Similarly, apparently discrepant observations were made regarding the role of endothelial PECAM-1 in leukocyte trafficking into the CNS. The PECAM-1 is localized outside of the structurally defined cell–cell contact zones (i.e. adherens junctions or tight junctions) on endothelial cells. Whereas blocking PECAM-1 was shown to inhibit the accumulation of antigen-specific T cells in the CSF after intraventricular antigen infusion (Qing *et al.*, 2001), it was also found to be a negative regulator of leukocyte diapedesis across the BBB in EAE. This conclusion was drawn from the observation that PECAM-1-deficient mice suffering from EAE exhibited increased cellular infiltration across the BBB (Graesser *et al.*, 2002). Enhanced leukocyte recruitment was accompanied by increased cerebrovascular permeability, linking the regulation of BBB permeability and leukocyte diapedesis at the level of PECAM-1.

Despite the evidence for the involvement of junctional proteins such as JAM-A and PECAM-1 in leukocyte migration across the BBB, ultrastructural studies investigating leukocyte diapedesis across the inflamed BBB into the CNS have mostly demonstrated transcellular diapedesis, as they have mostly shown leukocyte migration to occur through the endothelial cells, leaving the tight junctions morphologically intact (summarized in Engelhardt and Wolburg, 2004). Interestingly, neutrophil extravasation across the BBB during EAE was observed to occur through the BBB tight junctions in parallel to mononuclear cells migrating through the endothelium, suggesting that different leukocyte subpopulations might take different routes of diapedesis across the BBB (Cross and Raine, 1991). Using modern confocal imaging techniques, endothelial cells have been described to form a docking structure or transmigratory cup, where the endothelial cells embrace the leukocyte with cellular protrusions involving LFA-1/ICAM-1-interactions at least in vitro (Barreiro *et al.*, 2002; Carman and Springer, 2004). Although these studies provided no direct evidence for transcellular leukocyte diapedesis, engagement of endothelial ICAM-1 was recently shown to induce its redistribution to caveolae and to facilitate transcellular diapedesis of leukocytes in vitro (Millan *et al.*, 2006). Further evidence for distinct molecular pathways of paracellular versus transcellular leukocyte diapedesis was recently provided by a study demonstrating that macrophage

(Mac)–1-dependent leukocyte "crawling" on inflamed endothelium leads to paracellular diapedesis, whereas lack of Mac-1 resulted in loss of crawling and transcellular diapedesis (Phillipson *et al.*, 2006). Thus, transcellular diapedesis does occur under certain conditions and the unique molecular architecture of the BBB endothelium and of its tight junctions might favor this process.

The epithelial blood–cerebrospinal fluid barrier

How immune cells enter the cerebrospinal fluid (CSF)-filled ventricles is presently unknown. The CSF of a healthy individual contains between 1000 and 3000 leukocytes per milliliter, demonstrating active immune surveillance of this space in the healthy individual. Immune cell numbers in the CSF often increase significantly during MS. Interestingly, neither in the healthy state nor in MS does the cellular composition or the phenotype of the immune cells resemble that of the peripheral blood. Furthermore, the composition and phenotype of parenchymal inflammatory cells in MS is not necessarily identical to that of immune cells present in the CSF. These observations suggest that immune cell entry into the CSF is as stringently regulated as immune cell entry into the CNS parenchyma and that this may occur via a different pathway (Kleine and Benes, 2006). Direct access from the periphery into the CSF could be orchestrated via the choroid plexus. Interestingly, although several investigators had noted positive immunostaining for ICAM-1 and VCAM-1 – the adhesion molecules involved in inflammatory cell recruitment across the endothelial BBB – on choroid plexus epithelium during CNS inflammation (Deckert Schluter *et al.*, 1994; Steffen *et al.*, 1996), this site had not seriously been considered by many researchers as a possible entry site for immune cells into the CNS until recently (Carrithers *et al.*, 2002; Engelhardt *et al.*, 2001). Migration of leukocytes via the choroid plexus into the CSF under non-inflammatory conditions has been supported by the finding that fluorescently labeled lymphocytes are present in the choroid plexus stroma 2 h after intravenous injection in mice (Carrithers *et al.*, 2002). In human tissue, both P- and E-selectin immunoreactivity were detected in choroid plexus venules. As CD4[+] T cells in the CSF express high levels of PSGL-1, it is tempting to speculate that T cell recruitment into the choroid plexus involves selectin/PSGL-1 interactions (Kivisakk *et al.*, 2005). Whether constitutive expression of ICAM-1 and VCAM-1 on choroid plexus epithelium facilitates their penetration across this brain barrier into the CSF remains to be shown. During inflammatory conditions the choroid plexus epithelium up-regulates the expression of both VCAM-1 and ICAM-1 and de novo expresses mucosal adressin cell adhesion molecule (MAdCAM)-1 (Steffen *et al.*, 1996). All three adhesion molecules mediate binding of lymphocytes via their known ligands, α4β7-integrin (VLA-4), LFA-1 and α4β7-integrin, respectively, in vitro (Steffen *et al.*, 1996). Collectively, these findings suggest that the choroid plexus is involved in the communication between the immune system and CNS, probably by allowing the entry of immune cells directly into the CSF spaces.

Finally, the strategic localization of the CVOs, adjacent to the ventricular walls, suggests that CVOs, similar to the choroid plexus, might be involved in the recruitment of immune cells into the brain during EAE. There is evidence that CD45[+] inflammatory cells are recruited into these areas during EAE (Schulz and Engelhardt, 2005). One might therefore speculate that inflammatory cells can also access the CNS or the CSF space by penetrating the tanycytic barrier of the CVOs.

Entry of pathogens across the brain barriers

Although a relatively small number of pathogens account for most cases of CNS infections in humans, we still have an incomplete understanding of the strategies these pathogens have developed to bypass or disrupt the biological barriers between the blood and the brain and the CSF. In principle, pathogens can use three strategies to penetrate the brain barriers: firstly, as free pathogens they may breach a brain barrier by transcellular invasion; secondly, they can do so via paracellular entry after disruption of the barrier's tight junctions; and thirdly, pathogens may infect immune cells in the periphery and thus make use of the host cell trafficking machinery by entering the CNS through a so-called "Trojan horse" strategy (Kim, 2006). In this latter instance, the molecular mechanism involved in pathogen entry into the CNS would be identical to those involved in immune cell migration across the BBB, with a possible modification due to additional effects of virulence factors of the respective pathogens.

Transcellular passageways across brain barriers have been optimized by bacteria causing meningitis. However, although the molecular components of bacterial cell surfaces have been well-defined and their interactions with several receptor pathways have been described, our knowledge of how bacteria penetrate the BBB remains incomplete (reviewed by Huang and Jong, 2001; Kim, 2006). Based on our present knowledge, *Neisseria meningitidis* appears to have developed the most sophisticated strategy to pass the BBB. Its adhesion to the endothelium elicits the formation of membrane docking structures, resembling those induced by leukocytes, which allow for internalization and transcytosis of *N. meningitidis* across the endothelial cell (Doulet *et al.*, 2006). As the bacterial docking structures actively recruit ezrin and moesin, these molecules are no longer available for leukocyte–endothelial contacts, thus preventing the formation of the endothelial docking structures required for proper leukocyte diapedesis. *N. meningitidis* has thus developed a very successful strategy to penetrate the BBB and at the same time to inhibit the host's inflammatory response by hijacking the molecular pathway required for leukocyte diapedesis across the BBB. *Streptococcus pneumoniae* has also been suggested to cross the BBB by a transcellular pathway resembling transcytosis. Its interaction with brain endothelial cells was shown to lead to endothelial activation and increased expression of surface-expressed platelet activating factor (PAF) receptor. The endothelial PAF receptor was shown to provide a ligand for cell wall components of *S. pneumoniae* and to trigger its PFA receptor-dependent transcytosis (Ring *et al.*, 1998).

Clear evidence for paracellular penetration by pathogens is more elusive. *Toxoplasma gondii* can cross the BBB through tight junctions or, alternatively, by the Trojan horse mechanism. One study convincingly demonstrated that *T. gondii* can recruit CD11b[+] or CD11c[+] circulating leukocytes to cross the brain barrier in vivo (Courret *et al.*, 2006). Another study provided evidence for paracellular penetration of *T. gondii* through intercellular junctions involving endothelial ICAM-1 and the parasite adhesin, micronemal protein (MIC) 2 (Barragan *et al.*, 2005). Thus, this parasite could be able to use both pathways, interestingly both dependent on endothelial ICAM-1, to penetrate the BBB.

The Trojan horse mechanism has been optimized by the human immunodeficiency virus (HIV)-1 and the simian immunodeficiency virus (SIV) causing AIDS encephalitis (Banks *et al.*, 2006; MacLean *et al.*, 2004). HIV-1- or SIV-infected CD4[+] T cells and monocytes interact with brain endothelial cells leading to endothelial cell activation, as indicated by the up-regulated expression of adhesion molecules such as endothelial ICAM-1 and VCAM-1. Cell-associated virus is essential for this activation, which in turn increases immune cell entry across the BBB (MacLean *et al.*, 2004). In addition, proteins released by the HIV-1 virus such as gp120 or Tat have been shown to compromise BBB integrity at least in vitro and could therefore further enhance diapedesis of infected leukocytes across the BBB (Andras *et al.*, 2005; Kanmogne *et al.*, 2007).

A few studies have also addressed possible CNS entry of pathogens via the epithelial blood–CSF barrier. Experimental studies in mice revealed that choroid plexus epithelium is one target for *Listeria monocytogenes*, a relatively common cause of cerebral infections (Schluter *et al.*, 1999).

Conclusion

It is now well established that immune cells reach the CNS via the blood stream and can enter the CNS during both health and disease. Molecular signals that guide immune cells across the BBB appear to differ under physiological and pathological conditions and most probably even vary during different stages of inflammation, depending on the inflammatory stimulus and the CNS site involved. Current observations support the concept that there are even differences in endothelial signals utilized within meningeal versus parenchymal brain microvessels, which could well result in the recruitment of different leukocyte subpopulations into different sites within the CNS. Although not well characterized at the molecular level, it has already become quite evident that pathogens successfully exploit the natural host cell trafficking pathways to cross the brain barriers and reach the CNS parenchyma. Thus, in order to understand the molecular codes used by the different leukocyte subpopulations and different pathogens to breach the brain barriers, further research is necessary to delineate the role of adhesion and signaling molecules involved in this multi-step process.

References

Abbott NJ, et al. Astrocyte–endothelial interactions at the blood–brain barrier. *Nat Rev Neurosci* 2006; **7**: 41–53.

Adamson P, et al. Lymphocyte migration through brain endothelial cell monolayers involves signaling through endothelial ICAM-1 via a rho-dependent pathway. *J Immunol* 1999; **162**: 2964–73.

Allt G, Lawrenson JG. Is the pial microvessel a good model for blood–brain barrier studies? *Brain Res Brain Res Rev* 1997; **24**: 67–76.

Alt C, et al. Functional expression of the lymphoid chemokines CCL19 (ELClc) and CCL21 (SLC) at the blood–brain barrier suggests their possible involvement in lymphocyte recruitment into the central nervous system during experimental autoimmune encephalomyelitis. *Eur J Immunol* 2002; **32**: 2133–44.

Andras IE, et al. Signaling mechanisms of HIV-1 Tat-induced alterations of claudin-5 expression in brain endothelial cells. *J Cereb Blood Flow Metab* 2005; **25**: 1159–70.

Archelos JJ, et al. Inhibition of experimental autoimmune encephalomyelitis by an antibody to the intercellular adhesion molecule ICAM-1. *Ann Neurol* 1993; **34**: 145–54.

Banks WA, et al. The blood–brain barrier in neuroaids. *Curr HIV Res* 2006; **4**: 259–66.

Barragan A, Sibley LD. Migration of *Toxoplasma gondii* across biological barriers. *Trends Microbiol* 2003; **11**: 426–30.

Barragan A, et al. Transepithelial migration of *Toxoplasma gondii* involves an interaction of intercellular adhesion molecule 1 (ICAM-1) with the parasite adhesin MIC2. *Cell Microbiol* 2005; **7**: 561–8.

Barreiro O, et al. Dynamic interaction of VCAM-1 and ICAM-1 with moesin and ezrin in a novel endothelial docking structure for adherent leukocytes. *J Cell Biol* 2002; **157**: 1233–45.

Battistini L, et al. Cd8+ T cells from patients with acute multiple sclerosis display selective increase of adhesiveness in brain venules: A critical role for P-selectin glycoprotein ligand-1. *Blood* 2003; **101**: 4775–82.

Betz LA, et al. Blood brain–cerebrospinal fluid barriers. In Siegel GJ (Ed.), *Basic Neurochemistry: Molecular, Cellular, And Medical Aspects*. New York: Raven Press.

Bo L, et al. Distribution of immunoglobulin superfamily members ICAM-1, -2, -3, and the beta 2 integrin LFA-1 in multiple sclerosis lesions. *J Neuropathol Exp Neurol* 1996; **55**: 1060–72.

Bouchaud C, Bosler O. The circumventricular organs of the mammalian brain with special reference to monoaminergic innervation. *Int Rev Cytol* 1986; **105**: 283–327.

Brocke S, et al. Antibodies to Cd44 and integrin alpha4, but not L-selectin, prevent central nervous system inflammation and experimental encephalomyelitis by blocking secondary leukocyte recruitment. *Proc Natl Acad Sci USA* 1999; **96**: 6896–901.

Bullard DC, et al. Intercellular adhesion molecule-1 expression is required on multiple cell types for the development of experimental autoimmune encephalomyelitis. *J Immunol* 2007; **178**: 851–7.

Butcher EC, et al. Lymphocyte trafficking and regional immunity. *Adv Immunol* 1999; **72**: 209–53.

Cannella B, et al. Anti-adhesion molecule therapy in experimental autoimmune encephalomyelitis. *J Neuroimmunol* 1993; **46**: 43–55.

Carlos TM, Harlan JM. Leukocyte–endothelial adhesion molecules. *Blood* 1994; **7**: 2068–101.

Carman CV, Springer TA. A transmigratory cup in leukocyte diapedesis both through individual vascular endothelial cells and between them. *J Cell Biol* 2004; **167**: 377–88.

Carrithers MD, et al. Differential adhesion molecule requirements for immune surveillance and inflammatory recruitment. *Brain* 2000; **123**: 1092–101.

Carrithers MD, et al. Role of genetic background in P Selectin-dependent immune surveillance of the central nervous system. *J Neuroimmunol* 2002; **129**: 51–7.

Carvalho-Tavares J, et al. A role for platelets and endothelial selectins in tumor necrosis factor-alpha-induced leukocyte recruitment in the brain microvasculature. *Circ Res* 2000; **87**: 1141–8.

Cattelino A, et al. The conditional inactivation of the {beta}-catenin gene in endothelial cells causes a defective vascular pattern and increased vascular fragility. *J Cell Biol* 2003; **162**: 1111–22.

Columba-Cabezas S, et al. Lymphoid chemokines CCL19 And CCL21 are expressed in the central nervous system during experimental autoimmune encephalomyelitis: Implications for the maintenance of chronic neuroinflammation. *Brain Pathol* 2003; **13**: 38–51.

Courret N, et al. Cd11c- and Cd11b-expressing mouse leukocytes transport single *Toxoplasma gondii* tachyzoites to the brain. *Blood* 2006; **107**: 309–16.

Crone C, Olesen SP. Electrical resistance of brain microvascular endothelium. *Brain Res* 1982; **241**: 49–55.

Cross AH, Raine CS. Central nervous system endothelial cell–polymorphonuclear cell interactions during autoimmune demyelination. *Am J Pathol* 1991; **139**: 1401–9.

Deckert Schluter M, et al. Differential expression of ICAM-1, VCAM-1 and their ligands LFA-1, MAC-1, CD43, VLA-4, and MHC class II antigens in murine toxoplasma encephalitis: A light microscopic and ultrastructural immunohistochemical study. *J Neuropathol Exp Neurol* 1994; **53**: 457–68.

Del Maschio A, et al. Leukocyte recruitment in the cerebrospinal fluid of mice with experimental meningitis is inhibited by an antibody to junctional adhesion molecule (JAM). *J Exp Med* 1999; **190**: 1351–6.

Doulet N, *et al. Neisseria meningitidis* infection of human endothelial cells interferes with leukocyte transmigration by preventing the formation of endothelial docking structures. *J Cell Biol* 2006; **173**: 627–37.

Dzenko KA, *et al.* The chemokine receptor Ccr2 mediates the binding and internalization of monocyte chemoattractant protein-1 along brain microvessels. *J Neurosci* 2001; **21**: 9214–23.

Dziegielewska KM, *et al.* Development of the choroid plexus. *Microsc Res Tech* 2001; **52**: 5–20.

Ebnet K, *et al.* Junctional adhesion molecules (JAMs): More molecules with dual functions? *J Cell Sci* 2004; **117**: 19–29.

Engelhardt B. Development of the blood–brain barrier. *Cell Tissue Res* 2003; **314**: 119–29.

Engelhardt B, Ransohoff RM. The ins and outs of T-lymphocyte trafficking to the CNS: Anatomical sites and molecular mechanisms. *Trends Immunol* 2005; **26**: 485–95.

Engelhardt B, Wolburg H. Mini-review: Transendothelial migration of leukocytes – Through the front door or around the side of the house? *Eur J Immunol* 2004; **34**: 2955–63.

Engelhardt B, *et al.* Lymphocytes infiltrating the CNS during inflammation display a distinctive phenotype and bind to VCAM-1 but not to MADCAM-1. *Int Immunol* 1995; **7**: 481–91.

Engelhardt B, *et al.* E- and P-selectin are not involved in the recruitment of inflammatory cells across the blood–brain barrier in experimental autoimmune encephalomyelitis. *Blood* 1997; **90**: 4459–72.

Engelhardt B, *et al.* The development of experimental autoimmune encephalomyelitis in the mouse requires alpha4-integrin but not alpha4beta7-integrin. *J Clin Invest* 1998a; **102**: 2096–105.

Engelhardt B, *et al.* Adhesion molecule phenotype of T lymphocytes in inflamed CNS. *J Neuroimmunol* 1998b; **84**: 92–104.

Engelhardt B, *et al.* Involvement of the choroid plexus in central nervous system inflammation. *Microsc Res Tech* 2001; **52**: 112–29.

Engelhardt B, *et al.* PSGL-1 is not required for the development of experimental autoimmune encephalomyelitis in SJL and C57bl6 mice. *J Immunol* 2005; **175**: 1267–75.

Graesser D, *et al.* Altered vascular permeability and early onset of experimental autoimmune encephalomyelitis in PECAM-1-deficient mice. *J Clin Invest* 2002; **109**: 383–92.

Greenwood J, *et al.* Intracellular domain of brain endothelial intercellular adhesion molecule-1 is essential for T lymphocyte-mediated signaling and migration. *J Immunol* 2003; **171**: 2099–108.

Grewal IS, *et al.* Cd62l is required on effector cells for local interactions in the CNS to cause myelin damage in experimental allergic encephalomyelitis. *Immunity* 2001; **14**: 291–302.

Hickey WF, *et al.* T-lymphocyte entry into the central nervous system. *J Neurosci Res* 1991; **28**: 254–60.

Huang S, Jong AY. Cellular mechanisms of microbial proteins contributing to invasion of the blood–brain barrier. *Cell Microbiol* 2001; **3**: 277–87.

Johnson AK, Gross PM. Sensory circumventricular organs and brain homeostatic pathways. *FASEB J* 2003; **7**: 678–86.

Johnson-Léger C, Imhof BA. Forging the endothelium during inflammation: Pushing at a half-open door? *Cell Tiss Res* 2003; **314**: 93–105.

Kanmogne GD, *et al.* HIV-1 Gp120 compromises blood–brain barrier integrity and enhances monocyte migration across blood–brain barrier: Implication for viral neuropathogenesis. *J Cereb Blood Flow Metab* 2007; **27**: 123–34.

Kent SJ, *et al.* A monoclonal antibody to alpha 4 integrin suppresses and reverses active experimental allergic encephalomyelitis. *J Neuroimmunol* 1995; **58**: 1–10.

Kerfoot S, Kubes P. Overlapping roles of P-selectin and alpha 4 integrin to recruit leukocytes to the central nervous system in experimental autoimmune encephalomyelitis. *J. Immunol* 2002; **169**: 1000–6.

Kim KS. Microbial translocation of the blood–brain barrier. *Int J Parasitol* 2006; **36**: 607–14.

Kivisakk P, *et al.* Human cerebrospinal fluid central memory CD4+ T cells: Evidence for trafficking through choroid plexus and meninges via P-selectin. *Proc Natl Acad Sci USA* 2005; **100**: 8389–94. Epub 2003 Jun 26.

Kleine TO, Benes L. Immune surveillance of the human central nervous system (CNS): Different migration pathways of immune cells through the blood–brain barrier and blood–cerebrospinal fluid barrier in healthy persons. *Cytometry A* 2006; **69**: 147–51.

Laschinger M, Engelhardt, B. Interaction of alpha4-integrin with VCAM-1 is involved in adhesion of encephalitogenic T cell blasts to brain endothelium but not in their transendothelial migration in vitro. *J Neuroimmunol* 2000; **102**: 32–43.

Laschinger M, *et al.* Encephalitogenic T cells use LFA-1 during transendothelial migration but not during capture and adhesion in spinal cord microvessels in vivo. *Eur J Immunol* 2002; **32**: 3598–606.

Lechner F, *et al.* Antibodies to the junctional adhesion molecule cause disruption of endothelial cells and do not prevent leukocyte influx into the meninges after viral or bacterial infection. *J Infect Dis* 2000; **182**: 978–82.

Leonhardt H. Ependym und Circumventriculäre Organe. In Oksche A, Vollrath L (Eds.), *Handbuch der Mikroskopischen Anatomie des Menschen*. Berlin/Heidelberg/New York: Springer, 1980a.

Leonhardt H. *Ependym und Zirkumventrikuläre Organe*. Berlin: Springer, 1980b.

Luster AD, *et al.* Immune cell migration in inflammation: Present and future therapeutic targets. *Nat Immunol* 2005; **6**: 1182–90.

Lyck R, *et al.* T-cell interaction with ICAM-1/ICAM-2 double-deficient brain endothelium in vitro: The cytoplasmic tail of endothelial ICAM-1 is necessary for transendothelial migration of T cells. *Blood* 2003; **102**: 3675–83.

Maclean AG, *et al.* Activation of the blood–brain barrier by SIV (simian immunodeficiency virus) requires cell-associated virus and is not restricted to endothelial cell activation. *Biochem Soc Trans* 2004; **32**: 750–2.

Martin R, Mcfarland HF. Immunological aspects of experimental allergic encephalomyelitis and multiple sclerosis. *Crit Rev Clin Lab Sci* 1995; **32**: 121–82.

Martin-Padura I, *et al.* Junctional adhesion molecule, a novel member of the immunoglobulin superfamily that distributes at intercellular junctions and modulates monocyte transmigration. *J Cell Biol* 1998; **142**: 117–27.

Millan J, *et al.* Lymphocyte transcellular migration occurs through recruitment of endothelial ICAM-1 to caveola- and F-actin-rich domains. *Nat Cell Biol* 2006; **8**: 113–23. Epub 2006 Jan 22.

Muller WA. Leukocyte–endothelial cell interactions in leukocyte transmigration and the inflammatory response. *Trends Immunol* 2003; **6**: 327–34.

Nasdala I, *et al.* A transmembrane tight junction protein selectively expressed on endothelial cells and platelets. *J Biol Chem* 2002; **277**: 16294–303.

Osmers I, *et al.* PSGL-1 is not required for development of experimental autoimmune encephalomyelitis. *J Neuroimmunol* 2005; **166**: 193–6.

Padden M, *et al.* differences in expression of junctional adhesion molecule-A and beta-catenin in multiple sclerosis brain tissue: Increasing evidence for the role of tight junction pathology. *Acta Neuropathol (Berl)* 2007; **113**: 177–86. Epub 2006 Oct 6.

Pardridge WM. Blood–brain barrier delivery. *Drug Discov Today* 2007; **12**: 54–61.

Phillipson M, *et al.* Intraluminal crawling of neutrophils to emigration sites: A molecularly distinct process from adhesion in the recruitment cascade. *J Exp Med* 2006; **203**: 2569–75.

Piccio L, *et al.* Efficient recruitment of lymphocytes in inflamed brain venules requires expression of cutaneous lymphocyte antigen and fucosyltransferase-VII. *J Immunol* 2005; **174**: 5805–13.

Piccio L, *et al.* Molecular mechanisms involved in lymphocyte recruitment in inflamed brain microvessels: Critical roles for P-selectin glycoprotein ligand-1 and heterotrimeric G(I)-linked receptors. *J Immunol* 2002; **168**: 1940–9.

Plumb J, *et al.* Abnormal endothelial tight junctions in active lesions and normal-appearing white matter in multiple sclerosis. *Brain Pathol* 2002; **12**: 154–69.

Polman CH, *et al.* A randomized, placebo-controlled trial of Natalizumab for relapsing multiple sclerosis. *N Engl J Med* 2006; **354**: 899–910.

Qing Z, *et al.* Inhibition of antigen-specific T cell trafficking into the central nervous system via blocking PECAM1/CD31 molecule. *J Neuropathol Exp Neurol* 2001; **60**: 798–807.

Rascher G, Wolburg H. The tight junctions of the leptomeningeal blood–cerebrospinal fluid barrier during development. *J Hirnforsch* 1997; **38**: 525–40.

Reiss Y, *et al.* T cell interaction with ICAM-1-deficient endothelium in vitro: Essential role for ICAM-1 and ICAM-2 in transendothelial migration of T cells. *Eur J Immunol* 1998; **28**: 3086–99.

Ring A, *et al.* Pneumococcal trafficking across the blood–brain barrier. Molecular analysis of a novel bidirectional pathway. *J Clin Invest* 1998; **102**: 347–60.

Risau W, *et al.* Immune function of the blood–brain barrier: Incomplete presentation of protein (auto-) antigens by rat brain microvascular endothelium in vitro. *J Cell Biol* 1990; **110**: 1757–66.

Rudick RA, *et al.* Natalizumab plus interferon beta-1a for relapsing multiple sclerosis. *N Engl J Med* 2006; **354**: 911–23.

Schluter D, *et al.* Immune reactions to *Listeria monocytogenes* in the brain. *Immunobiology* 1999; **201**: 188–95.

Schulz M, Engelhardt B. The circumventricular organs participate in the immunopathogenesis of experimental autoimmune encephalomyelitis. *Cerebrospinal Fluid Res* 2005; **2**: 8.

Schulze C, Firth JA. Immunohistochemical localization of adherens junction components in blood–brain barrier microvessels of the rat. *JCell Sci* 1993; **104**: 773–82.

Sedgwick JD, *et al.* Antigen-specific damage to brain vascular endothelial cells mediated by encephalitogenic and nonencephalitogenic CD4+ T cell lines in vitro. *J Immunol* 1990; **145**: 2474–81.

Sixt M, *et al.* Endothelial cell laminin isoforms, laminins 8 and 10, play decisive roles in T cell recruitment across the blood–brain barrier in experimental autoimmune encephalomyelitis. *J Cell Biol* 2001; **153**: 933–46.

Sobel RA, *et al.* Intercellular adhesion molecule-1 (ICAM-1) in cellular immune reactions in the human central nervous system. *Am J Pathol* 1990; **136**: 1309–16.

Steffen BJ, *et al.* ICAM-1, VCAM-1, and MADCAM-1 are expressed on choroid plexus epithelium but not endothelium and mediate binding of lymphocytes in vitro. *Am J Pathol* 1996; **148**: 1819–38.

Steffen BJ, *et al.* Evidence for involvement of ICAM-1 and VCAM-1 in lymphocyte interaction with endothelium in experimental autoimmune encephalomyelitis in the central nervous system in the SJL/J mouse. *Am J Pathol* 1994; **145**: 189–201.

Ubogu EE, *et al.* The expression and function of chemokines involved in CNS inflammation. *Trends Pharmacol Sci* 2006; **27**: 48–55.

Vajkoczy P, *et al.* Alpha4-integrin-VCAM-1 binding mediates G protein-independent capture of encephalitogenic T cell blasts to CNS white matter microvessels. *J Clin Invest* 2001; **108**: 557–65.

Wekerle H, *et al.* Cellular immune reactivity within the CNS. *TINS* 1986; **9**: 271–7.

Welsh CT, *et al.* Augmentation of adoptively transferred experimental allergic encephalomyelitis by administration of a monoclonal antibody specific for LFA-1a. *J Neuroimmunol* 1993; **43**: 161–8.

Willenborg DO, *et al.* ICAM-1-dependent pathway is not critically involved in the inflammatory process of autoimmune encephalomyelitis or in cytokine-induced inflammation of the central nervous system. *J Neuroimmunol* 1993; **45**: 147–54.

Wolburg H, Lippoldt A. Tight junctions of the blood–brain barrier. Development, composition and regulation. *Vasc Pharmacol* 2002; **28**: 323–37.

Wolburg H, *et al.* Localization of claudin-3 in tight junctions of the blood–brain barrier is selectively lost during experimental autoimmune encephalomyelitis and human glioblastoma multiforme. *Acta Neuropathol (Berl)* 2003; **105**: 586–92.

Wolburg H, *et al.* Osp/claudin-11, claudin-1 and claudin-2 are present in tight junctions of choroid plexus epithelium of the mouse. *Neurosci Lett* 2001; **13**: 77–80.

Yednock TA, *et al.* Prevention of experimental autoimmune encephalomyelitis by antibodies against alpha 4 beta 1 integrin. *Nature* 1992; **356**: 63–6.

Yousry TA, *et al.* Evaluation of patients treated with Natalizumab for progressive multifocal leukoencephalopathy. *N Engl J Med* 2006; **354**: 924–33.

Zeine R, Owens T. Direct demonstration of the infiltration of murine central nervous system by PGP-1/Cd44 high Cd45rblow Cd4+ T cells that induce experimental allergic encephalomyelitis. *J Neuroimmunol* 1992; **40**: 57–70.

5 Immune effector heterogeneity in multiple sclerosis and related CNS inflammatory demyelinating disorders

Shanu F. Roemer and Claudia F. Lucchinetti

Introduction

Multiple sclerosis (MS) is an inflammatory demyelinating central nervous system (CNS) disorder, and the most common cause of non-traumatic disability in young adults. Pathological hallmarks include focal demyelinated white matter lesions associated with variable inflammation, "relative" axonal sparing and gliosis. Recent advances in immunology, molecular biology, genetics, experimental pathology, and neuro-imaging have expanded the traditional view of MS pathogenesis beyond a purely autoimmune CD4+ T cell-mediated disease, and contributed to the evolving concept that MS may be a pathogenetically heterogeneous disorder. Although the cause of the disease remains elusive, multiple potential effector mechanisms likely contribute to lesion initiation, evolution, and disease progression. This chapter focuses on pathogenic insights obtained via detailed analysis of MS neuropathology. Pathogenic and therapeutic implications will be discussed.

The inflammatory cell components in MS lesions

T lymphocytes

The inflammatory infiltrate in MS largely consists of activated mononuclear cells including lymphocytes, macrophages and activated microglia. Granulocytes may be present in lesions of acute Marburg MS and neuromyelitis optica (NMO). T cells are divided into subsets determined by the type of cytokines they produce. T helper cells 1 (Th1) secrete a spectrum of pro-inflammatory cytokines including interleukin-2 (IL-2), interferon-gamma (IFN-γ) and lymphotoxin

alpha (Martino *et al.*, 2000; Lassman *et al.*, 2001). Th1 cells also activate cytotoxic CD8+ T cells and macrophages. T helper 2 (Th2) cells secrete IL-4, -5, and -6, as well as stimulate B cell proliferation and immunoglobulin production (Martino *et al.*, 2000). Furthermore, a Th2 response can down-regulate Th1 cell responses as part of its anti-inflammatory effect. Both Th1 and Th2 cells are MHC II-restricted, whereas cytotoxic CD8+ T cells are MHC I-restricted. Chemokines play a role in polarizing the immune response of T cells and macrophages into either a type 1 or type 2 response. Chemokine receptors are differentially expressed on polarized Th cells. Th1 cells preferentially express CXCR3 and CCR5, whereas Th2 cells express CCR3, CCR4 and CCR8 (Mantovani *et al.*, 2004).

Multiple sclerosis has long been considered an autoimmune disease. Evidence for this is mainly derived from studies of experimental autoimmune encephalomyelitis (EAE), in which MHC II-restricted CD4+ T cells are the primary effector cells mediating autoimmunity (Steinman *et al.*, 1996; Lassmann and Ransohoff 2004; Gold and Lassman 2006). Lesions in EAE show a predominance of CD4+ T cells, and MHC II is identified on resting and activated microglia in MS lesions (Steinman, 1996; Conde and Streit 2006). Several clinical studies have suggested that some T cells are auto-reactive and stimulated by the recognition of specific CNS antigens (Ota *et al.*, 1990; Pette *et al.*, 1990; Steinman, 1996; de Rosbo *et al.*, 1998). Autoreactive T cells can be isolated from peripheral blood (Pette *et al.*, 1990; Kerlero de Rosbo *et al.*,1997), and in MS lesions, macrophages and microglia express antigenic T cell epitopes from the HLA-DR2 myelin peptide complex on their surface (Krogsgaard *et al.*, 2000), thus providing some evidence that HLA-DR2

Inflammatory Diseases of the Central Nervous System, ed. T. Kilpatrick, R. M. Ransohoff and S. Wesselingh. Published by Cambridge University Press. © Cambridge University Press 2010

molecules in MS lesions may present a myelin derived self-peptide. Additionally, inherited susceptibility to MS is associated with the HLA-DR2 haplotype (Fogdell *et al.*, 1997). Clonal expansion of T cells within MS lesions also suggests their antigen driven proliferation (Babbe *et al.*, 2000; Skulina *et al.*, 2004). However, the pathogenic role of autoreactive T cells in the majority of MS patients remains to be confirmed.

The role of MHC I CD8+ dependent tissue damage in MS has long been underestimated. Recently, experimental models have been developed in which EAE can be induced by adoptively transferring CD8+ T cells (Huseby *et al.*, 2001; Sun *et al.*, 2001). The transferred cells induce severe disease with brain lesions and pronounced demyelination that more closely resemble MS pathology. Since CD4+ T cells are not required to induce these models, MHC I-restricted CD8+ T cells act as the primary effector cells mediating tissue damage (Friese & Fugger, 2005). The majority of T cells in the inflammatory infiltrate of MS lesions consist of MHC I-restricted CD8+ cytotoxic T cells, and the CD8+ T-cell repertoire appears to be more antigen driven than that of the MHC II-restricted CD4+ T cells (Friese *et al.*, 2005). The close apposition of activated cytotoxic CD8+ T cells with degenerating oligodendrocytes, neurons, and axons can also be seen in some acute MS lesions, supporting a potential role for CD8-mediated tissue injury (Monteiro *et al.*, 1996; Babbe *et al.*, 2000; Jacobsen *et al.*, 2002; Neumann *et al.*, 2002). Recently, Hoftberger *et al.* examined MHC class I expression in MS lesions and found it is up-regulated on microglia, endothelial cells, neurons, axons, astrocytes and oligodendrocytes within active MS lesions, suggesting these cells could become targets of an MHC class I-restricted immune response (Hoftberger *et al.*, 2004).

B lymphocytes

B cells and antibody-producing plasma cells account for more than a quarter of the inflammatory cells found in CSF from MS patients (Corcione *et al.*, 2005), and the presence of CSF oligoclonal immunoglobulin bands is an important diagnostic hallmark of the disease (Kabat *et al.*, 1948). Elevated antibody titers to a number of self and foreign antigens are found in MS patients (Olsson *et al.*, 1990; Baig *et al.*, 1991; Martino *et al.*, 1991; Sun *et al.*, 1991), although none have proven pathogenic (Cross *et al.*, 2001). Serum antibodies targeting the myelin oligodendrocyte glycoprotein (MOG) have been described in MS patients;

however, reported frequencies vary between studies, and MOG antibodies are present in both patients with non-inflammatory neurological diseases and normal controls (Xiao *et al.*, 1991; Karni *et al.*, 1999; Lindert *et al.*, 1999; Reindl *et al.*, 1999; Egg *et al.*, 2001; Haase *et al.*, 2001; Gaertner *et al.*, 2004, Lampasona *et al.*, 2004; Mantegazza *et al.*, 2004). A recent study suggested that MOG IgM antibodies are associated with increased disease activity in MS, and could also be a predictor of early conversion to definite MS in patients with a clinically isolated syndrome (Berger *et al.*, 2003). However, a subsequent study could not confirm this finding (Lim *et al.*, 2005).

A prerequisite for pathogenicity of a demyelinating antibody is the recognition of a specific epitope at the outermost surface of the myelin sheath. Demyelination is often limited in T cell models of EAE; however, the presence of autoantibodies directed against MOG extensively amplifies the extent of demyelination (Lassmann *et al.*, 1988; Linington *et al.*, 1988; Burgoon and Owens, 2004). Autoantibodies can mediate their effector function either through activation of the classical complement cascade or through Fc receptor-mediated antibody-directed cell cytotoxicity (Urich *et al.*, 2006). The contribution of Fc receptor signaling is likely linked to accessory leukocytes residing within the systemic immune compartment, increasing the encephalitogenic potential of pathogenic lymphocytes (Urich *et al.*, 2006).

Although much attention has focused on MOG as a possible autoantigen, its role in MS pathogenesis remains uncertain. Small linear MOG peptides frequently used to induce EAE are not expressed on the surface of intact myelin or oligodendrocytes (Zhou *et al.*, 2006). Native MOG, on the other hand, is sequestered at the outermost surface of the myelin sheath, thereby making it a potential target of a pathogenic autoantibody. Immunoglobulin isolated from MS lesions recognized folded MOG, indicating binding of MOG in its native conformation, including glycosylation by Ig isolated from the lesions (O'Connor *et al.*, 2005). Several other studies suggested that antibodies can recognize native MOG, as well as fix complement (Bourquin *et al.*, 2000; Marta *et al.*, 2005a, 2005b). Furthermore, serum antibodies that bind to the extracellular domain of native MOG have been isolated from MS patients and can induce death of MOG-expressing target cells in vitro, further supporting a possible role for antibody-mediated pathogenicity to native MOG in MS (Lalive and Genain, 2006; Zhou *et al.*, 2006).

Pathologic studies have described the co-deposition of Ig and activated terminal lytic complement complex in active MS lesions (Storch *et al.*, 1998; Lucchinetti *et al.*, 2000). These findings, coupled with the presence in CSF of membrane attack complex-enriched membrane vesicles, also indicate a potential role for complement-mediated injury in MS (Hafler *et al.*, 2005). The deposition of immune complexes could partly be explained by the leakage of immune complexes through a disrupted blood–brain barrier (Kwon and Prineas, 1994), and/or by intrathecal production by infiltrating plasma cells (Tavolato, 1975). Both B cells and plasma cells are identified in acute MS lesions, but their density increases with disease chronicity. Interestingly, structures suggestive of lymphoid B cell follicles have been described in the meninges of some MS patients in the late, progressive phase of the disease, suggesting that the formation of ectopic lymphoid follicles could maintain humoral autoimmunity and contribute to disease severity in chronic MS (Serafini *et al.*, 2004). Furthermore, a co-stimulatory effect on autoreactive T cells (Cross *et al.*, 2001), a cytokine shift from Th1 toward Th2 (Saoudi *et al.*, 1995), the induction of T cell anergy (Hollsberg *et al.*, 1996) and enhancement of remyelination (Warrington *et al.*, 2000) are other potential roles for B cells, plasma cells and antibodies that could be relevant to MS pathogenesis (Cross *et al.*, 2001).

Macrophages/microglia

Hematogenous macrophages and activated CNS microglia are important antigen-presenting and myelin-phagocytosing cells involved in active demyelination (Schwartz *et al.*, 2006; Streit, 2006). Macrophages significantly outnumber lymphocytes within MS lesions (Ransohoff *et al.*, 2003; Mahad *et al.*, 2004). Brain parenchymal monocuclear phagocytes express chemokine receptors, including CCR1, CCR5, and to a lesser extent CCR2 (Balashov *et al.*, 1999; Sorensen *et al.*, 1999; Simpson *et al.*, 2000), which regulate the recruitment and activation of circulating monocytes into CNS tissue (Mahad *et al.*, 2006). A complement of CCR1+/CCR5+ mononuclear phagocytes is observed in brain perivascular regions only in inflammatory states and not in control tissue (Trebst *et al.*, 2001). Human monocyte maturation into tissue macrophages is accompanied by a loss of CCR2 expression and increased CCR1 and CCR5. This receptor switch could indicate that the CCL2–CCR2 axis is involved in initial recruitment, followed

by CCR1–CCR5-dependent positioning in the tissue (Mahad *et al.*, 2004).

The identification of different MS pathological subtypes has provided a framework within which to evaluate chemokine and chemokine receptor involvement in MS lesion pathogenesis (Lucchinetti *et al.*, 2000). Pattern II MS lesions are characterized by focal demyelinated lesions associated with sharp macrophage borders and antibody deposition and complement activation on myelin sheaths. CCR1+ mononuclear phagocytes in pattern II lesions localize to the plaque edge at sites of active demyelination, and CCR1 is down-regulated as monocytes transform into macrophages (Mahad *et al.*, 2004). The CCR5, on the other hand, is maintained on macrophages and microglia as demyelination proceeds. Pattern III lesions are characterized by ill-defined lesion borders, loss of MAG, and no evidence for antibody deposition or complement activation (Lucchinetti *et al.*, 2000). In contrast to pattern II, CCR1 and CCR5 are co-expressed within pattern III lesions and do not shift their expression throughout lesion evolution (Mahad *et al.*, 2004). These observations suggest the cytokine microenvironment differs between pattern II and III MS lesions.

Macrophages can potentially exert both beneficial and detrimental effects on MS lesion evolution (Boven *et al.*, 2006; Schwartz *et al.*, 2006), and are subclassified into two phenotypes. The M1 phenotype contributes to tissue damage, whereas the M2 phenotype promotes tissue repair. The M1 phenotype is characterized by the production of pro-inflammatory mediators and reactive oxygen species (ROS) (Hill *et al.*, 2004; Mantovani *et al.*, 2005), and is predominantly involved in Th1 cell responses. The M2 phenotype, on the other hand, is characterized by the production of anti-inflammatory mediators, and is associated with Th2 responses, tissue scavenging, tissue remodeling and repair and resolution of inflammation (Mantovani *et al.*, 2004). Additionally, M2-induced signals inhibit M1-induced chemokines (Mantovani *et al.*, 2002, 2004, 2005).

Active MS lesions contain numerous foamy macrophages, reflecting the ingestion and accumulation of myelin lipids within the macrophage cytoplasm (Bruck *et al.*, 1995). However, MS lesions are self-limiting, suggesting the presence of unidentified anti-inflammatory mechanisms. Subsets of macrophages/microglia could differ relative to their lesion topography and microenvironment. Foamy myelin-containing macrophages are concentrated at the expanding plaque edge and are mainly involved in myelin phagocytosis. However, foamy macrophages within the inactive lesion center could be more involved in down-regulating inflammation (Boven *et al.*, 2006). Foamy macrophages of both M1 and M2 phenotypes are identified in MS lesions, suggesting that macrophages are likely involved with functions in addition to antigen presentation and phagocytosis (Boven *et al.*, 2006). Macrophages also contribute to lesion repair and neuroprotection by promoting the clearance of cell debris (Schwartz *et al.*, 2006), as well as by the secretion of neurotrophic factors and cytokines (Kerchensteiner *et al.*, 1999; Stadelmann *et al.*, 2002).

Blood–brain barrier damage in MS

Pathologic evidence of vascular hyperpermeability and blood–brain barrier (BBB) disruption in active and inactive MS lesions was originally based on the observation that organic dyes leaked through open tight junctions (Broman *et al.*, 1964). The presence of gadolinium enhancement of active lesions on MRI provided further evidence of BBB damage in MS (Kermode *et al.*, 1994). However, Gd-enhancement becomes less frequent during the chronic progressive phase of MS, contributing to the assumption that BBB damage and inflammation are less pronounced during later disease stages (Rovaris *et al.*, 1999, 2006; Confavreux *et al.*, 2000). However, immunohistochemical studies of chronic MS lesions demonstrate persistent leakage of serum proteins, suggesting that the BBB may be permanently damaged in chronic MS, although to a degree that is undetectable with current Gd-MRI techniques (Kwon and Prineas, 1994).

The vascular changes associated with BBB breakdown include abnormalities in the tight junctions between endothelial cells. Abnormal expression of tight junction proteins, zonula occludens (ZO-1) and occludin have been demonstrated immunohistochemically in MS lesions, most pronounced in active lesions, but also evident in inactive lesions and in the normal-appearing white matter (NAWM) (Plumb *et al.*, 2005). This abnormal expression could lead to putatively open junctions resulting in BBB disruption, reflected on MRI as Gd-enhancement associated with active MS lesions, as well as possibly contributing to subtle non-enhancing NAWM abnormalities.

Increased expression of vascular endothelial growth factor (VEGF) is also detected in MS lesions (Proescholdt *et al.*, 2002). The VEGF induces vascular neogenesis, increased vascular permeability and is an important chemoattractant for mononuclear cells. Increased VEGF expression is associated with BBB breakdown in neoplasms and its increased expression in MS lesions suggests a possible role for VEGF in mediating BBB damage in MS.

In MS and EAE lesions, immunoreactivity against the muscle-specific protein dysferlin is induced in endothelial cells of inflamed CNS vessels associated with high trans-endothelial transport of inflammatory cells and vascular leakage of immunoglobulins (Hochmeister *et al.*, 2006). In MS, dysferlin expression in endothelial cells is not restricted to vessels with inflammatory cuffs, but is also present in non-inflamed vessels. In addition, many blood vessels with perivascular inflammatory infiltrates lack dysferlin expression in inactive lesions or in the NAWM. These observations suggest that dysferlin is not only a marker for leaky brain vessels, but also reveals dissociation of perivascular inflammatory infiltrates and BBB disturbance in MS (Hochmeister *et al.*, 2006). Inflammation in chronic MS is therefore not necessarily associated with either BBB damage or the formation of new active white matter lesions, and may reflect a compartmentalized immune reaction which, with disease chronicity, becomes trapped in the CNS behind a relatively intact BBB.

Additional effector mechanisms of tissue damage in MS

Nitric oxide

Nitric oxide (NO) is a membrane-permeable bioactive free radical and ubiquitous messenger molecule that exerts important physiological functions in intercellular signal transduction and neurotransmission, and is involved in glutamate-induced excitation with direct effects on BBB permeability, clearance of CNS inflammation, possibly via induction of encephalitogenic T cell apoptosis, and mediating demyelination, oligodendrocyte destruction and injury to axons (Smith *et al.*, 2002).

The NO is synthesized from L-arginine and oxygen by three types of NO synthases (NOS): the constitutively expressed synthase (cNOS), the inducible synthase (iNOS) and the mitochondrial NO synthase (mtNOS). In the brain, cNOS is found in neurons and endothelial cells, and is regulated predominantly at the post-transcriptional level by calmodulin, in a calcium-dependent manner (Brown *et al.*, 2002, 2006).

In contrast, iNOS is expressed in various cell types in response to a number of pro-inflammatory cytokines, including IL-1β, IFN-γ and TNF-α (Bo *et al.*, 1994; Forstermann *et al.*, 1995). During CNS inflammation, NO synthesis by ependymal cells, macrophages and astrocytes increases to concentrations that are neurotoxic to the CNS microenvironment. Detection of the by-product, nitrotyrosine, is indicative of oxidative cell membrane damage. Levels of NO within the CSF correlate with MS disease activity (Yamashita *et al.*, 1997).

Although not detected in the normal human CNS, iNOS is abundantly expressed by astrocytes in plaque areas analyzed from MS autopsies (Giovannoni *et al.*, 1998), as well as in a brain biopsy performed 33 days after onset of disseminated symptoms of fulminant MS (Bitsch *et al.*, 1999). In chronic active MS lesions, increased iNOS and nitrotyrosine expression can be detected in phagocytic macrophages at the active lesion edge, in and around perivascular lesions, and in periventricular ependymal cells (Hill *et al.*, 2004). Labeling with iNOS decreases as lesions age and become less active (Liu *et al.*, 2001). A study of brain biopsies from two acute cases of MS detected signal for iNOS in both reactive astrocytes and perivascular monocytes/macrophages, whereas no signal was found in chronic inactive MS lesions (Oleszak *et al.*, 1998). These observations support a potential role for iNOS in the initiation of MS lesions.

Cytotoxicity

MHC I molecules are not constitutively expressed in the CNS (Neumann *et al.*, 2002). However, their up-regulation in MS lesions, coupled with the close apposition of MHC I-restricted CD8+ T cells with cellular CNS targets strongly support a role for cytotoxic injury in MS. Furthermore, the number of cytotoxic CD8+ T cells outnumbers CD4+ T cells almost 10-fold in MS lesions (Booss *et al.*, 1983; Gay *et al.*, 1997). Interferon-γ, which is produced by macrophages in MS lesions, induces increased MHC I expression in vitro (Neumann *et al.*, 2002). Cell culture studies demonstrate that oligodendrocytes are highly susceptible to attack by perforin, liberated by CD8+ T cells, suggesting that oligodendrocytes are vulnerable to lysis and injury by this pore-forming T cell effector mechanism (Scolding *et al.*, 1990). There is an association between the number of gadolinium-enhancing brain lesions and perforin mRNA-expressing mononuclear cells in the CSF of MS patients, further supporting a role for perforin in MS pathogenesis

(Kivisakk *et al.*, 1999). Furthermore, granzyme-expressing CD8+ T cells are found in close contact with degenerating oligodendrocytes in acute MS lesions (Neumann *et al.*, 2002). CD8+ T cells can selectively transect neurites (Medana *et al.*, 2001; Neumann *et al.*, 2002) and destroy neurons by antigen-independent mechanisms (Nitsch *et al.*, 2004), possibly involving death receptors of the tumor necrosis factor family (Aktas *et al.*, 2005). Such death receptors are also expressed in actively demyelinating MS lesions, although their cellular location is still controversial (Dowling *et al.*, 1996; D'Souza *et al.*, 1996; Bonetti *et al.*, 1997). The extent of acute axonal injury in MS lesions is also associated with the density of CD8+ T cells within the lesions (Bitsch *et al.*, 2000). Within active MS lesions, granzyme B-expressing T cells are frequently found in close contact with injured axons. Confocal microscopy demonstrated that granzyme B cytotoxic granules are polarized toward the injured axon, suggesting direct cytotoxic injury (Neumann *et al.*, 2002). However, the number of granzyme B-positive CD8+ T cells diminishes with disease chronicity; therefore, it is uncertain as to what degree cytotoxicity contributes to tissue injury during later disease phases.

Hypoxia

Disturbances in microcirculation and excess liberation of inflammatory mediators such as reactive oxygen species (ROS) and NO can impair mitochondrial function, and result in a state of histiotoxic hypoxia (Abdoul-Enein *et al.*, 2005). Hypoxic brain damage often leads to the destruction of glial cells and neurons in the lesions. However, tissue preconditioning is often associated with hypoxia, and refers to a state in which temporary protection of adjacent tissue leads to increased tissue resistance to a subsequent hypoxic insult (Sharp *et al.*, 2004). This resistance is thought to occur as a result of the up-regulation of specific transcription factors, including hypoxia-inducible factors, HIF-1 alpha and HIF-1 beta, which induce gene expression of downstream molecules involved in neuroprotection, vasomotor control, angiogenesis, cell growth, and energy metabolism (Sharp *et al.*, 2004). Sublethal hypoxia at the border of a stroke lesion also induces the expression of stress proteins, especially heat shock protein (hsp) 70, a molecular chaperone that helps to refold damaged proteins and contributes to tissue protection (Vass *et al.*, 1988; Christians *et al.*, 2002).

The expression of these survival and stress proteins is not restricted to hypoxic or ischemic lesions. The expression of HIF can be induced or augmented by either pro- or anti-inflammatory cytokines, and denatured proteins in injured tissue induce expression of hsps. All these proteins are expressed at the border between active inflammatory lesions and the adjacent normal tissue. While *hsp70* is found at the edges of all inflammatory lesions in the CNS, the expression of HIF-1α is restricted to lesions which follow hypoxia-like tissue injury (Abdoul-Enein *et al.*, 2003). In a systematic study of over 80 cases of inflammatory and demyelinating CNS white matter diseases and 20 controls, HIF-1α expression was significantly associated with pattern III MS lesions, various viral encephalitides, metabolic encephalopathy and acute stroke lesions characterized by a preferential loss of MAG, and a distal oligodendrogliopathy with apoptotic oligodendrocyte cell death. The similar patterns of tissue injury and HIF-1α expression shared between these viral, demyelinating, and ischemic disorders suggests a shared pathogenic relationship related to energy failure.

Hypoxia-mediated tissue injury and tissue preconditioning are considered important mechanisms contributing to the pathogenesis of Balo's concentric sclerosis (BCS) (Stadelmann *et al.*, 2005). Both BCS and a subgroup of MS lesions display alternating layers of demyelination and myelin preservation (Lucchinetti *et al.*, 2000). The concentric pattern of demyelination in BCS is associated with pathological evidence of tissue preconditioning (Stadelmann *et al.*, 2005). Additional evidence for histiotoxic hypoxia in MS was described in a study comparing chemokine profiles in MS subtypes and infarcted tissue. Both MS pattern III lesions and acute infarcts are characterized by MAG loss and oligodendrocyte apoptosis, and share similar expression profiles for CCR1 and CCR5, further supporting a possible role for hypoxia-mediated tissue injury in a subset of MS lesions (Mahad *et al.*, 2004).

Excitotoxicity

Glutamate, the primary excitatory neurotransmitter in the CNS, is synthesized by all CNS cells as a key metabolite in the citric acid cycle. The BBB has a very low permeability to glutamate and essentially all glutamate is synthesized de novo in the brain (Nedergaard *et al.*, 2002). Glutamate is produced in high concentrations in neurons, packed into vesicles, and transported along the axon where it is stored in synaptic vesicles until release. This glutamate release is the major extracellular source in the normal brain. The low glutamate concentration in oligodendrocytes

and astrocytes, as well as the strategic location of astrocytes, makes the astrocyte the crucial cell in keeping glutamate levels low at the neuronal–glial synapse via enzymatic degradation of glutamate to glutamine (Nedergaard *et al.*, 2002). Recent data suggest that in the gray matter, astrocytes play a major role in glutamate uptake, whereas in the white matter, oligodendrocytes are primarily involved (Werner *et al.*, 2001; Pitt *et al.*, 2003). In addition to glutamate uptake and degradation, astrocytes release glutamate in response to molecules such as prostaglandin E2, ATP and bradykinin. This release is calcium-dependent and operates at physiological levels of intracellular calcium (Bezzi *et al.*, 1998, 2001). Excess levels of glutamate are found in MS lesions and occur when pro-inflammatory cytokines stimulate glutamate synthesis in macrophages (Werner *et al.*, 2001), or when there is reduced glutamate degradation by impaired astrocytes and oligodendrocytes. Glutamate transporters, EAAT1 and EAAT2, are virtually absent in active MS lesions that are depleted of oligodendrocytes (Pitt *et al.*, 2003), and EAAT2 is down-regulated in the periplaque white matter (PPWM) where oligodendrocytes are still present.

Excess glutamate leads to prolonged neuronal activation which may result in cytoskeletal degradation of axons and neurons via increased production of NOS, ROS, arachidonic acid, phospholipase A2, Ca^{2+} influx, as well as activation of calcium-dependent proteases such as calpain (Matute *et al.*, 2001). Macrophages immunoreactive for the glutamate-producing enzyme, glutaminase, colocalize with dystrophic axons in MS lesions (Werner *et al.*, 2001), suggesting a possible role for glutamate excitoxicity in contributing to axonal damage in MS lesions.

Adhesion molecules

Pro-inflammatory cytokines strongly promote trans-endothelial leukocyte migration by increasing the initial interactions between integrins expressed on leukocytes, and adhesion molecule receptors on vascular endothelial cells (Glabinski and Ransohoff, 1999a, 1999b). Leukocyte migration is further regulated by the concentration gradient of secreted chemokines (Mantovani *et al.*, 2004; Ambrosini *et al.*, 2005), which induce conformational changes in the integrins leading to increased receptor affinity (Luster, 1998), as well as selective recruitment and positioning of leukocytes (Ransohoff *et al.*, 2003).

Increased expression of vascular cell adhesion molecule-1 (VCAM-1), which interacts with the leukocyte integrin molecule α4 (Yednock *et al.*, 1992), is identified on activated endothelial cells in MS lesions (Washington *et al.*, 1994). Antibodies against integrin molecule α4 inhibit receptor binding and prevent the accumulation of leukocytes in CNS tissue in EAE (Yednock *et al.*, 1992). Natalizumab is a humanized IgG4k monoclonal antibody against α4B1 and α4B7 integrins, which are adhesion molecules expressed on the surface of all leukocytes, except neutrophils. It inhibits α4-mediated leukocyte adhesion to VCAM-1 receptor on vascular endothelial cells, and interferes with trafficking of activated T lymphocytes across the BBB (Rice *et al.*, 2005). Natalizumab is an FDA-approved therapeutic agent for the management of relapsing MS, which was initially withdrawn from the market due to its association with progressive multifocal leukoencephalopathy (PML). However, it has since been reintroduced to the market with specific safety, surveillance, and monitoring guidelines.

Metalloproteinases and proteases

Matrix metalloproteinases (MMPs) are proteolytic enzymes important in the remodeling of tissue, as they are capable of degrading basal lamina components, extracellular matrix and myelin proteins. In order to facilitate migration into the CNS, mononuclear inflammatory cells produce and secrete MMPs. The MMPs are found in active MS lesions where they may directly cause axonal transection (Anthony *et al.*, 1997; Linberg *et al.*, 2001). Foamy macrophages and ramified microglia in active MS lesions selectively express MMP-12 (Vos *et al.*, 2003) and MMP-19 (van Horssen *et al.*, 2006). The MMP-12 cleaves a broad spectrum of molecules including elastin, myelin basic protein (MBP), and collagen type IV. Its expression in active MS lesions suggests it could contribute to demyelination, as well as leukocyte migration across the BBB.

Increased levels of MMP-9 are associated with remyelination after lysolecithin-induced demyelination in mice, and are likely involved in the removal of inhibitory extracellular degradation products, such as proteoglycans, as well as facilitating recruitment of oligodendrocyte progenitors (Larsen *et al.*, 2003). The function of MMPs is in part regulated by the production by astrocytes of tissue inhibitors of metalloproteinases (TIMPs). Increased levels of TIMPs may reduce leukocyte trafficking as well as MMP production in macrophages (Crocker *et al.*, 2006).

The protease tissue plasminogen activator (tPA), secreted by macrophages, is also reportedly increased in MS and EAE, and induces neuronal apoptosis in vitro (Cuzner *et al.*, 1996; Flavin *et al.*, 1997, 2000; Lu *et al.*, 2002). Knockout mice deficient in tPA demonstrate delayed demyelination and axonal degeneration after EAE induction (Lu *et al.*, 2002). Therefore, proteases could contribute to axonal damage in MS.

Heterogeneity in MS pathology

Multiple sclerosis is a heterogeneous disorder with respect to its clinical, genetic, radiographic, and pathological features. Furthermore, as described above, multiple inflammatory effector mechanisms can potentially result in demyelination and tissue damage in MS. This could, in part, account for the variability in treatment response often observed among MS patients. Heterogeneity with respect to the character and extent of the inflammatory response, the pattern of demyelination, the nature of oligodendrocyte pathology, the extent of remyelination, and the degree of axonal injury and/or loss present in MS lesions is well recognized, and was initially thought to reflect the variable intensity of the inciting pathologic process. However, despite the pathologic heterogeneity found in MS lesions, there is a surprising degree of homogeneity with respect to many of these pathologic features within a single individual, when matched for demyelinating activity (Ozawa *et al.*, 1994; Brueck *et al.*, 1994; Lucchinetti *et al.*, 1999, 2000).

Although pathological studies reveal that the immune factors associated with diverse mechanisms of demyelination and tissue injury can be found in active MS lesions, whether there is a dominant immune effector pathway of lesion formation, or alternatively, whether multiple immune effector pathways occur in parallel or sequentially within a given patient, is a matter of debate. Prior MS immunopathological studies were largely based on few cases in which the staging of lesions was often inadequate, and the interpretation of the findings was in part biased by immunological concepts derived from EAE studies (Lassman, 2005). Over the last decade, the systematic analysis of MS lesions has provided novel insights into the immunopathogenesis of the disease. Detailed immunopathological studies have revealed a profound heterogeneity in the patterns of demyelination and tissue injury observed between different active MS lesions and, in particular, between active lesions from different patients, suggesting the pathogenesis of the disease could differ among patient subgroups

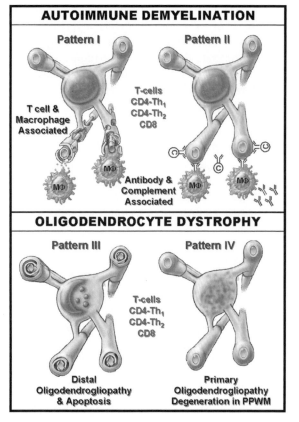

AUTOIMMUNE DEMYELINATION

Pattern I — T cell & Macrophage Associated

Pattern II — T-cells CD4-Th₁ CD4-Th₂ CD8 — Antibody & Complement Associated

OLIGODENDROCYTE DYSTROPHY

Pattern III — Distal Oligodendrogliopathy & Apoptosis

Pattern IV — T-cells CD4-Th₁ CD4-Th₂ CD8 — Primary Oligodendrogliopathy Degeneration in PPWM

Figure 5.1 MS immunopathologic patterns. Active Pattern I and II lesions are mainly associated with T cell and macrophage inflammation, suggesting that demyelination and tissue injury could be mediated by toxic products secreted from activated mononuclear cells. Active Pattern II lesions additionally demonstrate deposition of antibodies and complement. Active Pattern III lesions demonstrate ill-defined macrophage borders, oligodendrocyte apoptosis and early loss of MAG, which is located in the most distal oligodendrocyte processes. Active Pattern IV lesions are associated with activated mononuclear cells, near complete loss of oligodendrocytes in the lesion and profound non-apoptotic nuclear fragmentation of oligodendrocytes in the PPWM, suggesting a primary oligodendropathy. (Reprinted with permission from Lucchinetti *et al.*, 2005).

(Figure 5.1). It is therefore conceivable that immuno-pathogenic heterogeneity underlies the variable treatment response observed between MS patients.

Immunopathologic classification of active MS lesions

Investigations on immunopathogenic mechanisms involved in MS lesion formation must rely on a precise neuropathological definition of demyelinating activity. A variety of criteria for staging demyelinating activity in MS lesions have been proposed based on the density and activation states of lymphocytes and macrophages, the presence of MCH class II antigens, as well as the pattern of adhesion molecule or cytokine expression within the lesion. However, these approaches do not distinguish demyelinating activity from inflammatory activity, the latter of which could be present in the lesion in the absence of ongoing active demyelination. Bruck *et al.* (1995) proposed a staging scheme for demyelinating activity based on the composition and sequence of myelin degradation within macrophage lysozymes, in correlation with the expression of macrophage differentiation markers. Early active MS lesions contain macrophages expressing myeloid related protein (MRP14), a member of the S100 family of calcium-binding proteins, and 27E10, both distinct markers of macrophage activation and differentiation. Early active MS lesions also contain myelin degradation products immunoreactive for myelin oligodendrocyte glycoprotein (MOG) and myelin associated glycoprotein (MAG). These minor myelin proteins disappear within several days, whereas myelin debris immunoreactive for the major myelin proteins, myelin basic protein (MBP) and proteolipid protein (PLP), persist in the macrophages of a late active lesion for 1–2 weeks. Inactive areas no longer contain any minor or major myelin proteins, although PAS+ macrophages can still be present. Early remyelinating lesions are characterized by clusters of short, thin, irregularly organized myelin sheaths with greater MAG or CNPase reactivity relative to MOG or PLP. Macrophages positive for PAS can be present.

Using this staging scheme in order to identify actively demyelinating lesions, immunopathological analysis of a large number of active MS lesions suggested that the immune effector mechanisms resulting in demyelination and tissue injury can differ between MS patient subgroups (Lucchinetti *et al.*, 2000). Active MS lesions were classified into four different patterns based on plaque geography, myelin protein expression, pattern of oligodendrocyte pathology, and presence of immunoglobulin (Ig) deposition or complement activation (Figure 5.2). All active MS lesions were associated with a variable extent of T cell and macrophage infiltration; however, they were further classified into one of four patterns as follows. Pattern I: active lesions associated with T cells and macrophages; Pattern II: active lesions associated with deposition of immunoglobulin and complement activation products at sites of myelin breakdown (Figure 5.2A–F); Pattern III: active lesions associated with apoptotic

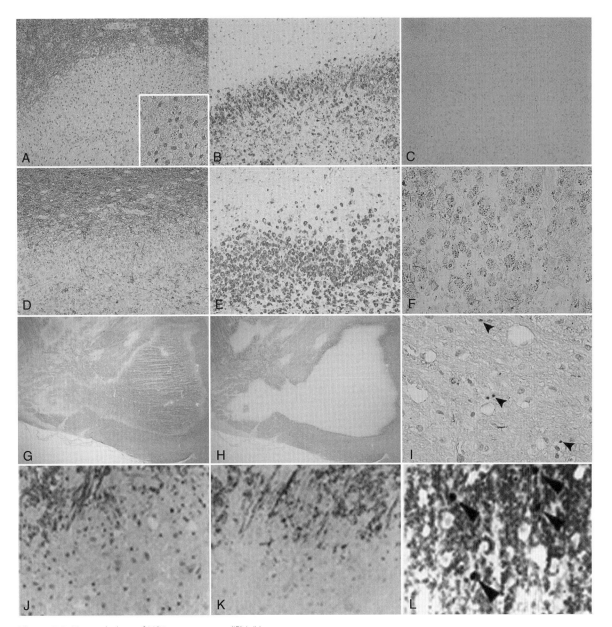

Figure 5.2 Histopathology of MS immunopattern (IP) I–IV.

A–C: **IP I**. A: A perivenous confluent active demyelinating lesion. Macrophages contain myelin debris within their cytoplasm (inset). B: Macrophages accumulate in a sharp rim at the lesion border. C: Complement deposition is absent.

D–F: **IP II**. D: A perivenous confluent active demyelinating lesion. Clustering of oligodendrocytes and labeling of delicate oligodendrocyte processes is suggestive of concurrent ongoing remyelination. E: Macrophages accumulate in a sharp rim at the lesion border. F: Macrophages contain complement positive myelin debris within their cytoplasm.

G–I: **IP III**. G: MOG overexpression within active MS lesion compared to adjacent NAWM. H: A striking loss of MAG is demonstrated within the lesion corresponding to the region of MOG overexpression.

I: Condensed oligodendrocyte nuclei suggestive of apoptosis (arrowheads). Note residual MAG immunoreactivity in the oligodendrocyte process at upper left corner.

J–L: **IP IV**. J/K: Distribution of myelin antigens MOG (J) and MAG (K) is similar in the lesions. L: DNA fragmentation of oligodendrocytes is seen in the periplaque white matter (double staining of *in-situ* tailing [DNA fragmentation] and CNPase [myelin and oligodendrocytes]. (J–L: Reprinted with permission from Lucchinetti *et al.*, 2000.)

oligodendrocytes, and a preferential loss of MAG and CNPase (Figure 5.2G–I); and Pattern IV: extensive oligodendrocyte degeneration in the periplaque white matter adjacent to the active lesion (Figure 5.2J–L). Pattern I and II lesions were characterized by sharp macrophage-rich plaque borders (Figure 5.2B,E) demarcating the plaque from the adjacent PPWM, and lesions were centered on blood vessels. Pattern III lesions demonstrated ill-defined plaque borders, and were often associated with myelin-sparing around blood vessels. Oligodendrocyte survival and remyelination was more extensive in Patterns I and II (Figure 5.2D), compared to Patterns III and IV.

The frequency of immunopathological patterns in 286 demyelinating disease cases (238 biopsies; 48 autopsies) analyzed to date revealed that Pattern II pathology was the most frequent, occurring in 58% of the cases, followed in decreasing frequency by Patterns III (26%), I (15%), and IV (1%) (Lucchinetti et al., 2004). Immunopathological patterns were identical in all the active MS lesions from a given patient, but differed between patients, suggesting that the pathogenesis of the disease may differ among patient subgroups.

Similarities between MS pathological patterns and MS animal models

Although the specific effector mechanism resulting in each immunopathological pattern remains speculative, there are similarities between each of these patterns and existing experimental models of MS. Pattern I (T cell–macrophage-associated demyelination) closely resembles myelin destruction in some mouse models of EAE in which toxic products of activated macrophages, such as TNF-α, and NO, can mediate destruction of myelin sheaths. Lesions similar to Pattern II (antibody/complement-associated demyelination) are found in models of EAE, induced by cooperation between encephalitogenic T cells and demyelinating anti-MOG antibodies. Although Pattern II lesions suggest that antibody (Ab)- and complement-mediated mechanisms may contribute to demyelination and tissue injury, definite proof is still lacking. Pattern III lesions suggest a pathological process at the level of the oligodendrocyte cell body. Both MAG and CNPase are localized to the most distal extension of the oligodendrocyte cell body – the periaxonal region. Their preferential loss preceding that of one of the major myelin proteins (MBP, PLP) possibly reflects the inability of the cell body to support the metabolic demands necessary to maintain the distal axon, resulting in a distal dying-back oligodendrogliopathy. Ultrastructurally, this pattern is characterized by alterations in the distal-most extensions of the oligodendroglial processes, the periaxonal region, with a uniform widening of inner myelin lamellae and degeneration of inner glial loops antedating destruction of the myelin sheaths. These pathological alterations have been described in certain experimental models of toxin- and viral-induced demyelination (Ludwin, 1981; Rodriguez, 1985), as well as in several stereotactic brain biopsies obtained for diagnosis in cases of early MS (Rodriguez and Scheithauer, 1994). Loss of MAG is also observed in acute white matter ischemia (Abdoul-Enein et al., 2003). Extensive oligodendrocyte damage resembling Pattern IV lesions has been described in ciliary neurotrophic factor (CNTF)-deficient animals with EAE (Linker et al., 2002).

Despite some similarities between these four MS immunopathological patterns and specific MS animal models, the reason for this complex pathology is unknown. It is possible that pathological heterogeneity reflects the involvement of different genetic factors influencing immune-mediated inflammation, as well as glial, axonal, and neuronal survival.

Is pathological heterogeneity stage- or patient-dependent?

A recent study has proposed that pathological heterogeneity observed in MS lesions reflects the stage of the disease, involving multiple sequential mechanisms operating within a given patient, thus disputing the concept of interindividual pathologic heterogeneity (Barnett and Prineas, 2004). The authors observed extensive oligodendrocyte apoptosis in the absence of inflammation or active demyelination in a brainstem lesion derived from a pediatric MS patient who died 9 months after disease onset, and 17 h after presentation with acute pulmonary edema. On the basis of this case, and 12 other cases which reportedly demonstrated similar pathological findings, the authors proposed that a primary injury to the oligodendrocyte represents the initial lesion in all relapsing–remitting MS (RRMS) patients. The basis for the oligodendrocyte apoptosis was not defined in this study, but could reflect a primary cell injury. This study raised the question as to whether inflammation is a prerequisite in MS pathogenesis and rejected the traditional belief that MS is an autoimmune disease (Barnett and

Prineas, 2004). Furthermore, the presence of additional lesions demonstrating complement activation and remyelination was interpreted as evidence of an overlap of pathological features within a given patient, thus challenging the hypothesis of MS immunopathogenic heterogeneity. However, myelin pallor and widespread oligodendrocyte apoptosis can also be seen in hypoxic and ischemic brain insults, and the index patient described in the study of Barnett and Prineas (2004) died in the setting of pulmonary edema likely associated with hypoxia. It therefore remains to be confirmed whether these apoptotic lesions represent pre-MS lesions, or alternatively represent another superimposed pathological process.

Clinical and therapeutic implications of heterogeneous MS pathology

Immunopathological MS studies focusing on pathogenesis require the analysis of lesions demonstrating ongoing early active demyelination, and as such are mainly based on cases that either died during a fulminant course of the disease, or were obtained from patients requiring brain biopsy during initial clinical presentation, when the diagnosis was still in question. Clinical and radiographic follow-up studies confirm that the majority of biopsied patients subsequently develop a clinical course and disability profile typical of multiple sclerosis, and resemble an MS population-based non-biopsied cohort (Pittock et al., 2005).

To date, correlations with clinical course reveal that Pattern IV has been seen exclusively in three patients with primary progressive MS (PPMS); however, Patterns I, II and III do not correlate with a specific clinical course (RR, SP, PP), or early disability. However, longer clinical follow-up is needed to determine whether immunopathological patterns differentially affect long-term clinical course and disability.

Despite the apparent lack of correlation between immunopathological patterns and prototypic MS clinical course in early MS, a striking correlation between therapeutic response to plasma exchange (PLEX) administered for steroid-unresponsive fulminant MS attacks and immunopathological pattern has been reported. Only Pattern II MS patients with lesions characterized by antibody and complement deposition responded to PLEX, in contrast to no response observed in either Pattern I or III patients (Keegan et al., 2005).

Since the mechanisms of MS lesion formation in chronic active plaques in late phases of the disease are not well understood, it is unknown how long these four immunopathological patterns persist into disease chronicity. Slowly expanding rims of low-grade active demyelination with microglial activation and limited inflammation have been described in MS during secondary progressive disease phases (Prineas et al., 2001); however, these lesions lack the degree of macrophage infiltration and active demyelination that characterize early, more acute MS lesions. It could be that once the highly active demyelinating phase of the disease subsides, a shared mechanism underlies disease progression common to all four pathological patterns. Studies to address the impact of these different pathological subtypes on long-term clinical and radiographic progression are ongoing.

The concept of immunopathogenic heterogeneity in MS could be important for future studies focusing on the etiology and therapy of the disease; however, the potential to apply these findings to MS patients requires the development of technologies that allow the stratification of MS pathologic subtypes without being dependent on brain biopsies. Studies to identify immunopathological pattern-specific clinical and paraclinical surrogate markers are ongoing.

Pathological heterogeneity in other CNS inflammatory demyelinating disorders

Neuromyelitis optica (NMO)

Neuromyelitis optica is an inflammatory, often relapsing, demyelinating disease, preferentially affecting the optic nerves and spinal cord. Acute spinal cord involvement is characterized by diffuse swelling and softening typically extending over multiple (>3) intervertebral segments, and occasionally involving the entire spinal cord in either a patchy or continuous distribution. Active NMO lesions are characterized by myelin loss associated with extensive macrophage infiltration, numerous eosinophils and granulocytes, and variable T cell inflammation (Lucchinetti et al., 2002). Axonal injury is prominent, often associated with necrosis involving both spinal cord gray and white matter. Chronic lesions are characterized by gliosis, cystic degeneration, cavitation, and atrophy of the spinal cord and optic nerves. The number and prominence of blood vessels with thickened and hyalinized walls is increased in NMO lesions (Mandler et al., 1993; Lucchinetti et al., 2002).

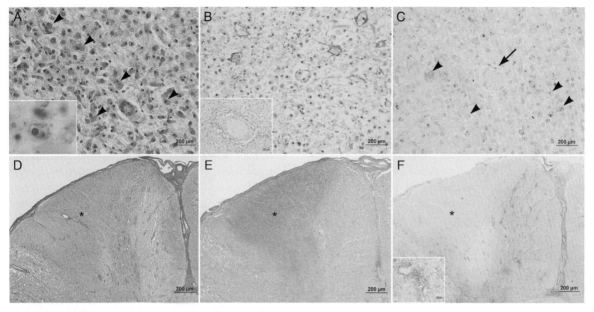

Figure 5.3 Histopathologic difference between MS IP II and NMO lesions.

A–C. **Active MS IP II lesion**. A: Macrophages contain myelin debris within their cytoplasm (arrowheads and inset). B: AQP4 expression is up-regulated on the surface of reactive astrocytes and in rosette pattern on penetrating blood vessel in the MS lesion. C: Macrophages contain complement positive myelin debris within their cytoplasm (arrowheads), but complement deposition is absent around blood vessels (arrow).

D–F. **Active NMO lesion**. D: Extensive demyelination involving both gray and white matter; asterisk indicates preserved myelin in the PPWM. E: AQP4 expression is lost in the NMO lesion but retained in the PPWM (*) and gray matter. F: Complement is deposited in a characteristic vasculocentric rim and rosette pattern within the active lesion, whereas, this is not detected in the PPWM (*). (Reprinted with permission from Roemer *et al.*, 2007.)

The pathogenic relationship between MS and NMO is uncertain; however, immunopathological studies suggest the effector mechanisms involved in NMO and MS are different. Unlike MS, NMO lesions are characterized by vasculocentric deposits of immunoglobulins and complement surrounding thickened hyalinized blood vessels, in a characteristic rim and rosette pattern (Lucchinetti *et al.*, 2002). Although Pattern II MS lesions also demonstrate immune complex deposition, it is present on degenerating myelin sheaths and within macrophages, but never in the perivascular rim–rosette pattern observed in NMO (Figure 5.3C), (Lucchinetti *et al.*, 2000; Roemer *et al.*, 2007). The rim–rosette vasculocentric pattern of immune complex deposition observed in NMO lesions (Figure 5.3F) suggests a role for humoral immunity targeting an antigen in the perivascular space, rather than reflecting an injury targeting myelin and/or oligodendrocytes, as described in MS (Lucchinetti *et al.*, 2002).

Further evidence that NMO and MS could be distinct pathogenic entities is supported by the recent discovery of a specific serum autoantibody biomarker, NMO-IgG, which distinguishes NMO from MS

(Lennon *et al.*, 2004). Binding at or near the BBB, NMO-IgG outlines CNS microvessels, pia, subpia and the Virchow–Robin spaces. The staining pattern of patients' serum IgG binding to mouse spinal cord is remarkably similar to the vasculocentric pathologic pattern of immunoglobulin and complement deposition seen in NMO lesions. Sensitivity and specificity for this autoantibody are 73% (95% CI=60–86%) and 91% (95%CI=79–100%), respectively, for NMO in North American patients, and 58% (95% CI=30–86%) and 100%, respectively, for optic–spinal multiple sclerosis in Japanese patients (Lennon *et al.*, 2004).

The NMO-IgG binds selectively to the mercurial-insensitive water channel protein aquaporin-4 (AQP4), which is concentrated in astrocytic foot processes at the BBB (Lennon *et al.*, 2005). The AQP4 is the predominant water channel in the brain, and is also expressed to a limited extent in stomach, kidney, lung, skeletal muscle and the inner ear (Amiry-Moghaddam *et al.*, 2003). The AQP4 has an important role in brain water homeostasis and, consistent with its location in the CNS, is involved in the development, function and integrity of the interface between the brain and blood and brain and cerebrospinal fluid

(Jung *et al.*, 1994). In contrast to MS lesions, which exhibit stage-dependent loss of AQP4, all NMO lesions demonstrate a striking loss of AQP4, regardless of the stage of demyelinating activity, extent of tissue necrosis, or site of CNS involvement (Roemer *et al.*, 2007). These data strongly suggest a pathogenic role for a complement-activating AQP4-specific autoantibody as the initiator of the NMO lesion, and further distinguish NMO from MS. A direct antibody-mediated injury against this astrocytic protein would be expected to disrupt essential homeostatic functions, including regulation of water flux, ions, and neurotransmitter levels, ultimately resulting in irreversible tissue damage.

Balo's concentric sclerosis

Balo's concentric sclerosis (BCS) shares some similarities with MS Pattern III lesions, and can be considered a hypoxic variant of CNS inflammatory demyelinating disease (Stadelman *et al.*, 2005). Pathological features consist of concentric alternating rims of demyelination and myelin preservation resembling the pattern of rings in a tree trunk (Figure 5.4). All actively demyelinating concentric lesions followed a pattern of demyelination suggesting hypoxia-like tissue injury, and were associated with high expression of iNOS in macrophages and microglia. Proteins involved in tissue preconditioning such as hsp70, HIF-1α and D-110, were up-regulated at the edge of actively demyelinating BCS lesions, as well as in the outermost myelinated layers of the concentric lesion. These results suggest that preconditioned oligodendrocytes may be resistant to further damage at the edge of radially expanding lesions, leading to the concentric preservation of myelin found in BCS (Stadelmann *et al.*, 2005).

Remyelination in MS

Recent studies demonstrate that extensive remyelination can be present both in acute (Lucchinetti *et al.*, 1999) and chronic MS lesions (Patrikios *et al.*, 2006) (Figure 5.5). Early in MS, remyelination can be extensive, and can occur simultaneously with demyelination (Figure 5.5A). During the early stage of remyelination, inflammation associated with macrophage infiltration can be prominent within the lesion (Figure 5.5B). The extent of remyelination at these early stages appears to depend on the availability of oligodendrocytes or their progenitor cells in the lesion. However, the remyelinating capacity varies among MS cases. This can range

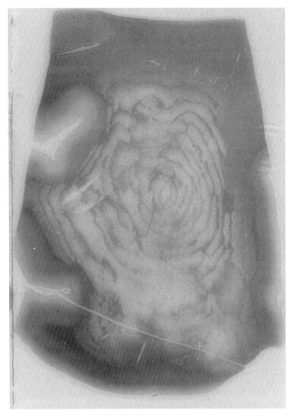

Figure 5.4 Balo's concentric sclerosis. Balo lesions are pathologically characterized by the concentric alternating layers of demyelination and myelin preservation reminiscent of a tree-trunk. (Courtesy of Professor Hans Lassmann).

from densities similar to or increased relative to the PPWM, to a near complete loss of oligodendrocytes (Lucchinetti *et al.*, 1999). Furthermore, some lesions demonstrate a variable oligodendrocyte loss in expanding actively demyelinating areas followed by their reappearance within the inactive plaque center, suggestive of recruitment of progenitor cells. However, other lesions demonstrate a gradual and progressive loss of oligodendrocytes in the course of lesion maturation, while in others, massive loss of oligodendrocytes occurs in the absence of any recruitment of progenitor cells. Although there is profound heterogeneity of oligodendrocyte damage between patients, lesions from a single individual exactly matched for stage of demyelinating activity show very similar oligodendrocyte densities. The profound heterogeneity in extent and topography of oligodendrocyte destruction in active demyelinating lesions suggests that myelin, mature oligodendrocytes and possibly oligodendrocyte progenitors are differentially

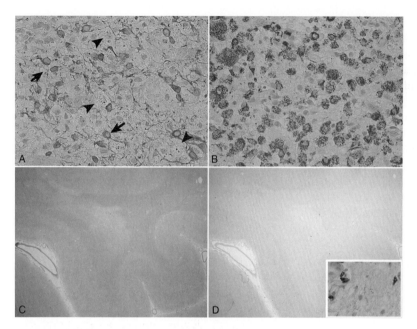

Figure 5.5 Remyelination in MS.
A,B. **Early active MS**. A: Clusters of oligodendrocytes that express minor myelin protein within their cytoplasm and processes (arrows) indicate ongoing remyelination. B: Macrophages contain myelin debris within their cytoplasm (arrowheads) indicative of concurrent demyelination. Numerous foamy macrophages are identified in the lesion.
C,D: **Chronic MS**. C: Myelin stain demonstrates an almost fully remyelinated lesion. D: Foamy macrophages are absent and ramified microglial cells are only identified at high magnification (inset).

affected in subsets of MS patients. Different mechanisms of myelin and/or oligodendrocyte injury can be operating in an individual MS patient, and could thereby influence the likelihood of effective remyelination in the early MS lesion.

The factors that influence the extent of remyelination could differ after several years' disease duration and in patients with chronic progressive disease, where mature oligodendrocyte numbers within the plaques are in general very low, and remyelination is generally less extensive. When present, remyelination in chronic MS lesions is often restricted to the plaque edge, or may extend throughout the lesion and form a shadow plaque representing a completely remyelinated lesion (Figure 5.5C). These late remyelinating lesions usually contain few macrophages (Figure 5.5D), and are typically associated with profound fibrillary gliosis. The inflammatory response can therefore provide a key stimulus promoting endogenous remyelination in early active MS lesions.

In vitro and in vivo data also demonstrate that inflammation can play an important role in promoting remyelination (Diemel *et al.*, 1998; Moalem *et al.*, 1999, 2000; Kotter *et al.*, 2001). The abundance of inflammation in inactive cases, together with observations demonstrating the local production of neurotrophic factors such as brain-derived neurotrophic factor (BDNF) by leukocytes, further support a potentially important role for inflammation in the repair of MS lesions (Kerschensteiner *et al.*, 1999).

Neurotrophin receptors are also expressed on glial cells and neurons in or near actively demyelinating MS lesions (Stadelmann *et al.*, 2002). Although transplanted oligodendrocyte progenitor cells (OPCs) can migrate to OPC-depleted areas of chronic demyelination, remyelination is dramatically enhanced only when the environment is made conducive to OPC expansion and differentiation (Franklin *et al.*, 2002). This is achieved by inducing acute inflammation, and thereby supports a clear relationship between acute inflammation and successful remyelination (Foote and Blakemore, 2005). Taken together, these observations raise the possibility that anti-inflammatory therapies might paradoxically contribute to the failure of remyelination during later progressive phases of the disease.

The presence of cells in very early stages of oligodendrocyte development identified in completely demyelinated plaques devoid of mature oligodendrocytes, as well as in chronic lesions devoid of remyelination (Wolswijk *et al.*, 1998), suggests that the failure of remyelination during these later disease phases is not due to a lack of oligodendrocyte progenitors, as is the case in early remyelinating MS lesions, but rather the lesion microenvironment may not be receptive to remyelination signals (Chang *et al.*, 2002). Whether this is due to an imbalance of growth factors, an abnormal composition of axons, impaired axon–oligodendrocyte interaction or glial scarring is uncertain. Mild astrogliosis is essential for maintaining tissue integrity in response to inflammation; however, when this results in a glial scar that is impermeable to chemical signals, remyelination could be inhibited (Blakemore et al., 2003; Holley et al., 2003).

A recent study demonstrated that there is significant interindividual heterogeneity in the extent of remyelination present in chronic MS cases (Patrikios et al., 2006). When the analysis was restricted to patients with large hemispheric or bi-hemispheric sections, patients segregated into two groups characterized either by extensive or low remyelinating capacity. This diverse capacity to form shadow plaques did not correlate with clinical subtype, age of disease onset or gender. Shadow plaques were not restricted to patients with early and relapsing MS, but were particularly prominent in patients with longstanding chronic disease, who died at an old age.

It is plausible that genetic factors could contribute to the variable extent of remyelination observed among MS patients. Recent studies on the Theiler's murine encephalomyelitis virus (TMEV) MS model demonstrate that hereditary factors exert a role upon remyelinating capacity following inflammatory demyelination. Crossing mice strains that lack spontaneous remyelination with strains that demonstrate extensive remyelination, leads to an inherited, dominant "reparative phenotype" (Bieber et al., 2005). Whether the extent of remyelination depends upon the genetic background in MS patients has yet to be determined.

The variable and patient-dependent extent of remyelination observed in MS needs to be considered in the design of future clinical trials aimed to promote CNS repair in MS. Human natural IgM antibodies have been shown to stimulate remyelination in TMEV-infected mice, an animal model of MS. Although the mechanisms responsible for promoting remyelination are unknown, a direct effect of the antibodies on oligodendrocytes could be involved. In addition, these naturally occurring antibodies could act indirectly by enhancing the clearance of myelin debris, altering cytokine expression, or inhibiting B cell differentiation, thereby optimizing the microenvironment for spontaneous remyelination to ensue (Warrington et al., 2000).

Axonal pathology in MS

Irreversible disability in MS patients cannot be explained by demyelination and inflammation alone. Demyelination can be clinically silent (Mew et al.,

1998), and secondary disease progression can occur in the absence of BBB breakdown and new lesion formation detected on MRI, suggesting the absence of overt inflammatory activity (Rovaris et al., 1999, 2006). Pathological MRI comparison studies correlate axonal damage and clinical disability with black holes on T1W images and reduction in N-acetylaspartate to creatine (NAA/Cr) ratio on MR spectroscopy (Bruck et al., 1997; van Walderveen et al., 1998; Bjartmar et al., 2000; Bitsch et al., 2001). However, acute axonal damage and transected axons are present even in the early disease phase and can be detected by the abnormal accumulation of axonally transported proteins, such as the amyloid precursor protein (β-APP) (Ferguson et al., 1997; Trapp et al., 1998; Bitsch et al., 2000). Acute axonal damage is most pronounced in the acute disease phase and decreases over time with diminishing inflammation (Kuhlmann et al., 2002). However, some β-APP positive axons can still be identified in inactive lesions and are thought to reflect a chronic "low-burning" axonal damage (Kornek et al., 2000), which accumulates and may contribute to late axonal degeneration in chronic MS (Kornek et al., 2000; Peterson and Trapp, 2005). Substantial reduction of axon densities ranging from 29 to 82% has been reported in chronic inactive MS lesions (Mew et al., 1998) and in the normal appearing white matter (NAWM) (Lovas et al., 2000).

The cause of axonal damage and loss in MS is unknown, but different mechanisms have been proposed (Figure 5.6). During acute demyelination, denuded axons are highly vulnerable to inflammatory mediators liberated from mononuclear cells. Close apposition of injured axons and macrophages–microglia and CD8+ T cells is identified within MS lesions, suggesting a direct immune attack on axons (Babbe et al., 2000; Kuhlman et al., 2002; Neumann et al., 2002). The macrophages/microglia secrete toxic levels of inflammatory cytokines, glutamate (Werner et al., 2001), proteases (van Horssen et al., 2006), ROS and NO (Hill et al., 2004). Nitric oxide induces a reversible conduction block in demyelinated axons (Redford et al., 1997), which becomes irreversible by repeated NO exposure or high NO concentrations. Irreversible conduction block eventually leads to axonal degeneration (Smith et al., 2001; Hill et al., 2004; Bechtold et al., 2005). The liberated NO impairs mitochondrial function and inhibits the respiratory chain and ATP production. The ubiquitous Na^+/K^+ ATPase serves to maintain intra- and extracellular ion

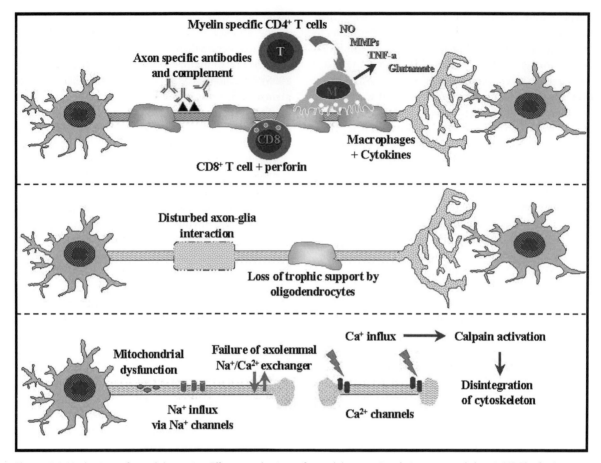

Figure 5.6 Mechanisms of axonal destruction. Effector mechanisms of axonal degeneration during acute and chronic MS. The final pathway of axon destruction is the result of mitochondrial dysfunction, ion influx, and proteolytic degradation. (Reprinted with permission from Lucchinetti *et al.*, 2005.)

levels by pumping Na$^+$ out of and K$^+$ into the cell in an energy-consuming active process driven by dephosphorylation of ATP (Skou, 1998). Inadequate ATP supply thus compromises Na$^+$ extrusion, increasing intra-axonal Na$^+$ levels and extracellular K$^+$, which triggers a reverse operation of the Na+/Ca^{2+} exchanger. This leads to increased intracellular Ca^{2+} levels and activation of Ca^{2+}- dependent proteases which degrade axonal cytoskeletal proteins (Waxman, 2006a, 2006b). Post-mortem micro-array analyses of MS lesions demonstrate a decrease of gene products specific for the mitochondrial electron transport chain, suggesting irreversible axonal damage could be mediated by the combined effect of direct NO toxicity, mitochondrial dysfunction, and energy failure in MS (Dutta *et al.*, 2006).

Abnormal levels of glutamate (Werner *et al.*, 2001) and metabotropic glutamate receptors are associated with damaged demyelinated axons in active MS lesions as well as in the PPWM and NAWM. Furthermore, abnormal glutamate immunoreactivity co-localizing with β-APP and non-phosphorylated axons suggests a potential direct role of glutamate in contributing to axonal damage (Geurts *et al.*, 2003).

Demyelinated axons suffer large current leaks through newly exposed K$^+$ channels and the large capacitance of the naked internodal axolemma. Compensatory redistribution of Na$^+$ channels along demyelinated axons restores conduction and neurologic function (Bostock and Sears, 1978; Foster *et al.*, 1980; Craner *et al.*, 2003a); however, this restoration is inefficient and increases energy demands that could render the axons more vulnerable to degeneration (Stys, 2004). Acute axonal injury leads to a disturbance in the axoplasmic membrane permeability and subsequent energy failure, leading to uncontrolled Na$^+$ influx into the axoplasm through the isoform of the voltage gated Na$^+$ channel Na$_v$1.6, which is the most abundant Na^+ channel at the node of Ranvier in normally myelinated axons. The $Na_v1.6$ contributes to the persistent current that drives the reversal of the Na^+/Ca^{2+} exchanger (NCX) (Craner et al., 2004b) and results in excess intraxonal calcium. This, in turn, activates Ca^{2+}-dependent proteases, which degrade cytoskeletal proteins, further impairing axonal transport. Voltage-gated calcium channels (VGCC) accumulate at sites of disturbed axonal transport, leading to further Ca^{2+} influx, and eventually disintegration of the axonal cytoskeleton (Lassmann, 2003). Co-localization of the NCX and $Na_v1.6$ with β-APP in MS lesions suggests increased expression and redistribution of Na^+ channels along acutely injured axons, implicating a contributory role for these channels in the pathogenesis of axonal degeneration in MS lesions (Craner et al., 2004b).

The cause of diffuse axonal loss in chronic MS that is not directly attributed to inflammation is uncertain, and several mechanisms have been proposed. Repeated demyelination within previously remyelinated lesions could contribute to axonal loss in chronic MS (Prineas, 1993). Chronically demyelinated axons could also degenerate due to the lack of trophic support from myelin and oligodendrocytes (Peterson and Trapp, 2005). Furthermore, anterograde Wallerian degeneration of transected axons could also contribute to diffuse axonal loss (Raff et al., 2002; Coleman, 2005) in the NAWM (Allen and McKeown, 1979; Evangelou et al., 2000). The identification of immunoglobulin and complement at the nodes of Ranvier suggests direct antibody binding to an axolemmal molecule (Hafer-Macko et al., 1996) and complement could also be involved in mediating axonal injury. Interestingly, anti-ganglioside antibodies are significantly higher in MS patients with PPMS compared to SPMS and RRMS (Sadatipour et al., 1998).

Cortical demyelination in MS

Advances in MR imaging and histologic techniques demonstrate that intrinsic NAWM and normal-appearing gray matter (NAGM) abnormalities are present in MS patients, suggesting that MS can result in global CNS tissue damage. Neuropathological studies have classified MS cortical lesions into three major subtypes based on their topographical location within the cortex: (i) subpial, (ii) intracortical, or (iii) compound leukocortical lesions located at the gray–white matter junction (Kidd et al., 1999; Peterson et al., 2001;

Bo et al., 2003a; Wegner et al., 2006; Albert et al., 2007). The degree of inflammation within all three lesion types is reportedly minimal (Bo et al., 2003b; Pomeroy et al., 2005). Whereas ramified microglia predominate in cortically demyelinated lesions, lymphocyte and macrophage infiltration is more extensive in white matter lesions. Quantitative studies suggest that inflammation in the gray matter component of a leukocortical lesion is lower than in the white matter component (Peterson et al., 2001; Bo et al., 2003b; Pomeroy et al., 2005; Albert et al., 2007). Subpial cortical lesions are often associated with meningeal inflammation (Bo et al., 2003b, Kutzelnigg et al., 2005), and the involvement of soluble myelinotoxic factors diffusing from the CSF has been proposed as a putative mechanism in the pathogenesis of the subpial cortical lesion (Bo et al., 2003b; Vercellino et al., 2005; Kutzelnigg et al., 2005).

The extent of cortical demyelination varies in relation to clinical subtypes, and is most prominent in secondary and primary progressive MS (Kutzelnigg et al., 2005; Vercellino et al., 2005), but infrequent and less pronounced in patients with an acute or relapsing course. These studies suggest that cortical demyelination, particularly the subpial type, accumulates with disease duration, and contributes to progressive irreversible disability in MS. The insular, temporobasal, and frontobasal cortex are predominantly involved (Kutzelnigg and Lassmann, 2006). The distribution of cortical plaques affecting the limbic circuit regions engaged in information processing could potentially result in cognitive deficits in MS patients. Furthermore, the extent of cortical demyelination does not appear to correlate with white matter lesion burden, suggesting that cortical demyelination could, in part, develop independently of white matter lesions. These findings might, in part, explain the poor correlation between clinical disability and white matter lesion load observed in progressive MS, as determined by conventional MRI.

Complete cortical demyelination is often associated with "relative" axon preservation (Peterson et al., 2001; Vercellino et al., 2005; Albert et al., 2007). Ubiquitin staining, which is considered indicative of derangement of axonal transport is identified in the periplaque and normal appearing white matter of MS specimens (Giordana et al., 2002), but is absent in demyelinated white matter lesions associated with axonal loss. On the other hand, diffuse ubiquitin staining has been observed with demyelinated gray matter lesions (Vercellino *et al.*, 2005), although a single study observed acute axonal damage and transected neuritis as well as the presence of TUNEL+ apoptotic neurons in these lesions (Peterson *et al.*, 2001). A subsequent study found no difference in synaptic densities in cortical lesions compared to the adjacent NAWM (Vercellino *et al.*, 2005). A quantitative assessment of neuronal density did, however, demonstrate a significant decrease in neurons within the demyelinated cortex compared to the adjacent normal cortex, although very few apoptotic neurons were identified when applying the more specific apoptotic marker caspase-3. These findings are not necessarily mutually exclusive given that apoptotic neurons are generally cleared within 24 h, and immunoreactivity for activated caspase-3 is detectable only for a limited period, whereas neuronal death would accumulate over time (Vercellino *et al.*, 2005). Another study reported a major reduction in synaptophysin within leukocortical lesions, when compared to the adjacent NAWM, as well as to normal control cortex (Wegner *et al.*, 2006). In Alzheimer's disease, a reduction in synaptophysin correlates with the severity of dementia. Although cognitive impairment and psychiatric manifestations are not uncommon among MS patients, dementia is rare. It is possible that variability in synaptophysin density could be a driver of clinical heterogeneity in MS patients.

A trend for an increased GAP-43 to synaptophysin ratio has also been described in leukocortical lesions (Wegner *et al.*, 2006). The GAP-43 is considered a marker of axonal sprouting, and the increased GAP-43/synaptophysin ratio may reflect the up-regulation of local remodeling and cortical reorganization in MS patients. It is uncertain whether this is clinically relevant, but identifying other possible repair mechanisms involved in cortical lesions could have therapeutic relevance. A recent study demonstrated evidence for extensive cortical remyelination, and found that remyelination of cortical lesions was greater than of white matter lesions, within a given patient. These data suggest that the propensity to remyelinate is high in cortical lesions (Albert *et al.*, 2007).

The mechanisms underlying cortical demyelination in MS are largely unknown. Both white matter and gray matter lesions are present in MOG-induced EAE in the common marmoset (Pomeroy *et al.*, 2005; Merkler *et al.*, 2006). The white matter lesions resemble antibody/complement-mediated demyelination described in MS Pattern II lesions (Merkler *et al.*,

2006); however, immunoglobulin and C9neo deposition are absent in subpial lesions. A similar pattern of complement deposition is also observed in MS lesions. Activation of the complete complement cascade is reportedly absent in the cortex, despite its presence in the actively demyelinated regions of adjacent white matter plaques (Schwab and McGeer, 2002; Brink *et al.*, 2005; Merkler *et al.*, 2006). This suggests that complete complement activation is important in a subset of MS white matter lesions but not in gray matter lesions. However, C4d, an activator of the classical, but not the alternative complement pathway, is observed on myelin and oligodendrocytes in small cortical lesions (Schwab and McGeer, 2002; Brink *et al.*, 2005) in a subset of MS cases. Deposition of C4d is associated with neurodegenerative disorders (Rostagno *et al.*, 2002; Yasojima *et al.*, 1999): whether this deposition is stage-dependent in MS gray matter lesion formation or rather represents evidence for ongoing neurodegeneration in a subset of MS patients is uncertain. Further studies examining actively demyelinating cortical lesions are needed in order to better understand the pathogenic mechanisms underlying cortical demyelination in MS. It is uncertain whether the same therapies used to limit white matter demyelination in MS influence gray matter pathology.

Conclusion and therapeutic implications

An improved understanding of the complexity of MS pathogenesis has led to the development of numerous therapeutic strategies aimed at targeting the diverse immune effector mechanisms that potentially contribute to disease activity and irreversible tissue damage in MS (Table 5.1). Some of these treatments are currently available, and others show promise at the experimental level. Although EAE and TMEV are important animal models for studying effector mechanisms in vivo, experimental results cannot always be successfully extrapolated to human disease. Whereas inhibition of IFN-γ and TNF-α ameliorated EAE, subsequent human clinical trials using these approaches resulted in triggering MS exacerbations, and worsening of the disease (Panitch *et al.*, 1987a, 1987b; The Lenercept Multiple Sclerosis Study Group (TNF) 1998).

Although several disease-modifying agents are currently available to treat relapsing MS, including β-interferon, glatiramer acetate, mitoxantrone, and

Table 5.1 Current and future MS therapies targeting potential pathogenic effectors

Effector mechanism	Effector "targets"	Possible therapeutic effect	Examples of current agents and future trials
BBB breakdown	Vascular permeability; mononuclear cell migration	Decreases edema; anti-inflammatory	Corticosteroids (FDA approved); phosphodiesterase-4 inhibitor
Trans-endothelial migration and CNS invasion	Inhibition of proteases and MMP activity	Prevents proteolytic degradation of basal lamina and extracellular components; decreases edema; anti-inflammatory	Minocycline; statins
Adhesion/ migration	Integrin antagonists	Blocks adhesion molecules and trans-endothelial T-cell migration; anti-inflammatory	Antibodies to α-4/β-1, α-4/β-7 integrins; natalizumab (FDA re-approved)
Chemokine system	Chemokine antagonists and receptor blockade	Anti-inflammatory	MCP-1, CXCR3, CCR5 receptor antagonist; CCR1, CCR2 inhibitors
Cytokines	Down-regulation of pro-inflammatory cytokines with cytokine inhibitors or antibodies; alter Th1–Th2 ratio	Anti-inflammatory	IFNs: IFN β-1a, IFN β-1b; IL-1 (anakrin), IL-2 (daclizumab), anti-IL-12p40
Inflammation	General immunosuppression	DNA interference and non-specific cytotoxic effects on inflammatory cells including APCs	Mitoxantrone; methotrexate, cyclophosphamide; azathioprine (FDA-approved)
T-cells (proliferation)	Antibodies against T cells	Immunosuppression, anti-inflammatory	Anti-CD3, anti-CD4, anti-CD52 (campath-1H, alemtuzumab)
Autoimmunity, molecular mimicry, immune response shift	Antigen-specific bystander suppression	MHC class II-restricted T cell binding to administered myelin derivative instead of patients myelin to induce Th1–Th2 shift	Glatiramer acetate (FDA approved)
Auto-antigens	Administration of specific antigens/ MHC molecules	Increasing tolerance to auto-antigens	Oral bovine myelin; synthetic myelin peptides (MBP peptides 82–98, 85–96); solubilized DR2: MBP84–102 complex
T cell autoreactivity	Antibodies against T cell receptors (TCRs); T cell vaccination	Immunity to autoreactive T cells	Antibodies against TCR V-β5.2/5.3; vaccination with TCR peptides (Vβ6 CDR2, BV6S2/6S5, autologous MBP-specific T cells)
B cells	B cell depletion/reduction	Inhibiting B cell proliferation, differentiation and migration; general immunosuppression	Anti-CD20 (rituximab); azathioprine
Pathogenic antibodies	Circulating humoral components	Serum depletion of pathogenic antibodies	Plasmapheresis
Repair-promoting antibodies	Human IgM autoantibody	Therapeutic antibodies promoting remyelination	Human studies planned
Autoimmunity	Fc-mediated tissue injury	Non-specific antibody substitution	Intravenous immunoglobulin
Stem cells	Autologous stem cells	Immune ablation, general immunosuppression	Hematopoietic autologous stem cell transplant

Table 5.1 (cont.)

Effector mechanism	Effector "targets"	Possible therapeutic effect	Examples of current agents and future trials
Free radicals/ nitrate groups	ROS, NOS	Antioxidants, NOS inhibition	Vitamins D, E and selenium; statins
Glutamate excitoxicity	AMPA receptor antagonists	Prevents glutamate-induced ion disturbances, neuroprotection of axons and neurons	Riluzole
Axonal damage	Axonal ion channels	Axon protection by Na^+ and VGCC channel inhibitors	Na^+: flecainide; phenytoin
Neuronal damage	Neurotrophic cytokines	Neuroprotection by modulation of neurotrophic cytokines	Leukemia inhibitory factor, ciliary neurotrophic factor, erythropoietin

natalizumab, their ability to slow disease progression is modest at best (Fox and Ransohoff, 2004; Hohlfeld and Werkele, 2004). Several possible explanations include that (i) the inciting antigen(s) is/are unknown; (ii) the B and T cell receptor (TCR) repertoire of the participating inflammatory cells could be more diverse in MS than in EAE; and (iii) that MS pathogenesis could be heterogeneous (Hohlfeld and Wekerle, 2004). Furthermore, it is important to recognize that MS pathogenesis has both an inflammatory and a degenerative phase. The advent of more sophisticated histological and molecular techniques to study MS pathology has provided new insights into the development and evolution of both focal and global tissue injury in MS. A better understanding of the diverse immune effector mechanisms and targets involved in MS pathogenesis will hopefully lead to more effective therapeutic strategies.

References

Abdoul-Enein F, *et al.* Preferential loss of myelin-associated glycoprotein reflects hypoxia-like white matter damage in stroke and inflammatory brain diseases. *J Neuropathol Exp Neurol* 2003; **62** (1): 25–33.

Abdoul-Enein F, *et al.* [Review] Mitochondrial damage and histotoxic hypoxia: A pathway of tissue injury in inflammatory brain disease? *Acta Neuropathol (Berl)* 2005; **109**(1): 49–55.

Aktas O, *et al.* Neuronal damage in autoimmune neuroinflammation mediated by the death ligand TRAIL. *Neuron* 2005; **46**(3): 421–32.

Albert M, *et al.* Extensive cortical remyelination in patients with chronic multiple sclerosis. *Brain Path Brain Pathol* 2007; **17**(2): 129–38.

Allen IV, McKeown SR. A histological, histochemical and biochemical study of the macroscopically normal white matter in multiple sclerosis. *J Neurol Sci* 1979; **41**(1): 81–91.

Ambrosini E, Aloisi F. Chemokines and glial cells: A complex network in the central nervous system. *Neurochem Res* 2004; **29**: 1017–38.

Amiry-Moghaddam M, *et al.* An alpha-syntrophin-dependent pool of AQP4 in astroglial end-feet confers bidirectional water flow between blood and brain. *Proc Natl Acad Sci USA* 2003; **100**(4): 2106–11.

Anthony DC, *et al.* Differential matrix metalloproteinase expression in cases of MS and stroke. *Neuropath Appl Neurobiol* 1997; **23**: 406–15.

Babbe H, *et al.* Clonal expansions of CD8(+) T cells dominate the T cell infiltrate in active multiple sclerosis lesions as shown by micromanipulation and single cell polymerase chain reaction. *J Exp Med* 2000; **192**(3): 393–404.

Baig S, *et al.* Multiple sclerosis: Cells secreting antibodies against myelin-associated glycoprotein are present in cerebrospinal fluid. *Scand J Immunol* 1991; **33**(1): 73–9.

Balashov KE, *et al.* CCR5(+) and CXCR3(+) T cells are increased in multiple sclerosis and their ligands MIP-1alpha and IP-10 are expressed in demyelinating brain lesions. *Proc Natl Acad Sci USA* 1999; **96**(12): 6873–8.

Barnett MH, Prineas JW. Pathological Heterogeneity in Multiple Sclerosis: A Reflection of Lesion Stage? *Ann Neurol* 2004; **56**(2): 309.

Bechtold DA, Smith KJ. Sodium-mediated axonal degeneration in inflammatory demyelinating disease. *J Neurol Sci* 2005; **233**(1–2): 27–35. Review.

Berger T, *et al.* Antimyelin antibodies as a predictor of clinically definite multiple sclerosis after a first demyelinating event. *N Engl J Med* 2003; **349**(2): 139–45.

Bezzi P, Volterra A. A neuron–glia signaling network in the active brain. *Curr Opin Neurobiol* 2001; **11**(3): 387–94.

Bezzi P, *et al.* Prostaglandins stimulate calcium-dependent glutamate release in astrocytes. *Nature* 1998; **391**(6664): 281–5.

Bjartmar CWJ, Trapp BD. Axonal loss in the pathology of MS: Consequences for understanding the progressive phase of the disease. *J Neurol Sci* 2003; **206**(2): 165–71.

Bieber A, *et al.* Genetically dominant spinal cord repair in a murine model of chronic progressive multiple sclerosis. *J Neuropathol Exp Neurol* 2005; **64**(1): 46–57.

Bitsch A, *et al.* Lesion development in Marburg's type of acute multiple sclerosis: From inflammation to demyelination. *Mult Scler* 1999; **5**: 138–46.

Bitsch A, *et al.* Acute axonal injury in multiple sclerosis. Correlation with demyelination and inflammation. *Brain* 2000; **123** (Pt 6): 1174–83.

Bitsch A, *et al.* A longitudinal MRI study of histopathologically defined hypointense multiple sclerosis lesions. *Ann Neurol* 2001; **49**(6): 793–6.

Blakemore WF, *et al.* The presence of astrocytes in areas of demyelination influences remyelination following transplantation of oligodendrocyte progenitors. *Exp Neurol* 2003; **184** (2): 955–63.

Bo L, *et al.* Induction of nitric oxide synthase in demyelinating regions of multiple sclerosis brains. *Ann Neurol* 1994; **36**(5): 778–86.

Bo L, *et al.* Subpial demyelination in the cerebral cortex of multiple sclerosis patients. *J Neuropathol Exp Neurol* 2003a; **62**(7): 723–32.

Bo L, *et al.* Intracortical multiple sclerosis lesions are not associated with increased lymphocyte infiltration. *Mult Scler* 2003b; **9**(4): 323–31.

Bonetti B, Raine CS. Multiple sclerosis: Oligodendrocytes display cell death-related molecules in situ but do not undergo apoptosis. *Ann Neurol* 1997; **42**(1): 74–84.

Booss J, *et al.* Immunohistological analysis of T lymphocyte subsets in the central nervous system in chronic progressive multiple sclerosis. *J Neurol Sci* 1983; **62**(1–3): 219–32.

Bostock H, Sears T. The internodal axon membrane: Electrical excitability and continuous conduction in segmental demyelination. *J Physiol (Lond)* 1978; **280**: 273–301.

Bourquin C, *et al.* Myelin oligodendrocyte glycoprotein-DNA vaccination induces antibody-mediated autoaggression in experimental autoimmune encephalomyelitis. *Eur J Immunol* 2000; **30**(12): 3663–71.

Boven LA, *et al.* Myelin-laden macrophages are anti-inflammatory, consistent with foam cells in multiple sclerosis. *Brain* 2006; **129**(2): 517–26.

Brink BP, *et al.* The pathology of multiple sclerosis is location-dependent: no significant complement activation is detected in purely cortical lesions. *J Neuropathol Exp Neurol* 2005; **64** (2): 147–55.

Broman T. Blood–brain barrier damage in multiple sclerosis supravital test-observations. *Acta Neurol Scand* 1964; **40**: 21–4.

Brown GC. Nitric oxide inhibition of mitochondrial respiration and its role in cell death. *Free Rad Biol Med* 2002; **33**(11): 1440–50.

Brown GC, *et al.* Interactions between nitric oxide, oxygen, reactive oxygen species and reactive nitrogen species. *Biochem Soc Trans* 2006; **34**(5): 953–6.

Bruck W, *et al.* Monocyte/macrophage differentiation in early multiple sclerosis lesions. *Ann Neurol* 1995; **38**(5): 788–96.

Bruck W, *et al.* Inflammatory central nervous system demyelination: Correlation of magnetic resonance imaging findings with lesion pathology. *Ann Neurol* 1997; **42**(5): 783–93.

Brueck W, *et al.* Oligodendrocytes in the early course of multiple sclerosis. *Ann Neurol* 1994; **35**(1): 65–73.

Burgoon MP, Owens GP. B cells in multiple sclerosis. *Front Biosci* 2004; **9**(3): 786–96.

Chang A, *et al.* Premyelinating oligodendrocytes in chronic lesions of multiple sclerosis. *N Engl J Med* 2002; **346**(3): 165–73.

Christians ES, *et al.* Heat shock factor 1 and heat shock proteins: Critical partners in protection against acute cell injury. *Crit Care Med* 2002; **30** (Suppl. 1): S43–50.

Coleman M. Axon degeneration mechanisms: Commonality amid diversity. *Nat Rev Neurosci* 2005; **6** (11): 889–98.

Conde JR, Streit WJ. Microglia in the aging brain. *J Neuropathol Exp Neurol* 2006; **65**(3): 199–203.

Confavreux C, *et al.* Relapses and progression of disability in multiple sclerosis. *N Engl J Med* 2000; **343** (20): 1430–8.

Corcione A, *et al.* Recapitulation of B cell differentiation in the central nervous system of patients with multiple sclerosis. *Proc Natl Acad Sci USA* 2004; **101**: 11064–9.

Craner MJ, *et al.* Co-localization of sodium channel Nav1.6 and the sodium–calcium exchanger at sites of axonal injury in the spinal cord in EAE. *Brain* 2004a; **127**(2): 294–303.

Craner, MJ, *et al.* Molecular changes in neurons in multiple sclerosis: Altered axonal expression of

Nav1.2 and Nav1.6 sodium channels and Na$^+$/Ca^{2+} exchanger. *Proc Natl Acad Sci USA* 2004b; **101** (21): 8168–73.

Crocker SJ, *et al.* Persistent macrophage/microglial activation and myelin disruption after experimental autoimmune encephalomyelitis in tissue inhibitor of metalloproteinase-1-deficient mice. *Am J Pathol* 2006; **169**: 2104–16.

Cross A, *et al.* B cells and antibodies in CNS demyelinating disease. *J Neuroimmunol* 2001; **112**: 1–14.

Cuzner M, *et al.* The expression of tissue-type plasminogen activator, matrix metalloproteinases and endogenous inhibitors in the central nervous system in multiple sclerosis: Comparison of stages in lesion evolution. *J Neuropathol Exp Neurol* 1996; **55**: 1194–204.

De Rosbo NK, Ben-Nun A. T-cell responses to myelin antigens in multiple sclerosis; relevance of the predominant autoimmune reactivity to myelin oligodendrocyte glycoprotein. *J Autoimmunol* 1998; **11**(4): 287–99.

Diemel LT, *et al.* Macrophages in CNS remyelination: Friend or foe? *Neurochem Res* 1998; **23**(3): 341–7.

Dowling P, *et al.* Involvement of the CD95 (APO-1/Fas) receptor/ligand system in multiple sclerosis brain. *J Exp Med* 1996; **184**(4): 1513–8.

D'Souza S, *et al.* Multiple sclerosis: Fas signaling in oligodendrocyte cell death. *J Exp Med* 1996; **184**: 2361–70.

Dutta R, *et al.* Mitochondrial dysfunction as a cause of axonal degeneration in multiple sclerosis patients. *Ann Neurol* 2006; **59**: 478–89.

Egg R, *et al.* Anti-MOG and anti-MBP antibody subclasses in multiple sclerosis. *Mult Scler* 2001; **7**(5): 285–9.

Evangelou N, *et al.* Quantitative pathological evidence for axonal loss in normal appearing white matter in multiple sclerosis. *Ann Neurol* 2000; **47**(3): 391–5.

Ferguson B, *et al.* Axonal damage in acute multiple sclerosis lesions. *Brain* 1997; **120**: 393–9.

Flavin MP, *et al.* Soluble macrophage factors trigger apoptosis in cultured hippocampal neurons. *Neuroscience* 1997; **80**: 437–448.

Flavin MP, *et al.* Microglial tissue plasminogen activator (tPA) triggers neuronal apoptosis in vitro. *Glia* 2000; **29**: 347–54.

Fogdell A, *et al.* Linkage analysis of HLA class II genes in Swedish multiplex families with multiple sclerosis. *Neurology* 1997; **48**(3): 758–62.

Foote AK, Blakemore WF. Inflammation stimulates remyelination in areas of chronic demyelination. *Brain* 2005; **128**(3): 528–39.

Forstermann U, *et al.* Nitric oxide synthase: Expression and expressional control of the three isoforms. *Naunyn Schmiedebergs Arch Pharmacol* 1995; **352**(4): 351–64.

Foster R, *et al.* Reorganization of the axon membrane in demyelinated peripheral nerve fibers: Morphological evidence. *Science* 1980; **210**: 661–3.

Franklin RJ. Why does remyelination fail in multiple sclerosis? *Nat Rev Neurosci* 2002; **3**(9): 705–14.

Friede RL, Bruck W. Macrophage functional properties during myelin degradation. *Adv Neurol* 1993; **59**: 327–36.

Friese M, *et al.* Humanized mouse models for organ-specific autoimmune diseases. *Curr Opin Immunol* 2006; **18**(6): 704–09.

Friese M, Fugger L. Autoreactive CD8+ T cells in multiple sclerosis: a new target for therapy? *Brain* 2005; **128** (8): 1747–63.

Gay FW, *et al.* The application of multifactorial cluster analysis in the staging of plaques in early multiple sclerosis. Identification and characterization of the primary demyelinating lesion. *Brain* 1997; **120**: 1461–83.

Gaertner S, *et al.* Antibodies against glycosylated native MOG are elevated in patients with multiple sclerosis. *Neurology* 2004; **63**(12): 2381–3.

Geurts JJ, *et al.* Altered expression patterns of group I and II metabotropic glutamate receptors in multiple sclerosis. *Brain* 2003; **126**(8): 1755–66.

Giordana MT, *et al*. Abnormal ubiquitination of axons in normally myelinated white matter in multiple sclerosis brain. *Neuropathol Appl Neurobiol* 2002; **28**(1): 35–41.

Giovannoni G, *et al*. The potential role of nitric oxide in multiple sclerosis. *Mult Scler* 1998; **4**: 212–6.

Glabinski AR, Ransohoff RM. Chemokines and chemokine receptors in CNS pathology. *J Neurovirol* 1999a; **5**(1): 3–12.

Glabinski AR, Ransohoff RM. Sentries at the gate: Chemokines and the blood–brain barrier. *J Neurovirol* 1999b; **5**(6): 623–34.

Gold R, *et al*. Understanding pathogenesis and therapy of multiple sclerosis via animal models: 70 years of merits and culprits in experimental autoimmune encephalomyelitis research. *Brain* 2006; **129**(8): 1953–71.

Hafler DA, *et al*. Multiple sclerosis. *Immunol Rev* 2005; **204**: 208–31.

Haase CG, *et al*. The fine specificity of the myelin oligodendrocyte glycoprotein autoantibody response in patients with multiple sclerosis and normal healthy controls. *J Neuroimmunol* 2001; **114**(1–2): 220–5.

Hill KE, *et al*. Inducible nitric oxide synthase in chronic active multiple sclerosis plaques: Distribution, cellular expression and association with myelin damage. *J Neuroimmunol* 2004; **151**(1–2): 171–9.

Hochmeister S, *et al*. Dysferlin is a new marker for leaky brain blood vessels in multiple sclerosis. *J Neuropathol Exp Neurol* 2006; **65**(9): 855–65.

Hoftberger R, *et al*. Expression of major histocompatibility complex class I molecules on the different cell types in multiple sclerosis lesions. *Brain Pathol* 2004; **14**: 43–50.

Hohlfeld R, Wekerle H. Autoimmune concepts of multiple sclerosis as a basis for selective immunotherapy: From pipe dreams to (therapeutic)

pipelines. *Proc Natl Acad Sci USA* 2004; **101**(Suppl 2): 14599–606.

Holley JE, *et al*. Astrocyte characterization in the multiple sclerosis glial scar. *Neuropathol Appl Neurobiol* 2003; **29**(5): 434–44.

Hollsberg P, *et al*. Induction of anergy in CD8 T cells by B cell presentation of antigen. *J Immunol* 1996; **157**(12): 5269–76.

Huseby ES, *et al*. A pathogenic role for myelin-specific CD8(+) T cells in a model for multiple sclerosis. *J Exp Med* 2001; **194**: 669–76.

Jung J, *et al*. Molecular characterization of an aquaporin cDNA from brain: Candidate osmoreceptor and regulator of water balance. *Proc Natl Acad Sci USA* 1994; **91**: 13052–6.

Kabat EA, *et al*. Quantitative estimation of albumin and gamma globulin in normal and pathological cerebrospinal fluid by immunochemical methods. *Am J Med* 1948; **4**: 653–62.

Karni A, *et al*. Elevated levels of antibody to myelin oligodendrocyte glycoprotein is not specific for patients with multiple sclerosis. *Arch Neurol* 1999; **56**(3): 311–5.

Keegan M, *et al*. Relation between humoral pathological changes in multiple sclerosis and response to therapeutic plasma exchange. *Lancet* 2005; **366**(9485): 579–82.

Kerlero De Rosbo N, *et al*. Predominance of the autoimmune response to myelin oligodendrocyte glycoprotein (MOG) in multiple sclerosis: Reactivity to the extracellular domain of MOG is directed against three main regions. *Eur J Immunol* 1997; **27**(11): 3059–69.

Kermode AG, *et al*. Heterogeneity of blood-brain barrier changes in multiple sclerosis. An MRI study with gadolinium-DTPA enhancement. *Neurology* 1990; **40**: 229.

Kerschensteiner M, *et al*. Activated human T cells, B cells, and monocytes produce brain-derived neurotrophic factor in vitro and in inflammatory brain lesions: A

neuroprotective role of inflammation? *J Exp Med* 1999; **189**(5): 865–70.

Kidd D, *et al*. Cortical lesions in multiple sclerosis. *Brain* 1999; **122** (Pt 1): 17–26.

Kivisakk P, *et al*. High numbers of perforin mRNA expressing CSF cells in MS with gadolinium-enhancing brain MRI lesions. *Acta Neurol Scand* 1999; **100**(1): 18–24.

Kornek B, *et al*. Multiple sclerosis and chronic autoimmune encephalomyelitis: A comparative quantitative study of axonal injury in active, inactive, and remyelinated lesions. *Am J Pathol* 2000; **157**(1): 267–76.

Kotter MR, *et al*. Macrophage depletion impairs oligodendrocyte remyelination following lysolecithin-induced demyelination. *Glia* 2001; **35**(3): 204–12.

Kuhlmann T *et al*. Acute axonal damage in multiple sclerosis is most extensive in early disease stages and decreases over time. *Brain* 2002; **125**(10): 2202–12.

Kutzelnigg A, Lassmann H. Cortical demyelination in multiple sclerosis: A substrate for cognitive deficits? *J Neurol Sci* 2006; **245**(1–2): 123–6.

Kutzelnigg A, *et al*. Cortical demyelination and diffuse white matter injury in multiple sclerosis. *Brain* 2005; **128**(11): 2705–12.

Kwon EE, Prineas JW. Blood–brain barrier abnormalities in longstanding multiple sclerosis lesions. An immunohistochemical study. *J Neuropathol Exp Neurol* 1994; **53**(6): 625–36.

Lalive PH, Genain CP. Antibodies to native myelin oligodendrocyte glycoprotein are serologic markers of early inflammation in multiple sclerosis. *Proc Natl Acad Sci USA* 2006; **103**(7): 2280–5.

Lampasona V, *et al*. Similar low frequency of anti-MOG IgG and IgM in MS patients and healthy subjects. *Neurology* 2004; **62**: 2092–4.

Lassmann H, *et al*. Experimental allergic encephalomyelitis: The balance between encephalitogenic T lymphocytes and demyelinating antibodies determines size and structure of demyelinated lesions. *Acta Neuropathol (Berl)* 1988; **75** (6): 566–76.

Lassmann H. Axonal injury in multiple sclerosis. *J Neurol Neurosurg Psychiatry* 2003; **74**: 695–7.

Lassmann H, Ransohoff RM. The CD4-Th1 model for multiple sclerosis: A critical re-appraisal. *Trends Immunol* 2004; **25**(3): 132–7.

Lassman H. Multiple sclerosis pathology: Evolution of pathogenetic concepts. *Brain Pathol* 2005; **15**(3): 217–22.

Lennon V, *et al.* A serum autoantibody marker of neuromyelitis optica: Distinction from multiple sclerosis. *Lancet* 2004; **364**(9451): 2106–12.

Lennon V, *et al.* IgG marker of optic-spinal multiple sclerosis binds to the aquaporin-4 water channel. *J Exp Med* 2005; **202**(4): 473–7.

Lim ET, *et al.* Anti-myelin antibodies do not allow earlier diagnosis of multiple sclerosis. *Mult Scler* 2005; **11**(4): 492–4.

Linberg RL, *et al.* The expression profile of matrix metalloproteinases and their inhibitors in lesions and normal appearing white matter of multiple sclerosis. *Brain* 2001; **124**: 1743–53.

Lindert RB, *et al.* Multiple sclerosis: B- and T-cell responses to the extracellular domain of the myelin oligodendrocyte glycoprotein. *Brain* 1999; **122** (Pt 11): 2089–100.

Linington C, *et al.* Augmentation of demyelination in rat acute allergic encephalomyelitis by circulating mouse monoclonal antibodies directed against a myelin/oligodendrocyte glycoprotein. *Am J Pathol* 1988; **130**(3): 443–54.

Linker RA, *et al.* CNTF is a major protective factor in demyelinating CNS disease: A neurotrophic cytokine as modulator in neuroinflammation. *Nat Med* 2002; **8**: 620–4.

Liu J, *et al.* Expression of inducible nitric oxide synthase and nitrotyrosine in multiple sclerosis lesions. *Am J Pathol* 2001; **158**: 2057–66.

Lovas G, *et al.* Axonal changes in chronic demyelinated cervical spinal cord plaques. *Brain* 2000; **123**(2): 308–17.

Lu W, *et al.* Involvment of tissue plasminogen activator in onset and effector phases of experimental allergic encephalomyelitis. *J Neurosci* 2002; **22**: 10781–9.

Lucchinetti C, *et al.* A quantitative analysis of oligodendrocytes in multiple sclerosis lesions. A study of 113 cases. *Brain* 1999; **122** (12): 2279–95.

Lucchinetti C, *et al.* Heterogeneity of multiple sclerosis lesions: Implications for the pathogenesis of demyelination. *Ann Neurol* 2000; **47**(6): 707–17.

Lucchinetti CF, *et al.* A role for humoral mechanisms in the pathogenesis of Devic's neuromyelitis optica. *Brain* 2002; **125**(7): 1450–61.

Lucchinetti CF, *et al.* Evidence for pathogenic heterogeneity in multiple sclerosis. *Ann Neurol* 2004; **56**(2): 308.

Lucchinetti CF, *et al.* The pathology of multiple sclerosis. *Neurol Clin* 2005; **23**(1): 77–105, vi.

Ludwin S, *et al.* Evidence of a "dying back" gliopathy in demyelinating disease. *Ann Neurol* 1981; **9**: 301–05.

Luster AD. Chemokines – chemotactic cytokines that mediate inflammation. *N Engl J Med* 1998; **338**(7): 436–45.

Mahad DJ, *et al.* Expression of chemokine receptors CCR1 and CCR5 reflects differential activation of mononuclear phagocytes in pattern II and pattern III multiple sclerosis lesions. *J Neuropathol Exp Neurol* 2004; **63**(3): 262–73.

Mahad D, *et al.* Modulating CCR2 and CCL2 at the blood–brain barrier: Relevance for multiple sclerosis pathogenesis. *Brain* 2006; **129**(Pt 1): 212–23.

Mandler RN, *et al.* Devic's neuromyelitis optica: A clinicopathological study of 8 patients. *Ann Neurol* 1993; **34**(2): 162–8.

Mantegazza R, *et al.* Anti-MOG autoantibodies in Italian multiple sclerosis patients: Specificity, sensitivity and clinical association. *Int Immunol* 2004; **16**(4): 559–65.

Mantovani A, *et al.* Macrophage polarization: Tumor-associated macrophages as a paradigm for polarized M2 mononuclear phagocytes. *Trends Immunol* 2002; **23**: 549–55.

Mantovani A, *et al.* The chemokine system in diverse forms of macrophage activation and polarization. *Trends Immunol* 2004; **25**(12): 677–86.

Mantovani A, *et al.* Macrophage polarization comes of age. *Immunity* 2005; **23**(4): 344–6.

Marta CB, *et al.* Pathogenic myelin oligodendrocyte glycoprotein antibodies recognize glycosylated epitopes and perturb oligodendrocyte physiology. *Proc Natl Acad Sci USA* 2005a; **102**(39): 13992–7.

Marta CB, *et al.* Signaling cascades activated upon antibody cross-linking of myelin oligodendrocyte glycoprotein: potential implications for multiple sclerosis. *J Biol Chem* 2005b; **280**(10): 8985–93.

Martino G, *et al.* Cells producing antibodies specific for myelin basic protein region 70–89 are predominant in cerebrospinal fluid from patients with multiple sclerosis. *Eur J Immunol* 1991; **12**: 2971–6.

Martino G, *et al*; Cytokines and immunity in multiple sclerosis: The dual signal hypothesis. *J Neuroimmunol* 2000; **109**(1): 3–9.

Matute C, *et al.* The link between excitotoxic oligodendroglial death and demyelinating diseases. *Trends Neurosci* 2001; **24**(4): 224–30.

Medana I, *et al.* Transection of major histocompatibility complex class I-induced neurites by cytotoxic T lymphocytes. *Am J Pathol* 2001; **159**(3): 809–15.

Merkler D, *et al.* Differential macrophage/microglia activation in neocortical EAE lesions in the marmoset monkey. *Brain Pathol* 2006; **16**(2): 117–23.

Mew I, *et al.* Oligodendrocyte and axon pathology in clinically silent multiple sclerosis lesions. *Mult Scler* 1998; **4**(2): 55–62.

Moalem G, et al. Autoimmune T cells protect neurons from secondary degeneration after central nervous system axotomy. Nat Med 1999; 5 (1): 49–55.

Moalem G, et al. Production of neurotrophins by activated T cells: Implications for neuroprotective autoimmunity. J Autoimmun 2000; 15(3): 331–45.

Nedergaard M, et al. Beyond the role of glutamate as a neurotransmitter. Nat Rev Neurosci 2002; 3(9): 748–55.

Neumann H, et al. Cytotoxic T lymphocytes in autoimmune and degenerative CNS diseases. Trends Neurosci 2002; 25(6): 313–9.

Nitsch R, et al. Direct impact of T cells on neurons revealed by two-photon microscopy in living brain tissue. J Neurosci 2004; 24(10): 2458–64.

Olsson T, et al. Antimyelin basic protein and antimyelin antibody-producing cells in multiple sclerosis. Ann Neurol 1990; 27(2): 132–6.

O'Connor KC, et al. Antibodies from inflamed central nervous system tissue recognize myelin oligodendrocyte glycoprotein. J Immunol 2005; 175(3): 1974–82.

Oleszak EL, et al. Inducible nitric oxide synthase and nitrotyrosine are found in monocytes/macrophages and/or astrocytes in acute, but not in chronic multiple sclerosis. Clin Diagn Lab Immunol 1998; 5: 438–45.

Ota K, et al. T-cell recognition of an immunodominant myelin basic protein epitope in multiple sclerosis. Nature 1990; 346(6280): 183–7.

Ozawa K, et al. Patterns of oligodendroglia pathology in multiple sclerosis. Brain 1994; 117: 1311–22.

Panitch HS, et al. Exacerbations of multiple sclerosis in patients treated with gamma interferon. Lancet 1987a; 1: 893–5.

Panitch HS, et al. Treatment of multiple sclerosis with gamma interferon: Exacerbations associated with activation of the immune system. Neurology 1987b; 37: 1097–102.

Patrikios P et al. Remyelination is extensive in a subset of multiple sclerosis patients. Brain 2006; 129 (12): 3165–72.

Peter H, et al. Matrix metalloproteinase-9 facilitates remyelination in part by processing the inhibitory NG2 proteoglycan. J Neurosci 2003; 23(35): 11127–35.

Peterson JW, et al. Transected neurites, apoptotic neurons, and reduced inflammation in cortical multiple sclerosis lesions. Ann Neurol 2001; 50(3): 389–400.

Peterson JW, rapp BD. Neuropathobiology of multiple sclerosis. Neurol Clin 2005; 23(1): 107–29.

Pette M, et al. Myelin basic protein-specific T lymphocyte lines from MS patients and healthy individuals. Neurology 1990; 40 (11): 1770–6.

Piddlesden S, et al. The demyelinating potential of antibodies to myelin oligodendrocyte glycoprotein is related to their ability to fix complement. Am J Pathol 1993; 143(2): 555–64.

Pitt D, et al. Glutamate uptake by oligodendrocytes: Implications for excitotoxicity in multiple sclerosis. Neurology 2003; 61(8): 1113–20.

Pittock SJ, et al. Clinical course, pathological correlations, and outcome of biopsy proved inflammatory demyelinating disease. J Neurol Neurosurg Psychiatry 2005; 76(12): 1693–7.

Plumb J, et al. Abnormal endothelial tight junctions in active lesions and normal-appearing white matter in multiple sclerosis. Brain Pathol 2002; 12(2): 154–69.

Pomeroy I, et al. Demyelinated neocortical lesions in marmoset autoimmune encephalomyelitis mimic those in multiple sclerosis. Brain 2005; 128(11): 2713–21.

Prineas JW, et al. Multiple sclerosis. Pathology of recurrent lesions. Brain 1993; 116(3): 681–93.

Prineas JW, et al. Immunopathology of secondary-progressive multiple sclerosis. Ann Neurol 2001; 50(5): 646–5.

Proescholdt MA, et al. Vascular endothelial growth factor is expressed in multiple sclerosis plaques and can induce inflammatory lesions in experimental allergic encephalomyelitis rats. J Neuropathol Exp Neurol 2002; 61: 914–25.

Raff M, et al. Axonal self-destruction and neurodegeneration. Science 2002; 296(5569): 868–71.

Ransohoff RM, et al. Three or more routes for leukocyte migration into the central nervous system. Nat Rev Immunol 2003; 3(7): 569–81.

Redford EJ, et al. Nitric oxide donors reversibly block axonal conduction: demyelinated axons are especially susceptible. Brain 1997; 120(12): 2149–57.

Reindl M, et al. Antibodies against the myelin oligodendrocyte glycoprotein and the myelin basic protein in multiple sclerosis and other neurological diseases: a comparative study. Brain 1999; 122 (11): 2047–56.

Rodriguez M. Virus-induced demyelination in mice: "Dying back" of oligodendrocytes. Mayo Clin Proc 1985; 60: 433–8.

Rodriguez M, Scheithauer B. Ultrastructure of multiple sclerosis. Ultrastruct Pathol 1994; 18(1–2): 3–13.

Roemer S, et al. Pattern-specific loss of aquaporin-4 immunoreactivity distinguishes neuromyelitis optica from multiple sclerosis. Brain 2007; 130(5): 1194–205.

Rostagno A, et al. Complement activation in chromosome 13 dementias. Similarities with Alzheimer's disease. J Biol Chem 2002; 277(51): 49782–90.

Rovaris M, et al. Correlation between MRI and short-term clinical activity in multiple sclerosis: Comparison between standard- and triple-dose Gd-enhanced MRI. Eur Neurol 1999; 41(3): 123–7.

Rovaris M, et al. Secondary progressive multiple sclerosis: current knowledge and future challenges. Lancet Neurol 2006; 5(4): 343–54.

Sadatipour BT, et al. Increased circulating antiganglioside antibodies in primary and secondary progressive multiple sclerosis. Ann Neurol 1998; 44: 980–3.

Saoudi A, *et al.* Prevention of experimental allergic encephalomyelitis in rats by targeting autoantigen to B cells: Evidence that the protective mechanism depends on changes in the cytokine response and migratory properties of the autoantigen-specific T cells. *J Exp Med* 1995; **182**(2): 335–44.

Schwab C, McGeer PL. Complement activated C4d immunoreactive oligodendrocytes delineate small cortical plaques in multiple sclerosis. *Exp Neurol* 2002; **174**(1): 81–8.

Schwartz M, *et al.* Microglial phenotype: Is the commitment reversible? *Trends Neurosci* 2006; **29**(2): 68–74.

Simpson J, *et al.* Expression of the beta-chemokine receptors CCR2, CCR3 and CCR5 in multiple sclerosis central nervous system tissue. *J Neuroimmunol* 2000; **108** (1–2): 192–200.

Serafini B, *et al.* Detection of ectopic B-cell follicles with germinal centers in the meninges of patients with secondary progressive multiple sclerosis. *Brain Pathol* 2004; **14**(2): 164–74.

Sharp FR, Bernaudin M. HIF1 and oxygen sensing in the brain. *Nat Rev Neurosci* 2004; **5**(6): 437–48.

Skou JC. Nobel Lecture. The identification of the sodium pump. *Biosci Rep* 1998; **18**(4): 155–69.

Skulina C, *et al.* Multiple sclerosis: Brain-infiltrating CD8+ T cells persist as clonal expansions in the cerebrospinal fluid and blood. *Proc Natl Acad Sci USA* 2004; **101** (8): 2428–33.

Smith KJ, *et al.* Electrically active axons degenerate when exposed to nitric oxide. *Ann Neurol* 2001; **49**(4): 470–6.

Smith KJ, *et al.* The role of nitric oxide in multiple sclerosis. *Lancet Neurol* 2002; **1**(4): 232–41.

Sorensen TL, *et al.* Expression of specific chemokines and chemokine receptors in the central nervous system of multiple sclerosis patients. *J Clin Invest* 1999; **103**(6): 807–15.

Stadelmann C, *et al.* BDNF and gp145trkB in multiple sclerosis brain lesions: Neuroprotective interactions between immune and neuronal cells? *Brain* 2002; **125**(1): 75–85.

Stadelmann C, *et al.* Tissue preconditioning may explain concentric lesions in Balo's type of multiple sclerosis. *Brain* 2005; **128** (5): 979–87.

Steinman L. Multiple sclerosis: A coordinated immunological attack against myelin in the central nervous system. *Cell* 1996; **85**(3): 299–302.

Storch MK, *et al.* Multiple sclerosis: In situ evidence for antibody- and complement-mediated demyelination. *Ann Neurol* 1998a; **43**(4): 465–71.

Storch MK, *et al.* Autoimmunity to myelin oligodendrocyte glycoprotein in rats mimics the spectrum of multiple sclerosis pathology. *Brain Pathol* 1998b; **8** (4): 681–94.

Streit W. Microglial senescence: Does the brain's immune system have an expiration date? *Trends Neurosci* 2006; **29**(9): 506–10.

Stys PK, *et al.* Axonal degeneration in multiple sclerosis: Is it time for neuroprotective strategies? *Ann Neurol* 2004; **55**(5): 601–3.

Sun J, *et al.* T and B cell responses to myelin-oligodendrocyte glycoprotein in multiple sclerosis. *J Immunol* 1991; **146**(5): 1490–5.

Tavolato BF. Immunoglobulin G distribution in multiple sclerosis brain. An immunofluorescence study. *Neurol Sci* 1975; **24**(1): 1–11.

The Lenercept Multiple Sclerosis Study Group and The University of British Columbia MS/MRI Analysis Group. TNF neutralization in MS: Results of a randomized, placebo-controlled multicenter study, 1998.

Trapp BD, *et al.* Axonal transection in the lesions of multiple sclerosis. *N Engl J Med* 1998; **338**(5): 278–85.

Trebst C, *et al.* CCR1+/CCR5+ mononuclear phagocytes accumulate in the central nervous system of patients with multiple sclerosis. *Am J Pathol* 2001; **159**(5): 1701–10.

Trebst C, *et al.* Chemokine receptors on infiltrating leucocytes in inflammatory pathologies of the central nervous system (CNS). *Neuropathol Appl Neurobiol* 2003; **29**(6): 584–95.

Urich E, *et al.* Autoantibody-mediated demyelination depends on complement activation but not activatory Fc-receptors. *Proc Natl Acad Sci USA* 2006; **103**(49): 18697–702.

Van Horssen J, *et al.* Matrix metalloproteinase-19 is highly expressed in active multiple sclerosis lesions. *Neuropathol Appl Neurobiol* 2006; **32**(6): 585–93.

van Walderveen MA, *et al.* Histopathologic correlate of hypointense lesions on T1-weighted spin-echo MRI in multiple sclerosis. *Neurology* 1998; **50**: 1282–8.

Vass K, *et al.* Localization of 70-kDa stress protein induction in gerbil brain after ischemia. *Acta Neuropathol (Berl)* 1988; **77**(2): 128–35.

Vercellino M, *et al.* Grey matter pathology in multiple sclerosis. *J Neuropathol Exp Neurol* 2005; **64** (12): 1101–7.

Vos CM, *et al.* Matrix metalloproteinase-12 is expressed in phagocytotic macrophages in active multiple sclerosis lesions. *J Neuroimmunol* 2003; **138**(1–2): 106–14.

Warrington AE, *et al.* Human monoclonal antibodies reactive to oligodendrocytes promote remyelination in a model of multiple sclerosis. *Proc Natl Acad Sci USA* 2000; **97**(12): 6820–5.

Washington R, *et al.* Expression of immunologically relevant endothelial cell activation antigens on isolated central nervous system microvessels from patients with multiple sclerosis. *Ann Neurol* 1994; **35**: 89–97.

Waxman SG. Ions, energy and axonal injury: Towards a molecular neurology of multiple sclerosis. *Trends Mol Med* 2006a; **12**(5): 192–5.

Waxman SG. Axonal conduction and injury in multiple sclerosis: The role of sodium channels. *Nat Rev Neurosci* 2006b; **7**(12): 932–41.

Wegner C, *et al.* Neocortical neuronal, synaptic, and glial loss in multiple sclerosis. *Neurology* 2006; **67**(6): 960–7.

Werner P, *et al.* Multiple sclerosis: Altered glutamate homeostasis in lesions correlates with oligodendrocyte and axonal damage. *Ann Neurol* 2001; **50**(2): 169–80.

Wolswijk G, *et al.* Chronic stage multiple sclerosis lesions contain a relatively quiescent population of oligodendrocyte precursor cells. *J Neuroscience* 1998; **18**(2): 601–9.

Xiao BG, *et al.* Antibodies to myelin-oligodendrocyte glycoprotein in cerebrospinal fluid from patients with multiple sclerosis and controls. *J Neuroimmunol* 1991; **31**(2): 91–6.

Yamashita T, *et al.* Changes in nitrite and nitrate (NO_2^-/NO_3^-) levels in cerebrospinal fluid of patients with multiple sclerosis. *J Neurol Sci* 1997; **153**(1): 32–4.

Yasojima K, *et al.* Up-regulated production and activation of the complement system in Alzheimer's disease brain. *Am J Pathol* 1999; **154**(3): 927–36.

Yednock TA, *et al.* Prevention of experimental autoimmune encephalomyelitis by antibodies against alpha 4 beta 1 integrin. *Nature* 1992; **356**(6364): 63–6.

Zhou D, *et al.* Identification of a pathogenic antibody response to native myelin oligodendrocyte glycoprotein in multiple sclerosis. *Proc Natl Acad Sci USA* 2006; **103**(50): 19057–62.

Multiple sclerosis: neuro-immune cross-talk in acute and progressive stages of the disease

Martin Kerschensteiner and Reinhard Hohlfeld

Introduction

Interactions between infiltrating immune cells and resident cells of the central nervous system play a crucial role in the pathogenesis of multiple sclerosis (MS). In recent years, the interactions between immune cells and neurons in particular have moved into the focus of MS research. This is largely based on recent reports suggesting that the outcome of the neuro-immune interaction determines the clinical outcome of MS patients (De Stefano *et al.*, 1998; van Waesberghe *et al.*, 1999; Bjartmar *et al.*, 2000). However, the interplay between immune cells and neurons during CNS inflammation is complex, as a growing body of evidence suggests that, in addition to orchestrating well-documented neurotoxic effects, inflammation in the CNS can also convey neuroprotection (Rapolino *et al.*, 1998; Moalem *et al.*, 1999; Serpe *et al.*, 1999; Hammarberg *et al.*, 2000). A possible molecular explanation for these findings is that the nervous and immune systems engage in an intense cross-talk (Kerschensteiner *et al.*, 2003). Both systems produce a range of factors (e.g. cytokines for the immune system and neurotrophic factors for the CNS) that modulate cell growth and differentiation. Interestingly, the factors expressed by immune and nervous system cells overlap, and neither cytokines nor neurotrophic factors are completely exclusive to either system (Kerschensteiner *et al.*, 2003).

In this chapter we examine the contribution of neuro-immune cross-talk to the pathogenesis of MS. We first describe which molecules can mediate the communication between immune cells and neurons and assess potential functional neuroprotective effects of immune cells. Finally, we summarize the neuro-immune interactions during the acute and chronic stages of MS and explore how the outcome of these interactions could be influenced by present and future immunomodulatory treatment strategies.

Molecular mediators of neuroimmune cross-talk

The communication of infiltrating immune cells and their neuronal counterparts is likely based on shared molecules with overlapping expression patterns in the immune and nervous systems; the subsequent discussion highlights examples of these shared mediators which can convey signals from immune cells to neurons or vice versa.

Neurotrophic factors

Neurotrophic factors comprise a family of proteins that are essential for the development of the CNS in vertebrates. Neurotrophic action is pleiotropic; in addition to mediating neuronal survival, neurotrophic factors regulate a host of neuronal and glial cell activities, including axonal and dendritic growth, synaptic structure and plasticity, neurotransmitter expression, and long-term potentiation (Lewin and Barde, 1996; Thoenen and Sendtner, 2002; Lu, 2004). Furthermore, many neurotrophic factors can influence immune cell functions, such as migration, activation, differentiation, and local antigen presentation (Torcia *et al.*, 1996; Neumann *et al.*, 1998; Villoslada *et al.*, 2000; Flugel *et al.*, 2001). Families of neurotrophic factors that have been characterized include: (1) the NGF-related neurotrophic factors, called "neurotrophins", namely NGF, BDNF, neurotrophin-3 (NT-3) and neurotrophin-4/5 (NT-4/5); (2) the glial cell line-derived neurotrophic factor (GDNF) family ligands, namely GDNF, neurturin, artemin, and persephin; (3) the neuropoietic cytokines, such as ciliary neurotrophic factor and leukemia inhibitory factor; and (4) miscellaneous other factors that can also exert neurotrophic effects.

BDNF

BDNF is a member of the NGF-related neurotrophin family. It plays an essential role in neuronal plasticity

Inflammatory Diseases of the Central Nervous System, ed. T. Kilpatrick, R. M. Ransohoff and S. Wesselingh. Published by Cambridge University Press. © Cambridge University Press 2010.

and survival and also regulates neurotransmitter release and dendritic growth (Lewin and Barde, 1996; Lu, 2004). Further, BDNF can prevent neuro-axonal damage in animal models following various pathologic insults and injuries (Thoenen and Sendtner, 2002). These actions affect key cell populations, including sensory, cerebellar, and spinal neurons. The BDNF binds preferentially to the TrkB receptor (gp145trkB), which is expressed on neuronal cells. Like other neurotrophins, BDNF also binds to the p75 neurotrophin receptor. Although neurons were considered to be the main cellular source of BDNF, work from our group and others has demonstrated that various immune cells secrete BDNF in vitro (Braun *et al.*, 1999; Besser and Wank, 1999; Kerschensteiner *et al.*, 1999; Moalem *et al.*, 2000). Specifically, BDNF expression is increased following antigen stimulation in T helper (Th)1 and Th2 CD4[+] cell lines specific for myelin autoantigens such as myelin basic protein (MBP) and myelin oligodendrocyte glycoprotein (Kerschensteiner *et al.*, 1999; Ziemssen *et al.*, 2002). The neurotrophin was bioactive, as it supported neuronal survival in vitro. Moreover, inflammatory cells in brain lesions and perivascular locations in patients with acute disseminated encephalomyelitis and MS also expressed BDNF (Kerschensteiner *et al.*, 1999; Stadelmann *et al.*, 2002). Notably, lesion areas with high numbers of demyelinating macrophages showed enhanced BDNF immunoreactivity. Subsequently, Stadelmann and colleagues found that the BDNF receptor gp145trkB is also expressed by neurons adjacent to MS lesions and in reactive astrocytes within plaques (Stadelmann *et al.*, 2002). However, neurotrophin signaling may engage other pathways and produce a more complex response. Precursor proteins, known as proneurotrophins, are cleaved proteolytically to produce mature BDNF, NGF, NT3, and NT4 (Lu *et al.*, 2005). Although mature neurotrophins bind with high affinity to cognate Trk receptors to foster neuronal cell survival, pro-neurotrophins bind preferentially to the p75 neurotrophin receptor to promote cell death. The predisposition to produce both pro- and anti-apoptotic responses has been described as the "yin and yang" of neurotrophin action (Lu *et al.*, 2005). In this concept, the particular effect depends on the form of the activated neurotrophin (pro- or mature) and the class of targeted receptor (Trk or p75). In addition to BDNF, other members of the neurotrophin family such as NGF, neurotrophin 3 and neurotrophin4/5

are also widely expressed in the immune system (Ehrhard *et al.*, 1993; Torcia *et al.*, 1996; Besser and Wank, 1999; Moalem *et al.*, 2000). Members of the neurotrophin family are thus likely to contribute to neuro-immune communication and due to their dual properties could contribute to both neuroprotective and neurodestructive effects of inflammation.

GDNF

Ligands of the GDNF family (GFL) – GDNF, neurturin, artemin, and persephin – promote central and peripheral neuronal growth and differentiation (Airaksinen and Saarma, 2002). The GDNF protects dopaminergic neurons in animal models of Parkinson's disease and promotes motor neuron survival in vivo (Tomac *et al.*, 1995; Wang *et al.*, 2002). This factor also has a number of important non-neural functions, which range from regulating kidney development to mediating spermatogonal differentiation (Airaksinen and Saarma, 2002). Neuroprotective effects in animal models of ischemia have also been identified for the GFL persephin (Tomac *et al.*, 2002). The GFLs signal through the RET ("rearranged during transfection" proto-oncogene) receptor tyrosine kinase. To activate this pathway, GFLs must first link with a second protein class, the GDNF family receptor-α (GFRα) receptors, which in turn bind to the RET plasma membrane. Four such GFRα receptors that determine the ligand specificity have been characterized: GDNF binds to GFRα1, neurturin to GFRα2, artemin to GFRα3, and persephin to GFRα4. In addition to these high-affinity interactions, more promiscuous bindings between GFLs and GFRαs have been observed (Airaksinen and Saarma, 2002). Like the NGF family ligands, GFLs also function in the immune system and are expressed by immune cells. Vargas-Leal *et al.* (2005) reported that human CD4[+] and CD8[+] T cells, B cells, and monocytes express neurturin transcript and protein. These immune cells also express RET and GFRα2, allowing the formation of the GFRα2–RET complex. The addition of GDNF or neurturin to activated peripheral blood mononuclear cells reduced the amount of detectable tumor necrosis factor (TNF) protein without altering its transcription (Vargas-Leal *et al.*, 2005). These findings suggest that intercellular communication between immune cell populations could be mediated by neurturin.

Cytokines

A large number of studies have now shown that cytokines that were primarily known to mediate communication between different cell types within the immune system are also expressed by neurons and glial cells. Expression in the nervous system has now been described for cytokines of many families including interleukins, interferons, and members of the tumor necrosis factor (TNF) family (Neumann *et al.*, 1997; Knoblach *et al.*, 1999; Krumbholz *et al.*, 2005; Liu *et al.*, 2005).

BAFF

Family members of the TNF regulate many aspects of immune cell survival, differentiation, and effector function. Their secretion in the CNS could thus provide important signals to infiltrating immune cells. One particularly interesting example is the TNF family member BAFF (B cell-activating factor of the tumor necrosis factor family), which is required for peripheral B cell survival and homeostasis (Kalled, 2006). It was long believed that immune cells such as monocytes, macrophages, and neutrophils were the only source of BAFF. However, Krumbholz and colleagues found that BAFF is also expressed in the normal human brain and that its production by reactive astrocytes could foster B cell survival in MS (Krumbholz *et al.*, 2005). Specifically, the level of BAFF expression in normal human brain was approximately 10% of the level observed in lymphatic tissues (e.g. tonsils and adenoids). Immunohistochemical analysis of CNS tissue revealed astrocytes as a major source of CNS-derived BAFF. In MS plaques, BAFF expression was strongly up-regulated to levels observed in lymphatic tissues (Krumbholz *et al.*, 2005). The BAFF was localized in astrocytes close to BAFF receptor-expressing immune cells, suggesting that astrocyte-derived BAFF can directly act on the B cells. Furthermore, in-vitro studies showed that stimulation of cultured human astrocytes with interferon-gamma and TNF-alpha induced the secretion of functionally active BAFF via a furin-like protease-dependent pathway. In these experiments, BAFF secretion per cell was substantially higher in activated astrocytes than in monocytes and macrophages. Taken together, these observations identified astrocytes as a major "non-immune" source of BAFF. It is tempting to speculate that CNS-derived BAFF supports B cell survival in and around inflammatory lesions. This mechanism would offer one plausible explanation for the notorious persistence of the intrathecal oligoclonal immunoglobin response in MS patients (Meinl *et al.*, 2006).

Chemokines

Chemokines guide the migration of immune cells throughout the body and are central to the immigration of immune cells into the CNS. The expression of chemokines in the nervous system would thus allow resident CNS cells to directly influence the immune infiltration of their environment. One chemokine that has recently been shown to participate in the neuronal regulation of CNS inflammation is fractalkine (Cardona *et al.*, 2006).

Fractalkine

Fractalkine or CX3CL1 is the only member of the δ-family of chemokines and the exclusive ligand for the chemokine receptor CX3CR1 (Bazan *et al.*, 1997; Imai *et al.*, 1997). Fractalkine and its receptor show a peculiar expression pattern: while fractalkine is predominantly expressed in CNS neurons, its receptor CX3CR1 is primarily expressed by monocytes and dendritic cells in the immune system and microglial cells in the CNS (Harrison *et al.*, 1998). This expression pattern strongly suggests that fractalkine can relay neuronal signals to the immune system. Indeed, a recent study demonstrates that fractalkine is a crucial regulator of inflammatory neurotoxicity in the brain (Cardona *et al.*, 2006). The authors used CX3CR1-deficient mice to investigate how the lack of fractalkine receptor expression affects microglial function. The induction of systemic inflammation by peripheral injections of lipopolysaccharide in mice lacking the CX3CR1 receptor lead to a massive activation of microglial cells and subsequently to neuronal cell death. Interestingly, the increased activation of microglial cells in these mice appears to be a cell-autonomous process and can be transferred by the injection of CX3CR1$^{-/-}$ microglia into the cortex of wild-type recipients. In line with these findings, CX3CR1-deficient mice also show increased microglial neurotoxicity in animal models of Parkinson's disease and amyotrophic lateral sclerosis. In summary, these results suggest that neurons can regulate the activation of microglial cells through the release of fractalkine. The constitutive expression of neuronal fractalkine in the CNS indicates that it provides a tonic signal that limits microglial activation in the healthy nervous system. To what extent fractalkine signaling can also contribute to the control of autoimmune inflammation is not yet fully understood. It seems likely, however, that the neuronal expression of fractalkine is unaltered both in MS and its animal model EAE

(Hulshof *et al.*, 2003; Sunnemark *et al.*, 2005). The functional role of fractalkine signaling in EAE was recently studied using CX3CR1-deficient mice (Huang *et al.*, 2006). Interestingly, CX3CR1 deficiency affected the recruitment of NK cells into the CNS, but did not affect the recruitment of macrophages. The impaired infiltration of NK cells was associated with increased disease severity, suggesting a regulatory role for NK cells in this scenario.

Further studies will be necessary to fully understand how fractalkine signaling regulates CNS inflammation. With regard to the dual nature of immune responses in the brain, it is interesting to note that fractalkine-deficient mice which show an increased activation of microglial cells are partially protected from focal ischemic stroke (Soriano *et al.*, 2002).

Functional evidence of neuro-immune cross-talk

The production of both neurotoxic as well as neuroprotective mediators by immune cells supports the notion that neuro-immune cross-talk can, in principle, have both beneficial as well as destructive consequences. While the destructive capability of neuroinflammation has long been documented, evidence for its beneficial properties has emerged only recently. Experimental evidence for "protective autoimmunity" has been provided by the work of Schwartz and colleagues, who showed that T cells specific to a CNS self-antigen, such as myelin basic protein (MBP), can protect damaged neurons from secondary degeneration (Moalem *et al.*, 1999). Although anti-MBP T cells are encephalitogenic in rodent animals models, these cells are also found in the immune systems of healthy subjects (Burns *et al.*, 1983; Pette *et al.*, 1990). To determine whether accumulating T cells exert a beneficial or deleterious effect following axonal injury, Moalem and colleagues injected anti-MBP T cells into rats that experienced injury to the optic nerve (Moalem *et al.*, 1999). Compared with control rats, anti-MBP-injected rats maintained more than twice as many retinal ganglion cells with functional axons. Electrophysiological analysis suggested that the neuroprotective effect of the anti-MBP cell clones was due to a transient reduction in energy requirements, which caused a temporary state of inactivity in the damaged nerve. However, the investigators also considered other explanations, such as the expression of growth factors by anti-MBP cells which has been shown, for example, to be the case for members of the NGF and GDNF neurotrophin families (Besser and Wank, 1999; Kerschensteiner *et al.*, 1999; Moalem *et al.*, 2000; Vargas-Leal *et al.*, 2005). Subsequent studies, mainly in Lewis rats with spinal cord injury (SCI), provided further support for the neuroprotective role of CNS autoreactive T lymphocytes (Hauben *et al.*, 2000; Yoles *et al.*, 2001). In addition, Hammarberg *et al.* reported that T and natural killer (NK) cells in the spinal cord of rats with EAE produced BDNF, NT-3, and GDNF, and can reduce the extent of neuronal injury after ventral root avulsion (Hammarberg *et al.*, 2000). They also found that bystander recruited NK and T cells displayed comparable or increased neurotrophic factor levels, compared with the anti-MBP T cell populations. Recently, Ziv *et al.* (2006) showed that hippocampal neurogenesis could be restored in mice with SCI by the transfer of CNS-reactive T cells. These regulatory T lymphocytes were also necessary for the completion of spatial learning and memory tasks and, notably, for BDNF expression in the dentate gyrus.

It is important to note, however, that a series of studies by Jones and colleagues challenged the notion that autoreactive T lymphocytes can minimize neuronal and glial cell death following CNS injury (Jones *et al.*, 2002, 2004). These authors reported that TCR transgenic mice in which more than 95% of CD4$^+$ T cells are reactive to MBP experienced impaired recovery of locomotor and reflex function after spinal cord injury compared with non-transgenic mice. This impairment correlated with aggravated demyelination and axonal loss, along with the increased expression of pro-inflammatory cytokines (Jones *et al.*, 2002). Likewise, the immunization of rats with MBP enhanced tissue damage and functional disability after SCI (Jones *et al.*, 2004). The investigators were unable to observe neuroprotection or functional improvement in MBP-immunized rats and thus concluded that myelin-reactive T cells are pathologic effector cells that impair recovery and exacerbate tissue injury at and beyond traumatic sites.

The discrepancies between these studies and previous work illustrate an important point: namely, that the net effect of inflammation crucially depends on the respective experimental setting. Immunostimulation in one setting may lead to net neuroprotection while immunostimulation in a slightly different setting or genetic background that favors an encephalitogenic immune response leads to net neurodestruction. This notion should also caution us about the naive use of

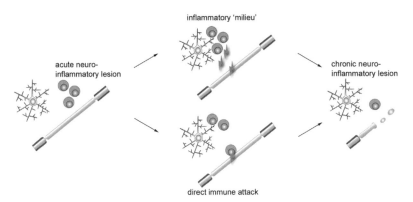

inflammatory 'milieu'

acute neuro-inflammatory lesion

chronic neuro-inflammatory lesion

direct immune attack

Figure 6.1 The neuro-immune balance. Immune cells produce both mediators that can result in neuronal damages as well as neuroprotection. The net effect of inflammation in a particular pathologic situation is determined by which process outweighs the other. (Adapted, with permission, from Kerschensteiner *et al.*, Neurotrophic cross-talk between the nervous and immune systems: implications for neurological diseases. *Ann Neurol*, 2003; **52**(3): 292–304.)

immunostimulatory treatment strategies for human CNS disease given its complexity and heterogeneity. A concept that can reconcile these discrepancies is illustrated by the "neuro-immune balance" (Figure 6.1). This concept emphasizes that immune cells can, in principle, release both neuroprotective and neurodestructive mediators. The net effect of the immune reaction – the position of the balance – can vary with the nature as well the particular stage of the underlying disease process.

Neuro-immune cross-talk in acute and chronic multiple sclerosis

Inflammation of the CNS is, in essence, a double-edged process, that can have both protective and destructive effects. In MS, several lines of evidence indicate that the net effect of CNS inflammation is destructive, at least in the acute stage of the disease. Animal models of MS like experimental autoimmune encephalomyelitis (EAE) illustrate that an inflammatory reaction against myelin targets can lead to the formation of destructive CNS lesions which reflect the pathological hallmarks of multiple sclerosis (Storch *et al.*, 1998; Kornek *et al.*, 2000). As immune reactivity against myelin proteins – albeit certainly more diverse than in the EAE model – can also be detected in MS patients (Burns *et al.*, 1983; Soriano *et al.*, 2002), it is likely that anti-myelin autoimmunity contributes to tissue destruction in multiple sclerosis. Experimental studies further suggest that antigen-independent activation of immune cells, in particular macrophages, can lead to CNS damage (Newman *et al.*, 2001). In line with these findings, the histopathological analysis of MS lesions reveals close contacts between infiltrating immune cells and damaged axons (Trapp *et al.*, 1998). Furthermore, the extent of axonal

damage in a given lesion correlates with the number of both macrophages and CD8$^+$ T cells present in these lesions (Bitsch *et al.*, 2000). The most conclusive evidence in support of a damaging role of the immune response in MS, however, stems from MS therapy. A number of immunosuppressive and immunomodulatory treatment strategies have proven to improve the clinical outcome in multiple sclerosis (Hohlfeld, 1997). The most direct evidence is probably that the inhibition of immune cell infiltration in the CNS using the anti-integrin antibody natalizumab dramatically reduces the number of relapses and limits disease progression (Polman *et al.*, 2006). This clinical benefit is paralleled by a reduction of apparent tissue damage, as assessed by MRI measurements. In summary, these findings suggest that immune cell infiltration leads to tissue damage in the acute stages of MS. It is, however, currently unclear as to how infiltrating immune cells mediate CNS damage and, in particular, how the devastating loss of axonal connections emerges. As outlined above, histopathological data strongly suggest that immune cells, in particular macrophages and CD8$^+$ T cells, participate in the process that ultimately leads to axonal damage (Trapp *et al.*, 1998; Bitsch *et al.*, 2000). How precisely this destructive interaction of immune cells and axons evolves in MS plaques is not yet understood. At least two different scenarios are possible (Figure 6.2): first, the infiltration of immune cells (and influx of antibodies) could primarily lead to the demyelination of the axon. Loss of the protective myelin cover would then render axons susceptible to toxic mediators in the neuro-inflammatory environment. Recent evidence suggests that this indirect path contributes to axon damage in EAE models and could also be operative in MS. Elegant studies by the groups of Ken Smith and Stephen Waxman show that through exposure, the demyelination of axons in

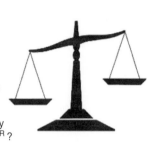

Pro-inflammatory and neurotoxic factors	Anti-inflammatory and neuroprotective factors
TH1 cytokines	TH2 cytokines
TNF	TGF
IL-1	TNF ?
osteopontin	soluble TNF receptor
leukotrienes	soluble IL-1 receptor
MMP	IL-1 receptor antagonist
plasminogen activators	some prostaglandins
nitric oxide	lipoxins
reactive oxygen species	TIMP
glutamate	antithrombin
antibody + complement	
cell-mediated cytotoxicity	BDNF
neurotrophins via p75^{NTR} ?	NGF
	NT3 neurotrophic
	NT4/5 factors
	GDNF
	LIF

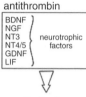

Destruction   Protection

Figure 6.2 Pathogenesis of immune-mediated axonal damage. Two distinct scenarios can explain how immune cells damage axons in neuro-inflammatory lesions. One possibility (above) is that axons are damaged indirectly as a consequence of immune-mediated demyelination and their subsequent exposure to the noxious inflammatory environment. An alternative possibility (below) is that immune cells damage axons through direct cell–cell contact. It is difficult to differentiate between these two possibilities based on the analysis of either acute (left) or chronic (right) lesions. (Adapted, with permission, from Misgeld and Kerschensteiner, In vivo imaging of the diseased nervous system. Nat Rev Neurosci 2006; **7**(6): 449–63.)

conjunction with the effect of nitric oxide alters the distribution and function of ion channels and exchangers, which in turn leads to an increased influx of sodium and ultimately calcium ions into the axonal cytoplasm (Smith *et al.*, 2001; Kapoor *et al.*, 2003; Waxman 2003). Intra-axonal calcium overload can then trigger the activation of proteolytic degradation cascades that lead to axonal destruction. In line with this concept, the therapeutic application of sodium channel blockers which prevent the intra-axonal accumulation of sodium ions abrogates axon damage and clinical signs of disease in several EAE models (Bechtold *et al.*, 2004; Black *et al.*, 2006). In this model, immune cells would thus damage axons indirectly by removing their myelin sheaths and exposing them to the noxious mediators present in the inflammatory environment. In contrast, it is also plausible that immune cells could directly contact axons and induce their transection, e.g. by the secretion of cytotoxic granules in the case of CD8$^+$ T cells or by the secretion of proteases in the case of macrophages or microglial cells (Figure 6.2). Evidence for a direct path to axon damage is provided, on the one hand, by histopathological studies which reveal the presence of immune cells in direct contact with damaged axons (Trapp *et al.*, 1998) and, on the other hand, by experimental studies which indicate that axonal destruction can evolve in response to direct immune attacks (Medana *et al.*, 2001). Future studies will be necessary to determine whether the indirect or direct path or a combination of both is responsible for immune-mediated axon damage in the acute stages of MS.

While it seems established that CNS inflammation is destructive in the acute stages of MS, the net effect of the inflammation in the chronic stages of the disease is more difficult to assess. In particular, recent studies suggest that neurodegenerative and not neuro-inflammatory mechanisms drive disease progression in the advanced stages of MS (Bjartmar and Trapp, 2001; Hauser and Oksenberg, 2006). Histopathological and neuro-imaging studies support the view that axonal damage in the chronic disease stages evolves with a slow constant progression compatible with a neurodegenerative mechanism (Losseff *et al.*, 1996; Bjartmar *et al.*, 2000; Kornek *et al.*, 2000). Likewise, the clinical course of MS follows a more uniform progression pattern in the chronic, compared to the acute stages of the disease (Confavreux *et al.*, 2000), and a neurodegenerative mechanism would explain why many of the established immunomodulatory or immunosuppressive therapies fail in the chronic stages of the disease (Killestein and Polman, 2005). However, proof of autonomous neurodegeneration in chronic MS is still lacking, and an alternative hypothesis has been provided by the group of Hans Lassmann (Kutzelnigg *et al.*, 2005). The alternative hypothesis is one of "smoldering inflammation", and implies that CNS inflammation is still driving the disease process in the chronic, as well as the acute stages of MS. However, the type of CNS inflammation has been observed to change as the disease progresses. While focal demyelinated lesions densely infiltrated by macrophages and T cells dominate the histopathological presentation of acute MS, chronic MS is primarily

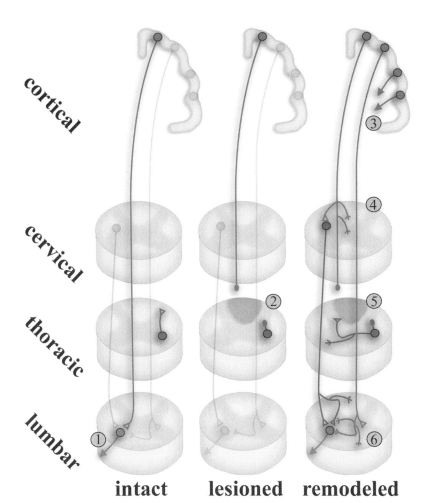

cortical

cervical

thoracic

lumbar

intact   **lesioned**   **remodeled**

Figure 6.3 Remodeling of axonal connections in an animal model of multiple sclerosis

A spinal neuro-inflammatory lesion induces the remodeling of axonal connections on multiple anatomical levels. (1) The hind limb corticospinal tract (CST) (green) forms a direct connection to lumbar motor neurons (blue) in the intact spinal cord. A targeted neuro-inflammatory lesion in the dorsal column (2, orange) interrupts the hind limb CST, as well as local spinal circuits (red). Extensive remodeling is induced in response to the inflammatory lesion. Near the lesion, local interneurons sprout (5, red). In parallel, the descending CST is remodeled in two ways. Below the lesion, spared hindlimb CST fibers increase their branching (6) and contact more target cells. (4) Above the lesion, damaged CST fibers form new collaterals and contact preserved spinal interneurons (PSNs) (e.g. long PSNs (red) that relay to lumbar motor circuits). (3) The intraspinal remodeling is complemented by reorganization of the cortical motor representation. (Adapted, with permission, from Kerschensteiner *et al.*, Remodeling of axonal connections contributes to recovery in an animal model of multiple sclerosis. *J Exp Med* 2004; **200**(8): 1027–38.)

characterized by a disseminated activation of microglial cells, which are postulated to induce widespread axonal damage. In this model, the minor role of immune cell infiltration from the blood stream could also explain why many immunomodulatory and immunosuppressive therapies fail, despite the underlying inflammatory pathogenesis. It is of obvious importance for the evolution and focus of future MS therapeutic strategies to clarify the extent to which either neurodegeneration or neuro-inflammation are responsible for the devastating progression of axonal loss and clinical disability that occur in chronic MS. If, indeed, neurodegeneration dominates chronic MS, one could argue that it is worthwhile to explore neuroprotective strategies as the principal therapeutic modality. The relevance of endogenous repair strategies has also been highlighted by a recent study that investigated axonal repair in a targeted animal model of MS, and this applies independent of whether either

primary neuronal damage or inflammation is the principal pathogenetic mechanism (Kerschensteiner *et al.*, 2004). Multiple tracing techniques revealed that axonal connections are remodeled on multiple anatomical levels in response to a single neuro-inflammatory lesion (Figure 6.3) and behavioral testing indicated that this remodeling contributed to the functional recovery of the animals. Interestingly, the comparison of inflammatory and traumatic lesions of the spinal cord suggested that axonal sprouting around the lesion site was more prominent in inflammatory lesions while remodeling processes distant to the lesion site evolved similarly after traumatic and inflammatory lesions (Bareyre *et al.*, 2004; Kerschensteiner *et al.*, 2004). These results are compatible with the notion that inflammatory cells can first damage CNS tissue and at a later stage of the disease induce self-repair.

In any event, neuroprotection by endogenous or exogenous mechanisms is increasingly appreciated as a valid therapeutic goal in both acute and chronic multiple sclerosis. It is reasonable to assume that all of the currently used immunomodulatory therapies, including interferon-beta, glatiramer acetate, natalizumab, and mitoxantrone, have some indirect neuroprotective effect by reducing the extent of immune-mediated injury of myelin, which in turn protects axons and neurons.

Primary neuroprotective therapies are increasingly studied in animal models of MS, but with respect to human MS, these therapies are still in their infancy (Kapoor, 2006). In addition, it seems possible that some of the currently used immunomodulatory agents might have a neuroprotective component, for example by enhancing the expression of neurotrophic factors in the CNS. Such a scenario has first been suggested for glatiramer acetate (Ziemssen *et al.*, 2002; Aharoni *et al.*, 2003). Treatment with glatiramer acetate shifts the cytokine profile towards an anti-inflammatory Th2 type and increases the activation threshold of monocytes (Farina *et al.*, 2005). In addition, glatiramer acetate could support the local production of neurotrophic factors by supporting the reactivation of drug-specific T cell lines within the CNS (Ziemssen *et al.*, 2002; Aharoni *et al.*, 2005; Farina *et al.*, 2005).

Conclusion and therapeutic implications

The complexity of neuro-immune cross-talk illustrates that it might be possible to develop new therapies based on the beneficial components of CNS inflammation. This might be achieved by either modulating the endogenous expression of protective factors in immune cells or, more directly, by using immune cells as genetically engineered therapeutic vehicles (Kramer *et al.*, 1995; Neumann, 2006). In the long run, it should become possible to identify the molecular switches that govern the balance between the production of destructive and protective immune mediators (Figure 6.1). Therapies that modulate these switches could then enable us to shift the neuro-immune balance to promote beneficial immune effects and at the same time to limit immune-mediated tissue destruction.

Acknowledgments

This chapter is in part reprinted, with permission from Hohleld R., Kerschensteiner M., Meinl E. Dual role of inflammation in CNS disease. *Neurology* **68** (22), Suppl. 58–63.

References

Aharoni R, *et al*. Glatiramer acetate-specific T cells in the brain express T helper 2/3 cytokines and brain-derived neurotrophic factor in situ. *Proc Natl Acad Sci* USA 2003; **100**(24): 14157.

Aharoni R, *et al*. The immunomodulator glatiramer acetate augments the expression of neurotrophic factors in brains of experimental autoimmune encephalomyelitis mice. *Proc Natl Acad Sci* USA 2005; **102**(52): 19045.

Airaksinen MS, Saarma M. The GDNF family: Signaling, biological functions and therapeutic value. *Nat Rev Neurosci* 2002; **3**(5): 383.

Bareyre FM, *et al*. The injured spinal cord spontaneously forms a new intraspinal circuit in adult rats. *Nat. Neurosci* 2004; **7**(3): 269.

Bazan JF, *et al*. A new class of membrane-bound chemokine with a CX3C motif. *Nature* 1997; **385**(6617): 640.

Bechtold DA, Kapoor R, Smith KJ. Axonal protection using flecainide in experimental autoimmune encephalomyelitis. *Ann Neurol* 2004; **55**(5): 607.

Besser M, Wank R. Cutting edge: clonally restricted production of the neurotrophins brain-derived neurotrophic factor and neurotrophin-3 mRNA by human immune cells and Th1/Th2-polarized expression of their receptors. *J Immunol* 1999; **162**(11): 6303.

Bitsch A, *et al*. Acute axonal injury in multiple sclerosis. Correlation with demyelination and inflammation. *Brain* 2000; **123**(6): 1174.

Bjartmar C, Trapp BD. Axonal and neuronal degeneration in multiple sclerosis: Mechanisms and functional consequences. *Curr Opin Neurol* 2001; **14**(3): 271.

Bjartmar C, *et al*. Neurological disability correlates with spinal cord axonal loss and reduced N-acetyl aspartate in chronic multiple sclerosis patients. *Ann Neurol* 2000; **48**(6): 893.

Black JA, *et al*. Long-term protection of central axons with phenytoin in monophasic and chronic-relapsing EAE. *Brain* 2006; **129**(12): 3196.

Braun A, *et al*. Cellular sources of enhanced brain-derived neurotrophic factor production in a mouse model of allergic inflammation. *Am J Respir Cell Mol Biol* 1999; **21**(4): 537.

Burns J, Rosenzweig A, Zweiman B, Lisak RP. Isolation of myelin-basic protein-reactive T cell lines from normal human blood. *Cell Immunol* 1983; **81**(2): 435–440.

Cardona AE, *et al*. Control of microglial neurotoxicity by the fractalkine receptor. *Nat Neurosci* 2006; **9**(7): 917.

Confavreux C, *et al*. Relapses and progression of disability in multiple sclerosis. *N Engl J Med* 2000; **343**(20): 1430.

De Stefano N, *et al*. Axonal damage correlates with disability in patients with relapsing–remitting multiple sclerosis. Results of a longitudinal magnetic resonance spectroscopy study. *Brain* 1998; **121**(8): 1469.

Ehrhard PB, *et al*. Expression of nerve growth factor and nerve growth factor receptor tyrosine kinase Trk in activated CD4-positive T-cell clones. *Proc Natl Acad Sci USA* 1993; **90**(23): 10984.

Farina C, *et al*. Glatiramer acetate in multiple sclerosis: Update on potential mechanisms of action. *Lancet Neurol* 2005; **4**(9): 567.

Flugel A, *et al*. Anti-inflammatory activity of nerve growth factor in experimental autoimmune encephalomyelitis: Inhibition of monocyte transendothelial migration. *Eur J Immunol* 2001; **31**(1): 11.

Hammarberg H, *et al*. Neuroprotection by encephalomyelitis: Rescue of mechanically injured neurons and neurotrophin production by CNS-infiltrating T and natural killer cells. *J Neurosci* 2000; **20**(14): 5283.

Harrison JK, *et al*. Role for neuronally derived fractalkine in mediating interactions between neurons and CX3CR1-expressing microglial. *Proc Natl Acad Sci USA* 1998; **95**(18): 10896.

Hauben E, *et al*. Passive or active immunization with myelin basic protein promotes recovery from spinal cord contusion. *J Neurosci* 2000; **20**(17): 6421.

Hauser SL, Oksenberg JR. The neurobiology of multiple sclerosis: Genes, inflammation, and neurodegeneration. *Neuron* 2006; **52**(1): 61.

Hohlfeld R. Biotechnological agents for the immunotherapy of multiple sclerosis. Principles, problems and perspectives. *Brain* 1997; **120**(5): 865.

Huang D, *et al*. The neuronal chemokine CX3CL1/fractalkine selectively recruits NK cells that modify experimental autoimmune encephalomyelitis within the central nervous system. *FASEB J* 2006; **20**(7): 896.

Hulshof S, *et al*. CX3CL1 and CX3CR1 expression in human brain tissue: Noninflammatory control versus multiple sclerosis. *J Neuropathol Exp Neurol* 2003; **62**(9): 899.

Imai T, *et al*. Identification and molecular characterization of fractalkine receptor CX3CR1, which mediates both leukocyte migration and adhesion. *Cell* 1997; **91**(4): 521.

Jones TB, *et al*. Pathological CNS autoimmune disease triggered by traumatic spinal cord injury: Implications for autoimmune vaccine therapy. *J Neurosci* 2002; **22**(7): 2690.

Jones TB, *et al*. Passive or active immunization with myelin basic protein impairs neurological function and exacerbates neuropathology after spinal cord injury in rats. *J Neurosci* 2004; **24**(15): 3752.

Kalled SL. Impact of the BAFF/BR3 axis on B cell survival, germinal center maintenance and antibody production. *Semin Immunol* 2006; **18**(5): 290.

Kapoor R. Neuroprotection in multiple sclerosis: Therapeutic strategies and clinical trial design. *Curr Opin Neurol* 2006; **19**(3): 255.

Kapoor R, *et al*. Blockers of sodium and calcium entry protect axons from nitric oxide-mediated degeneration. *Ann Neurol* 2003; **53**(2): 174.

Kerschensteiner M, *et al.* Activated human T cells, B cells, and monocytes produce brain-derived neurotrophic factor in vitro and in inflammatory brain lesions: A neuroprotective role of inflammation? *J Exp Med* 1999; **189**(5): 865.

Kerschensteiner M, *et al.* Neurotrophic cross-talk between the nervous and immune systems: Implications for neurological diseases. *Ann Neurol* 2003; **53**(3): 292.

Kerschensteiner M, *et al.* Remodeling of axonal connections contributes to recovery in an animal model of multiple sclerosis. *J Exp Med* 2004; **200**(8): 1027.

Killestein J, Polman CH. Current trials in multiple sclerosis: Established evidence and future hopes. *Curr Opin Neurol* 2005; **18**(3): 253.

Knoblach SM *et al.* Early neuronal expression of tumor necrosis factor-alpha after experimental brain injury contributes to neurological impairment. *J Neuroimmunol* 1999; **95**(1–2): 115.

Kornek B, *et al.* Multiple sclerosis and chronic autoimmune encephalomyelitis: A comparative quantitative study of axonal injury in active, inactive, and remyelinated lesions. *Am J Pathol* 2000; **157**(1): 267.

Kramer R, *et al.* Gene transfer through the blood-nerve barrier: NGF-engineered neuritogenic T lymphocytes attenuate experimental autoimmune neuritis. *Nat Med* 1995; **1**(11): 1162.

Krumbholz M, *et al.* BAFF is produced by astrocytes and up-regulated in multiple sclerosis lesions and primary central nervous system lymphoma. *J Exp Med* 2005; **201**(2): 195.

Kutzelnigg A, *et al.* Cortical demyelination and diffuse white matter injury in multiple sclerosis. *Brain* 2005; **128**(11): 2705.

Lewin GR, Barde YA. Physiology of the neurotrophins. *Annu Rev Neurosci* 1996; **19**: 289.

Liu L, *et al.* S100B-induced microglial and neuronal IL-1 expression is mediated by cell type-specific transcription factors. *J Neurochem* 2005; **92**(3): 546.

Losseff NA, *et al.* Progressive cerebral atrophy in multiple sclerosis. A serial MRI study. *Brain* 1996; **119**(6): 2009.

Lu B, Acute and long-term synaptic modulation by neurotrophins. *Prog Brain Res* 2004; **146**: 137.

Lu B, Pang PT, Woo NH. The yin and yang of neurotrophin action. *Nat Rev Neurosci* 2005; **6**(8): 603.

Medana I, *et al.* Transection of major histocompatibility complex class I-induced neurites by cytotoxic T lymphocytes. *Am J Pathol* 2001; **159**(3): 809.

Meinl E, Krumbholz M, Hohlfeld R. B lineage cells in the inflammatory central nervous system environment: Migration, maintenance, local antibody production, and therapeutic modulation. *Ann Neurol* 2006; **59**(6): 880.

Moalem G, *et al.* Autoimmune T cells protect neurons from secondary degeneration after central nervous system axotomy. *Nat Med* 1999; **5**(1): 49.

Moalem G, *et al.* Production of neurotrophins by activated T cells: Implications for neuroprotective autoimmunity. *J Autoimmun* 2000; **15**(3): 331.

Neumann H. Microglia: A cellular vehicle for CNS gene therapy. *J Clin Invest* 2006; **116**(11): 2857.

Neumann H, *et al.* Interferon gamma gene expression in sensory neurons: Evidence for autocrine gene regulation. *J Exp Med* 1997; **186**(12): 2023.

Neumann H, *et al.* Neurotrophins inhibit major histocompatibility class II inducibility of microglia: Involvement of the p75 neurotrophin receptor. *Proc Natl Acad Sci U SA* 1998; **95**(10): 5779.

Newman TA, *et al.* T-cell- and macrophage-mediated axon damage in the absence of a CNS-specific immune response: involvement of metalloproteinases. *Brain* 2001; **124**(11): 2203.

Pette M, *et al.* Myelin autoreactivity in multiple sclerosis: Recognition of myelin basic protein in the context of HLA-DR2 products by T lymphocytes of multiple-sclerosis patients and healthy donors. *Proc Natl Acad Sci USA* 1990; **87**(20): 7968.

Polman CH, *et al.* A randomized, placebo-controlled trial of natalizumab for relapsing multiple sclerosis. *N Engl J Med* 2006; **354**(9): 899.

Rapalino O, *et al.* Implantation of stimulated homologous macrophages results in partial recovery of paraplegic rats. *Nat Med* 1998; **4**(7): 814.

Serpe CJ, *et al.* Exacerbation of facial motoneuron loss after facial nerve transection in severe combined immunodeficient (scid) mice. *J Neurosci* 1999; **19**(11): RC7.

Smith KJ, *et al.* Electrically active axons degenerate when exposed to nitric oxide. *Ann Neurol* 2001; **49**(4): 470.

Soriano SG, *et al.* Mice deficient in fractalkine are less susceptible to cerebral ischemia–reperfusion injury. *J Neuroimmunol* 2002; **125**(1–2): 59.

Stadelmann C, *et al.* BDNF and gp145trkB in multiple sclerosis brain lesions: Neuroprotective interactions between immune and neuronal cells? *Brain* 2002; **125**(1): 75.

Storch MK, *et al.* Autoimmunity to myelin oligodendrocyte glycoprotein in rats mimics the spectrum of multiple sclerosis pathology. *Brain Pathol* 1998; **8**(4): 681.

Sunnemark D, *et al.* CX3CL1 (fractalkine) and CX3CR1 expression in myelin oligodendrocyte glycoprotein-induced experimental autoimmune encephalomyelitis: kinetics and cellular origin. *J Neuroinflamm* 2005; **2**: 17.

Thoenen H, Sendtner M. Neurotrophins: From enthusiastic expectations through sobering experiences to rational therapeutic approaches. *Nat Neurosci* 2002; **5**(Suppl): 1046.

Tomac A, *et al.* Protection and repair of the nigrostriatal dopaminergic system by GDNF in vivo. *Nature* 1995; **373**(6512): 335.

Tomac AC, *et al.* Effects of cerebral ischemia in mice deficient in Persephin. *Proc Natl Acad Sci USA* 2002; **99**(14): 9521.

Torcia M, *et al.* Nerve growth factor is an autocrine survival factor for memory B lymphocytes. *Cell* 1996; **85**(3): 345.

Trapp BD, *et al.* Axonal transection in the lesions of multiple sclerosis. *N Engl J Med* 1998; **338**(5): 278.

van Waesberghe JH, *et al.* Axonal loss in multiple sclerosis lesions: Magnetic resonance imaging insights into substrates of disability. *Ann Neurol* 1999; **46**(5): 747.

Vargas-Leal V, *et al.* Expression and function of glial cell line-derived neurotrophic factor family ligands and their receptors on human immune cells. *J Immunol* 2005; **175**(4): 2301.

Villoslada P, *et al.* Human nerve growth factor protects common marmosets against autoimmune encephalomyelitis by switching the balance of T helper cell type 1 and 2 cytokines within the central nervous system. *J Exp Med* 2000; **191**(10): 1799.

Wang LJ, *et al.* Neuroprotective effects of glial cell line-derived neurotrophic factor mediated by an adeno-associated virus vector in a transgenic animal model of amyotrophic lateral sclerosis. *J Neurosci* 2002; **22**(16): 6920.

Waxman SG. Nitric oxide and the axonal death cascade. *Ann Neurol* 2003; **53**(2): 150.

Yoles E, *et al.* Protective autoimmunity is a physiological response to CNS trauma. *J Neurosci* 2001; **21**(11): 3740.

Ziemssen T, *et al.* Glatiramer acetate-specific T-helper 1- and 2-type cell lines produce BDNF: Implications for multiple sclerosis therapy. Brain-derived neurotrophic factor. *Brain* 2002; **125**(11): 2381.

Ziv Y, *et al.* Immune cells contribute to the maintenance of neurogenesis and spatial learning abilities in adulthood. *Nat Neurosci* 2006; **9**(2): 268.

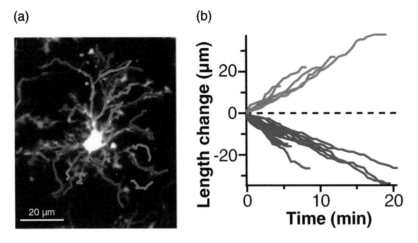

(a)

20 μm

(b)

Figure 2.1 A. Transcranial time-lapse recording of a single microglial cell expressing EGFP in the mouse cortex *in situ*. Processes marked in green represent their formation while processes marked in red represent retraction of processes over a 20-min period. B. Plot of length changes amongst the processes depicted in the upper panel as a function of time. (Modified from Nimmerjahn *et al.* (2005). Reprinted with permission from AAAS.)

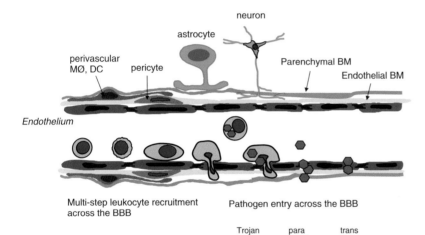

Figure 4.1 Immune cell and pathogen penetration across the endothelial BBB. Immune cells penetrate the endothelial BBB by a multi-step recruitment cascade involving the molecular mechanisms outlined in the text. Tethering and rolling is followed by chemokine mediated activation of secondary leukocyte adhesion molecules, which mediate the firm adhesion of the leukocyte to the endothelium and finally its diapedesis across the BBB probably via a transcellular route. Pathogens (pink hexagon) can penetrate the BBB via a Trojan horse mechanism inside immune cells or traverse as free pathogens using a paracellular route through the BBB tight junction or a transcellular route through the endothelial cell. BBB = blood brain barrier BM = basement membrane, MØ = macrophage DC = dendritic cell.

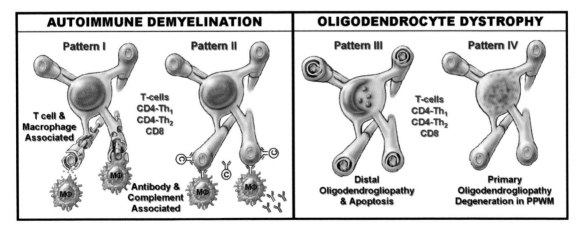

Figure 5.1 MS immunopathologic patterns. Active Pattern I and II lesions are mainly associated with T cell and macrophage inflammation, suggesting that demyelination and tissue injury could be mediated by toxic products secreted from activated mononuclear cells. Active Pattern II lesions additionally demonstrate deposition of antibodies and complement. Active Pattern III lesions demonstrate ill-defined macrophage borders, oligodendrocyte apoptosis and early loss of MAG, which is located in the most distal oligodendrocyte processes. Active Pattern IV lesions are associated with activated mononuclear cells, near complete loss of oligodendrocytes in the lesion and profound non-apoptotic nuclear fragmentation of oligodendrocytes in the PPWM, suggesting a primary oligodendropathy. (Reprinted with permission from Lucchinetti *et al.*, 2005).

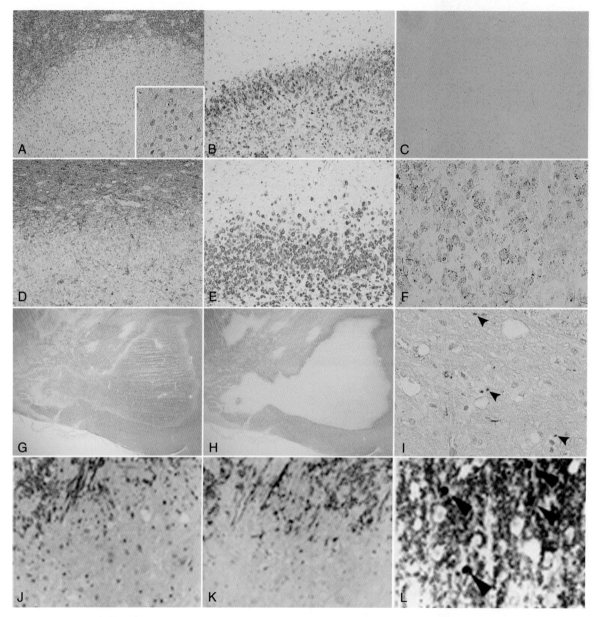

Figure 5.2 Histopathology of MS immunopattern (IP) I–IV.

    A–C: **IP I**. A: A perivenous confluent active demyelinating lesion. Macrophages contain myelin debris within their cytoplasm (inset).
B: Macrophages accumulate in a sharp rim at the lesion border. C: Complement deposition is absent.

    D–F: **IP II**. D: A perivenous confluent active demyelinating lesion. Clustering of oligodendrocytes and labeling of delicate oligodendrocyte processes is suggestive of concurrent ongoing remyelination. E: Macrophages accumulate in a sharp rim at the lesion border. F: Macrophages contain complement positive myelin debris within their cytoplasm.

    G–I: **IP III**. G: MOG overexpression within active MS lesion compared to adjacent NAWM. H: A striking loss of MAG is demonstrated within the lesion corresponding to the region of MOG overexpression.

    I: Condensed oligodendrocyte nuclei suggestive of apoptosis (arrowheads). Note residual MAG immunoreactivity in the oligodendrocyte process at upper left corner.

    J–L: **IP IV**. J/K: Distribution of myelin antigens MOG (J) and MAG (K) is similar in the lesions. L: DNA fragmentation of oligodendrocytes is seen in the periplaque white matter (double staining of *in-situ* tailing [DNA fragmentation] and CNPase [myelin and oligodendrocytes]. (J–L: Reprinted with permission from Lucchinetti *et al.*, 2000.)

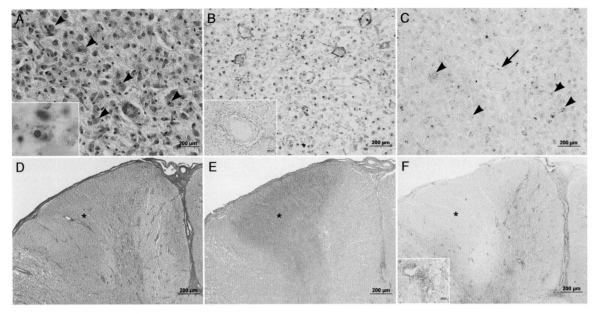

Figure 5.3 Histopathologic difference between MS IP II and NMO lesions.

A–C. **Active MS IP II lesion**. A: Macrophages contain myelin debris within their cytoplasm (arrowheads and inset). B: AQP4 expression is up-regulated on the surface of reactive astrocytes and in rosette pattern on penetrating blood vessel in the MS lesion. C: Macrophages contain complement positive myelin debris within their cytoplasm (arrowheads), but complement deposition is absent around blood vessels (arrow).

D–F. **Active NMO lesion**. D: Extensive demyelination involving both gray and white matter; asterisk indicates preserved myelin in the PPWM. E: AQP4 expression is lost in the NMO lesion but retained in the PPWM (*) and gray matter. F: Complement is deposited in a characteristic vasculocentric rim and rosette pattern within the active lesion, whereas, this is not detected in the PPWM (*). (Reprinted with permission from Roemer *et al.*, 2007.)

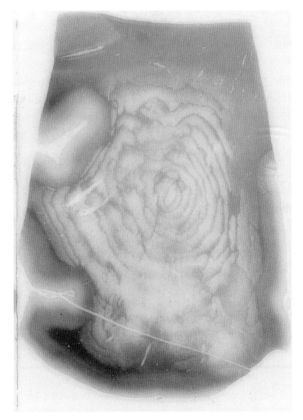

Figure 5.4 Balo's concentric sclerosis. Balo lesions are pathologically characterized by the concentric alternating layers of demyelination and myelin preservation reminiscent of a tree-trunk. (Courtesy of Professor Hans Lassmann).

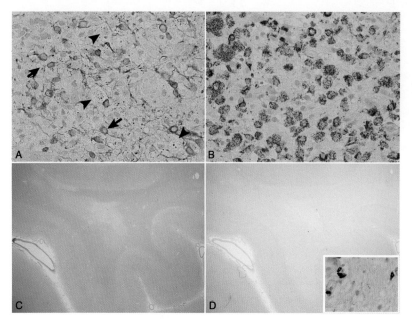

Figure 5.5 Remyelination in MS.
A,B. **Early active MS**. A: Clusters of oligodendrocytes that express minor myelin protein within their cytoplasm and processes (arrows) indicate ongoing remyelination. B: Macrophages contain myelin debris within their cytoplasm (arrowheads) indicative of concurrent demyelination. Numerous foamy macrophages are identified in the lesion.
C,D: **Chronic MS**. C: Myelin stain demonstrates an almost fully remyelinated lesion. D: Foamy macrophages are absent and ramified microglial cells are only identified at high magnification (inset).

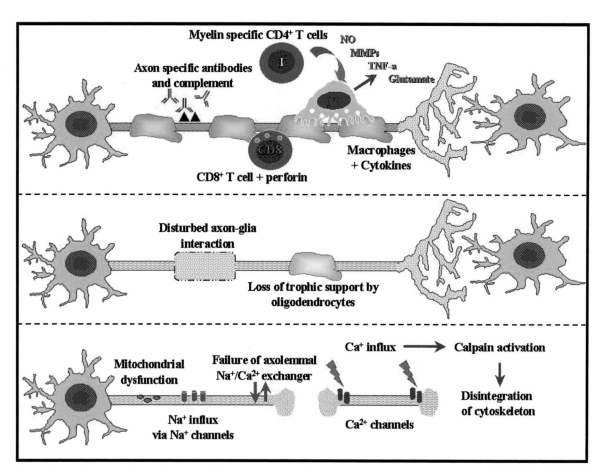

Figure 5.6 Mechanisms of axonal destruction. Effector mechanisms of axonal degeneration during acute and chronic MS. The final pathway of axon destruction is the result of mitochondrial dysfunction, ion influx, and proteolytic degradation. (Reprinted with permission from Lucchinetti *et al.*, 2005.)

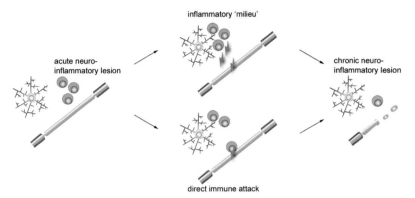

Figure 6.1 The neuro-immune balance. Immune cells produce both mediators that can result in neuronal damages as well as neuroprotection. The net effect of inflammation in a particular pathologic situation is determined by which process outweighs the other. (Adapted, with permission, from Kerschensteiner *et al.*, Neurotrophic cross-talk between the nervous and immune systems: implications for neurological diseases. *Ann Neurol*,2003; **52**(3): 292–304.)

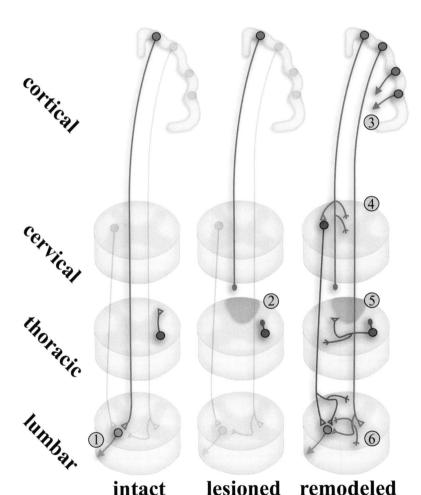

Figure 6.3 Remodeling of axonal connections in an animal model of multiple sclerosis

A spinal neuro-inflammatory lesion induces the remodeling of axonal connections on multiple anatomical levels. (1) The hind limb corticospinal tract (CST) (green) forms a direct connection to lumbar motor neurons (blue) in the intact spinal cord. A targeted neuro-inflammatory lesion in the dorsal column (2, orange) interrupts the hind limb CST, as well as local spinal circuits (red). Extensive remodeling is induced in response to the inflammatory lesion. Near the lesion, local interneurons sprout (5, red). In parallel, the descending CST is remodeled in two ways. Below the lesion, spared hindlimb CST fibers increase their branching (6) and contact more target cells. (4) Above the lesion, damaged CST fibers form new collaterals and contact preserved spinal interneurons (PSNs) (e.g. long PSNs (red) that relay to lumbar motor circuits). (3) The intraspinal remodeling is complemented by reorganization of the cortical motor representation. (Adapted, with permission, from Kerschensteiner *et al.*, Remodeling of axonal connections contributes to recovery in an animal model of multiple sclerosis. *J Exp Med* 2004; **200**(8): 1027–38.)

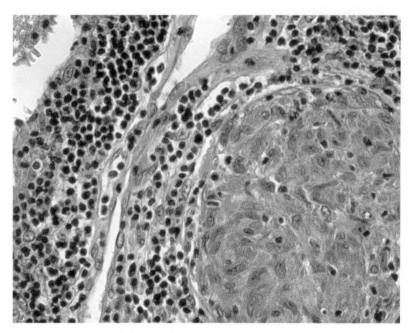

Figure 9.3 Marked mononuclear inflammatory infiltrate in a cortical vessel with a well-formed perivascular granuloma. Magnification ×200. (With permission from Calabrese LH. Vasculitis of the central nervous system. *Rheum Dis Clin North Am*1995; **21**: 1059–76.)

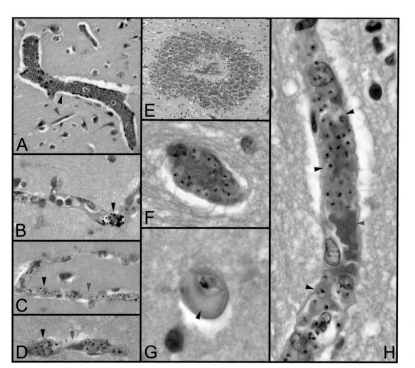

Figure 13.1 Cerebral sequestration within brain tissue obtained from pediatric patients in Africa. Sequestration can be extremely variable, being dense in some blood vessels (Panel A, black arrow) but sparse in others (Panel A, red arrow). Pigment-laden macrophages are important in the removal of *P. falciparum* from sequestered sites in the body but can become greatly enlarged with masses of pigment (Panel B, black arrow). Within a single segment of vessel (Panels C, D, black arrow) sequestration can be focal and adjacent to segments that are apparently unaffected (Panels C, D, red arrow). Ring hemorrhages are a classic finding (Panel E) that usually include fibrin thrombi within the core in and around the damaged vessel. Larger vessels with sequestration appear to maintain blood flow through the center (Panel F). Fibrin thrombi are occasionally seen without ring hemorrhages (Panel G, black arrow). In a given specimen, a mixture of PRBC with pathogens at different stages of development and with different levels of hemoglobin loss (Panel H, black arrows) can be identified when compared to unaffected cells (Panel H, red arrow).

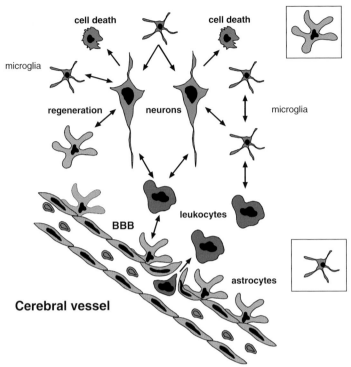

Activated astrocytes

Anisomorphic:
Localized at the glial scar
Release of neurotoxic molecules:
TNF, NO, oxygen radicals.
Killing of neurons, oligodendrocytes

Isomorphic:
Distant from the injury site
glutamate uptake
release of energy substrates,
neurotrophic factors, anti-oxidants,
extracellular matrix, anti-
inflammatory cytokines.
BBB restoration and tissue repair

Activated microglia

M1: stimulated by TNF, LPS or
IFN_γ = cytotoxicity

M2: stimulated by IL-4, IL-13,
IL-10 = immune suppression and
tissue remodeling

Figure.14.2 Modes of activation of astrocytes and microglia.

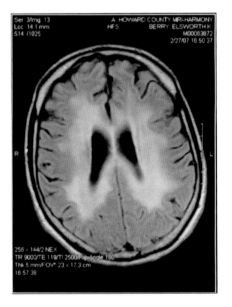

Figure 15.2 FLAIR MRI image of HIV-D. Lesions are symmetric, diffuse and loosely circumscribed, sparing the U-fibers.

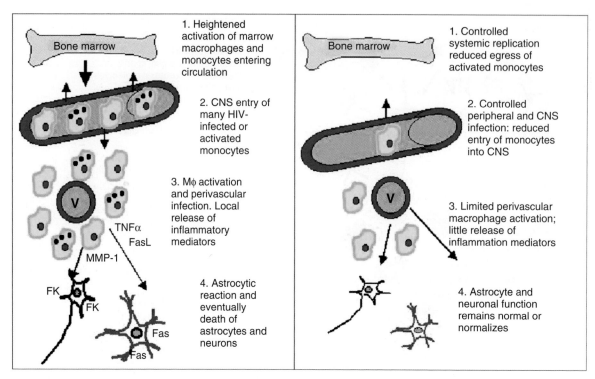

Figure 15.3 Theoretical differences in the pathological features of CNS HIV infection between untreated and HAART-treated subjects. From McArthur JC, with permission. (MØ= macrophages, TNF-α= Tumor necrosis factor α, FasL = Fas Ligand, MMP-1 = matrix metalloprotease-1, FK = Fractalkine/ CX3CL1.

CD8$^+$ T cell-mediated autoimmune diseases of the CNS

Lisa Walter and Matthew L. Albert

Introduction

Cytotoxic CD8$^+$ T lymphocytes (CTLs) are an important component of the adaptive immune response and are critical for the eradication of virally infected and malignant cells. While beneficial in protecting the host, CD8$^+$ T cells are also responsible for mediating certain autoimmune disorders, including those in the central nervous system (CNS). This chapter addresses the cellular mechanisms by which CD8$^+$ T cells can be primed towards CNS antigens. It also focuses on two examples of CNS autoimmunity – the paraneoplastic neurologic diseases (PNDs) and multiple sclerosis (MS) (Walter and Santamaria, 2005). In addition, a model for how antigen presenting cells (APCs) could initiate disease pathogenesis is explored.

CNS "immune privilege"

The CNS, which consists of the brain and spinal cord, is considered to be relatively "immune-privileged" – a concept that is supported by the presence of the blood–brain barrier (BBB), the lack of conventional lymphatics and the paucity of endogenous dendritic cells (DCs). Nonetheless, antigen presentation and immune surveillance of the CNS do occur, although with some unique modifications compared with other tissues. First, the BBB is important in regulating cellular transmigration (Fabry *et al.*, 1994; Ransohoff *et al.*, 2003). Major components of the BBB include endothelial cells that form tight junctions, astrocytes, pericytes and neurons (Reese and Karnovsky, 1967; Hawkins and Davis, 2005). Under inflammatory conditions, the BBB becomes more accessible to lymphocytes, and immune cells can access the CNS via the BBB (Hickey, 1991; Tsukada *et al.*, 1993). Second, the brain parenchyma is a highly specialized site in which the anatomy, cellular composition, and microenvironment of soluble factors can influence the immune response (Fabry *et al.*, 1994). For example, the brain parenchyma is hostile for CD8$^+$ T cell immune function (Gordon *et al.*, 1998). Finally, there are no draining lymphatic vessels for the CNS, but outflow of antigens from the brain occurs by interstitial fluid and cerebrospinal fluid (CSF) drainage to lymphoid organs via the blood to the spleen, or by escape along cranial nerves into the nasal lymphatics and subsequent draining to the cervical lymph nodes (LNs) (Bradbury *et al.*, 1981; Yamada *et al.*, 1991; Walter *et al.*, 2006a, 2006b).

Despite the "immune-privileged" characteristics of the CNS, CD8$^+$ T cell responses to CNS antigens are a major component of human disease pathogenesis in PND and MS. Over the past few decades, much information has been discovered concerning the handling of CNS antigens by the immune system for the activation of CD8$^+$ T cells. By definition, this activation is occurring via an indirect pathway, whereby CNS-restricted antigen (expressed by neurons or glia) are captured and presented by APCs. This mechanism for antigen presentation is called cross-presentation (so named given that it crosses the classically defined restriction for MHC I presenting peptides that are normally derived from endogenously synthesized cellular proteins). In vivo, the relative contributions of different APC populations and signaling molecules have been difficult to ascertain because it is almost impossible to manipulate these parameters individually without global activation of the immune system or gross changes in CNS physiology. Keeping these challenges in mind, this chapter focuses on the likely events, as determined by clinical data and experimental models, that initiate and perpetuate CD8$^+$ T cell priming towards CNS antigens, focusing on PND and MS.

Inflammatory Diseases of the Central Nervous System, ed. T. Kilpatrick, R. M. Ransohoff and S. Wesselingh. Published by Cambridge University Press. © Cambridge University Press 2010

The paraneoplastic neurologic degenerations

The PNDs are defined as a set of neurologic syndromes that occur as an indirect result of a malignancy; in other words, they are not due to direct tumor invasion (Darnell, 1996). The mechanisms underlying this indirect effect between the neoplasm and the neurologic syndromes are not well understood, yet it is known that the immune system plays a key role. For example, in paraneoplastic cerebellar degeneration (PCD), previously healthy patients present with loss of motor control that evolves over days to months, due to loss of Purkinje neurons. After diagnosis, careful inspection often reveals that these patients harbor(ed) occult breast or ovarian carcinomas. The recognition that PND patients have high titer autoantibodies, specific for now defined "onconeural" antigens, was a critical insight into the pathogenesis of PND and helped establish an early model for how the disease progressed. Patients are believed to first develop the systemic cancer (breast, ovarian and small cell lung cancer are known to associate with the various PNDs), which initiates an immune response specific for the onconeural antigen (expressed by the tumor), thus leading to the observed tumor immunity. Following this immune response, it was believed that a "cross-over" reaction, not well defined, led to neuronal degeneration specific to the subset of neurons expressing the onconeural antigen (Darnell, 1996).

While the findings of autoantibodies in conjunction with neurologic symptoms is pathognomonic for the specific PND, several data suggest that they are not responsible for the disease pathogenesis and that, instead, CD8$^+$ T cells play a critical role in the observed tumor immunity and neuronal degeneration. Specifically, the antibody-mediated hypothesis for PND pathogenesis suffered from failure to reproduce the disease in animals by either passive transfer or active antibody immunization and from clinical data that demonstrated little benefit to patients receiving therapy aimed at reducing autoantibody levels in the cerebrospinal fluid (Furneaux et al., 1990). Furthermore, cloning of the genes encoding the PND onconeural antigens revealed that the proteins were intracellular, and in some cases intranuclear, thus making it hard to understand how antibodies might target tumor cells and neurons for immune-mediated destruction. For PCD, the onconeural protein is called cerebellar degeneration related protein-2 (cdr2) and protein expression is restricted to the cytosol of Purkinje neurons and is aberrantly expressed by breast and ovarian cancer patients. Based on these observations, a role for T cells was examined and, indeed, increased numbers of cdr2-specific CD8$^+$ T cells could be identified in patients with PCD. These studies were initiated by the identification of a patient who presented with acute neurologic disease and a small mass in her axillary lymph node: she was found to have activated T cells in her blood (able to lyze target cells presenting the cdr2 antigen in the absence of ex-vivo re-stimulation) (Albert et al., 1998). Subsequent studies in other chronically ill patients have used autologous APCs such as DCs to re-stimulate memory CTL responses to the cdr2 antigen; such responses have been found in all PCD patients studied (Albert et al., 1998, 2000a). These studies have been complemented by additional reports of limited Vβ chain T cell repertoire in patients with the Hu syndrome (Voltz et al., 1998) – this PND is initiated by expression of Hu-D in small cell lung cancer and a subsequent immune attack of neurons in the dorsal root ganglia and the hippocampus. More recently, the presence of Hu-D specific T cells has been described in such patients (Rousseau et al., 2005). Together, it appears that an important part of the tumor immunity consists of CD8$^+$ T cell responses to the PND antigens, and this helps to explain the effectiveness of the immune response to intracellular antigens.

While it remains unclear whether CD8$^+$ class I-restricted T cells mediate the neuronal degeneration observed in patients with PCD, some evidence suggests that this may indeed be the case. Activated T cells have been identified in the CSF of PCD patients, and this correlated with cdr2-specific T cells in the peripheral blood (Albert et al., 200b). While it has been difficult to quantify the lack of progression clinically (due to the variable clinical course of patients and the small population of affected individuals), it has been possible to demonstrate a role for immunosuppressive agents in eliminating activated T$_H$1 cells from the CNS in patients with progressive disease. While it was initially believed that all neurons lacked major histocompatibility complex (MHC) I expression, it is now clear that inflammatory cytokines such as interferon-γ (IFN-γ) and tumor necrosis factor-α (TNF-α) up-regulate the expression of MHC I and B2-microglobulin (β2-m), offering the possibility that CD8$^+$ T cells are the effectors responsible for the neuronal degeneration (Albert et al., 200b). The establishment of a mouse model for PCD will help to establish a causal link between the cdr2-specific CTLs and the lysis of the Purkinje cells.

Multiple sclerosis and CD8$^+$ T cell models of experimental autoimmune encephalitis (EAE)

Multiple sclerosis is a chronic disease of the CNS of unknown etiology, characterized by a wide spectrum of neurological symptoms believed to be a result of multi-focal inflammatory infiltrates within discrete zones of demyelination, called plaques (Steinman, 1996; Traugott et al., 1983; Hauser et al., 1986; Gay et al., 1997). To classify the CNS lesions, four pathologic categories have been posited to occur and are defined based on the extent of myelin loss, the location and extent of the lesion, the pattern of oligodendrocyte destruction, and the nature of the immune infiltrate (Luchinetti et al., 2000) (see also Chapter 5). With respect to the inflammatory cell profile, active lesions are characterized by perivascular infiltration of oligo-clonal CD4$^+$ and CD8$^+$ αβ T cell populations, as well as γδ T cells (Oksenberg et al., 1990; Babbe et al., 2000). Importantly, two of the four posited patterns match lesions predictive of T cell-mediated autoimmiune encephalomyelitis (the other two being suggestive of vasculopathy or primary oligodendrocyte dystrophy). These observations, combined with an uncertain role for antibodies in the pathogenesis of disease and an overwhelming amount of data from experimental auto-immune encephalomyelitis (EAE), suggesting the importance of T cells in pathogenesis, have resulted in a model in which autoreactive T cells are considered responsible for both the initiation and the relapsing–remitting attacks during disease progression.

The CD4$^+$ T cells are a defined component of the immune infiltrate in the CNS of patients; MHC II haplotypes have been mapped as disease-associated alleles (Ebers et al., 1996; Haines et al., 1996; Sawcer et al., 1996); and clinical studies aimed at depleting CD4$^+$ T cells through the use of humanized monoclonal antibodies have shown small but significant improvements in relapse rate and the level of CNS inflammation (Lindsey et al., 1994; Van Oosten et al., 1997). That said, effector CD4$^+$ T cells likely reflect only a component of the immune pathogenesis of MS. In particular, it must be considered that models of CD4$^+$ T cell-mediated EAE have failed to recapitulate the CNS lesions characteristic of MS (Steinman, 1999). In addition, there is a striking disparity between many of the immunologic changes observed in EAE and the influence that modulating these factors has on the human disease (e.g. the effects of systemic IFNγ or treatment with anti-TNF-α in mouse and man) (Steinman, 1999). Thus, it could be the case that small animal models have been chasing the wrong effector cell and that CD4$^+$ T cells are playing a different role than was originally believed.

More recently, there has been greater attention given to CD8$^+$ T cells. Pathologic reports indicate that CD8$^+$ T cells are observed in close proximity to demyelinated axons in MS brain tissue (Neumann et al., 2002) and that they are potentially enriched at the site of actively demyelinating MS lesions (Babbe et al., 2000; Bitsch et al., 2000). Within such active lesions, the CD8$^+$ T cells were found to express granzyme-B, with their cytotoxic granules polarized towards the axons, suggestive of a directed cytotoxic attack (Neumann et al., 2002). Moreover, some studies have suggested that CD8$^+$ T cells outnumber CD4$^+$ T cells almost 10-fold within MS lesions (Booss et al., 1983; Gay et al., 1997). There is also evidence of linkage disequilibrium for MHC I alleles (Bugawan et al., 2000). Antigen-presenting cells have also been reported to harbor myelin antigens in the lymph nodes of MS patients (De Vos et al., 2002). Strikingly, there are now two models of CD8$^+$ T cell-mediated EAE, and in one of them, the brain lesions are closer to what is seen in MS patients than in the classical CD4 models. Governman and colleagues have shown that, in vitro, activated myelin basic protein-reactive CD8$^+$ T cell clones can be transferred into normal C3H mice, traffic to the CNS and induce severe EAE (Huseby et al., 2001). Interestingly, significant differences between CD4$^+$ and CD8$^+$ T cell-mediated EAE were seen when attempts were made to modulate the disease. In the latter model, anti-IFNγ mAbs reduced disease pathogenesis – a finding consistent with MS studies where recombinant IFNγ treatment resulted in accelerated disease progression.

Major questions still remain concerning the immune pathogenesis of MS: how are the CD8$^+$ T cells primed, and where? Do the CD4$^+$ T cells, instead of being effector cells, play an active role in the priming and/or maintenance of the CD8$^+$ T cells? Does epitope spreading play an important role in disease relapse? If so, what APCs are responsible for capturing CNS antigen and where do they engage naive CNS-reactive CD8$^+$ T cells?

The role of dendritic cells in CD8$^+$ T cell activation

Given the role of CD8$^+$ T cells in the PNDs and MS, it is important to consider how and where they are becoming activated. Prior to becoming effector cells, CD8[+] T cells must be primed by specialized APCs, namely DCs. These DCs must harbor the T cells' cognate epitope in MHC I and classically, it was believed that only antigen synthesized endogenously could have access to the MHC I presentation pathway, thus excluding the possibility of generating immunity to tissue-restricted antigens. However, it is now accepted that exogenous antigen can be captured by resident DCs that in turn migrate to draining lymph nodes (LNs) for the engagement of CD8[+] T cells. In fact, DCs are unique in their ability to present endocytosed or phagocytosed exogenous antigen onto their own MHC I molecules for the priming of CD8[+] T cells (Albert et al., 1998). This mechanism of T cell activation has been termed "cross-priming" for the crossing of the classically defined restriction of MHC I to endogenously synthesized proteins (Heath and Carbone, 2001); and this accounts for the activation of T cells specific for tissue-derived tumor, viral, donor and self antigen. The CNS likely behaves as do other organs in terms of cross-priming CD8[+] T cells (Walter and Albert, 2007) – antigen is captured within the CNS and is trafficked to regional lymph nodes, in particular the submandibular cervical nodes, where naive CD8[+] T cells are activated and undergo the initial rounds of cell division.

Autoimmune responses directed towards onconeural antigens are believed to be critical for neuronal degeneration in the PNDs. Here, the presence of aberrantly expressed CNS antigen allows for the priming of CD8[+] T cells. Most likely, this occurs in tumor-draining lymph nodes, and once activated, the effector cells are capable of trafficking into the tumor. It remains unclear if these activated T cells are also capable of trafficking into the CNS or if an additional event (e.g. viral infection) is necessary for up-regulation of adhesion molecules on the BBB, thus permitting the T cells to enter the brain and spinal cord. For MS, it has been suggested that myelin components are key antigens for immune priming; however, the anatomical site of antigen presentation and the features of the APC involved remain to be clarified. The myelin sheath is formed by Schwann cells in the peripheral nervous system and by oligodendrocytes in the CNS, and it is feasible that CD8[+] T cell priming towards myelin epitopes is initiated from DCs coming from either anatomical site. As lymphatic drainage of the peripheral nervous system is even less well characterized than that of the CNS, it

remains to be seen if there are links between these two sites in terms of disease initiation, perpetuation, and epitope spreading.

Experimental rodent models that have addressed the paradox of CD8[+] T cells gaining access to "immune privileged" CNS antigen indicate that it is indeed possible to elicit a CD8[+] T cell immune response specific to CNS antigen (Huseby et al., 2001; Karman et al., 2004). However, these results, as well as those obtained from injection of antigen into the CNS, must be evaluated keeping in mind that CNS antigen could also be expressed in other tissues such as the peripheral nervous system or, alternatively, leaked into the blood, and it is not yet possible by current techniques to fully explore the contributions of each of these sites to the immune response. Additionally, both DCs and resting B cells can present MBP epitopes endogenously expressed by these cell types in lymphoid tissues, perhaps contributing to the tolerization of CD8[+] T cells (Seamons et al., 2006).

In-situ presentation of CNS antigens

While we favor a model in which CD8[+] T cells are primed outside the CNS, there is a critical requirement for the capture and trafficking of cell-associated antigen, thus implicating a role for APCs within the CNS. Moreover, there is an intriguing and likely possibility that to achieve effector function, primed T cells require secondary or tertiary engagement with tissue APCs. If this is so, then CNS antigen must be presented in situ. That said, the "immune-privileged" qualities of the CNS include a paucity of DCs. Microglia are clearly the dominant immune cell population in healthy brain. However, monocytes, macrophages, and small numbers of DCs have been reported to be present. One clue as to which cell type is presenting antigen comes from studies in the healthy CNS, where invading CD8[+] T cells can find constitutive MHC I-expressing target cells presenting antigen in the meninges, the choroid plexus, the perivascular space, but notably, not in the CNS parenchyma (Vass and Lassmann, 1990).

As discussed above, DCs remain the best candidate for the APC uniquely responsible for the capture and presentation of brain antigen to T cells (Greter et al., 2005; McMahon et al., 2005; Lauterbach et al., 2006). Evidence suggests that brain DCs can originate from several different places in the body. The DCs can develop from microglia in the brain (Santambrogio et al., 2001); they may be found as resident cells in the CNS (Pashenkov and Link, 2002); or, alternatively, infiltrate into the CNS from blood (Greter *et al.*, 2005). Both resident and infiltrating DCs are candidates for the APCs that are responsible for initiating T cell immunity (Carson *et al.*, 1999; Karman *et al.*, 2004; Hatterer *et al.*, 2006). Under steady-state conditions, DCs are present in the CSF, meninges, and choroid plexus (Pashenkov and Link, 2002). Under inflammatory conditions, DCs with a mature, activated phenotype also appear in the brain parenchyma (Fischer and Bielinsky, 1999; Serafini *et al.*, 2000; Fischer and Reichmann, 2001; Reichmann *et al.*, 2002). This latter situation could be important in mediating the phenomenon of epitope or determinant spreading, a critical step in the pathogenesis of MS and possibly some PNDs (e.g. Hu syndrome)(Albert and Darnell, 2004).

Other cell types have been proposed to be implicated. The adult brain has two microglial subsets: resting parenchymal microglia and perivascular microglia (Hickey and Kimura, 1988). They are derived from CD45[+] bone marrow precursors of the myeloid lineage. Parenchymal microglia are ubiquitously distributed in the CNS (Lawson *et al.*, 1990). They are relatively inefficient at eliciting CD8[+] T cell responses (Bergmann *et al.*, 1999), but there is some evidence that parenchymal microglia are uncommitted myeloid progenitors of immature DCs and macrophages (Santambrogio *et al.*, 2001). It has also been proposed that glial cell types and neurons are capable of expressing MHC I (Neumann, 2001), and there exists the possibility that either astrocytes or oligodendrocytes present antigen to CD8[+] T cells in the CNS for re-stimulation (Kort *et al.*, 2006).

It is also important to point out that under inflammatory situations, especially chronic disease, there is the possibility of lymphoid structures emerging within the CNS. Such organized lymphoid structures have been observed to resemble secondary lymphoid organs (Aloisi and Pujol-Borrell, 2006). The presence of these so-called tertiary lymphoid tissues suggests that lymphoid neogenesis could also have a role in maintaining immune responses against antigens (Aloisi and Pujol-Borrell, 2006), and that it could even contribute to the priming of T cells during secondary waves of antigen presentation. In fact, it has been shown that encephalitogenic CD4[+] T cells can migrate into the CNS, recognize their antigen locally presented by CNS-resident APCs, and cause disease even in the absence of a functional peripheral lymphoid system (Greter *et al.*, 2005).

Priming of CNS antigen-specific CD8[+] T cells and subsequent migration into the CNS

Given the requirement for naive T cells to be primed in secondary lymphoid tissue, and based on what is known regarding disease pathogenesis, it has been proposed for both PND and MS that the priming of CNS-reactive T cells occurs outside of the nervous system. Although there is more limited trafficking of CD8[+] T cells into the CNS compared with other tissues (Hickey, 1999), once CD8[+] T cells are activated they can enter the brain parenchyma. This is supported by several studies that investigated priming of antigen-specific T cells following targeted, including intracerebral, injection of antigen (Karman *et al.*, 2004; Calzascia *et al.*, 2005; Lang and Nikolich-Zugich *et al.*, 2005). Furthermore, adoptive transfer experiments indicated that effector T cells can traffic to the brain, but only those cells recognizing locally expressed antigen that is presented in situ are retained (Calzascia *et al.*, 2005). In addition to changes in the expression of adhesion molecules and homing receptors on the T cell, inflammation alters the endothelium of the BBB in a manner that permits increased cellular traffic into the CNS (Hickey *et al.*, 1991).

While we argue that the antigen involved in the initiation of disease was captured from a peripheral source – the tumor in the case of PNDs, and an unknown site for MS – there could still be an important role for T cells primed by APCs that have captured antigen within the CNS. This is likely the mechanism by which epitope spreading occurs. This broadening of the autoimmune response during chronic MS (Tuohy *et al.*, 1997, 1999) occurs when T cell reactivity is directed initially toward a narrow set of myelin epitopes, but then spreads to other epitopes in the same antigen (intramolecular spreading). The pathogenic significance of this process has been demonstrated in CD4[+] T cell-mediated models of EAE in mice (McRae *et al.*, 1995; Miller *et al.*, 1995; Yu *et al.*, 1996), but whether this also occurs for CD8[+] T cells remains to be investigated. The mechanism underlying epitope spreading is thought to involve APCs that present degraded myelin derived from the inflammatory process in the CNS, and it is likely this presentation occurs in the draining cervical LNs, as DCs presenting myelin antigens have been found there in a simian model of EAE and in human MS patients (De Vos *et al.*, 2002). The initial CNS inflammation could also trigger the spreading of immune activation to distinct CNS antigens (intermolecular spreading). Regarding this form of feed-forward immunity, it has been shown that the injection of anti-proteolipid protein (PLP)-specific CD4[+] T cells against one epitope triggers the activation of PLP-specific CD4[+] T cells towards a second epitope (McMahon *et al.*, 2005). In other tissues, presentation of a vast repertoire of heteroclitic epitopes to the immune system can enhance the generation of adaptive immune responses to self antigens (Engelhorn *et al.*, 2006).

Attention must also be given to the cross-presentation of antigen under non-inflammatory conditions. Clones of CD8[+] T cells specific for myelin antigens have been isolated from the periphery of normal donors (Tsuchida *et al.*, 1994; Dressel *et al.*, 1997), suggesting that this is a constitutive process. While it is not surprising that cross-presentation results in the priming of CD8[+] T cells after brain injury, it is unclear if a constitutive pathway for cross-tolerance exists. In a CD4[+] T cell-mediated model of EAE, tolerance towards myelin basic protein results in decreased responses to other CNS antigens (Al-Sabbagh *et al.*, 1994). Dendritic cells could also play a tolerogenic role under steady-state conditions in the brain (Serot *et al.*, 2000). In a CD4[+] T cell-mediated model of EAE, brain-resident DCs have been shown to induce tolerance against autoantigens after the onset of disease (Suter *et al.*, 2003). Other possibilities for tolerance come from central tolerance in the thymus during T cell development and peripheral tolerance from LN stromal cells (Lee *et al.*, 2007).

CD4[+] T cell help in generating CD8[+] T cell-mediated CNS disease

While much of this discussion has focused on the activation of CD8[+] T cells, it is important to recognize the role of CD4[+] T cells in determining the outcome of DC–CD8[+] T cell interactions. For certain, CD4[+] T cells are a critical determinant of when antigen is being cross-presented and in their absence, cross-presentation results in the tolerization of T cells, a phenomenon termed "cross-tolerance" (Heath *et al.*, 1998; Steinman *et al.*, 2000). This was first demonstrated in a model for peripheral tolerance using a neo-self antigen, chicken ovalbumin protein (OVA), expressed specifically in the β cells of the pancreas (Kurts *et al.*, 1996). When OVA-specific, MHC I-restricted TCR transgenic CD8[+] T cells were adoptively transferred into these mice, the T cells accumulated and expanded in the draining lymph node.

These T cells were responding to antigen cross-presented by bone marrow-derived cells and not to the islet cells themselves. Following the observed proliferation, the T cells died via apoptosis, suggestive of peripheral tolerance or deletion of self-reactive CTLs (Heath *et al.*, 1998; Kurts *et al.*, 1996, 1998, 1999). In contrast, when both OVA-specific MHC I- and MHC II-restricted TCR transgenic T cells were transferred into the same mice, the CD8[+] T cells became effector cells and lysed the OVA-expressing islet cells, resulting in diabetes (Bennett *et al.*, 1997; Kurts *et al.*, 1997). It was therefore proposed that a bone marrow-derived cell captures exogenous antigens for both class I and class II presentation, transports these antigens to the lymph node and cross-presents them to CD4[+] and CD8[+] T cells.

For CNS antigen, it has been recently demonstrated that, as for antigen captured from the pancreas, cross-priming requires CD4[+] T cell help (Walter and Albert, 2007). In particular, CD40 engagement on the cross-presenting DC is critical, a pathway reminiscent of the "licensing" model that has been proposed for other tissue-restricted antigen (Lanzavecchia *et al.*, 1998). It is interesting to note that many of the defined genetic susceptibility determinants of MS map to the MHC II locus (Ebers *et al.*, 1996; Haines *et al.*, 1996; Sawcer *et al.*, 1996). Perhaps these genetic susceptibility loci relate to the role of CD4[+] T cells as the gatekeepers for cross-priming brain antigen-reactive CD8[+] T cells. This mechanism could also play a role in the PNDs as well; however, HLA association has yet to be defined.

Conclusion

The CD8[+] T cells are highly potent cells that are capable of cytotoxicity. They can provide defense against viral and microbial infections of the CNS by direct cytotoxicity or by limiting their spread by killing infected cells. They can also participate in the detection and clearance of neoplastic cells. In addition, CD8[+] T cells are important effectors in autoimmune and degenerative CNS diseases such as PND and MS, but CD8[+] T cells that react to brain autoantigens are a regular feature of the healthy immune repertoire. After CD8[+] T cells are primed in LNs, they can enter the CNS where, in lesional or inflamed tissue, CNS cells can be recognized by the invading autoimmune CD8[+] T cells. Treatment to eliminate or modulate antigen-specific CD8[+] T cells in PND and MS should be considered as a therapeutic approach.

It remains unclear whether the development of CNS pathologies such as MS is due to a failure to tolerize T cells to CNS antigens, or alternatively, to the activation of leukocytes outside the CNS by similar antigens expressed in the peripheral nervous system or by other tissues, or from T cell priming selectively in the cervical LNs that drain the CNS. Studies of early cases of MS favor the former possibility because initial demyelinating lesions are composed primarily of activated microglia and macrophages and not lymphocytes (Barnett and Prineas, 2004). Although, to date, there have been no clinical trials that uniquely target CD8$^+$ T cell immune responses, manipulation of CD8$^+$ T cells could provide ways to induce suppression of the cells that otherwise mediate pathogenic effects in a cell- and antigen-specific manner. Understanding the cascade of events resulting in CD8$^+$ T cell-mediated CNS disease is important to treating a range of CD8$^+$ T cell-mediated disorders.

References

Albert ML, Darnell RB. Paraneoplastic neurological degenerations: keys to tumour immunity. *Nat Rev Cancer* 2004; **4**(1): 36–44.

Albert ML, *et al*. Tumor-specific killer cells in paraneoplastic cerebellar degeneration. *Nat Med* 1998; **4**(11): 1321–4.

Albert ML, *et al*. Detection and treatment of activated T cells in the cerebrospinal fluid of patients with paraneoplastic cerebellar degeneration. *Ann Neurol* 2000; **47**: 9–17.

Aloisi F, Pujol-Borrell R. Lymphoid neogenesis in chronic inflammatory diseases. *Nat Rev Immunol* 2006; **6**(3): 205–17.

Al-Sabbagh A, *et al*. Antigen-driven tissue-specific suppression following oral tolerance: Orally administered myelin basic protein suppresses proteolipid protein-induced experimental autoimmune encephalomyelitis in the SJL mouse. *Eur J Immunol* 1994; **24**(9): 2104–9.

Babbe H, *et al*. Clonal expansions of CD8(+) T cells dominate the T cell infiltrate in active multiple sclerosis lesions as shown by micromanipulation and single cell polymerase chain reaction. *J Exp Med* 2000; **192**(3): 393–404.

Barnett MH, Prineas JW. Relapsing and remitting multiple sclerosis: Pathology of the newly forming lesion. *Ann Neurol* 2004; **55**(4): 458–68.

Bennett SR, *et al*. Induction of a CD8+ cytotoxic T lymphocyte response by cross-priming requires cognate CD4+ T cell help. *J Exp Med* 1997; **186**(1): 65–70.

Bergmann CC, *et al*. Microglia exhibit clonal variability in eliciting cytotoxic T lymphocyte responses independent of class I expression. *Cell Immunol* 1999; **198**(1): 44–53.

Bitsch A, *et al*. Acute axonal injury in multiple sclerosis. Correlation with demyelination and inflammation. *Brain* 2000; **123**(6): 1174–83.

Booss J, *et al*. Immunohistological analysis of T lymphocyte subsets in the central nervous system in chronic progressive multiple sclerosis. *J Neurol Sci* 1983; **62**(1–3): 219–32.

Bugawan TL, *et al*. High-resolution HLA class I typing in the CEPH families: Analysis of linkage disequilibrium among HLA loci. *Tissue Antigens* 2000; **56**(5): 392–404.

Calzascia T, *et al*. Homing phenotypes of tumor-specific CD8 T cells are predetermined at the tumor site by crosspresenting APCs. *Immunity* 2005; **22**(2): 175–84.

Carson MJ, *et al*. Disproportionate recruitment of CD8+ T cells into the central nervous system by professional antigen-presenting cells. *Am J Pathol* 1999; **154**(2): 481–94.

Darnell RB. Onconeural antigens and the paraneoplastic neurologic disorders: At the intersection of cancer, immunity, and the brain. *Proc Natl Acad Sci USA* 1996; **93**(10): 4529–36.

De Vos AF, *et al*. Transfer of central nervous system autoantigens and presentation in secondary lymphoid organs. *J Immunol* 2002; **169**(10): 5415–23.

Dressel A, *et al*. Autoantigen recognition by human CD8 T cell clones: Enhanced agonist response induced by altered peptide ligands. *J Immunol* 1997; **159**(10): 4943–51.

Ebers GC, *et al*. A full genome search in multiple sclerosis. *Nat Genet* 1996; **13**(4): 472–6.

Engelhorn ME, *et al*. Autoimmunity and tumor immunity induced by immune responses to mutations in self. *Nat Med* 2006; **12**(2): 198–206.

Fabry Z, *et al*. Nervous tissue as an immune compartment: The dialect of the immune response in the CNS. *Immunol Today* 1994; **15**(5): 218–24.

Furneaux HF, *et al*. Autoantibody synthesis in the central nervous system of patients with paraneoplastic syndromes. *Neurology* 1990; **40**(7): 1085–91.

Gay FW, *et al*. The application of multifactorial cluster analysis in the staging of plaques in early multiple sclerosis. Identification and characterization of the primary demyelinating lesion. *Brain* 1997; **120**(8): 1461–83.

Gordon LB, *et al*. Normal cerebrospinal fluid suppresses the in vitro development of cytotoxic T cells: Role of the brain microenvironment in CNS immune regulation. *J Neuroimmunol* 1998; **88**(1–2): 77–84.

Greter M, *et al*. Dendritic cells permit immune invasion of the CNS in an animal model of multiple sclerosis. *Nat Med* 2005; **11**(3): 328–34.

Hatterer E, *et al*. How to drain without lymphatics? Dendritic cells migrate from the cerebrospinal fluid to the B-cell follicles of cervical lymph nodes. *Blood* 2006; **107**(2): 806–12.

Hawkins BT, Davis TP. The blood–brain barrier/neurovascular unit in health and disease. *Pharmacol Rev* 2005; **57**(2): 173–85.

Heath WR, Carbone FR. Cross-presentation, dendritic cells, tolerance and immunity. *Annu Rev Immunol* 2001; **19**: 47–64.

Heath WR, *et al*. Cross-tolerance: A pathway for inducing tolerance to peripheral tissue antigens. *J Exp Med* 1998; **187**(10): 1549–53.

Hickey WF. Migration of hematogenous cells through the blood–brain barrier and the initiation of CNS inflammation. *Brain Pathol* 1991; **1**(2): 97–105.

Hickey WF. Leukocyte traffic in the central nervous system: The participants and their roles. *Semin Immunol* 1999; **11**(2): 125–37.

Hickey WF, Kimura H. Perivascular microglial cells of the CNS are bone marrow-derived and present antigen in vivo. *Science* 1988; **239**(4837): 290–2.

Hickey WF, *et al*. T-lymphocyte entry into the central nervous system. *J Neurosci Res* 1991; **28**(2): 254–60.

Huseby ES, *et al*. A pathogenic role for myelin-specific CD8(+) T cells in a model for multiple sclerosis. *J Exp Med* 2001; **194**(5): 669–76.

Karman J, et al. Initiation of immune responses in brain is promoted by local dendritic cells. *J Immunol* 2004; **173**(4): 2353–61.

Kort JJ, et al. Efficient presentation of myelin oligodendrocyte glycoprotein peptides but not protein by astrocytes from HLA-DR2 and HLA-DR4 transgenic mice. *J Neuroimmunol* 2006; **173**(1–2): 23–34.

Kurts C, et al. Constitutive class I-restricted exogenous presentation of self antigens in vivo. *J Exp Med* 1996; **184**(3): 923–30.

Kurts C, et al. CD4+ T cell help impairs CD8+ T cell deletion induced by cross-presentation of self-antigens and favors autoimmunity. *J Exp Med* 1997; **186**(12): 2057–62.

Kurts C, et al. CD8 T cell ignorance or tolerance to islet antigens depends on antigen dose. *Proc Natl Acad Sci USA* 1999; **96**(22): 12703–7.

Lang A, Nikolich-Zugich J. Development and migration of protective CD8+ T cells into the nervous system following ocular herpes simplex virus-1 infection. *J Immunol* 2005; **174**(5): 2919–25.

Lanzavecchia A. Immunology. Licence to kill [news; comment]. *Nature* 1998; **393**(6684): 413–14.

Lauterbach H, et al. Adoptive immunotherapy induces CNS dendritic cell recruitment and antigen presentation during clearance of a persistent viral infection. *J Exp Med* 2006; **203**(8): 1963–75.

Lawson LJ, et al. Heterogeneity in the distribution and morphology of microglia in the normal adult mouse brain. *Neuroscience* 1990; **39**(1): 151–70.

Lee JW, et al. Peripheral antigen display by lymph node stroma promotes T cell tolerance to intestinal self. *Nat Immunol* 2007; **8**(2): 181–90.

Lindsey JW, et al. Repeated treatment with chimeric anti-CD4 antibody in multiple sclerosis. *Ann Neurol* 1994; **36**(2): 183–9.

Lucchinetti C, et al. Heterogeneity of multiple sclerosis lesions: Implications for the pathogenesis

of demyelination. *Ann Neurol* 2000; **47**(6): 707–17.

McMahon EJ, et al. Epitope spreading initiates in the CNS in two mouse models of multiple sclerosis. *Nat Med* 2005; **11**(3): 335–9.

McRae BL, et al. Functional evidence for epitope spreading in the relapsing pathology of experimental autoimmune encephalomyelitis. *J Exp Med* 1995; **182**(1): 75–85.

Miller SD, et al. Blockade of CD28/B7–1 interaction prevents epitope spreading and clinical relapses of murine EAE. *Immunity* 1995; **3**(6): 739–45.

Neumann H. Control of glial immune function by neurons. *Glia* 2001; **36**(2): 191–9.

Neumann H, et al. Cytotoxic T lymphocytes in autoimmune and degenerative CNS diseases. *Trends Neurosci* 2002; **25**(6): 313–19.

Oksenberg JR, et al. Limited heterogeneity of rearranged T-cell receptor V alpha transcripts in brains of multiple sclerosis patients. *Nature* 1990; **345**(6273): 344–6.

Pashenkov M, Link H. Dendritic cells and immune responses in the central nervous system. *Trends Immunol* 2002; **23**(2): 69–70.

Ransohoff RM, et al. Three or more routes for leukocyte migration into the central nervous system. *Nat Rev Immunol* 2003; **3**(7): 569–81.

Reese TS, Karnovsky MJ. Fine structural localization of a blood–brain barrier to exogenous peroxidase. *J Cell Biol* 1967; **34**(1): 207–17.

Reichmann G, et al. Dendritic cells and dendritic-like microglia in focal cortical ischemia of the mouse brain. *J Neuroimmunol* 2002; **129**(1–2): 125–32.

Rousseau A, et al. T cell response to Hu-D peptides in patients with anti-Hu syndrome. *J Neurooncol* 2005; **71**(3): 231–6.

Santambrogio L, et al. Developmental plasticity of CNS microglia. *Proc Natl Acad Sci USA* 2001; **98**(11): 6295–300.

Sawcer S, et al. A genome screen in multiple sclerosis reveals susceptibility loci on chromosome

6p21 and 17q22. *Nat Genet* 1996; **13**(4): 464–8.

Seamons A, et al. Endogenous myelin basic protein is presented in the periphery by both dendritic cells and resting B cells with different functional consequences. *J Immunol* 2006; **177**(4): 2097–106.

Serafini B, et al. Intracerebral recruitment and maturation of dendritic cells in the onset and progression of experimental autoimmune encephalomyelitis. *Am J Pathol* 2000; **157**(6): 1991–2002.

Serot JM, et al. Monocyte-derived IL-10-secreting dendritic cells in choroid plexus epithelium. *J Neuroimmunol* 2000; **105**(2): 115–9.

Steinman L. Multiple sclerosis: A coordinated immunological attack against myelin in the central nervous system. *Cell* 1996; **85**(3): 299–302.

Steinman L. Assessment of animal models for MS and demyelinating disease in the design of rational therapy. *Neuron* 1999; **24**(3): 511–4.

Steinman RM, et al. The induction of tolerance by dendritic cells that have captured apoptotic cells. *J Exp Med* 2000; **191**(3): 411–6.

Suter T, et al. The brain as an immune privileged site: Dendritic cells of the central nervous system inhibit T cell activation. *Eur J Immunol* 2003; **33**(11): 2998–3006.

Tsuchida T, et al. Autoreactive CD8+ T-cell responses to human myelin protein-derived peptides. *Proc Natl Acad Sci USA* 1994; **91**(23): 10859–63.

Tsukada N, et al. Adhesion of cerebral endothelial cells to lymphocytes from patients with multiple sclerosis. *Autoimmunity* 1993; **14**(4): 329–33.

Tuohy VK, et al. Diversity and plasticity of self recognition during the development of multiple sclerosis. *J Clin Invest* 1997; **99**(7): 1682–90.

Tuohy VK, et al. Spontaneous regression of primary autoreactivity during chronic progression of experimental autoimmune encephalomyelitis and multiple sclerosis. *J Exp Med* 1999; **189**(7): 1033–42.

Van Oosten BW, *et al.* Treatment of multiple sclerosis with the monoclonal anti-CD4 antibody cM-T412: Results of a randomized, double-blind, placebo-controlled, MR-monitored phase II trial. *Neurology* 1997; **49**(2): 351–7.

Vass K, Lassmann H. Intrathecal application of interferon gamma. Progressive appearance of MHC antigens within the rat nervous system. *Am J Pathol* 1990; **137**(4): 789–800.

Voltz R, *et al.* T-cell receptor analysis in anti-Hu associated paraneoplastic encephalomyelitis. *Neurology* 1998; **51**(4): 1146–50.

Walter BA, *et al.* The olfactory route for cerebrospinal fluid drainage into the peripheral lymphatic system. *Neuropathol Appl Neurobiol* 2006b; **32**(4): 388–96.

Walter L, Albert ML. Cross-presented intracranial antigen primes CD8+ T cells. *J Immunol* 2007; **178**(10): 6038–42.

Walter U, Santamaria P. CD8+ T cells in autoimmunity. *Curr Opin Immunol* 2005; **17**(6): 624–31.

Yamada S, *et al.* Albumin outflow into deep cervical lymph from different regions of rabbit brain. *Am J Physiol* 1991; **261**(4 Pt 2): H1197–204.

Yu M, *et al.* A predictable sequential determinant spreading cascade invariably accompanies progression of experimental autoimmune encephalomyelitis: A basis for peptide-specific therapy after onset of clinical disease. *J Exp Med* 1996; **183**(4): 1777–88.

Chapter 8

Acute disseminated encephalomyelitis: determinants and manifestations

Eppie M. Yiu and Andrew J. Kornberg

Introduction

Acute disseminated encephalomyelitis (ADEM) is classically a monophasic inflammatory condition of the CNS that usually presents in children and young adults. It typically occurs following a viral prodrome with multifocal neurologic disturbance and altered conscious state. The majority of children make a full recovery. In recent years, a number of series describing the clinical and radiological features of childhood ADEM have been published (Dale *et al.*, 2000; Hynson *et al.*, 2001; Murthy *et al.*, 2002; Tenembaum *et al.*, 2002) with a focus on the differentiation between ADEM and multiple sclerosis (MS) at first presentation (Brass *et al.*, 2004; Dale and Branson, 2005).

Epidemiology

Acute disseminated encephalomyelitis is uncommon (Dale *et al.*, 2000; Hynson *et al.*, 2001; Tenembaum *et al.*, 2002), with a reported incidence of approximately 0.4 per 100,000, based on a retrospective analysis of medical records (Leake *et al.*, 2004) Most studies have not demonstrated a gender bias, although an Argentinian study reported a male predominance (Tenembaum *et al.*, 2002). Peak incidence occurs in children aged 4–8 years (Dale *et al.*, 2000; Hynson *et al.*, 2001; Murthy *et al.*, 2002; Tenembaum *et al.*, 2002).

Three-quarters of patients have a history of a prodromal illness or vaccination within the 4–6 weeks prior to symptom onset, with a mean latency of 2 weeks (Dale *et al.*, 2000; Hynson *et al.*, 2001; Murthy *et al.*, 2002; Tenembaum *et al.*, 2002). Not surprisingly, seasonal variation is seen, with ADEM being more common in the winter months.

Upper respiratory tract infections are the commonest associated prodromal illness, although either serological or culture evidence of the organism is often absent. Preceding gastroenteritis or varicella infection is not uncommon, with the incidence of ADEM following varicella infection estimated to be 1 in 10,000 cases (Stuve and Zamvil, 1999). Other specific organisms associated with ADEM include measles, mumps, herpes simplex virus (HSV), including post-HSV encephalitis, human herpes virus-6, Epstein–Barr virus, cytomegalovirus, influenza, enterovirus, *Mycoplasma pneumoniae*, Group A Streptococcus, *Chlamydia pneumoniae*, hepatitis A, and Coxsackie virus (Pasternak *et al.*, 1980; Kaji *et al.*, 1996; Kamei *et al.*, 1997; Heick and Skriver, 2000; Revel-Vilk *et al.*, 2000; Dale *et al.*, 2000, 2001; Hynson *et al.*, 2001; Tenembaum *et al.*, 2002; Saitoh *et al.*, 2004; Tan *et al.*, 2004).

Acute disseminated encephalomyelitis has also been documented post-vaccination. Implicated vaccines include hepatitis B, measles, pertussis, BCG, Japanese B encephalitis, smallpox, rabies, and the oral polio vaccine (Ohtaki *et al.*, 1992; Apak *et al.*, 1999; Dale *et al.*, 2000; Ozawa *et al.*, 2000; Hynson *et al.*, 2001; Tenembaum *et al.*, 2002).

Pathophysiology

Acute disseminated encephalomyelitis is thought to have an autoimmune basis. Pathologic similarities to experimental allergic encephalomyelitis (EAE), an animal model of inflammatory demyelination, support this theory (Stonehouse *et al.*, 2003). It is postulated that a common antigen shared by an infectious agent and a myelin epitope results in an autoimmune response. Proposed myelin autoantigens include myelin basic protein (MBP), proteolipid protein and myelin oligodendrocyte protein (Stuve and Zamvil, 1999). Studies of children with ADEM have shown that blood lymphocytes, particularly Th2 cells, have increased reactivity to MBP compared to those with encephalitis or normal controls (Pohl-Koppe *et al.*, 1998).

Inflammatory Diseases of the Central Nervous System, ed. T. Kilpatrick, R. M. Ransohoff and S. Wesselingh. Published by Cambridge University Press. © Cambridge University Press 2010

Expression of cellular adhesion molecules such as ICAM-1 and selectins are thought to mediate lymphocyte migration across the blood–brain barrier (Hartung *et al.*, 1995). These adhesion molecules are over-expressed in EAE and multiple sclerosis, implying a role in brain inflammatory processes, with elevated soluble forms of these molecules detected in the serum and cerebrospinal fluid of MS patients (Hartung *et al.*, 1995; Lee and Benveniste, 1999). A study showing increased expression of soluble adhesion molecules such as soluble E-selectin and soluble ICAM-1 in the serum of children with ADEM suggests similar involvement of these molecules in the pathogenesis of ADEM (Martino *et al.*, 2005).

Histologic findings include demyelination with relative axonal sparing, perivascular lymphocytic cuffing and an abundant inflammatory infiltrate of lymphocytes and lipid-laden macrophages containing myelin degradation products. Gliosis and astrocyte hyperplasia can also be seen (Dale *et al.*, 2000; Hynson *et al.*, 2001).

Clinical features

At present, there are no accepted diagnostic criteria for the diagnosis of ADEM. The clinical findings are often diverse, multifocal, and variable between patients.

Progression to maximal neurologic deficit occurs over 4–7 days, on average. However, variations are seen, with acute and rapid progression within a day in some patients, to a more indolent course of up to 45 days in others (Dale *et al.*, 2000; Hynson *et al.*, 2001; Tenembaum *et al.*, 2002). Children that present more indolently usually have symptoms such as a change in behavior and withdrawal (Dale *et al.*, 2000; Hynson *et al.*, 2001). Ongoing deterioration after admission to hospital is not uncommon, occurring in up to one-third of patients (Hynson *et al.*, 2001; Murthy *et al.*, 2002).

Systemic symptoms are often a prominent feature, with fever present in 40–50% of patients (Hynson *et al.*, 2001; Murthy *et al.*, 2002). Headache is present in up to 40% of patients, vomiting in a third, and meningism in 5–40%. Seizures occur in 10–30% of children and may be generalized or focal, and sometimes associated with fever (Hynson *et al.*, 2001; Murthy *et al.*, 2002; Tenembaum *et al.*, 2002).

Neurological signs are variable and depend on the location of the demyelinating lesions. Motor deficits and impaired consciousness are the most common features (Dale *et al.*, 2000; Hynson *et al.*, 2001;

Murthy *et al.*, 2002; Tenembaum *et al.*, 2002). Recently published consensus definitions propose that for a diagnosis of ADEM, there should be evidence of encephalopathy, as well as a polysymptomatic presentation. Encephalopathy can manifest as an alteration in consciousness such as somnolence or coma, or behavioral change such as irritability or lethargy (Krupp *et al.*, 2007). In recent childhood series, impaired consciousness was present in 45–70% of children and irritability in 40% (Dale *et al.*, 2000; Hynson *et al.*, 2001; Murthy *et al.*, 2002; Tenembaum *et al.*, 2002). Motor deficits were seen in up to 85% of patients, and consisted of hemiparesis, paraparesis, monoparesis and ataxia. Upper motor neuron signs were common. Ataxia was present in 50–60% of patients and was the commonest presenting feature in two series (Hynson *et al.*, 2001; Gupte *et al.*, 2003), and is generally present at the onset of the illness rather than developing later on (Hynson *et al.*, 2001).

Cranial nerve abnormalities are seen in 20–50% of children and include facial weakness, ophthalmoplegia, visual disturbance and, less commonly, swallowing difficulties (Dale *et al.*, 2000; Hynson *et al.*, 2001; Murthy *et al.*, 2002; Tenembaum *et al.*, 2002). Optic neuritis was present in 23% of children in one series, being bilateral in all cases with significant impairment of visual acuity (Dale *et al.*, 2000). This tendency for bilateral rather than unilateral optic neuritis has also been found in other series (Tenembaum *et al.*, 2002; Richer *et al.*, 2005). Language disturbance manifesting as mutism, aphasia or other language disturbance is an interesting and not uncommon presenting feature, occurring in 5–26% of children. It occurs in children with left, right and bilateral motor dysfunction (Hynson *et al.*, 2001; Murthy *et al.*, 2002; Tenembaum *et al.*, 2002).

Admission to intensive care for ventilation occurs in up to 30% of patients (Dale *et al.*, 2000; Murthy *et al.*, 2002; Tenembaum *et al.*, 2002).

Concurrent spinal cord involvement or myelitis is also relatively common (3–25%) (Dale *et al.*, 2000; Hynson *et al.*, 2001; Tenembaum *et al.*, 2002) and reflects the multifocal nature of demyelination seen in ADEM. Whilst it can be difficult to differentiate clinically if some symptoms and signs arise from brain or spinal cord demyelination, bladder or bowel disturbance such as urinary retention or constipation, areflexia, a discrete sensory level or absent abdominal reflexes indicate spinal cord involvement (Yiu *et al.*, 2009). Sensory deficits occur in 3–30% of cases, generally in children with evidence of spinal cord disease (Dale *et al.*, 2000; Hynson *et al.*, 2001; Murthy *et al.*, 2002; Tenembaum *et al.*, 2002).

Despite the often frequent deep gray matter involvement seen on neuro-imaging, there is a relatively low frequency (up to 12%) of extrapyramidal features clinically. Cogwheel rigidity, athetosis, choreoathetosis, hemidystonia, paroxysmal hemidystonia and hemichorea have been described (Dale *et al.*, 2000; Tenembaum *et al.*, 2002). Post-streptococcal ADEM appears to have a higher frequency of extrapyramidal symptoms (up to 50%), with prominent basal ganglia involvement on MRI (Dale *et al.*, 2001). Other more unusual clinical manifestations of ADEM include transient amaurosis (Aydin *et al.*, 2005), acute psychosis (Nasr *et al.*, 2000) and Landau Kleffner syndrome (Perniola *et al.*, 1993).

Adults with ADEM share similar clinical features, however lower rates of preceding infection, fever and meningism are seen (Schwarz *et al.*, 2001).

Investigations

Laboratory investigations

Investigations of the peripheral blood often show non-specific findings of inflammation. A raised white cell count (especially lymphocytosis) is very common, and is seen in up to two-thirds of patients (Dale *et al.*, 2000; Murthy *et al.*, 2002). The erythrocyte sedimentation rate and C-reactive protein are also often raised.

The CSF is often abnormal with a raised protein or pleocytosis in 70% of patients (Dale *et al.*, 2000; Hynson *et al.*, 2001; Tenembaum *et al.*, 2002). Lymphocytes are usually the predominant cell type in the CSF, with a mean count of 40–50 white cells/mm^3. Cell counts of up to 600 white cells/mm^3 have been reported (Murray *et al.*, 2000).

The presence of intra-thecal synthesis of oligoclonal bands ranges from 0 to 29% of ADEM cases in paediatric series (Dale *et al.*, 2000; Hynson *et al.*, 2001; Murthy *et al.*, 2002; Tenembaum *et al.*, 2002). The series by Dale *et al.* where 29% had true CSF oligoclonal bands showed that none of these children developed further episodes of demyelination at a mean of 6.5 years follow up (Dale *et al.*, 2000). In adults, CSF oligoclonal bands are reported in 58% of ADEM patients in one large series (Schwarz *et al.*, 2001). Oligoclonal bands are also seen in other conditions such as CNS infections and inflammatory conditions (Zeman *et al.*, 1993).

Neurophysiology

Electroencephalograms often show non-specific diffuse or less commonly focal slowing of the background activity, reflecting the encephalopathic process. Epileptiform discharges are much less common (Dale *et al.*, 2000; Hynson *et al.*, 2001; Murthy *et al.*, 2002; Tenembaum *et al.*, 2002).

Visual evoked potentials are abnormal in children with optic neuritis, but occasionally are also abnormal in children without visual symptoms or signs (Dale *et al.*, 2000).

Nerve conduction studies are normal in ADEM (Dale *et al.*, 2000), however cases of ADEM associated with Guillain-Barré syndrome (GBS) and polyradiculitis, with either electrophysiologic or pathologic confirmation have been described (Amit *et al.*, 1986; Kinoshita *et al.*, 1996). Concurrent transverse myelitis and polyradiculitis has also been described in the literature (Martens-Le Bouar and Korinthenberg, 2002; Yiu *et al.*, 2009).

Imaging findings

Abnormalities on computer tomography (CT) scans are reported in 11–78% of patients (Dale *et al.*, 2000; Murthy *et al.*, 2002; Tenembaum *et al.*, 2002; Gupte *et al.*, 2003), although in our experience this is more in the order of 5–10%. This could reflect the lower radiation doses now used in our center for CT scans due to concerns about malignancy risk, particularly in children (Brenner *et al.*, 2001; de Campo *et al.*, 2003). The CT findings usually consist of hypodense lesions in the white matter, often in patients with corresponding large demyelinating lesions on magnetic resonance imaging (MRI). Smaller subtle lesions tend not to be seen (Tenembaum *et al.*, 2002).

Magnetic resonance imaging is the investigation of choice. Lesions are seen much more readily on T2-weighted and FLAIR (fluid-attenuated inversion recovery) sequences than T1-weighted images. Lesions are typically bilateral but asymmetric, and are highly variable in terms of number, size, and location of lesions, although some typical features of ADEM have been described.

White matter abnormalities are almost universal, occurring in 90% of patients (Kesselring *et al.*, 1990; Hynson *et al.*, 2001; Murthy *et al.*, 2002; Tenembaum *et al.*, 2002) with subcortical white matter involvement being the most common (in up to 90% of cases) (see Figure 8.1a). There is a predilection for the frontal, parietal and occipital regions (Hynson *et al.*, 2001;

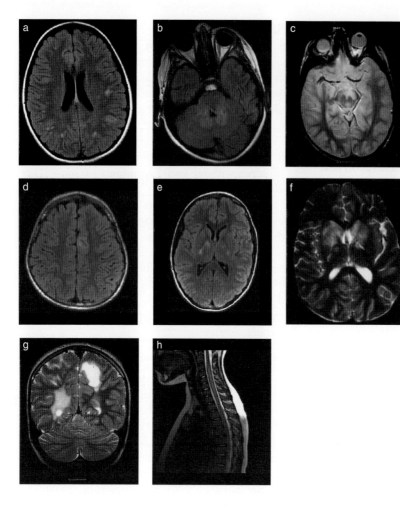

Figure 8.1 *a*. Axial FLAIR image of a 12-year-old boy with ADEM. Multiple areas of hyperintensity are seen in the subcortical white matter of the parietal and occipital regions, bilaterally. *b*. Axial FLAIR image of the same 12-year-old boy as in part (a), showing hyperintensity in the cerebellar white matter and peduncles, bilaterally. *c*. Axial FLAIR image showing hyperintensity in the pons. *d*. Axial FLAIR image of a 9-year-old boy with ADEM showing an area of hyperintensity involving cortical gray matter of the inferior frontal lobe. *e*. Axial FLAIR image of a 14-year-old boy with ADEM showing bilateral involvement of the basal ganglia. *f*. Axial T2 image of another child with ADEM, also showing bilateral but asymmetric hyperintensity in the basal ganglia. *g*. Coronal FLAIR image of a 7-year-old boy with ADEM showing large confluent areas of demyelination in the white matter, bilaterally. *h*. Sagittal T2 image of the spine of the 12-year-old boy in (a) and (b) who also had spinal cord involvement (myelitis). Contiguous T2 hyperintensity is seen involving the cervical and upper thoracic cord, with cord swelling in the cervical region.

Gupte *et al.*, 2003). Periventricular white matter lesions are less common (seen in 30–60%; Dale *et al.*, 2000; Hynson *et al.*, 2001; Murthy *et al.*, 2002; Richer *et al.*, 2005), and it has been suggested that relative sparing of periventricular compared to subcortical white matter is predictive of ADEM compared to MS (Dale *et al.*, 2000; Hynson *et al.*, 2001; Murthy *et al.*, 2002). Involvement of the cerebellum, including the cerebellar peduncles, is seen in up to 40% of cases (Caldemeyer *et al.*, 1994; Dale *et al.*, 2000) (Figure 8.1b). Brainstem involvement is also frequent, seen in 40–60% of cases (Dale *et al.*, 2000; Hynson *et al.*, 2001; Khong *et al.*, 2002) (Figure 8.1c). Demyelination of the corpus callosum is relatively uncommon and seen in 7–30% of children, as is involvement of the internal capsule, seen in only 7–28% of cases (Caldemeyer *et al.*, 1994; Dale *et al.*, 2000; Murthy *et al.*, 2002).

Although ADEM is typically described as affecting white matter, gray matter involvement is not unusual because it also contains myelin. Cortical gray lesions can be seen in 10–80% of cases (Baum *et al.*, 1994; Dale *et al.*, 2000; Khong *et al.*, 2002; Murthy *et al.*, 2002), often adjacent to subcortical white matter lesions (Richer *et al.*, 2005) (Figure 8.1d). Several series have also noted that deep gray matter involvement is common, with lesions in the thalamus and basal ganglia seen in up to 60% and 40% of patients, respectively (Baum *et al.*, 1994; Hynson *et al.*, 2001; Khong *et al.*, 2002). It is felt that this is a useful imaging feature distinguishing ADEM from MS, as overt MRI-based involvement of deep gray structures, particularly the thalami, are uncommon in MS (Baum *et al.*, 1994; Hynson *et al.*, 2001). Basal ganglia and thalamic lesions are often bilateral, but asymmetric (Dale *et al.*, 2000; Tenembaum *et al.*, 2002) (Figure 8.1e, f).

Lesions often have poorly defined margins (Dale et al., 2000) and are highly variable in size, with most up to 1 × 1 cm in diameter, with some lesions up to 5 cm in diameter (Khong et al., 2002; Murthy et al., 2002). An average of 17 lesions per patient has been reported (Murthy et al., 2002). More confluent large white matter lesions are also described (Khong et al., 2002; Tenembaum et al., 2002) (Figure 8.1g). Occasionally, ADEM presents as a single, large tumor-like lesion with or without mass effect and gadolinium enhancement (tumefactive demyelination) (Kepes, 1993; Miller et al., 1993; Hynson et al., 2001; Tenembaum et al., 2002). In these cases, brain biopsy is often performed to exclude a tumor.

Tenembaum classified ADEM patients into four groups according to the abnormalities seen on MRI in the acute stage of the disease. Group A (62%) consisted of ADEM with small lesions (<5mm); Group B (24%) ADEM with large confluent white matter lesions; Group C (12%) ADEM with symmetric bithalamic involvement and small or large white matter lesions; and Group D (2%) acute hemorrhagic encephalomyelitis with haemorrhage into large demyelinating lesions (Tenembaum et al., 2002).

Contrast enhancement can occur in lesions where there is a breakdown of the blood–brain barrier, generally seen in the acute phase of ADEM. In theory, all new lesions should enhance with gadolinium, but in practice, gadolinium enhancement is only seen in about one-third of cases (Hynson et al., 2001; Murthy et al., 2002; Richer et al., 2005).

Concurrent spinal cord involvement is seen in up to 30% of cases of ADEM (Dale et al., 2000), although it is difficult to determine the true frequency of involvement as the cord is often not routinely imaged. Axial T2 images are the most sensitive for detecting spinal cord abnormalities. Typically there is quite extensive cord involvement, with lesions involving many spinal segments (average of 11 spinal segments) in a contiguous manner (Figure 8.1h). It is not uncommon for the entire spinal cord to be involved. On axial images, involvement of the whole cord (holocord) or gray matter of the cord are the most common findings. Cord swelling is often seen in the cervical region. Gadolinium enhancement is seen in about 50% of cases (Yiu et al., 2009).

Despite the often dramatic MRI findings in ADEM, initial normal MRI scans despite significant neurological deficit have been described, with a lag of subsequent imaging-based changes of up to 3–4 weeks (Murray et al., 2000; Khurana et al., 2005). New lesions can also evolve over a few weeks, even in the presence of clinical improvement (Kesselring et al., 1990; Pradhan et al., 1999; Khurana et al., 2005).

Follow-up imaging

Tenembaum's large study of 84 children, all of whom had regular follow-up MRIs, showed that most had complete or almost complete resolution of lesions between 3 and 24 months (with a mean of 7.2 months) after treatment (Tenembaum et al., 2002). Nevertheless, it is well documented that lesions can persist for up to many years, despite clinical recovery (Kesselring et al., 1990; Dale et al., 2000; Hynson et al., 2001), although they tend to decrease in size, and any enhancement or mass effect present acutely also resolves over time (Hynson et al., 2001). In some patients there is no change in the imaging findings (Apak et al., 1999; Dale et al., 2000; Hynson et al., 2001; Murthy et al., 2002). Atrophy of the cerebrum or spinal cord can also be seen (Khong et al., 2002). Importantly, however, patients with a diagnosis of monophasic ADEM do not develop new demyelinating lesions after 3–6 months of onset.

Treatments

As many children with ADEM present with fever, meningeal signs and encephalopathy, treatment with broad spectrum antibiotics and acyclovir is often the initial treatment until an infectious etiology is excluded.

Although spontaneous improvement without treatment is well documented (Kimura et al., 1996), treatment with high-dose intravenous methylprednisolone followed by a course of oral prednisolone is now the mainstay of treatment, although there are no randomized controlled trials to support this (Dale et al., 2000). Early reports on the use of steroids and/or ACTH were based on cases of measles encephalitis and other acute meningoencephalitides, often showing no benefit in outcome or recovery (Karelitz and Eisenberg, 1961; Ziegra, 1961; Boe et al., 1965). This was unlikely a pure ADEM population, and probably included cases of infective encephalitis. Steroid dosages and duration were also variable.

Pasternak reported benefit from the use of steroids in a small series of children with parainfectious encephalomyelitis. These patients showed a temporally related improvement in neurological status soon after commencement of steroids, and good outcome, overall (Pasternak *et al.*, 1980). This has also been noted in more recent larger series, where clinical improvement within 24 h of the first dose of methylprednisolone was demonstrated in children who had no sign of improvement or deterioration prior to the commencement of steroids (Hynson *et al.*, 2001). Other case reports of ADEM responding to steroids have also been published (Straub *et al.*, 1997; Hawley, 1998). The more recent series of children with ADEM show that most have a good long-term outcome after treatment with steroids (Dale *et al.*, 2000; Hynson *et al.*, 2001; Tenembaum *et al.*, 2002), supporting the generally accepted opinion that steroids improve prognosis. It has also been suggested that a prolonged weaning regimen of 6 weeks or more could decrease the risk of relapse and a multiphasic course of the illness (Dale *et al.*, 2000).

Whilst steroids are the mainstay of treatment, other immunomodulatory therapies have been tried, including immunoglobulin and plasmapheresis. Immunoglobulin has been reported to be successful in a case report in a child with ADEM (Kleiman and Brunquell, 1995), and also in other case reports or small series of adults and children who did not appear to respond to steroids (Pradhan *et al.*, 1999; Sahlas *et al.*, 2000). Plasmapheresis has also been reported to be successful in more severe cases of ADEM not responsive to steroids and/or immunoglobulin (Kanter *et al.*, 1995; Keegan *et al.*, 2002; Khurana *et al.*, 2005). It is difficult to prove which immunomodulatory treatment resulted in clinical improvement in these cases.

Supportive care is paramount. This includes ventilatory support, bladder catherization for patients with spinal cord involvement, use of gastric protection for steroids, and involvement of physiotherapy, occupational therapy, and speech therapy, as required.

Outcome

In the past, the mortality of ADEM has been described to be as high as 10–30%, related, in particular, to postinfectious measles ADEM which is now uncommon due to immunization (Epperson *et al.*, 1988; Rust, 2000). More recent childhood series document survival rates of 100% (Dale *et al.*, 2000; Hynson *et al.*, 2001; Murthy *et al.*, 2002; Tenembaum *et al.*, 2002), whilst an adult series had a mortality rate of 3% (Schwarz *et al.*, 2001).

Despite the often dramatic presentation of ADEM, the overall long-term outcome is good, particularly in children, with 57–89% of children making a full recovery (Dale *et al.*, 2000; Hynson *et al.*, 2001; Murthy *et al.*, 2002; Tenembaum *et al.*, 2002). Time to full recovery ranged between 0.25 and 6 months in one series (Dale *et al.*, 2000), with a mean hospitalization time of 1–2 weeks (Hynson *et al.*, 2001; Schwarz *et al.*, 2001; Murthy *et al.*, 2002). Adults with ADEM appear to have a poorer outcome, with only 46% showing complete recovery, excluding those that progressed to an ultimate diagnosis of MS (Schwarz *et al.*, 2001).

Sequelae from ADEM include motor impairment in up to 17%, behavioral problems in up to 11%, significant cognitive deficits in up to 11%, visual impairment in up to 11%, epilepsy in up to 9%, limb parasthesias, recurrent headache, and urinary problems in those who had spinal cord involvement (Dale *et al.*, 2000). In most children, these sequelae are mild. More severe sequelae are uncommon, but include some children requiring a wheelchair long-term (up to 8% in one series). This is more common in children with concurrent myelitis at presentation (Dale *et al.*, 2000). Rarely, patients remain ventilator-dependent: this also appears to occur predominantly in those with spinal cord involvement (O'Riordan *et al.*, 1999; Khong *et al.*, 2002).

More recently, there has been concern regarding long-term mild neurocognitive deficits in children with ADEM who have apparent full clinical recovery, as well as complete resolution of MRI changes. In addition, children who develop ADEM before five years of age appear to have a higher risk of cognitive deficits as well as social, behavioral, and emotional problems in comparison to children affected at older ages (Hahn *et al.*, 2003; Jacobs *et al.*, 2004). This raises the question of the long-term impact on cognition, academic achievement, and vocation, and the need for long-term follow-up (Hahn *et al.*, 2003).

In general, prognostic factors are not well established. It has been suggested that there is a correlation between complete resolution of MRI changes within 6 months and a normal neurologic outcome, whilst incomplete resolution or progression to atrophy is associated with a poorer outcome (Khong *et al.*, 2002; Richer *et al.*, 2005). These studies are small, however, and other series do not suggest this same finding (Hynson *et al.*, 2001). Interestingly, the extent and site of the initial lesions on MRI does not appear to affect clinical outcome (Khong *et al.*, 2002; Tenembaum *et al.*, 2002). One study demonstrated that children with ADEM who presented with optic neuritis tend to have a poorer outcome (Tenembaum *et al.*, 2002).

Recurrent ADEM, biphasic disseminated encephalomyelitis, multiphasic ADEM and multiple sclerosis

Although ADEM is generally regarded as a monophasic illness, further demyelinating events are well described in up to 25% of children (Dale *et al.*, 2000) and 35% of adults (Schwarz *et al.*, 2001). Debate remains around the significance of further demyelinating events, especially in children, in whom MS is relatively uncommon.

Children with an initial diagnosis of ADEM who develop a second episode of demyelination are labelled with a variety of diagnoses, including recurrent ADEM, biphasic disseminated encephalomyelitis, multiphasic disseminated encephalomyelitis as well as MS, depending on the timing of the second episode, the clinical and radiological features at the time, and the presence or absence of further episodes of demyelination on long-term follow-up. The lack of clear diagnostic criteria for the diagnosis of ADEM and the alternative diagnostic possibilities add to the confusion.

It is clear that some children relapse within 2–3 months of the initial episode, often during or soon after steroid wean. Some 25% of children in the series by Dale *et al.* relapsed within 8 weeks of stopping steroid treatment, and subsequently remained relapse-free for a mean follow-up period of 5.3 years. These children were described as having multiphasic disseminated encephalomyelitis rather than MS. In contrast, children with an ultimate diagnosis of MS in the same series relapsed at a mean of 1.1 years (range 0.2–6 years) (Dale *et al.*, 2000). In other series where children have relapsed relatively early, the relapse was regarded more as a protracted course or flare-up of the initial monophasic disease rather than a new episode (Hynson *et al.*, 2001).

Tenembaum's study of 84 children with ADEM reported a group of children with a second polysymptomatic episode of demyelination between 2 months and 8 years following the initial attack. The lack of further clinical events, lack of new lesions on repeat MRIs during the mean follow-up period of 8.2 years, and lack of oligoclonal bands in the CSF were felt to argue against a diagnosis of MS. These children were described as having biphasic disseminated encephalomyelitis (Tenembaum *et al.*, 2002).

Others feel that the occurrence of relapses with clear dissemination in time and space from the initial episode should raise the diagnosis of MS, although the time interval required from the initial episode is not well-defined (Menge *et al.*, 2005). A series of 40 adult ADEM patients reported a 35% progression to a diagnosis of MS, with the second episode of demyelination occurring within the first year of the initial presentation (Schwarz *et al.*, 2001).

Mikaeloff's recent large study of 296 French children who presented with their first episode of CNS demyelination showed that progression to MS is probably more common than previously thought. In this series, 57% of all children with a first episode of demyelination (including clinically isolated syndromes) progressed to a diagnosis of MS, which included 29% of children with an initial diagnosis of ADEM (Mikaeloff *et al.*, 2004b). The median latency to the second attack for children with an initial diagnosis of ADEM was 4 years (range 0.2 to 9.4 years). For patients with onset before age 10, the median latency to a second attack was 6 years compared with 1 year for those older than 10 years at the time of the first demyelinating event. This study has highlighted the fact that prolonged follow-up is necessary in these children in whom a second event could occur many years after the first.

Clear diagnostic criteria for ADEM, as well as for ADEM with further episodes of demyelination, and their differentiation from MS are required if we are to clarify the long-term outcome of ADEM. Recently published consensus definitions aim to provide this framework, and will benefit future prospective studies (Krupp *et al.*, 2007). These guidelines provide definitions for monophasic ADEM, recurrent ADEM, and multiphasic ADEM. Symptoms that vary during periods of steroid taper within 3 months of the initial event, or less than 30 days after discontinuation of steroids are considered part of the initial course of monophasic ADEM. Recurrent ADEM refers to when there is recurrence of *similar* symptoms, signs and neuro-imaging findings more than 3 months after the first ADEM attack and at least 1 month after completing steroid therapy. Multiphasic ADEM, however, refers to *new* symptoms, signs and MRI findings compared to the first ADEM episode more than 3 months after the first attack and at least 1 month after steroid completion (Krupp *et al.*, 2007).

In a child with an initial diagnosis of ADEM, a second demyelinating event that does not meet the criteria for recurrent or multiphasic ADEM is felt to be insufficient for the diagnosis of MS. In order to reach a diagnosis of MS there must be additional evidence of further dissemination in time, either on MRI or clinically, at least 3 months from the second event. This conservative approach is preferred to avoid the potential of incorrectly labeling a child with a diagnosis of MS (Krupp *et al.*, 2007).

Differentiating between ADEM and those at risk of MS at initial presentation

Of prognostic importance at the first episode of demyelination is the diagnostic differentiation between ADEM and a first demyelinating event (FDE) with features typical of an attack of MS, as children with ADEM generally have a good outcome, whereas children in the latter category are more likely to develop subsequent events and disability in the long term (Dale and Branson, 2005). Whilst there are differences, some also regard the two conditions as being on a spectrum of demyelinating disorders (Hartung and Grossman, 2001; Dale and Branson, 2005). These differences are summarized in Table 8.1.

As MS is uncommon in children, with 2.7–4.4% of cases presenting before age 16 (Mikaeloff *et al.*, 2004b), it is not surprising that children with a first presentation of MS are older than those with monophasic ADEM (Dale *et al.*, 2000; Brass *et al.*, 2003; Mikaeloff *et al.*, 2004b). Mikaeloff's large series of children showed a mean age of 7.1 years in children with ADEM compared to 12 years in children with MS. This same series demonstrated that age at onset of a first demyelinating episode of ≥10 years was an adverse prognostic factor for a second episode (Mikaeloff *et al.*, 2004b). Similarly, Rust reported a <6% risk of MS for children who presented with ADEM at age <12 years, compared to a 50% risk for children older than 12 (Rust, 2000).

A preceding infection or vaccination is also more common in ADEM. Although infections are known to precipitate relapse in MS, prodromal infections occur in only 16–38% of children with MS (Dale *et al.*, 2000; Brass *et al.*, 2003; Mikaeloff *et al.*, 2004b).

Encephalopathy is seen in 40–75% of ADEM patients (Dale *et al.*, 2000; Hynson *et al.*, 2001; Murthy *et al.*, 2002; Tenembaum *et al.*, 2002; Mikaeloff *et al.*, 2004b), compared to 13–15% of MS patients (Dale *et al.*, 2000; Mikaeloff *et al.*, 2004b) and is now felt to be an essential diagnostic criterion for NOEM. In addition, non-focal systemic symptoms

Table 8.1 Comparison of characteristic features of ADEM and MS

Characteristic	ADEM	MS
Age at first attack	<10 years	>10 years
Preceding viral infection/ vaccination	Usually present	Less likely
Symptoms and signs	Polysymptomatic	Monosymptomatic
Encephalopathy	Present	Absent
Fever, meningism, headache	Common	Uncommon
Seizures	Not uncommon	Rare
Optic neuritis	Bilateral	Unilateral
CSF lymphocytic pleocytosis	Common	May be present but usually <50 cells/mm^3
CSF oligoclonal bands	0–29% (Dale *et al.*, 2000; Hynson *et al.*, 2001; Murthy *et al.*, 2002; Tenembaum *et al.*, 2002)	40–92% (Dale *et al.*, 2000; Mikaeloff *et al.*, 2004b; Pohl *et al.*, 2004)
MRI features	Ill-defined lesions Extensive lesion load Subcortical white matter lesions Bilateral deep gray matter lesions Cortical gray matter lesions	Well-defined lesions (Dale *et al.*, 2000; Mikaeloff *et al.*, 2004a) Periventricular lesions Callosal lesions especially perpendicular to long axis (Mikaeloff *et al.*, 2004a)
Follow-up MRI	Resolution or no change in lesions	New lesions

and signs such as fever, vomiting, meningism and headache are more common in ADEM, as is a poly-symptomatic presentation (multiple symptoms and signs) (Dale *et al.*, 2000; Brass *et al.*, 2003; Mikaeloff *et al.*, 2004b). Pyramidal signs were felt to be more common in ADEM in one series (Dale *et al.*, 2000), but this was not seen in others (Mikaeloff *et al.*, 2004b). Posterior column dysfunction is uncommon in ADEM (Rust, 1999). Brainstem and cerebellar signs are seen in both and are non-discriminatory (Dale *et al.*, 2000; Brass *et al.*, 2003; Mikaeloff *et al.*, 2004b). Although seizures are not a prominent feature of ADEM, they are rare in MS (Rust, 1999).

True CSF oligoclonal bands are positive in 40–92% of children with MS (Dale *et al.*, 2000; Mikaeloff *et al.*, 2004b; Pohl *et al.*, 2004), often at the first demyelinating episode (Pohl *et al.*, 2004), but only in 0–29% of ADEM patients (Dale *et al.*, 2000; Hynson *et al.*, 2001; Murthy *et al.*, 2002; Tenembaum *et al.*, 2002). A large study of adults by Schwarz *et al.* (2001) did not find the presence of oligoclonal bands useful in discriminating ADEM from MS. Hence the presence of oligoclonal bands does not, on its own, herald a high risk for the development of multiple sclerosis, and other factors must be taken into account.

Magnetic resonance imaging (MRI) features of ADEM have already been discussed, but the main discriminatory features are that the abnormalities are poorly defined compared to MS lesions, there is often a large lesion load, white matter lesions tend to occur in the subcortical white matter with sparing of the periventricular region, and involvement of gray matter (both cortical and deep gray) is common. A recent MRI study of 116 children with a first episode of demyelination showed that lesions perpendicular to the axis of the corpus callosum, and the consistent presence of well-defined lesions, were the greatest risk factors for relapse (Mikaeloff *et al.*, 2004a).

Follow-up MRI is useful in the differentiation of ADEM/MS, as new lesions should not occur in ADEM. Repeat MRI is generally not routinely performed after an episode of ADEM unless clinically indicated. It has been suggested that a latency of 6 months after presentation would be an appropriate time for repeat scanning, as too early a repeat scan could cause diagnostic confusion/uncertainty if new lesions are present (Dale and Branson, 2005).

Acute hemorrhagic leukoencephalitis (AHLE)

Acute haemorrhagic encephalomyelitis (AHEM) is probably best regarded as a severe form of ADEM, rather than as a distinct condition (Rosman *et al.*, 1997; Lee *et al.*, 2005). It was first described by Hurst in 1941 in two adults who developed a fatal acute encephalopathy with focal neurological signs after a respiratory illness (Hurst, 1941). Uncommon in childhood, AHLE was present in only 2% of Tenembaum's large ADEM series based on radiological features (Tenembaum *et al.*, 2002). If anything, AHLE is seen most frequently in young adults (Kuperan *et al.*, 2003; Leake *et al.*, 2003), but it remains uncommon, with most cases identified in the literature representing either small series or case reports. Prior to neuroimaging, the diagnosis was based on typical pathological findings, and there are only a few reports in the literature where MRI features are described in pathologically confirmed cases (Kuperan *et al.*, 2003; Leake *et al.*, 2003; Hofer *et al.*, 2005).

Typical pathological features include the presence of perivascular hemorrhages, fibrinoid vessel wall necrosis, and a neutrophilic perivascular infiltrate which are not classically seen in ADEM.

Clinically, AHLE tends to present more acutely and severely, often with asymmetric neurological deficits such as a hemiparesis (Rosman *et al.*, 1997; Hofer *et al.*, 2005; Alemdar *et al.*, 2006). The CSF often shows a polymorphonuclear rather than lymphocytic pleocytosis and red cells can be present (Leake *et al.*, 2002; Lee *et al.*, 2005). Cases have been reported with a normal CSF, however (Mader *et al.*, 2004). A predominantly polymorphonuclear blood leukocytosis is also common, as is a raised erythrocyte sedimentation rate (ESR) (Rosman *et al.*, 1997; Leake *et al.*, 2002).

Imaging-based features are similar to those in ADEM; however edema and mass effect can be more prominent (Kuperan *et al.*, 2003). Areas of hemorrhage in regions of demyelination can be seen (Tenembaum *et al.*, 2002; Mader *et al.*, 2004; Lee *et al.*, 2005), but this is not a consistent feature (Rosman *et al.*, 1997; Leake *et al.*, 2002). Recent case reports have also described diffusion-weighted and apparent diffusion coefficient changes, with areas of true restricted diffusion seen, indicating cytotoxic edema (Mader *et al.*, 2004; Lee *et al.*, 2005; Alemdar *et al.*, 2006). Some consider that these changes could be due to an acute vasculitis with subsequent vessel occlusion (Mader *et al.*, 2004). Follow-up imaging can show evolving encephalomalacia (Leake *et al.*, 2002; Lee *et al.*, 2005).

Treatment for AHLE is the same as ADEM, with reports of good response to steroids (Rosman *et al.*, 1997), although fatalities still occur (Kuperan *et al.*, 2003; Hofer *et al.*, 2005).

Summary/conclusion

In summary, ADEM is a predominantly childhood post-infectious demyelinating condition characterized by multifocal neurologic symptoms and signs associated with encephalopathy. Concurrent cord involvement (myelitis) is not uncommon, resulting in spinal neurologic disturbances, such as sphincter dysfunc-tion. Typical MRI features include multifocal areas of T2/FLAIR hyperintensity involving subcortical white matter, cerebellum, brainstem, spinal cord, and cortical and deep gray matter. High-dose intravenous steroids, followed by a slow weaning course of oral steroids is the treatment of choice, with most children having a good to excellent outcome.

Considerable interest revolves around the differentiation between ADEM and MS, particularly from a prognostic perspective, and whilst most children have a clear monophasic illness, some develop ongoing episodes of demyelination that can occur many years after the initial event. Recently published consensus definitions on ADEM and other demyelinating conditions of childhood should provide a framework for ongoing research in this area.

References

Alemdar M, *et al.* The importance of EEG and variability of MRI findings in acute hemorrhagic leukoencephalitis. *Eur J Neurol* 2006; **13**(11): e1–3.

Amit R, *et al.* Acute, severe, central and peripheral nervous system combined demyelination. *Pediatr Neurol* 1986; **2**(1): 47–50.

Apak RA, *et al.* Acute disseminated encephalomyelitis in childhood: Report of 10 cases. *J Child Neurol* 1999; **14**(3): 198–201.

Aydin A, *et al.* Acute disseminated encephalomyelitis presenting with bilateral transient amaurosis. *Pediatr Neurol* 2005; **32**(1): 60–3.

Baum PA, *et al.* Deep gray matter involvement in children with acute disseminated encephalomyelitis. *Am J Neuroradiol* 1994; **15**(7): 1275–83.

Boe J, *et al.* Corticosteroid treatment for acute meningoencephalitis: A retrospective study of 346 cases. *Br Med J* 1965; **5442**: 1094–5.

Brass SD, *et al.* Multiple sclerosis vs acute disseminated encephalomyelitis in childhood. *Ped Neurol* 2003; **29**(3): 227–31.

Brenner D, *et al.* Estimated risks of radiation-induced fatal cancer from pediatric CT. *Am J Roentgenol* 2001; **176**(2): 289–96.

Caldemeyer KS, *et al.* MRI in acute disseminated encephalomyelitis. *Neuroradiology* 1994; **36**(3): 216–20.

Dale RC, Branson JA. Acute disseminated encephalomyelitis or multiple sclerosis: Can the initial presentation help in establishing a correct diagnosis? *Arch Dis Childhood* 2005; **90**(6): 636–9.

Dale RC, *et al.* Acute disseminated encephalomyelitis, multiphasic disseminated encephalomyelitis and multiple sclerosis in children. *Brain* 2000; **123**(Pt 12): 2407–22.

Dale RC, *et al.* Poststreptococcal acute disseminated encephalomyelitis with basal ganglia involvement and auto-reactive antibasal ganglia antibodies. *Ann Neurol* 2001; **50**(5): 588–95.

de Campo JF, *et al.* Is informed consent necessary for paediatric computed tomography? *J Paed Child Hlth* 2003; **39**(6): 399–400.

Epperson LW, *et al.* Cranial MRI in acute disseminated encephalomyelitis. *Neurology* 1988; **38**(2):332–3.

Gupte G, *et al.* Acute disseminated encephalomyelitis: A review of 18 cases in childhood. *J Paed Child Hlth* 2003; **39**(5): 336–342.

Hahn CD, *et al.* Neurocognitive outcome after acute disseminated encephalomyelitis. *Ped Neurol* 2003; **29**(2): 117–23.

Hartung HP, Grossman RI. ADEM: Distinct disease or part of the MS spectrum? *Neurology* 2001; **56**(10): 1257–60. [Erratum appears in *Neurology* 2001; **57**(6): 1146.]

Hartung HP, *et al.* Circulating adhesion molecules and inflammatory mediators in demyelination: A review. *Neurology* 1995; **45**(6 Suppl. 6): S22–32.

Hawley RJ. Early high-dose methylprednisolone in acute disseminated encephalomyelitis. *Neurology* 1998; **51**(2): 644–5.

Heick A, Skriver E. *Chlamydia pneumoniae*-associated ADEM. *Eur J Neurol* 2000; **7**(4): 435–8.

Hofer M, *et al.* Acute hemorrhagic leukoencephalitis (Hurst's disease) linked to Epstein–Barr virus infection. *Acta Neuropathol* 2005; **109**(2): 226–30.

Hurst E. Acute haemorrhagic leucoencephalitis: A previously unidentified entity. *Med J Aust* 1941; **1**: 1–6.

Hynson JL, *et al.* Clinical and neuroradiologic features of acute disseminated encephalomyelitis in children. *Neurology* 2001; **56**(10): 1308–12.

Jacobs RK, *et al.* Neuropsychological outcome after acute disseminated encephalomyelitis: Impact of age at illness onset. *Ped Neurol* 2004; **31**(3): 191–7.

Kaji M, *et al.* Survey of herpes simplex virus infections of the central nervous system, including acute disseminated encephalomyelitis, in the Kyushu and Okinawa regions of Japan. *Mult Scler* 1996; **2**(2): 83–7.

Kamei A, *et al.* Acute disseminated demyelination due to primary human herpesvirus-6 infection. *Eur J Pediatr* 1997; **156**(9): 709–12.

Kanter DS, *et al.* Plasmapheresis in fulminant acute disseminated encephalomyelitis. *Neurology* 1995; **45**(4): 824–7.

Karelitz S, Eisenberg M. Measles encephalitis. Evaluation of treatment with adrenocorticotropin and adrenal corticosteroids. *Pediatrics* 1961; **27**: 811–18.

Keegan M, *et al.* Plasma exchange for severe attacks of CNS demyelination: predictors of response. *Neurology* 2002; **58**(1): 143–6.

Kepes JJ. Large focal tumor-like demyelinating lesions of the brain: Intermediate entity between multiple sclerosis and acute disseminated encephalomyelitis? A study of 31 patients. *Ann Neurol* 1993; **33**(1): 18–27.

Kesselring J, *et al.* Acute disseminated encephalomyelitis. MRI findings and the distinction from multiple sclerosis. *Brain* 1990; **113**(Pt 2): 291–302.

Khong P-L, *et al.* Childhood acute disseminated encephalomyelitis: The role of brain and spinal cord MRI. *Ped Radiol* 2002; **32**(1): 59–66.

Khurana DS, *et al.* Acute disseminated encephalomyelitis in children: Discordant neurologic and neuro-imaging abnormalities and response to plasmapheresis. *Pediatrics* 2005; **116**(2): 431–6.

Kimura S, *et al.* Serial magnetic resonance imaging in children with postinfectious encephalitis. *Brain Dev* 1996; **18**(6): 461–5.

Kinoshita A, *et al.* Inflammatory demyelinating polyradiculitis in a patient with acute disseminated encephalomyelitis (ADEM). *J Neurol Neurosurg Psychiatry* 1996; **60**(1): 87–90.

Kleiman M, Brunquell P. Acute disseminated encephalomyelitis: Response to intravenous immunoglobulin. *J Child Neurol* 1995; **10**(6): 481–3.

Krupp LB, *et al.* Consensus definitions proposed for pediatric multiple sclerosis and related childhood disorders. *Neurology* 2007; **68**(16 Suppl. 2): S7–12.

Kuperan S, *et al.* Acute hemorrhagic leukoencephalitis vs ADEM: FLAIR MRI and neuropathology findings. *Neurology* 2003; **60**(4): 721–2.

Leake JA, *et al.* Acute disseminated encephalomyelitis in childhood: Epidemiologic, clinical and laboratory features. *Pediatr Infect Dis J* 2004; **23**(8): 756–64.

Leake JAD, *et al.* Pediatric acute hemorrhagic leukoencephalitis: Report of a surviving patient and review. *Clin Infect Dis* 2002; **34**(5): 699–703.

Lee HY, *et al.* Serial MR imaging findings of acute hemorrhagic leukoencephalitis: A case report. *Am J Neuroradiol* 2005; **26**(8): 1996–9.

Lee SJ, Benveniste EN. Adhesion molecule expression and regulation on cells of the central nervous system. *J Neuroimmunol* 1999; **98**(2): 77–88.

Mader I, *et al.* Acute haemorrhagic encephalomyelitis (AHEM): MRI findings. *Neuropediatrics* 2004; **35**(2): 143–6.

Martens-Le Bouar H, Korinthenberg R. Polyradiculoneuritis with myelitis: A rare differential diagnosis of Guillain–Barre syndrome. *Neuropediatrics* 2002; **33**(2): 93–6.

Martino D, *et al.* Soluble adhesion molecules in acute disseminated encephalomyelitis. *Pediatr Neurol* 2005; **33**(4): 255–8.

Menge T, *et al.* Acute disseminated encephalomyelitis: An update. *Arch Neurol* 2005; **62**(11): 1673–80.

Mikaeloff Y, *et al.* MRI prognostic factors for relapse after acute CNS inflammatory demyelination in childhood. *Brain* 2004a; **127**(Pt 9): 1942–7.

Mikaeloff Y, *et al.* First episode of acute CNS inflammatory demyelination in childhood: Prognostic factors for multiple sclerosis and disability. *J Pediat* 2004b; **144**(2): 246–52.

Miller DH, *et al.* Acute disseminated encephalomyelitis presenting as a solitary brainstem mass. *J Neurol Neurosurg Psychiatry* 1993; **56**(8): 920–2.

Murray BJ, *et al.* Severe acute disseminated encephalomyelitis with normal MRI at presentation. *Neurology* 2000; **55**(8): 1237–8.

Murthy SNK, *et al.* Acute disseminated encephalomyelitis in children. *Pediatrics* 2002; **110**(2 Pt 1): e21.

Nasr JT, *et al.* ADEM: literature review and case report of acute psychosis presentation. *Pediatr Neurol* 2000; **22**(1): 8–18.

O'Riordan JI, *et al.* Long term MRI follow-up of patients with post infectious encephalomyelitis: Evidence for a monophasic disease. *J Neurol Sci* 1999; **167**(2): 132–6.

Ohtaki E, *et al.* Acute disseminated encephalomyelitis after Japanese B encephalitis vaccination. *Ped Neurol* 1992; **8**(2): 137–9.

Ozawa H, *et al.* Acute disseminated encephalomyelitis associated with poliomyelitis vaccine. *Ped Neurol* 2000; **23**(2): 177–9.

Pasternak JF, *et al.* Steroid-responsive encephalomyelitis in childhood. *Neurology* 1980; **30**(5): 481–6.

Perniola T, *et al.* A case of Landau-Kleffner syndrome secondary to inflammatory demyelinating disease. *Epilepsia* 1993; **34**(3): 551–6.

Pohl D, *et al.* CSF characteristics in early-onset multiple sclerosis. *Neurology* 2004; **63**(10): 1966–7.

Pohl-Koppe A, *et al.* Myelin basic protein reactive Th2 T cells are found in acute disseminated encephalomyelitis. *J Neuroimmunol* 1998; **91**(1–2): 19–27.

Pradhan S, *et al.* Intravenous immunoglobulin therapy in acute disseminated encephalomyelitis. *J Neurol Sci* 1999; **165**(1): 56–61.

Revel-Vilk S, *et al.* Recurrent acute disseminated encephalomyelitis associated with acute cytomegalovirus and Epstein–Barr virus infection. *J Child Neurol* 2000; **15**(6): 421–4.

Richer LP, *et al.* Neuro-imaging features of acute disseminated encephalomyelitis in childhood. *Ped Neurol* 2005; **32**(1): 30–6.

Rosman NP, *et al.* Acute hemorrhagic leukoencephalitis: Recovery and reversal of magnetic resonance imaging findings in a child. *J Child Neurol* 1997; **12**(7): 448–54.

Rust RS. Multiple sclerosis, acute disseminated encephalomyelitis, and related conditions. *Semin Pediatr Neurol* 2000; **7**(2): 66–90.

Sahlas DJ, *et al.* Treatment of acute disseminated encephalomyelitis with intravenous immunoglobulin. *Neurology* 2000; **54**(6): 1370–2.

Saitoh A, *et al.* Acute disseminated encephalomyelitis associated with enteroviral infection. *Ped Infect Dis J* 2004; **23**(12): 1174–5.

Schwarz S, *et al.* Acute disseminated encephalomyelitis: A follow-up study of 40 adult patients. *Neurology* 2001; **56**(10): 1313–8.

Stonehouse M, *et al.* Acute disseminated encephalomyelitis: Recognition in the hands of general paediatricians. *Arch Dis Childhood* 2003; **88**(2): 122–4.

Straub J, *et al.* Early high-dose intravenous methylprednisolone in acute disseminated encephalomyelitis: A successful recovery. *Neurology* 1997; **49**(4): 1145–7.

Stuve O, Zamvil SS. Pathogenesis, diagnosis, and treatment of acute disseminated encephalomyelitis. *Curr Opin Neurol* 1999; **12**(4): 395–401.

Tan H, *et al.* Acute disseminated encephalomyelitis following hepatitis A virus infection. *Ped Neurol* 2004; **30**(3): 207–9.

Tenembaum S, *et al.* Acute disseminated encephalomyelitis: A long-term follow-up study of 84 pediatric patients. *Neurology* 2002; **59**(8): 1224–31.

Yiu E, *et al.* Acute transverse myelitis and acute disseminated encephalomyelitis in childhood: Spectrum or separate entities? *J Child Neurol* 2009; **24**(3); 287–96

Zeman A, *et al.* The significance of serum oligoclonal bands in neurological diseases. *J Neurol Neurosurg Psychiatry* 1993; **56**(1): 32–5.

Ziegra SR. Corticosteroid treatment for measles encephalitis. *J Pediat* 1961; **59**: 322–3.

Primary angiitis of the CNS and its mimics

Tina Chadha, George F. Duna and Leonard H. Calabrese

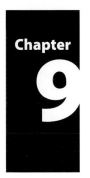

Introduction

The identification of primary angiitis of the central nervous system (PACNS) as a discrete entity dates back to the late 1950s, with the elegant description of several patients with a progressive and fatal form of vasculitis limited to the central nervous system (CNS) and characterized by a rich granulomatous pathology. The disease was named granulomatous angiitis of the CNS (GACNS), and remained a diagnosis of extreme rarity, with fewer than 40 cases reported over the next 25 years (Calabrese and Mallek, 1988). The 1970s and 1980s witnessed an increased use of cerebral angiography and an increase in reported cases. However, many of these newly reported cases lacked histologic confirmation. The next major change in the approach to PACNS came in the early 1980s with reports of successful therapy using a combination of cyclophosphamide and glucocorticoids. In retrospect, overreliance on angiography without biopsy confirmation led to some patients being treated with prolonged and intensive immunosuppressive regimens without clearcut evidence of a progressive and fatal form of granulomatous arteritis. Then, in the 1990s, we and others (Calabrese et al., 1992b; Hankey, 1991) began to question whether all cases of PACNS diagnosed solely on the basis of cerebral angiography were indeed equivalent to those diagnosed by ante-mortem biopsy. It was suggested then that within the spectrum of angiographically diagnosed PACNS existed a subset of patients with a predictably less ominous outcome. This subset was labeled benign angiopathy of the central nervous system (BACNS), emphasizing the term *angiopathy* as opposed to *angiitis* to indicate the uncertainty concerning the nature of the underlying vascular pathology. However, given that BACNS often does *not* necessarily have a benign prognosis, we believe that BACNS should be more appropriately renamed "reversible vasoconstrictive disorders", or RVDs. The last several years have witnessed an increasing appreciation of the complexity of PACNS and the need for a multidisciplinary approach to diagnosis and management (Calabrese et al., 1997).

Primary angiitis of the CNS

Diagnostic criteria

In 1988, Calabrese and Mallek proposed three working criteria for the diagnosis of PACNS. Although imperfect and not validated by controlled investigation, these criteria have been useful for both the clinical management of suspected patients, and assisting in nosologic classification. The criteria proposed are as follows.

1. A history of a neurologic deficit that remains unexplained after a vigorous diagnostic work up, including lumbar puncture and neuro-imaging.
2. Either classic angiographic evidence (high probability) of vasculitis or, preferably, histopathologic demonstration of vasculitis within the CNS.
3. No evidence of systemic vasculitis or of any other condition to which the angiographic or pathologic evidence can be attributed. These conditions include but are not limited to those in Table 9.1.

Following the diagnosis of PACNS, all attempts should be made to categorize the patient into one of the recognized subsets or clinical variants, as described below. These subsets appear to have important prognostic and therapeutic implications.

Of note, given that numerous conditions can mimic PACNS, it is critical that a thorough history and physical examination be performed in each case (Duna and Calabrese, 2005). A detailed history from either the patient or family, including the use of prescription and illicit drugs, is a key starting point. Signs

Inflammatory Diseases of the Central Nervous System, ed. T. Kilpatrick, R. M. Ransohoff and S. Wesselingh. Published by Cambridge University Press. © Cambridge University Press 2010

Table 9.1 Conditions resembling PACNS excluded by the preliminary diagnostic criteria

Systemic vasculitides
Polyarteritis nodosa
Allergic granulomatosis
Hypersensitivity vasculitis group disorders
Vasculitis with connective tissue disease
Wegener's granulomatosis
Temporal arteritis
Takayasu's arteritis
Behçet's disease
Lymphomatoid granulomatosis
Cogan's syndrome
Infections
Viral, bacterial, mycobacterial, fungal, spirochetes, rickettsial
Neoplasm
Primary CNS lyphoma
Angioimmunoproliferative disorders
Carcinomatous meningitis
Infiltrating glioma
Malignant angioendotheliomatosis
Drug use
Amphetamines
Ephedrine
Phenylpropanolamine
Cocaine
Ergotamine
Reversible cerebral vasoconstrictive disorders
Sympathomimetic drugs
Post partum angiopathy
Eclampsia
Pheochromocytoma or other uncontrolled hypertensive states
Following head trauma, neurovascular surgery
Subarachnoid hemorrhage
Migraine and exertional headache
Other vasculopathies
Atherosclerosis
Fibromuscular dysplasia
Moyamoya disease
Thrombotic thrombocytopenic purpura
Sickle cell anemia

Table 9.1 (cont.)

Neurofibromatosis
Demyelinating disease
Sarcoidosis
Emboli (i.e. bacterial endocarditis, cardiac myxoma, paradoxical emboli)
Hypercoaguable states, including antiphospholipid antibody syndrome
Acute posterior placoid pigment epitheliopathy and cerebral vasculitis
CADASIL (cerebral autosomal dominant arteriopathy with subcortical infarcts and leukoencephalopathy)
MELAS syndrome (myopathy, encephalopathy, lactic acidosis and stroke-like episodes)
Retinocochleocerebral vasculopathy (Susac syndrome)

of other diseases (i.e. zoster rash, malar rash, synovitis) or infections (Roth spots, splinter hemorrhages) can guide the workup into entirely different avenues.

Clinical subsets

Granulomatous angiitis of the CNS

Granulomatous angiitis of the central nervous system (GACNS) represents approximately 20% of all patients fulfilling the diagnostic criteria for PACNS. The epidemiology of the disease is poorly understood, but it does appear to be male-predominant and can occur at virtually any age. Examples of an acute onset have been reported, but it is far more commonly subacute or chronic in its presentation, often lasting 6 months or longer. The most common clinical manifestations of GACNS are headache and mental status changes. In addition to these features, the majority of patients develop additional neurologic symptoms and signs during the course of their illness, including transient ischemic episodes, varying degrees of paresis, seizures, ataxia, visual changes, aphasia, and, in rare situations, coma. It is the combination of evolving focal and diffuse neurologic dysfunction that is the hallmark of GACNS.

A number of less-common clinical manifestations of GACNS have also been reported, including either acute or subacute encephalopathy and pure dementia. It is far more common to experience fluctuating levels of consciousness during the course of the illness. A pseudo multiple sclerosis-like presentation has also been described. Of note is the fact that signs and symptoms of systemic vasculitis, such as peripheral neuropathies, fever, weight loss, and rash are rarely, if ever, part of GACNS. Wasting and low-grade fever can occasionally be observed, but this is generally believed to be due to disability secondary to neurologic dysfunction rather than direct manifestations of the primary disorder.

In a review of 136 reported cases of GACNS, Younger and colleagues (1997) identified a number of associated conditions, including lymphoproliferative diseases, varicella zoster infection, amyloidosis, sarcoidosis and several others. Whether such cases are equivalent to primary GACNS is unclear. Further analysis is needed to determine whether such confounded cases need to be approached differently. Several of these disorders are discussed below.

Etiology

Given the presence of granulomas in GACNS, it seems logical to search for an occult infectious agent as the causative agent (Duna and Calabrese, 2005). However, no organism has clearly emerged as a possible trigger for the disease. Associations with varicella zoster virus (VZV) (discussed below) and other viruses such as human immunodeficiency virus (HIV) and cytomegalovirus (CMV) have been proposed but not clearly proven (Duna and Calabrese, 2005).

Diagnosis and treatment

There are no diagnostic or characteristic blood tests for PACNS. In particular, there are no characteristic autoantibodies. Acute phase reactants such as erythrocyte sedimentation rate (ESR) or C-reactive protein (CRP) can be normal and are not specific (Duna and Calabrese, 2005).

The most critical initial elements in securing the diagnosis of GACNS are the lumbar puncture and neuroradiographic studies, in particular magnetic resonance imaging (MRI). Examination of the cerebrospinal fluid is essential, given that it is abnormal in approximately 90% of patients with GACNS. Thus, a totally normal lumbar puncture argues against this diagnosis (Calabrese et al., 1992a; Stone et al., 1994). In addition, the lumbar puncture is essential for ruling out malignancies and infection, which may mimic CNS vasculitis. The characteristic findings of the lumbar puncture in GACNS are those of aseptic meningitis. The white count averages 77 cells/mm^3 and

rarely exceeds 250 cells/mm^3; the protein count averages 177 mg/dl and rarely exceeds 500 mg/dl (Duna and Calabrese, 2005). Because the disease is chronic, the lumbar puncture remains abnormal in the untreated patient over many weeks to months. Of note, although an abnormal CSF is almost a prerequisite for GACNS, it is certainly not specific for the disease, with the positive predictive value of an abnormal CSF for a diagnosis of PACNS averaging 37% (Duna and Calabrese, 2005).

Neuro-imaging studies are vital in the diagnostic workup, and MRI is generally the initial test to be performed (Wynne et al., 1997). There are no specific or diagnostic MRI findings, but the most suggestive ones are those of multifocal cerebral ischemic lesions occurring over time. These lesions are generally multiple and bilateral and located within the cortex, deep white matter and/or leptomeninges. Gray–white matter lesions are generally more suspicious for vasculitis, as the disease is rarely confined to the white matter. Enhancement, particularly in the leptomeninges, can occasionally be observed and serves to increase the sensitivity of a biopsy guided to the affected area. Collectively, abnormalities of the MRI and CSF analysis are noted in close to 100% of patients. Conversely, the combination of a normal MRI and CSF make the diagnosis of GACNS unlikely.

Angiography has a critical role in the diagnosis of GACNS, but is limited by a lack of specificity. The literature has suggested that angiography can be normal in up to 40% of GACNS cases (Calabrese et al., 1992a), but in our recent experience only 10–20% of such patients have abnormal studies. Although the specificity of angiography is extremely low in securing the diagnosis of PACNS (Duna and Calabrese, 1995), a high-probability angiogram in the setting of a chronic meningitis workup is highly suspicious for vasculitis if infection can be effectively ruled out. Unfortunately, this is not always possible, and thus biopsy is often required. The most characteristic angiographic findings in PACNS include the presence of alternating areas of stenosis and ectasia in multiple vascular distributions (Duna and Calabrese, 2005).

The gold standard for the diagnosis of GACNS is biopsy of the CNS. The histology of GACNS has been well described (Lie, 1992b), and the gross findings consist of multiple small, but occasionally large, foci of infarction or hemorrhage. At the microscopic level, GACNS is characterized by segmental necrotizing

111

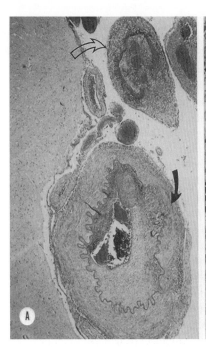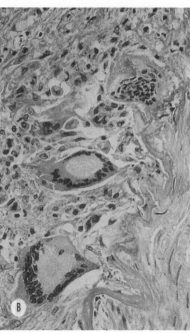

Figure 9.1 Granulomatous vasculitis. (a) Brain biopsy findings of granulomatous vasculitis side by side with a polyarteritis-type necrotizing arteritis (open arrow). (b) High-power view of (a) showing foreign body giant cells in granulomatous vasculitis. Hematoxylin and eosin, (magnification × 64 and × 400, respectively). (With permission from Calabrese *et al.*, 1997.)

granulomatous inflammation of small and medium-sized arteries affecting predominantly the leptomeninges and underlying cortical blood vessels. Veins are affected in about half the cases. The majority of the inflammatory infiltrate is composed of small lymphocytes, with an admixture of epithelioid cells, plasma cells, macrophages and giant cells of both the Langerhans and foreign body types (Figure 9.1). Importantly, acute lesions often coexist with more chronic and repaired lesions (Duna and Calabrese, 2005). Clearly, not all features are present in every patient, and the presence of giant cells is variable. Well-formed granulomas are rarely seen. More commonly, there is loose granuloma formation. Lastly, lymphocytic-predominant lesions without prominent granulomas can be seen in up to 20% of biopsy-proven cases of PACNS, and it is unclear whether these cases, which are similar to GACNS in every other respect, are clinically equivalent or whether they represent a distinct nosologic entity. These will be discussed later under "atypical forms."

The differential diagnosis of GACNS primarily includes those conditions considered within the differential diagnosis of chronic meningitis (Gripshover and Ellner, 1998). Infections are the most important category of illness to rule out in this setting. Infections of particular importance, which may be overlooked,

include HIV, *Borrelia burgdorferi* and VZV. As discussed later, VZV may confound the diagnosis of GACNS, as CNS vasculitis can occur in the wake of either clinical or asymptomatic VZV infection. VZV can also be detected within vasculitic lesions (Gilden *et al.*, 2000). In general, given the gravity of the diagnosis and the therapeutic implications, we favor CNS biopsy as the preferred diagnostic technique, not only to secure the diagnosis of GACNS, but also to rule out the many mimicking conditions noted in Table 9.1 (Moore, 1994).

Based on the historical literature, there is little doubt that GACNS is a progressive and potentially fatal disorder. Although there are no controlled clinical therapeutic trials in GACNS, informal therapeutic guidelines have been proposed, based on the assumption of its progressive and fatal nature (Grade C evidence). In general, the majority of patients with documented GACNS should be treated with a combination regimen consisting of oral cyclophosphamide and glucocorticoids. Originally, it was felt that oral cyclophosphamide needed to be continued for approximately 1 year after the patient achieved clinical remission, but more recently (applying the treatment paradigm of antineutrophile cytoplasmic antibody (ANCA)-associated vasculitis), prevailing wisdom has shifted thinking to limiting the patient's exposure to alkylating agents. It is now our practice to treat with oral cyclophosphamide for 3–6 months, and once the patient is in clinical remission to switch to an anti-metabolite such as azathioprine or methotrexate for the duration of therapy. As in systemic vasculitides, oral glucocorticoids are used starting with 1 mg/kg of oral prednisone and gradually tapering to a small daily dose over 8–12 weeks. The use of long-term glucocorticoid therapy and/or the addition of cytotoxic drugs should be reserved for those patients with biopsy-proven disease or those with progressive clinical findings (Grade C evidence). Given the debilitating nature of the disease and the intensity of the immunosuppressive regimen, we also advocate anti-microbial prophylaxis with trimethoprim–sulfamethoxazole to prevent *Pneumocystis carinii* pneumonia (Calabrese, 1997).

One of the most critical problems in the management of GACNS is assessing disease activity over time. Clinical symptoms and signs of neurologic damage are slow to improve, similar to any other ischemic event in the brain. Furthermore, certain neurologic events such as seizures can be related to an irreversibly damaged focus rather than active disease. In addition to clinical follow-up, serial MRI examinations at 3–4-month intervals should be performed during the first year. These are not primarily performed to look for radiographic resolution, but rather to search for silent progression (i.e. new ischemic lesions) during the tapering of the immunosuppressive regimen. The MRI changes should improve, but are likely to leave residual scars, and thus can be difficult to interpret. In our experience, improvement in CSF abnormalities serves as a useful indicator of decreased disease activity and should be documented after 8–12 weeks of therapy. Similar to the treatment of other forms of systemic necrotizing vasculitis with high-intensity immunosuppressive regimens, PACNS patients treated with cyclophosphamide and prednisone need to be carefully monitored to prevent or limit treatment-related morbidity (Calabrese, 1997).

Atypical PACNS

A majority of patients (80%) with either angiographically or histopathologically documented PACNS do not fall neatly within the diagnostic categories of GACNS or RVDs and thus are considered atypical. Given our limited knowledge of the spectrum of PACNS, it is quite possible that further subclassifications will be developed in the future. Most patients falling within this category have either clinical features

such as abnormal spinal fluid that preclude the diagnosis of RVDs, or a more subacute to chronic presentation than one generally sees. Also represented are those rare cases of patients with a reversible cerebral vasoconstrictive-like presentation (see the next section) who upon repeat angiography fail to show dynamic improvement. As stated previously, we believe that most of these patients have non-arteritic forms of disease, but we cannot preclude the possibility that some have refractory forms of CNS vasculitis requiring more aggressive therapy. Other atypical cases would include presentations with a GACNS-like syndrome but where biopsies reveal non-granulomatous pathology. Alternative patterns of histopathology include either a predominantly lymphocytic angiitis (Figure 9.2) or, occasionally, eosinophilic or even leukocytoclastic variants.

Also included within the atypical category are those patients with unusual anatomic presentations. Spinal cord involvement is uncommon in PACNS but has been well documented (Calabrese *et al.*, 1997). Spinal cord involvement may or may not coincide with cortical involvement, and when isolated poses a formidable diagnostic challenge. The vast majority of reported cases with spinal cord involvement have been diagnosed post-mortem, with only rare examples of ante-mortem diagnosis described. The presentation of spinal cord variant PACNS is non-specific and similar to any other vascular and/or inflammatory myelopathy. The most common clinical presentation is that of progressive paraparesis. Other unusual presentations include the presence of multiple aneurysms leading to acute spinal subdural hemorrhage. Several cases of spinal cord vasculitis have also been described in association with lymphoproliferative diseases. Neuroimaging studies are not specific but can reveal enhancement within the cord or an appearance consistent with infiltrative disease (Giovanini *et al.*, 1994). Most cases of spinal cord vasculitis have a granulomatous pathology. There is no way of diagnosing PACNS within the spinal cord without biopsy. Surgical exploration for tissue confirmation is essential. Treatment is similar to that for GACNS.

Another poorly appreciated variant of PACNS is the presentation with mass lesions. This has been observed in about 15% of our cases. As always, a patient presenting with a mass lesion should be suspected of having either an infection or neoplasm until proven otherwise. Virtually all cases of PACNS with mass lesions are diagnosed only at biopsy.

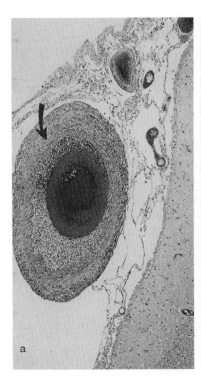
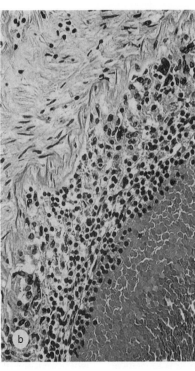

Figure 9.2 Brain biopsy findings of lymphocytic vasculitis in a patient with PACNS with thrombosis. (b) High-power view of the region arrowed in (a), demonstrating lymphocytic infiltrate in vessel wall. Hematoxylin and eosin, magnification × 64 and × 400, respectively. (With permission from Calabrese *et al.*, 1997.)

Angiograms are generally normal except for a possible mass effect if the lesion has achieved a critical size. Neuro-imaging of these mass lesions by CT or MRI demonstrates variable degrees of enhancement, but offers no specific features to suspect the diagnosis. In our experience, a mass lesion presentation is the sole indication for stereotactic biopsy, which has rarely been successful in diagnosing PACNS. A sizable percentage of such lesions display non-granulomatous lesions, often with leukocytoclastic features (Calabrese *et al.*, 1997). The optimal therapy for such patients is unclear, but rare reports of excisional cure have been documented. We generally treat patients with high-dose glucocorticoids, following them frequently with neuro-imaging, and add in cyclophosphamide only if the condition fails to respond (Grade C evidence). As always, it is essential to provide adequate tissue for special analysis, such as for clonality, particularly when there is a lymphocyte-predominant infiltrate.

PACNS associated with varicella zoster infection (VZV)

It would seem that PACNS associated with an infection like VZV would most likely be considered a form of secondary CNS vasculitis; however, the relationship between VZV and cerebral vasculitis is highly complex and often subtle. The association of VZV infection with CNS vascular disease has been well described (Gilden *et al.*, 2002) and there is a broad range of CNS vascular pathology described in the literature. Varicella zoster infection causes chicken pox, usually in childhood, with most children manifesting none or only minimal neurologic sequelae. After chicken pox resolves, the virus becomes latent in the neurons and the spinal ganglia of nearly all infected individuals. In immunocompetent patients with reactivated virus, the most common spread is a centrifugal pattern, manifesting as the dermatomal rash of shingles. Less commonly, the spread from the ganglia is centripetal, with migration towards the spinal cord or brain, resulting in a variety of neurologic signs and symptoms. The virus can spread to the proximal nerve roots, including the cranial nerves, or even more centrally to the spinal cord and its meninges. Alternatively, the virus can also spread to the large vessels at the base of the brain, causing one of several distinct syndromes.

The best-described neurovascular syndrome associated with VZV follows infection of the trigeminal nerve, particularly when it involves its ophthalmic division (Calabrese *et al.*, 1997; Gilden *et al.*, 2000). In this syndrome, several weeks to months following VZV infection, the patient suffers an ischemic event secondary to vasculitis of the middle cerebral artery, several of its branches, and occasionally the internal

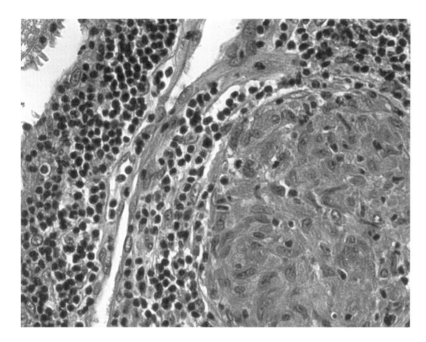

Figure 9.3 Marked mononuclear inflammatory infiltrate in a cortical vessel with a well-formed perivascular granuloma. Magnification ×200. (With permission from Calabrese LH. Vasculitis of the central nervous system. *Rheum Dis Clin North Am* 1995; **21**: 1059–76.)

carotid artery. The mechanism appears to be due to retrograde spread of VZV to the cerebral circulation via anastomotic branches of the gasserian ganglion (Calabrese *et al.*, 1997; Gilden *et al.*, 2000). In general, the disease remains anatomically localized (i.e. angiographically) and monophasic in course, but the mortality in such patients can approach 25%. We do not consider patients with this typical monophasic illness limited to the ipsilateral side of brain to have true PACNS, as they are readily differentiated on clinical and/or angiographic grounds. A more complex VZV-associated vascular syndrome of the CNS has been described in patients who are frequently elderly or who have other alterations in their host defenses. In this instance, the syndrome can become indistinguishable from classic GACNS (Lie, 1992b). Interestingly, this disease can evolve in the setting of VZV infection of either the trigeminal nerve or a somatic dermatome, or even in the absence of clinical VZV infection (i.e. zoster sine herpete). In each of these vascular syndromes, VZV has been occasionally isolated in inflamed vascular tissues. Anatomically, the VZV has been found in the outer layers of the vessel, as opposed to the endothelium. It has also been occasionally isolated in the CSF by polymerase chain reaction (Calabrese *et al.*, 1993), although its presence in CSF can be only transient. Pathologically, a spectrum of vascular involvement exists, ranging from frank necrotizing vasculitis to moderate vascular inflammation, to thrombosis without inflammation, or rarely an intimal proliferative lesion indistinguishable from atherosclerosis. Given that the clinical suspicion for VZV infection has traditionally been low in suspected cases of PACNS that lack the classic dermatomal rash, an unanswered question is how many patients could have clinically unrecognized VZV disease. The treatment of such cases is problematic, but probably requires a combination of prolonged antiviral therapy and varying degrees of immunosuppression, as well as antiplatelet and/or anticoagulant therapy (Category C evidence). There are no controlled therapeutic trials in this disease.

CNS sarcoid vasculitis

Another complex subgroup of patients comprises those with sarcoidosis and a clinical and histologic picture indistinguishable from that of GACNS (Younger *et al.*, 1997). As shown in Figure 9.3, GACNS at times can display well-formed nonnecrotizing perivascular granulomas indistinguishable from sarcoidosis. In several of these cases, including the one illustrated, there was no evidence of sarcoidosis outside the CNS. Classification of such patients is problematic (Calabrese, 2003). Similar pathology in a patient with well-documented systemic sarcoidosis would clearly warrant the diagnosis of CNS sarcoid vasculitis. In the absence of such systemic disease, such patients would probably best be classified as GACNS.

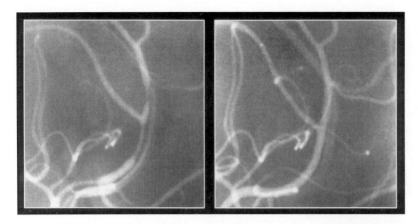

Figure 9.4 Angiographic findings in a patient with reversible cerebral vasoconstrictive disease. (a) Prior to therapy, demonstrating alternating areas of stenosis in branches of the middle cerebral artery. (b) Angiographic findings in the same patient approximately four weeks into therapy, demonstrating total resolution of the deficits. (With permission from Hajj-Ali *et al.*, 2002.)

The therapy of such patients is similar to that outlined under GACNS.

CNS amyloidosis

There are growing numbers of case reports of patients with cerebral amyloid and features similar to GACNS. In their review, Younger and colleagues (1997) expressed the belief that such patients were clinically and pathologically inseparable from others with GACNS. Clinically, headache, mental status changes, multifocal cerebral signs and gait disturbances were noted in 70% of patients and progressive neurologic dysfunction was common. Post-mortem findings revealed an admixture of diffuse granulomatous angiitis of the CNS and cerebral amyloid angiopathy (Schwab *et al.*, 2003).

From a pathophysiologic perspective, the question has been raised as to whether these conditions are linked or merely coincidental. In a recent detailed report by Anders and colleagues (1997) describing six patients with GACNS and cerebral amyloid, these authors pointed out that the inflammatory infiltrate in their series was somewhat atypical for GACNS. They noted that mononuclear cells were only found in the outer portion of the vessels and surrounding brain parenchyma and not in a transmural distribution. These authors also demonstrated the presence of β-amyloid deposition in the thickened media of vessels and within the cytoplasm of multinucleated giant cells. These authors proposed that the granulomatous angiitis most likely represented a foreign body response to amyloid proteins, with a secondary destruction of the vessel wall. Optimal therapy of this variant is unclear, but the condition has been rarely reported to respond to aggressive therapy similar to that used for GACNS.

Conditions that mimic PACNS and secondary causes of CNS vasculitis

Reversible vasoconstrictive disease states (previously called benign angiopathy of the CNS)

History

Cerebral vasoconstrictive syndromes are an important cause of stroke in young adults and are often clinically and angiographically indistinguishable from CNS vasculitis. In addition, the nosology of these RVDs is confusing and the field suffers from a lack of validated diagnostic criteria. The differentiation from PACNS is important since these disorders generally carry a far better prognosis, and patients should be spared exposure to unnecessary immunosuppressive therapies. Since the 1960s, numerous case reports have established that reversible cerebral vasoconstriction is an underlying mechanism for a number of acute neurologic syndromes generally characterized by sudden onset, severe headache with or without stroke (Calabrese *et al.*, 1997; Hajj-Ali *et al.*, 2002). Reversibility of vascular constriction has been demonstrated directly by cerebral angiography (Fig. 9.4) or indirectly by magnetic imaging angiography (MRA), CT angiography, or transcranial Doppler ultrasound in many of these reports (Singhal, 2004). Conditions that have been associated with reversible cerebral vasoconstriction include a number of complex headaches such as migraine, thunderclap headache, effort-induced headache, pre-eclampsia, eclampsia, the post partum state, the use of sympathomimetic drugs such as cocaine, head trauma, subarachnoid hemorrhage, neurosurgical or vascular procedures, uncontrolled blood pressure, and/or other metabolic conditions (Singhal, 2004). Collectively, these reports have demonstrated that such patients often have a distinctive clinical, neuro-imaging, and angiographic picture that should allow clinical recognition and appropriate therapy.

As the above reports of RVDs were appearing, individual cases and small series of CNS vasculitis were described whereby the diagnosis was made by cerebral angiography as the sole invasive diagnostic procedure: with time, these cases were defined by some as BACNS. The lack of histologic evidence of vasculitis led authors to use the term "angiopathy" to denote an abnormal vascular state but of uncertain pathology. We now believe, based on growing clinical experience, that these cases should no longer be included within the PACNS spectrum. Since the outcome is not always favorable (e.g. in the context of intracranial hemorrhage), we prefer the term RVDs over that of BACNS. Given the frequency of this condition, we believe that it is the most clinically important mimic to rule out when entertaining the diagnosis of PACNS.

Clinical features

Most cases of RVDs are seen in 20- to 50-year-old women. The most important feature that often distinguishes this condition from CNS vasculitis is that the onset is frequently hyperacute and intense. When headache is present, it is frequently, although not necessarily, of the thunderclap variety which crescendos to the "worst headache" of the patient's life in less than a minute. It is often precipitated by exercise or sexual activity and accompanied by nausea, vomiting, and photophobia. Interestingly, the headache can abate either with or without therapy but then recurs repeatedly over the period of a few weeks. It is not uncommon for such patients to be evaluated in an emergency room for subarachnoid bleeding with CT and lumbar puncture, only to be discharged with analgesics when such testing is unrevealing. In our experience (heavily influenced by the referral bias of seeing patients with suspected vasculitis), many patients unfortunately then go on to develop focal neurologic abnormalities due to transient ischemic attacks or frank stroke. Patients can also develop seizures presumably due to ischemia, or global cortical visual impairment due to a reversible posterior leukoencephalopathy (Dodick et al., 2003). When stroke occurs, it is often hemorrhagic. Blood pressures can be markedly elevated or relatively normal.

Laboratory tests in this disorder are generally normal and there is no elevation of acute-phase reactants and no pathologic autoantibodies are present. Importantly, the lumbar puncture should be normal or near normal, although a few patients with post partum forms of this disease have been noted to have moderately elevated protein levels. The presence of this benign CSF picture is important in differentiating RVDs from vasculitis of the atypical variety, in which CSF inflammation is far more common, or from GACNS, where it is almost universal.

Neuro-imaging results vary and are governed mostly by whether a stroke has occurred or not. Computerized axial tomography and MRI can be normal or can show single or multifocal ischemic or hemorrhagic infarcts. When ischemia is present, it is frequently identified in the "watershed areas" or border zone regions tending to spare the cortical ribbon (Singhal, 2004). At times, reversible posterior white matter changes can occur (Dodick et al., 2003). The hallmark of RVDs, however, is the presence of diffuse angiographic changes generally characterized by multifocal areas of stenosis and ectasia, often accompanied by long areas of smooth symmetric narrowing in multiple vascular beds (Figure 9.4). Unfortunately, identical findings can be seen in a wide variety of other vascular conditions including CNS vasculitis, atherosclerosis, and infectious arteritis. The clinical course of most patients with RVDs is monophasic and benign, but can be debilitating and even fatal if cerebral hemorrhage occurs. We believe that prompt recognition and treatment (see below) offers the best chance for a benign outcome.

In a recently reported cohort of patients with RVDs (Hajj-Ali et al., 2002), the mean age was 40 years, with a female to male ratio of 4.3:1. Headache was the most common presenting symptom, observed in 88% of cases, followed by focal symptoms in 63% and diffuse symptoms in 44%. All patients had highly abnormal cerebral angiography and MRI abnormalities were present in 77%. Severe CSF abnormalities were present in only a single patient. Interestingly and importantly, 12 of their patients underwent follow-up cerebral angiography over a period ranging from 4 weeks to 8 months, revealing total or near-total resolution of prior changes (Figure 9.4). These investigators proposed that follow-up angiography (or alternatively some indirect form of assessment of reversible compromise of vascular flow) is essential to secure the diagnosis of RVDs. Also reported

Table 9.2 Differentiating reversible cerebral vasoconstrictive disease from PACNS

	Reversible cerebral vasoconstrictive disease	PACNS
Sex	5:1 female to male	1:1 female to male
Age	20 to 50 most common	Any age
Clinical onset	Acute to hyperacute	Insidious
Common presentations	Severe headache with or without Hemorrhagic stroke	Chronic headache plus focal and diffuse neurologic dysfunction
CSF in majority	Normal	Abnormal
MRI in majority	Normal or abnormal	Abnormal
Angiography	High probability of abnormality	Frequently normal in GACNS
Associated features	History of sympathomimetic drug use, uncontrolled hypertension, post partum state, thunderclap headache	
Reversibility	Vascular lesions reverse in 4–12 weeks or sooner	Variable response

in this study was a prospective evaluation of long-term morbidity, demonstrating that 94% of the patients experienced significant recovery, with 71% showing no evidence of long-term disability.

Diagnosis and treatment

There are several important clinical points that help differentiate reversible vasoconstriction from true vasculitis based on angiographic abnormalities (Table 9.2). In most cases, the differentiation is not difficult, particularly when there are associated clinical or epidemiologic features associated with the RVDs. Otherwise, the clinician could have to rely on the observation of relatively rapid dynamic improvement (occurring over days to weeks), as well as documentation of reversibility either by direct visualization (i.e. cerebral angiography) or by indirect methods (i.e. MRA, CT angiography or transcranial Doppler ultrasound) (Hajj-Ali et al., 2002).

Treatment

There are no controlled therapeutic studies of patients with RVDs but, at present, there seems little justification for the use of immunosuppressive therapies other than glucocorticoids (see below). In our experience (Hajj-Ali et al., 2002), no patient was treated with more than 6 months of oral glucocorticoids and the majority were treated with adjunctive calcium channel blockers. We generally initiate therapy with a calcium channel blocker, alone, if the presentation is one of isolated headache without associated focal ischemic events (Grade C evidence). Based on long-term experience, we generally use verapamil, starting at 240 mg/day. If symptoms such as headaches are not controlled,

the dose of verapamil is increased, as needed. We add prednisone 1 mg/kg/day, if (a) there is associated evidence of ischemia (i.e. TIA or stroke), or (b) the patient does not respond promptly to calcium channel blockade. In patients presenting with more catastrophic clinical manifestations such as stroke, hemorrhagic stroke, or marked focal neurologic deficits, intravenous methylprednisolone pulse therapy is initiated. The rationale for the use of high-dose glucocorticoids is based not only on their anti-inflammatory properties but also their application in the treatment of experimentally induced vasoconstriction in animal models. As noted above, it is essential that when clinical signs and symptoms have abated repeat cerebral angiography (or other indirect technique either visualizing the cerebral vasculature or assessing cerebral blood flow) be performed to document total or near total resolution of the underlying abnormalities. We believe that this can be done as early as 4 weeks, but we generally perform this between 6 and 12 weeks after initiating therapy, depending upon the clinical situation. The absence of improvement or the occurrence of angiographic progression should warrant complete diagnostic re-evaluation. In particular, the absence of dynamic angiographic change on therapy suggests either atherosclerotic disease, embolic disease, or a hypercoaguable state, and only rarely, the possibility that this is an aggressive form of true angiitis which is being undertreated.

Infection

In evaluating CNS vasculitis, it is essential to search for infections, as the clinical and angiographic presentations of infection-related cerebral arteritis can mimic those of

Table 9.3 Infectious etiologies of CNS vasculitis

Viruses (HIV-1, varicella zoster virus, hepatitis C virus, others)
Syphilis
Borrelia burgdorferi
Bartonella
Mycobacterium tuberculosis
Fungi (*Aspergillus, Coccidioides*, others)
Bacteria (multiple)
Rickettsiae

PACNS. Complicating this evaluation is the fact that infection can be occult when neurovascular complications arise. Several pathogens have been described in association with either focal or diffuse cerebral vasculitis (Table 9.3) (Calabrese *et al.*, 1997). The search for a specific pathogen begins with an assessment of the epidemiologic features and individual risk factors in the suspected patient. Among viral pathogens that have been implicated in the development of CNS vasculitis, VZV has already been discussed in detail. Human immunodeficiency virus has been incriminated in a number of cases of CNS vasculitis, although the precise mechanism of its involvement is, as yet, unclear. More recently, hepatitis C virus has been associated with several cases both with and without the presence of associated cryoglobulinemia (Petty *et al.*, 1996). Ruling out infectious causes is particularly important in patients presenting with inflammatory changes in their spinal fluid. Certain pathogens, such as *Mycobacterium tuberculosis*, are notoriously difficult to identify and can take long periods of time to culture. Advances in molecular detection have minimized but not eliminated this problem.

Drugs

The relationship between drug use and CNS vasculitis is complex and has recently been reviewed (Calabrese and Duna, 1996; Buxton and McConachie, 2000). The most commonly implicated drugs in the development of CNS vasculitis are oral and intravenous amphetamines, cocaine, ephedrine, phenylpropanolamine, and heroin. It should be noted that most reported cases of "drug-induced CNS vasculitis" have been defined by cerebral angiography in the absence of pathologic confirmation. Because most of the implicated drugs are capable of inducing vasospasm, some or most of these cases could represent further examples of RVDs rather than true angiitis. For example, a

post-mortem study of patients dying of cerebral events with detectable cocaine in their system failed to demonstrate vasculitis in any (Nolte *et al.*, 1996). Despite these findings, well-documented cases of drug-associated vasculitis have been reported, with pathology ranging from perivascular cuffing to frank vasculitis either with or without vascular necrosis.

A high index of suspicion leading to prompt withdrawal of the offending drug is clearly the cornerstone of treatment. In addition, we recommend the use of a calcium channel blocker and a short course of glucocorticoids.

Malignancy-associated CNS vasculitis

Central nervous system vasculitis has been reported in association with Hodgkin's lymphoma, non-Hodgkin's lymphoma, angioimmunolymphoproliferative lesions (AIL), and intravascular B cell lymphoma (Calabrese *et al.*, 1997; Rosen *et al.*, 2000). In view of the recent data incriminating VZV as a possible etiologic agent in cases of widespread CNS vasculitis in immune-compromised hosts, we believe all cases of CNS vasculitis occurring in the setting of lymphoproliferative disease should be carefully screened for VZV. Clinical features of CNS vasculitis in association with lymphoproliferative disease are similar to those found in idiopathic PACNS. Reported presentations have included mass lesions, spinal cord involvement, and CNS hemorrhage. In most cases, therapy should be directed at the underlying lymphoproliferative disease and can consist of combination chemotherapy and/or radiotherapy. Favorable neurologic responses have been reported.

Systemic vasculitides

Central nervous system vasculitis can occur with any of the systemic vasculitides, but it is most commonly reported in polyarteritis nodosa, Behçet's syndrome, and in the ANCA-associated vasculitides (Moore and Calabrese, 1994). The true prevalence of CNS vasculitis in the systemic vasculitides is problematic to estimate as the diagnosis is frequently presumptive. In the setting of the systemic vasculitides, the new onset of neurologic signs or symptoms should raise the possibility of arteritic involvement of the CNS: however, the possibility of intercurrent complications such as opportunistic infections or the sequelae of other comorbidities such as hypertension also need to be considered. Treatment of CNS disease is generally directed at the underlying systemic vasculitis and generally consists of high doses of glucocorticoids in combination with a cytotoxic drug, particularly cyclophosphamide.

Central nervous system complications of giant cell arteritis (GCA) deserve special consideration. In general, CNS vasculitis is an uncommon complication of GCA. Hence, when CNS signs or symptoms arise in the setting of GCA, atherosclerosis should first and foremost be considered as the potential etiology. When CNS vasculitis does occur, extracranial vascular involvement, particularly of the carotid artery, is commonly seen. Rarely, the proximal intracranial segments of both the carotid and vertebral arteries can be affected (Rhodes et al., 1995; Ronthal et al., 2003). Among pathologically documented cases of GCA with intracranial involvement, inflammation has been generally limited to the proximal segments of the major arteries to the brain, and in a single example, a branch of the circle of Willis (Caselli and Hunder, 1993). Small vessel involvement in the setting of GCA is distinctly uncommon.

Miscellaneous mimicking conditions

As described in Table 9.1, there are numerous conditions capable of mimicking either the clinical and/or the angiographic characteristics of CNS vasculitis. Perhaps one of the most common and difficult to differentiate is cerebral atherosclerosis. Because of the ability of atherosclerosis to mimic the angiographic findings of vasculitis, the use of angiography as the sole diagnostic modality in elderly patients or those with multiple cardiovascular risk factors is particularly problematic.

Another condition that could at times be difficult to differentiate is demyelinating disease. The MRI appearance of demyelinating plaques, particularly when large, can resemble ischemic lesions (Finelli et al., 1997; Provenzale et al., 1994). The anatomic configuration of these lesions, confinement to the white matter, and characteristic CSF findings are helpful in the diagnosis of demyelinating disease, but equivocal cases can require biopsy.

The antiphospholipid (APL) antibody syndrome can at times be difficult to distinguish from CNS arteritis, as it is clearly associated with CNS ischemic events related to arterial thrombosis. An angiographic study of a series of APL patients revealed that 59% had solely intracranial lesions, of which 60% were solitary arterial occlusions and 40% were suggestive of vasculitis (Provenzale et al., 1994). This is potentially misleading,

as the occurrence of true CNS vasculitis in the APL syndrome is distinctly unusual.

Other conditions that can pose diagnostic problems include intravascular neoplasms, such as malignant angioendotheliomatosis, a neoplasm of B-cell origin which can be confined to the CNS and which can be associated with both inflammatory CSF and angiographic abnormalities (Lie, 1992a). Carcinomatous meningitis can present as chronic meningitis and can be problematic to identify. Multiple lumbar punctures with high-volume CSF analysis are sometimes required to secure this diagnosis. Radiation vasculitis can also be problematic to differentiate from CNS vasculitis unless a careful history reveals an exposure to therapeutic irradiation in the appropriate anatomic areas (Alfonso et al., 1997).

Diagnostic approach

As can be seen from Table 9.1, the differential diagnosis of PACNS is extensive and complex. The optimal approach to PACNS requires a well-constructed multidisciplinary team. Ideally, this should include a rheumatologist or immunologist interested in vascular inflammatory disease and a neurologist subspecializing in cerebrovascular disease with expertise in the broad differential of non-inflammatory acquired CNS vascular disorders. To secure the diagnosis, the team should also include a neurosurgeon experienced in the biopsy of CNS tissues, a neuroradiologist who understands the roles and limitations of neurodiagnostic techniques such as angiography, and a neuropathologist with experience and interest in such unusual cases.

Neuro-imaging modalities such as CT and MRI are important in the diagnosis of PACNS in its varying subsets. It can be stated again that MRI is more sensitive than CT and is the preferred initial diagnostic imaging technique when CNS vasculitis is suspected. Common MRI findings in PACNS include multiple, and often bilateral, infarcts, including lesions in the cortex, deep white matter and/or leptomeninges. Occasionally, such lesions demonstrate increased signal intensity with contrast enhancement, but this is a non-specific finding. Contrast enhancement in the leptomeninges, although not specific for arteritis, provides an ideal place for biopsy and may increase the yield of this technique. Atypical neuroradiographic presentations of PACNS have been reported, including white matter disease mimicking multiple sclerosis. More advanced neuroradiographic techniques, such as

SPECT and PET scanning, merely increase the sensitivity for detecting abnormalities of cerebral vascular flow while limiting specificity even further. The diagnosis of CNS vasculitis should never be made on the basis of non-vascular neuro-imaging studies.

In patients presenting acutely, such as described for those with suspected RVDs, an exhaustive search for emboli and hypercoagulability is essential. If none is found, cerebral angiography is generally the next logical step. Magnetic resonance angiography (MRA) is a poor substitute for high-quality cerebral angiography given its lower spatial resolution, even though it is easier to perform and associated with less risk (Calabrese et al., 1997). Critical in the interpretation of cerebral angiography is the appreciation that virtually no findings, regardless of how "classic", can alone secure the diagnosis of cerebral arteritis. Cerebral vasospasm, intravascular tumor, thromboembolism, atheromas, and vascular inflammation secondary to infection can all at times be indistinguishable from the findings in idiopathic PACNS. As with all diagnostic tests, cerebral angiography must be interpreted in the context of the clinical presentation. Even in a highly biased referral population for suspected CNS vasculitis, we have found that the specificity of cerebral angiography was only about 26% (Duna and Calabrese, 1995). These data emphasize that the greatest pitfall in the diagnosis of CNS angiitis is overreliance on the specificity of neuroradiographic studies.

The relationship between MRI and cerebral angiography is complex. In one study, the MRI was abnormal in 100%, but interestingly enough, there was only a modest correlation between MRI abnormalities and lesions noted on angiography (Pomper et al., 1999). However, other studies of patients with angiographically documented PACNS have revealed that MRIs can occasionally be normal. Thus, a normal MRI by itself does not exclude the diagnosis if the pre-test probability is high.

Perhaps the most important caveat in the diagnostic workup of suspected CNS vasculitis is that most patients will have a disease other than arteritis. A thoughtful differential diagnosis, accompanied by the appropriate use of cerebral angiography and/or biopsy, remains the gold standard. Given the lack of specificity of angiographic findings, we support advocating brain and/or leptomeningeal biopsies if alternative diagnoses cannot be eliminated.

The disturbing lack of correlation between angiography and brain biopsy results was recently highlighted in a retrospective review of 38 patients who had undergone cerebral angiography followed by cortical and leptomeningeal biopsy over an 8-year period (Kadkhodayan et al., 2004). Fourteen patients had typical angiographic findings of vasculitis (isolated multiple cerebral arterial segmental narrowings) but none had PACNS (transmural inflammation of small and medium sized blood vessels of meninges and/or cortex and fibrinoid necrosis of vessel walls) at brain biopsy. Six patients had specific pathologic diagnoses other than PACNS based on the brain biopsy and the remaining eight had non-diagnostic biopsies. Conversely, of the remaining 24 patients who also had both angiography and brain biopsy performed, 2 had PACNS diagnosed by biopsy but did *not* have typical angiographic findings. The authors noted that the changes in small vessels (arterioles and venules) seen in PACNS are below the resolution capabilities of conventional angiographic techniques, thus reducing the sensitivity of angiography. This study also confirms the lack of specificity of angiography for PACNS given that numerous other conditions can cause similar cerebral arterial stenoses.

When brain biopsy is indicated, the preferred technique is an open biopsy of the temporal tip of the non-dominant hemisphere, including both leptomeninges and underlying cortex (Parisi and Moore, 1994). Unfortunately, from a diagnostic perspective, lesions can be distributed in a patchy manner throughout the CNS, leading to the possibility of skipped lesions and false negative biopsies. Premortem brain biopsy has a sensitivity of 75% compared to autopsy results, representing a gold standard (Duna and Calabrese, 2005).

Sampling of the basilar meninges is important when attempting to exclude certain indolent infections or sarcoidosis. In the presence of leptomeningeal enhancement, a directed biopsy to involved areas is the preferred approach. Sterotactic biopsy is probably not indicated unless approaching a mass lesion. Regardless of the technique, tissue samples should be stained and cultured for microorganisms, with an effort being made to preserve frozen tissues for further investigations (i.e. immunohistochemistry, molecular analysis, etc.) as needed. In general, temporal artery biopsy has no role in the diagnosis of PACNS.

Another important reason to perform brain and leptomeningeal biopsies is that alternative diagnoses can often be determined only by this method. A review of 61 patients over a 7-year period who underwent brain biopsy to assess for possible PACNS yielded biopsies consistent with PACNS in 22 (36%), but also yielded alternative diagnoses even more often (39%) (Alrawi *et al.*, 1999). The most common alternative diagnoses determined were infectious encephalitis and primary CNS lymphoma. Of note, of the biopsy-proven cases of PACNS who also underwent angiography, a remarkable 64% had normal angiograms.

Monitoring disease activity

Regardless of the clinical subset or the specific therapy applied to a given patient with PACNS, a major problem for the clinician is how to monitor such therapy from the perspective of disease activity. The CNS, once injured, is slow to regenerate (if it ever does), and thus improvement in signs or symptoms caused by fixed tissue ischemia and necrosis is problematic. Other signs or symptoms such as headache, transient ischemic attacks, seizures, and weakness are only crude and non-specific markers of activity. Furthermore, we have found that many patients with PACNS will long complain of new and occasionally severe headaches that persist after the acute phase of the illness has been treated, and these may not be true indicators of disease activity. In our experience, calcium channel blockers are frequently helpful in treating this associated symptom.

Serial MRI examinations reveal that signs of tissue necrosis are often slow to resolve. On the other hand, serial MRIs are extremely valuable in identifying silent progression of ischemia, particularly during periods when immunusuppressive agents are being tapered. The appearance of new infarcts is strong evidence of increased disease activity even in the absence of symptoms or signs. For patients with GACNS, confirmation that CSF inflammation is subsiding is reassuring evidence that a treatment is effective. We generally perform repeat lumbar punctures soon after initiating treatment and after approximately 2–3 months of therapy to ensure declining cell counts and protein.

For patients with abnormal cerebral angiograms, repeating this study is an option to assure oneself that there is improvement. In patients with RVDs, documenting angiographic reversibility is essential, not only to assess the adequacy of therapy but also to verify the underlying diagnosis (Giovanini *et al.*, 1994). Failure to reverse angiographic findings suggests an alternative diagnosis. The optimal timing of repeat angiography is uncertain but, in general, we wait 6–12 weeks. Non-invasive assessments of cerebral blood flow, such as transcranial Doppler ultrasound and SPECT scanning, can also be useful, but, at present, there are no data regarding these applications.

Conclusion

In summary, the diagnosis of PACNS requires an extensive evaluation for mimicking conditions and a thorough workup including lumbar puncture, MRI, selective application of angiography, and more likely than not, a brain/leptomeningeal biopsy. Once the diagnosis of GACNS is comfortably made, treatment involves corticosteroids and other immunosuppressive drugs such as cyclophosphamide. For cases that fall within the RVDs category, we recommend calcium channel blockers, with the addition of corticosteroids when necessary. Although more studies are needed to determine optimal diagnostic and therapeutic modalities, much progress has been made in classifying and treating these disorders that only decades ago were thought to carry a uniformly fatal prognosis.

References

Alfonso ER, *et al*. Radiation myelopathy in over-irradiated patients: MR imaging findings. *Eur Radiol* 1997; **7**: 400–40.

Alrawi A, *et al*. Brain biopsy in primary angiitis of the central nervous system. *Neurology* 1999; **53**: 858–60.

Anders KH, *et al*. Giant cell arteritis with cerebral amyloid angiopathy: immunohistochemical and molecular studies. *Hum Pathol* 1997; **28**: 1237–46.

Buxton N, McConachie NS. Amphetamine abuse and intracranial haemorrhage. *J R Soc Med* 2000; **93**(9): 472–7.

Calabrese LH. Therapy of systemic vasculitis. *Neurol Clin* 1997; **15**(4): 973–91. [Erratum appears in *Neurol Clin* 1998; 16(3): x.]

Calabrese LH. A headache and a mass lesion: Vasculitis or CNS sarcoid? *Clin Exp Rheumatol* 2003; **21**(6 Suppl 32): S131–2.

Calabrese LH, Duna GF. Drug-induced vasculitis. *Curr Opin Rheumatol* 1996; **8**(1): 34–40.

Calabrese LH, Mallek JA. Primary angiitis of the central nervous system. Report of 8 new cases, review of the literature, and proposal for diagnostic criteria. *Medicine (Baltimore)* 1988; **67**(1): 20–39.

Calabrese LH, *et al*. Primary angiitis of the central nervous system: Diagnostic criteria and clinical approach. *Cleveland Clin J Med* 1992; **59**: 293–306.

Calabrese LH, *et al*. Benign angiopathy: A distinct subset of angiographically defined primary angiitis of the central nervous system. *J Rheumatol* 1993; **20**(12): 2046–50.

Calabrese LH, *et al*. Vasculitis in the central nervous system *Arthr Rheum* 1997; **40**(7): 1189–201.

Caselli RJ, Hunder GG. Neurologic aspects of giant cell (temporal) arteritis. *Rheum Dis Clin N Am* 1993; **19**(4): 941–53.

Dodick DW, *et al*. Thunderclap headache associated with reversible vasospasm and posterior leukoencephalopathy syndrome. *Cephalalgia* 2003; **23**(10): 994–7.

Duna GF, Calabrese LH. Limitations of invasive modalities in the diagnosis of primary angiitis of the central nervous system. *J Rheumatol* 1995; **22**(4): 662–7.

Duna GF, Calabrese LH. Primary angiitis of the central nervous system. In *Pathology and Genetics: Cerebrovascular Diseases*. Basel: ISN Neuropath Press; 2005: 147–51.

Finelli PF, *et al*. Idiopathic granulomatous angiitis of the CNS manifesting as diffuse white matter disease. *Neurology* 1997; **49**(6): 1696–9.

Gilden DH, *et al*. Neurologic complications of the reactivation of varicella-zoster virus. *N Engl J Med* 2000; **342**(9): 635–45. [Erratum appears in *N Engl J Med* 2000; 342 (14): 1063.]

Gilden DH, *et al*. The protean manifestations of varicella-zoster virus vasculopathy. *J Neurovirol* 2002; **8**(Suppl 2): 75–9.

Giovanini MA, *et al*. Granulomatous angiitis of the spinal cord: A case report. *Neurosurgery* 1994; **34**(3): 540–3.

Gripshover BM, Ellner JJ. Chronic meningitis. In Mandell GL, *et al*., (Eds). *Principles and Practice of Infectious Diseases*. 4th edn. Philadelphia: Churchill Livingstone, 1998.

Hajj-Ali RA, *et al*. Benign angiopathy of the central nervous system: Cohort of 16 patients with clinical course and long-term followup. *Arthr Rheum* 2002; **47**(6): 662–9.

Hankey GJ. Isolated angiitis/angiopathy of the central nervous system. *Cerebrovasc Dis* 1991; **1**: 2–15.

Kadkhodayan BA, *et al*. Primary angiitis of the central nervous system at conventional angiography. *Radiology* 2004; **233** (3): 878–82.

Lie JT. Malignant angioendotheliomatosis (intravascular lymphomatosis) clinically simulating primary angiitis of the central nervous system. *Arthr Rheum* 1992a; **35**(7): 831–4.

Lie JT. Primary (granulomatous) angiitis of the central nervous system: A clinicopathologic analysis of 15 new cases and a review of the literature. *Hum Pathol* 1992b; **23**(2): 164–71.

Moore PM. Vasculitis of the central nervous system. *Semin Neurol* 1994; **14**(4): 307–12.

Moore PM, Calabrese LH. Neurologic manifestations of systemic vasculitides. *Semin Neurol* 1994; **14**(4): 300–6.

Nolte KB, *et al*. Intracranial hemorrhage associated with cocaine abuse: A prospective autopsy study. *Neurology* 1996; **46**(5): 1291–6.

Parisi JE, Moore PM. The role of biopsy in vasculitis of the central nervous system. *Semin Neurol* 1994; **14**(4): 341–8.

Petty GW, *et al*. Cerebral ischemia in patients with hepatitis C virus infection and mixed cryoglobulinemia. *Mayo Clin Proc* 1996; **71**(7): 671–8. [Erratum appears in *Mayo Clin Proc* 1996; **71**(8): 824.]

Pomper MG, *et al*. CNS vasculitis in autoimmune disease: MR imaging findings and correlation with angiography. *Am J Neuroradiol* 1999; **20**(1): 75–85.

Provenzale JM, *et al*. Antiphospholipid antibodies in patients without systemic lupus erythematosus: Neuroradiologic findings. *Radiology* 1994; **192**(2): 531–7.

Rhodes RH, *et al*. Primary angiitis and angiopathy of the central nervous system and their relationship to systemic giant cell arteritis. *Arch Pathol Lab Med* 1995; **119**(4): 334–49.

Ronthal M, *et al*. Case records of the Massachusetts General Hospital. Weekly clinicopathological exercises. Case 21–2003. A 72-year-old man with repetitive strokes in the posterior circulation *N Engl J Med* 2003; **349**(2): 170–80.

Rosen CL, *et al*. Primary angiitis of the central nervous system as a first presentation in Hodgkin's disease: A case report and review of the literature. *Neurosurgery* 2000; **46**(6): 1504–8.

Schwab C, *et al*. Familial British dementia: Colocalization of furin and ABri amyloid. *Acta Neuropathol* 2003; **106**(3): 278–84.

Singhal AB. Cerebral vasoconstriction syndromes. *Top Stroke Rehab* 2004; **11**(2): 1–6.

Stone JH, *et al*. Sensitivities of noninvasive tests for central nervous system vasculitis: A comparison of lumbar puncture, computed tomography, and magnetic resonance imaging. *J Rheumatol* 1994; **21**(7): 1277–82.

Wynne PJ, *et al*. Radiographic features of central nervous system vasculitis. *Neurol Clin* 1997; **15**(4): 779–804.

Younger DS, *et al*. Granulomatous angiitis of the nervous system. *Neurol Clin* 1997; **15**(4): 821–34.

Acute viral encephalitis: role of the immune system in viral clearance from the CNS and in the generation of pathology

David N. Irani and Natalie Prow

Introduction

Viral infections of the central nervous system (CNS) are uncommon but potentially devastating clinical events. As a group, these infections range from benign, self-limited forms of meningitis, to full-blown and often fatal cases of acute encephalitis to chronic, persistent diseases. The relative inaccessibility of the CNS to circulating components of the immune system renders the brain and spinal cord particularly susceptible to persistent viral infection, and the CNS has evolved unique ways to modulate local immune responses during these diseases. Furthermore, the longevity and lack of regenerative capacity of many neural cells pose unique challenges to viral clearance efforts, as the cytolytic elimination of virus-infected cells could be more detrimental to the infected host than the effects of the pathogen itself. Still, many viruses are effectively cleared from the CNS without causing significant neurological damage, and studies in animal models are now elucidating the non-cytolytic clearance mechanisms that serve to accomplish this task. Likewise, the contribution of host responses to the generation of neuropathology in these diseases is also being increasingly understood, and interventions designed to target these detrimental responses could eventually prove to be an important adjunctive strategy for the treatment of some of these infections. This chapter reviews how the immune system mounts a response to infection, clears virus from the CNS, and sometimes contributes to tissue injury during acute viral encephalitis. It will focus primarily on immunological mechanisms elucidated in animal models of these diseases.

Viruses that cause acute encephalitis in humans and animals

Acute viral encephalitis in humans

Nearly 100 different viruses are known to infect the human CNS (Johnson, 1998), although a much smaller number of these pathogens cause most cases of acute viral encephalitis. Infections caused by both DNA and RNA viruses can produce this syndrome (Table 10.1). Because DNA viruses have a nuclear phase during their replication cycle, they can establish latency (either by integrating into the host genome or by persisting in an episomal form) and thus evade detection or elimination by the immune system. As such, these viruses sometimes cause significant CNS disease in the immunocompromised host only when they reactivate as antiviral defenses fail. Most RNA viruses, on the other hand, replicate only in the cytoplasm and therefore are susceptible to different mechanisms of immune-mediated control. Although these pathogens do not typically enter a true latent state (i.e. where no infectious virus is produced), they can still cause persistent CNS infection, whereby low-level production of infectious virus or viral RNA can occur. In this setting, the immune response may not actually have to completely eradicate the pathogen to meet the needs of the host, but instead simply suppresses viral replication to a level where clinically apparent disease subsides. In considering the concept of non-cytolytic clearance from the CNS, a state of suppressed viral replication (even though it falls short of full viral eradication) can sometimes be the best result the host can achieve without causing immune-mediated injury.

Inflammatory Diseases of the Central Nervous System, ed. T. Kilpatrick, R. M. Ransohoff and S. Wesselingh. Published by Cambridge University Press. © Cambridge University Press 2010.

Table 10.1 Important causes of viral meningoencephalitis in humans

Virus	Tropism	Geographical distribution
DNA viruses		
Herpes simplex virus	Neurons	Worldwide
Cytomegalovirus	Neurons	Worldwide
Human herpesvirus 6	Oligodendrocytes	Worldwide
JC virus	Oligodendrocytes	Worldwide
Adenovirus	Neurons, ependyma	Worldwide
RNA viruses		
Poliovirus	Neurons*	Africa, India
Coxsackie virus	Meninges	Worldwide
ECHO virus	Meninges	Worldwide
Enterovirus 71	Neurons	Asia, Australia
Japanese encephalitis virus	Neurons	Asia, Australia
West Nile virus	Neurons	Africa, Europe, Americas
St. Louis encephalitis virus	Neurons	USA
Eastern equine encephalitis virus	Neurons	Americas
Venezuelan equine encephalitis virus	Neurons	Americas
LaCrosse virus	Neurons	USA
Lymphocytic choriomeningitis virus	Meninges	Worldwide
Rabies virus	Neurons	Africa, Asia, Americas
Human immunodeficiency virus	Microglia	Worldwide

*Cranial and spinal motor neurons, in particular.

Animal models of acute viral encephalitis

Most of our current understanding of the immune responses elicited during acute viral encephalitis comes from the study of a few well-characterized infections (mostly caused by RNA viruses) that occur in rodent models (Table 10.2). In several of these experimental systems, viral clearance from the CNS is more complete and recovery ensues after the acute phase of disease subsides. In others, full viral clearance is not achieved or viral tropism changes and a chronic phase of infection develops. Some of these infections elicit a host immune response that actually contributes to CNS injury. In others, virus–host cell interactions are the main determinant of outcome, with little contribution from the associated inflammation. Still, across all these model systems, host factors (primarily age and genetic background) and viral determinants (viral strain differences) both contribute to the fate of infected animals. Here, immune responses typically progress through a stage where innate defense mechanisms in the CNS recognize the presence of the pathogen, followed thereafter by an influx of lymphocytes and monocytes from the periphery as the adaptive immune response becomes engaged. Partial or complete control of virus replication and/or viral clearance is achieved, and finally, regulatory mechanisms act to terminate any local inflammation that persists within the CNS.

Cellular targets of encephalitic viruses

Neurons

Many viruses that infect the CNS target cells of the leptomeninges covering the brain and spinal cord and cause meningitis. This scenario is rarely of long-term significance to the host, since the pathogen is accessible to the immune system and because damaged cells can be renewed. A less common, but potentially more severe, situation arises when viruses directly infect neurons in the underlying CNS parenchyma, causing encephalitis or encephalomyelitis. These terminally differentiated and non-renewable cells present formidable challenges to the immune system, both in terms of recognizing and coping with an intracellular pathogen. Further, not all populations of neurons are equally susceptible to different viruses; tropism depends on the surface expression of viral receptors, the route of viral entry into the CNS, and mechanisms of intercellular viral spread. Many neurotropic viruses spread within the CNS by subverting axonal transport mechanisms as they pass from cell to cell across their connecting synapses (Ehrengruber *et al.*, 2002). Others can disseminate via the cerebrospinal fluid (CSF) (Griffin, 2003). The neuronal response to infection is one primary determinant of clinical outcome from many forms of acute viral encephalitis.

Table 10.2 Common animal models of CNS viral infection

Virus*	Disease	Tropism	Phase	Clearance
LCMV	Immune-mediated choriomeningitis	Meninges, neurons, choroid plexus	Acute	Yes
TMEV	Encephalitis	Neurons, glial cells	Acute	Yes[†]
TMEV	Demyelinating encephalomyelitis	Astrocytes, microglia, oligodendrocytes	Chronic	Gray matter only
MHV	Encephalomyelitis microglia, astrocytes	Oligodendrocytes	Acute	Yes
MHV	Demyelinating encephalomyelitis	Oligodendrocytes	Chronic	Unclear
SV	Encephalomyelitis	Neurons	Acute	Yes
RV	Encephalomyelitis	Neurons	Acute	Yes

* LCMV, lymphocytic choriomeningitis virus; TMEV, Theiler's murine encephalomyelitis virus; MHV, mouse hepatitis virus; SV, Sindbis virus; RV, rabies virus.
† From resistant host strains only.

Glial cells

Other encephalitic viruses target glial cells instead of, or in addition to, neurons. Direct infection of oligodendrocytes can result in demyelination, while viruses that damage astrocytes often disrupt critical homeostatic processes such as the production of neurotrophic factors, the removal of extracellular toxins, or the support of the blood–brain barrier (BBB). Infection of microglia can subvert the phagocytic or antigen-presenting properties of these cells, or result in excessive activation to the point where the cells themselves produce neurotoxic substances. Accordingly, viruses that target glial cells can also cause severe forms of acute encephalitis by producing local changes that indirectly injure neurons. From the standpoint of immune clearance mechanisms, the tropism of a given pathogen (neuronal versus glial) is an important factor in determining how the host response detects and responds to CNS viral infection.

Induction of immune responses to CNS viral infection

Immunological quiescence of the normal CNS

In the absence of infection, the CNS is relatively devoid of immunological activity. Although T cells provide some low-level surveillance of certain CNS compartments (Ransohoff et al., 2003), the BBB normally excludes most circulating immune cells and there are few cell adhesion and major histocompatibility (MHC) molecules that are expressed in the absence of disease. Likewise, highly reactive microglial cells are

kept in a quiescent state via the synaptic activity of normal neurons (Hoek et al., 2000), and astrocytes and meningeal cells both constitutively produce anti-inflammatory substances such as transforming growth factor-beta (TGF-β) that serve to suppress the activation of endothelial cells and further inhibit leukocyte migration into the normal CNS (Johnson et al., 1992). The older idea of the CNS as an "immunologically privileged" site (i.e. one where immune cells have highly restricted access and where inflammation is never supposed to occur) has given way to the more modern concept that the CNS simply maintains a set of more active immunoregulatory properties than most other tissues that can be rapidly disengaged, such as with acute viral infection, as the need arises.

Induction of the interferon response

When neural cells become infected with viral pathogens, rapid cellular changes in the CNS initiate a cascade of neuroprotective responses. As in other tissues, one of the first events to occur with CNS viral infection is the induction of type I interferon (IFN) molecules. Not only do IFN-α/β have direct actions to constrain virus replication and slow virus spread in response to a variety of neurotropic viruses (Muller et al., 1994; Greider and Vogel, 1999; Byrnes et al., 2000), but these substances also induce the local production of neurotrophic factors and immunoregulatory cytokines such as interleukin (IL)-10 by astrocytes and microglial cells (Boutros et al., 1997; Chabot and Yong, 2000). The IFN-β is the main type I IFN produced within the CNS by neurons and glial cells during viral infection (Sandberg et al., 1994). Several reports suggest that IFN-α can actually have unwanted CNS toxicity in response to certain neurotropic viruses (Akwa *et al.*, 1998). From the standpoint of the pathogen, viruses encoding proteins that inhibit IFN production or that block IFN activity have emerged with a greater capacity to avoid full clearance from the CNS (van Pesch *et al.*, 2001). In terms of outcome for the host, the central importance of type I IFN in the innate defense against many different CNS viral infections is most clearly demonstrated in experimental studies showing that susceptibility to fatal disease is markedly increased in animals lacking IFN-α/β receptors (Muller *et al.*, 1994; Fiette *et al.*, 1995; Greider and Vogel, 1999; Byrnes *et al.*, 2000). Indeed, despite some lingering concerns about neurotoxicity (Akwa *et al.*, 1998), IFN-α has now actually been investigated as a therapeutic agent in both animal models and in human cases of flavivirus encephalitis (Brooks and Phillpotts, 1999; Solomon *et al.*, 2003).

Activation of other innate immune pathways

A number of mediators besides IFN-β can also be produced by neurons stressed or damaged from viral infection that then activate nearby astrocytes and microglia. These activated glial cells, in turn, can respond directly to the neurons from which the stress signals originated, or they can release factors that increase MHC molecule expression and enhance the recruitment of circulating leukocytes into the CNS. While the soluble factors produced by neurons in response to viral-mediated injury remain incompletely characterized, they certainly include inflammatory cytokines (IFN-γ, IL-6) and chemokines (CX3CL1, CCL21). The CX3CL1 (fractalkine), in particular, is a membrane-bound chemokine constitutively expressed by a subset of neurons that is cleaved from the cell surface following a variety of injuries (Chapman *et al.*, 2000). The soluble form of the molecule can interact with local microglial cells expressing the CX3CL1 receptor (CX3CR1), resulting in their proliferation, chemotaxis, and further cytokine and chemokine release (Harrison *et al.*, 1998; Maciejewski-Lenoir *et al.*, 1999; Neumann, 2001). Although specific cytokines and chemokines made by glial cells in response to CNS viral infection can vary with the specific pathogen involved, commonly induced mediators include IL-1, IL-6, IL-12, tumor necrosis factor-alpha (TNF-α), CCL2 (MCP-1), CCL4 (MIP-1β), CCL5 (RANTES), CCL7 (MCP-3), and CXCL10 (IP-10) (Wesselingh *et al.*, 1994; Asensio and Campbell, 1997; Parra *et al.*, 1997; Lane *et al.*, 1998).

Local production of these factors in the CNS results in the induction of MHC molecules on microglia, the up-regulation of adhesion molecules on vascular endothelial cells, and the influx of lymphocytes and monocytes into perivascular spaces and then into the CNS parenchyma itself. For many experimental forms of acute viral encephalitis in rodents, these changes evolve over a period of several days to a week after infection and typically before adaptive immune mechanisms become fully engaged.

Activation of the adaptive immune response to CNS viral infection

Priming of antigen-specific immune responses

While cells within the CNS can present antigens to previously activated T cells, it is generally agreed that most naive T and B lymphocytes must be primed in secondary lymphoid organs before they migrate into the CNS (Cserr and Knopf, 1992; Fisher and Reichmann, 2001). Because most naturally occurring CNS viral infections emerge on the heels of a gastrointestinal or respiratory phase of disease, or develop following the bite of an infected mosquito or animal vector, it is likely that exposure of viral antigens to the immune system occurs in the periphery before CNS involvement develops. Even for antigens delivered experimentally into the CNS, the most effective presentation to the immune system occurs after their passage into deep cervical lymph nodes (Cserr and Knopf, 1992), and for viruses inoculated directly into CSF, robust systemic and CNS inflammatory responses are clearly elicited (Stevenson *et al.*, 1997). Thus, the induction of virus-specific immune responses during acute encephalitis likely occurs via the transport of viral antigens to peripheral lymphoid tissue where antigen presentation as well as immune priming and expansion most effectively occur. The homing of activated immune effectors into the CNS then allows for cognate antigens to be recognized on neural cells.

Development of CNS inflammation

Infiltration of mononuclear inflammatory cells into CNS parenchyma during acute viral encephalitis typically begins several days after infection and evolves rapidly thereafter. All cellular components of the adaptive immune system can be found in these infiltrates; natural killer (NK) cells and CD4+ and CD8+ T cells are usually detected first, followed soon thereafter by B cells and monocyte/macrophages (Irani and Griffin, 1992; Hatalski *et al.*, 1998; Haring *et al.*, 2001; Tschen *et al.*, 2002). The number of inflammatory cells may peak within the CNS one to two weeks after infection, and then cells gradually disappear unless viral clearance is incomplete (Tyor *et al.*, 1992; Marten *et al.*, 2000). Activated T cells traffic non-specifically into the CNS during acute viral encephalitis, but only antigen-specific T cells are selectively retained at that site (Irani and Griffin, 1996). Tissue-infiltrating T cells locally produce multiple cytokines including IFN-γ, IL-4, and IL-10, but rarely IL-2 (Pearce *et al.*, 1994; Wesselingh *et al.*, 1994; Parra *et al.*, 1997; Hatalski *et al.*, 1998; Chang *et al.*, 2000). These mediators can either participate in the control of virus replication or serve to regulate other local immune effectors (Binder and Griffin, 2001; Patterson *et al.*, 2002). The B cells that infiltrate the CNS can produce significant amounts of antibody, mainly of the immunoglobulin (Ig) A and IgG subclasses (Griffin, 1981). In some cases, long-term production of virus-specific antibody is found within the CNS, even well after the active stage of infection has subsided (Tyor *et al.*, 1992). This persistent humoral response in both the brain and CSF may be required to prevent any late reactivation of viruses that were suppressed but incompletely cleared.

Antigen presentation within the CNS

Anti-viral T cells responding to infections in the CNS require MHC molecules in order to recognize their cognate antigens, but expression of these molecules in the brain and spinal cord is tightly controlled. While there is no constitutive expression of MHC class I molecules within the CNS, endothelial cells and certain glial cell populations rapidly up-regulate these proteins during the early phases of several experimental viral infections (Kimura and Griffin, 2000). Neurons, however, rarely express detectable MHC class I proteins, and suppression of these molecules on these cells appears to be regulated at both a transcriptional and a post-transcriptional level (Jarosinski *et al.*, 2001). A few in-vivo studies, however, have reported that the mRNAs encoding MHC class I heavy chain, β$_2$-microglobulin, and transporter associated with antigen processing (TAP)-1 and TAP-2 are induced in neurons with CNS viral infection (Kimura and Griffin, 2000). Still, it remains controversial whether functional MHC class I molecules are ever expressed on the neuronal cell surface during these diseases (Periera and Simmons, 1999; Kimura and Griffin, 2000). The MHC class II

molecules are also absent from the normal CNS, but they, too, can be induced following viral infection. Perivascular macrophages and parenchymal microglia express MHC class II proteins during acute viral encephalitis (Pope *et al.*, 1998), and these cells are likely the only ones in the CNS that truly present antigens to CD4+ T cells. Astrocytes can be induced to express MHC class II molecules in vitro, but this is rarely observed in vivo (Pope *et al.*, 1998).

Regulation of local immune responses during CNS viral infection

Immunological effects of CNS glycolipids

Several lines of evidence suggest that the CNS actively regulates immune responses during acute viral encephalitis beyond just controlling the passage of leukocytes across the BBB and limiting the local expression of MHC molecules. In particular, the brain can also directly influence the effector functions and survival of infiltrating immune cells via tissue-specific regulatory mechanisms that have implications for the recovery from infection. Indeed, once T cells traverse the BBB and pass through perivascular spaces into the CNS parenchyma, they encounter a local immunological environment that actively inhibits their proliferation and that strongly favors the production of T helper 2 (Th2)-type cytokines. Brain gangliosides, glycolipids that are highly expressed on neural cells compared to parenchymal cells of other tissues, directly inhibit IL-2 production and proliferation of T cells in the CNS without altering their production of IL-4, IL-5, or IL-10 (Irani *et al.*, 1996, 1997). Resistance of T cells to this local immunoregulatory effect in certain inbred strains of mice predisposes these animals to the development of immune-mediated CNS injury following alphavirus encephalitis (Irani, 1998).

Immunoregulatory effects of CNS microglial cells

Another immunoregulatory mechanism unique to the CNS relates to the local antigen-presenting capacity of microglial cells. While microglia can stimulate antigen-specific CD4+ T cells to produce IFN-γ in a MHC class II-dependent manner, these cells cannot trigger IL-2 production or proliferation by T cells (Ford *et al.*, 1996). Conversely, peripheral macrophages that infiltrate the CNS but that tend to remain localized around blood vessels can support full T cell activation, including clonal expansion (Ford *et al.*, 1996). This difference is not attributed to altered expression of co-stimulatory molecules (Ford *et al.*, 1996), and it has been proposed to represent a unique mechanism through which the CNS can limit local inflammatory responses. Whether this results from some unique intrinsic property of microglia or has to do with effects of the CNS microenvironment on antigen-presenting cells (APC) is somewhat unclear; astrocytes, however, have been identified as a source of soluble factors that can deactivate the stimulatory capacity of brain paren-chymal APCs (Hailer *et al.*, 1998)

Control of T cell survival in the CNS

Induction of apoptosis is an important means used by the CNS to limit the survival of activated T cells that leave the perivascular space and invade the brain parenchyma. Indeed, the CNS microenvironment may be considerably pro-apoptotic for infiltrating lympho-cytes in several ways. Thus, in addition to death signals that are delivered to T cells by CNS APCs (Ford *et al.*, 1996), there also are apoptosis-inducing mechanisms that do not occur at the time of antigen presentation (Bauer *et al.*, 1998). Neurons, in particular, can express Fas ligand (CD95L) on their cell surfaces, and these molecules serve to limit the survival of adjacent Fas (CD95)-expressing activated T cells (Flugel *et al.*, 2000; Medana *et al.*, 2001). In addition, gangliosides can induce apoptosis in activated T cells (Irani, 1998), and their abundance within the CNS also contributes to the control of local inflammation. Indeed, T cells that resist the apoptotic effects of these glycolipids can persist within the CNS and are more likely to result in immune-mediated injury (Irani, 1998). Thus, failure to induce T cell apoptosis within the CNS during acute viral encephalitis can have significant detrimental con-sequences for the infected host.

Mechanisms of immune-mediated clearance of viruses from the CNS

General considerations and strategies

Clearing viruses from the CNS is a complex process that varies with both the target cell infected and with the nature of the pathogen involved. As in all tissues, successful viral clearance involves both the eradication of cell-free extracellular virus and the elimination (or at least the permanent suppression) of virus-infected cells. Indeed, if infected cells such as neurons are to survive, then clearance mechanisms need to inhibit the intracellular synthesis of viral proteins and nucleic acids without significantly altering cellular function. Short of fully cleansing all viral genomes from each cell, host responses must be able to prevent the resumption of viral replication over the long term in order to avoid persistent or recurrent disease (Tyor *et al.*, 1992; Hawke *et al.*, 1998; Marten *et al.*, 2000). Experimental data suggest that, in general, antibody responses have a central role in clearing viruses from neurons, while T cell responses are more important in viral clearance from glial cells. As with other complex biological processes, however, overlapping and redun-dant mechanisms clearly exist.

Viral clearance from neurons

Anti-viral antibodies play a central role in clearing alphaviruses, rhabdoviruses, coronaviruses, and picor-naviruses from the neurons of infected mice (reviewed in Griffin, 2003). Many of the specific antibodies that mediate disease protection or CNS viral clearance are directed against viral surface proteins, and most are also capable of inhibiting virus replication in primary neurons in vitro (Levine *et al.*, 1991). The precise molecular mechanisms by which such large mole-cules act to inhibit an intracellular process such as viral replication remain incompletely characterized, but they are perhaps best studied for the murine alphavirus, Sindbis virus (SV). Here, bivalent antibo-dies against a viral envelope glycoprotein bind the infected cell surface to inhibit replication; monovalent fragments are ineffective implying that crosslinking of surface viral proteins is required (Ubol *et al.*, 1995). Antibody treatment restores normal cellular processes such as the maintenance of membrane polarity and host cell protein synthesis that are shut off by infection (Depres *et al.*, 1995a), and it also directly inhibits the synthesis of viral proteins (Levine *et al.*, 1991; Ubol *et al.*, 1995). Type I IFN can synergize with anti-viral antibodies to control SV replication in vitro (Depres *et al.*, 1995b), and this combination of host factors is crucial to CNS clearance of SV in vivo (Levine *et al.*, 1991; Byrnes *et al.*, 2000). Still, "clearance" in this model is an incomplete process, as viral RNA can be amplified from the brains of mice many months after clinical recovery has occurred (Levine and Griffin, 1992). Indeed, long-term production of anti-viral anti-bodies within the brains of these recovered animals suggests the continued need for local immunological control over the life of the host (Tyor *et al.*, 1992; Tschen *et al.*, 2002).

In other animal models of CNS viral infection, both CD4+ and CD8+ T cells have been shown to play a role in viral clearance from neurons. The CD8+ T cells are important for the rapid control of rabies virus and herpes simplex virus replication in neurons (Hooper *et al.*, 1998; Liu *et al.*, 2001), and these cells can exert their anti-viral effector functions either through direct cytolysis of infected targets or via non-cytolytic, cytokine-mediated clearance pathways (Bilzer and Stitz, 1994; Patterson *et al.*, 2002). It is generally assumed that non-cytolytic mechanisms would result in a more favorable clinical outcome for the host, and among T cell-derived cytokines, IFN-γ in particular has been shown to be important for clearance of SV, measles virus, and mouse hepatitis virus (MHV) from neurons (Pearce *et al.*, 1994; Binder and Griffin, 2001; Patterson *et al.*, 2002). In the SV system, different neuronal populations vary in their responsiveness to the anti-viral effects of IFN-γ; spinal motor neurons are highly responsive and clear virus in the complete absence of antibody, while cortical neurons require anti-viral antibodies for full clearance to be achieved (Binder and Griffin, 2001). It is not known whether this difference relates to the ability of these different neuronal populations to bind IFN-γ or to respond to this mediator. Neurons, to a much greater extent than glial cells, widely express the IFN-γ receptor (Robertson *et al.*, 2000). Beyond IFN-γ, other T cell-derived factors that directly control viral replication in neurons include granzyme A (Periera *et al.*, 2000), while other cytokines can facilitate viral clearance from neurons indirectly via the induction of nitric oxide (Komatsu *et al.*, 1999).

Viral clearance from glial cells

The clearance of viruses from glial cells likely involves multiple overlapping mechanisms, in part because glia are more capable than neurons of expressing MHC molecules and thus being directly recognized by virus-specific T cells. Still, in two well-studied animal models of encephalitis where the viruses cause prominent infection of glial cells, incomplete viral clearance results in a chronic disease accompanied by immune-mediated demyelination in susceptible strains of mice. Intracerebral challenge with Theiler's murine encephalomyelitis virus (TMEV) causes infection of both neurons and glia, and the recovery of host strains that are resistant to chronic disease follows complete viral clearance from both cell populations. When clearance from astrocytes, oligodendrocytes, and microglia is incomplete, particularly in the cerebral white matter (Njenga *et al.*, 1997), chronic disease develops in susceptible hosts.

Among resistant mice, deletion of either CD4+ or CD8+ T cells (Murray *et al.*, 1998), or genetic deficiency of perforin (Rossi *et al.*, 1998), results in incomplete viral clearance and chronic disease. These findings strongly implicate both T cell cytotoxicity (perforin) and non-cytolytic mechanisms (cytokine production by CD4+ T cells) in viral clearance and recovery. Antibody can also contribute to clearance from glia in this model, as the transfer of immune serum from vaccinated animals reduces the number of infected CNS cells in otherwise susceptible mice (Rossi *et al.*, 1998). Despite these observations, it is not fully understood why susceptible hosts are unable to clear TMEV from the CNS.

Intracerebral inoculation of mice with the JHM strain of mouse hepatitis virus (JHMV) results mainly in the infection of glial cells. Here, too, virus-specific CD4+ or CD8+ T cells help to control CNS viral replication (Sussman *et al.*, 1989), and measurable anti-viral antibody titers are not detected until after CNS clearance is achieved (Lin *et al.*, 1997). Furthermore, the mechanism of JHMV clearance from glia is cell type-specific; IFN-γ is important for clearance from oligodendrocytes (Parra *et al.*, 1999), while perforin-dependent CD8+ T cell-mediated cytolysis eradicates virus from astrocytes and microglia (Lin *et al.*, 1997). The CD4+ T cells can provide help in the viral clearance process by facilitating the survival and effector function of CNS-infiltrating CD8+ T cells (Stohlman *et al.*, 1998). Although antibody does not appear to participate in the initial clearance of JHMV from the CNS, antibody-producing B cells persist in the brain and are essential to prevent reactivation after initial clearance has been achieved (Ramakrishna *et al.*, 2002; Tschen *et al.*, 2002).

Role of the immune response in generating neuropathology

Injurious innate immune responses

While innate immune responses activated by CNS viral infection can serve various protective functions, these responses may also have negative consequences for the host. Viral spread to the CNS occurs early in the course of systemic infection with either human or simian immunodeficiency virus (HIV or SIV), often leading to the development of neurological symptoms and characteristic neuropathological changes over time. Microglia are the main neural cells infected by these pathogens, and there is little to no direct infection of neurons despite extensive damage to these cells.

An explanation for this neuronal pathology therefore requires that some indirect or bystander injury mechanism be invoked. While it is clear that viral proteins can themselves be neurotoxic (Li *et al.*, 2005; Rumbaugh and Nath, 2006), there is also strong evidence that the products of activated microglial cells play an important role in the generation of clinical symptoms and neuronal and axonal damage (Glass and Wesselingh, 2001; Wesselingh and Thompson, 2001). In HIV infection, brain levels of TNF-α and inducible nitric oxide synthase (iNOS) correlate with the severity of neurological impairment (Wesselingh *et al.*, 1993; Adamson *et al.*, 1996). In SIV-infected macaques that develop a rapid neurological syndrome with a high CNS viral load, treatment of animals with drugs that suppress microglial activation reduces axonal injury and renders infected cells less hospitable to virus replication (Zink *et al.*, 2005). Furthermore, activated monocytes trafficking into the CNS of these SIV-infected animals directly contribute to neuronal injury, albeit via poorly defined mechanisms (Williams *et al.*, 2005). Nevertheless, these cells and the soluble products they generate become additional therapeutic targets in these diseases.

In the SV model of alphavirus encephalomyelitis, mice deficient in the pro-inflammatory cytokine, IL-1β, are highly resistant to paralysis and death when challenged with a lethal viral strain (Liang *et al.*, 1999). This suggests that IL-1β is a central mediator of disease pathogenesis in this model. Subsequent studies using two completely unrelated compounds have shown that pharmacological inhibitors of microglial activation that also suppress local IL-1β production in the CNS can directly protect mice and their vulnerable neuronal populations from the damaging effects of this pathogen without altering virus tropism, replication, or clearance from CNS tissues (N. Prow and D. Irani, unpublished observations). Related studies now demonstrate that these innate immune responses activate a non-cell-autonomous pathway that results in glutamate-mediated damage of both infected and non-infected neurons (Darman *et al.*, 2004). Cytokines such as IL-1β derived from activated microglial cells are suspected of acting on astrocytes to diminish their physiological capacity to buffer extracellular levels of glutamate, an excitatory amino acid neurotransmitter that actually kills neurons at supra-therapeutic levels. Indeed, pharmacological blockade of glutamate receptors also protects mice from lethal SV infection without altering CNS virus replication or spread (Nargi-Aizenman *et al.*, 2004).

Detrimental adaptive immunity

In several well-characterized animal models of viral encephalitis, part of the T cell response elicited consequent to infection actually contributes to the neuropathology and the adverse clinical outcome from disease. Lymphocytic choriomeningitis virus (LCMV) infection of adult mice is perhaps the best studied example of this phenomenon; the pathogen itself is non-cytopathic and the fatal choriomeningitis that animals develop is fully mediated by the same virus-specific CD8+ T cells that promote viral clearance (Cole *et al.*, 1972; Buchmeier *et al.*, 1980). Furthermore, a seminal paper demonstrated that clinical disease in this model depends entirely on CD8+ T cell expression of the cytotoxic granule protein, perforin, implying that pathogenic T cells enter the CNS and cause disease in a cell contact-dependent manner (Kagi *et al.*, 1994). More recently, however, this result has been challenged; one study showed that perforin-deficient CD8+ T cells still can mediate fatal choriomeningitis, despite impaired cytotoxic activity and reduced cytokine production (Storm *et al.*, 2006). Nevertheless, a requirement for these T cells to access the CNS to cause disease was shown (Storm *et al.*, 2006). As such, a definitive role for CD8+ T cells in the generation of LCMV-induced neuropathology, despite some unanswered questions about the actual molecular mechanisms of neural injury, appears secure.

During murine TMEV infection of certain susceptible host strains, viral clearance from the CNS in the acute stages of encephalitis is incomplete and for infected animals there is a transition into a chronic phase of the disease characterized by immune-mediated demyelination (Lipton and Dal Canto, 1976). Here, CD4+ T cells are the cellular element responsible for the destruction of oligodendrocytes and the myelin loss (Pope *et al.*, 1996). Although initially directed against viral antigens in this chronic phase of disease, CD4+ T cells specific for various myelin peptides later emerge in infected animals through a process referred to as epitope spreading (Miller *et al.*, 1997). The working hypothesis is that the anti-viral immune response acting within the brain against persistently infected cells exposes otherwise cryptic myelin epitopes that then results in priming to these self-antigens. Indeed, the finding that induction of peripheral tolerance among T cells to TMEV epitopes prevents the subsequent demyelinating phase of disease supports the idea that this myelin-reactive T cell autoimmunity is a direct result of the virus-specific T cell immunity (Karpus *et al.*, 1995). Again, however, the exact molecular mechanisms of neural injury in this model remain to be fully elucidated.

A potential role for antigen-specific humoral immune responses in the generation of neuropathology either during or following CNS viral infection has been posited, but never rigorously confirmed. As already discussed, anti-viral antibodies, when immunologically active, generally clear viruses from infected neurons and glial cells in a non-cytolytic manner and thus do not affect the survival of the host cell. There are no reported experimental examples of antibodies exacerbating clinical disease or the neuropathology of viral encephalitis. From a clinical standpoint, however, there are a few reports describing the detection of antibodies against neuronal antigens in the CSF of patients with various CNS viral infections (Gisslen *et al.*, 2000), including several papers that suggest the local presence of such antibodies is associated with more severe clinical disease progression (Fokina *et al.*, 1991; Desai *et al.*, 1994). Still, whether such humoral responses are causally related to the worsening of clinical disease is unknown. In one circumstance, a patient with West Nile virus (WNV) fever developed stiff-person syndrome soon after infection (Hassin-Baer *et al.*, 2004). This rare autoimmune disorder is associated with autoantibodies against glutamic acid decarboxylase (GAD) that are hypothesized to cause the neurological findings by targeting inhibitory spinal interneurons. In this case, a database search revealed a stretch of 12 amino acids in the NS1 protein of WNV that has a high homology to GAD (Hassin-Baer *et al.*, 2004). As a result, a cross-reactive antibody response through the process of molecular mimicry was proposed. Again, however, a cause-and-effect relationship between the two events remains unproven.

Conclusion

While the immune response to viral infections of the CNS has been the focus of active study in a number of experimental models, important unanswered questions persist. For example, in some circumstances, full viral clearance from the CNS is achieved and recovery ensues. While immune components involved in the clearance of non-cytolytic viruses from neurons are understood to some degree, the precise molecular mechanisms underlying this event remain ill-defined. Another important observation that demands further investigation is that different inbred strains of mice infected with the same encephalitic virus exhibit very different clinical outcomes over time (i.e. viral clearance versus persistent infection and survival versus death). Thus, further clarification of the genetic basis for variability in host determinants that control inflammation, viral persistence within the CNS, and susceptibility to fatal virus- and immune-mediated disease is required. Knowing the mechanisms of viral clearance from the CNS as well as the injury of underlying neural cells could allow for the passive transfer of immune components or the use of neuroprotective agents as adjunctive therapies until more effective antiviral agents are developed. Proper preclinical testing in animals will allow the best quality clinical trials in humans to be performed.

References

Adamson DC, et al. Immunologic NO synthase: Elevation in severe AIDS dementia and induction by HIV-1 gp41. *Science* 1996; **274**: 1917–21.

Akwa Y, et al. Transgenic expression of IFN-α in the central nervous system of mice protects against lethal neurotropic viral infection but induces inflammation and neurodegeneration. *J Immunol* 1998; **161**: 5016–26.

Asensio VC, Campbell IL. Chemokine gene expression in the brains of mice with lymphocytic choriomeningitis. *J Virol* 1997; **71**: 7832–40.

Bauer J, et al. T cell apoptosis in inflammatory brain lesions: Destruction of T cells does not depend on antigen recognition. *Am J Pathol* 1998; **153**: 715–24.

Bilzer T, Stitz L. Immune-mediated brain atrophy. CD8+ T cells contribute to tissue destruction during borna disease. *J Immunol* 1994; **153**: 818–23.

Binder GK, Griffin DE. Interferon-γ-mediated site-specific clearance of alphavirus from CNS neurons. *Science* 2001; **293**: 303–6.

Boutros T, et al. Interferon-β is a potent promoter of nerve growth factor production by astrocytes. *J Neurochem* 1997; **69**: 939–46.

Brooks TJ, Phillpotts RJ. Interferon-alpha protects mice against lethal infection with St. Louis encephalitis virus delivered by the aerosol and subcutaneous routes. *Antiviral Res* 1999; **41**: 57–64.

Buchmeier MJ, et al. The virology and immunobiology of lymphocytic choriomeningitis virus infection. *Adv Immunol* 1980; **30**: 275–331.

Byrnes AP, et al. Control of Sindbis virus infection by antibody in interferon-deficient mice. *J Virol* 2000; **74**: 3905–8.

Chabot S, Yong VW. Interferon-β1b increases interleukin-10 in a model of T cell-microglia interactions: Relevance to MS. *Neurology* 2000; **55**: 1497–505.

Chang JR, et al. Differential expression of TGF-β, IL-2, and other cytokines in the CNS of Theiler's murine encephalomyelitis virus-infected susceptible and resistant strains of mice. *Virology* 2000; **278**: 346–60.

Chapman GA, et al. Fractalkine cleavage from neuronal membranes represents an acute event in the inflammatory response to excitotoxic brain damage. *J Neurosci* 2000; **20**: 1–5.

Cole GA, et al. Requirement for θ-bearing cells: Lymphocytic choriomeningitis virus induced central nervous system disease. *Nature* 1972; **238**: 335–7.

Cserr HF, Knopf PM. Cervical lymphatics, the blood brain barrier, and the immunoreactivity of the brain: A new view. *Immunol Today* 1992; **13**: 507–12.

Darman JS, et al. Viral-induced spinal motor neuron death is non cell-autonomous and involves glutamate excitoxicity. *J Neurosci* 2004; **24**: 7566–75.

Depres P, et al. Effects of anti-E2 monoclonal antibody on Sindbis virus replication in AT3 cells expressing Bcl-2. *J Virol* 1995a; **69**: 7006–14.

Depres P, et al. Antiviral activity of α-interferon in Sindbis virus-infected cells is restored by anti-E2 monoclonal antibody treatment. *J Virol* 1995b;**69**: 7345–8.

Desai A, et al. Detection of autoantibodies to neural antigens in the CSF of Japanese encephalitis patients and correlation of findings with the outcome. *J Neurol Sci* 1994; **122**: 109–16.

Ehrengruber MU, et al. Measles virus spreads in rat hippocampal neurons by cell-to-cell contact and in a polarized fashion. *J Virol* 2002; **76**: 5720–8.

Fiette L, et al. Theiler's virus infection of 129Sv mice that lack the interferon-alpha/beta or interferon-gamma receptors. *J Exp Med* 1995; **181**: 2069–76.

Fisher HG, Reichmann G. Brain dendritic cells macrophages/microglia in central nervous system inflammation. *J Immunol* 2001: **166**: 2717–26.

Flugel A, et al. Neuronal FasL induces the death of encephalitogenic T lymphocytes. *Brain Pathol* 2000; **10**: 353–64.

Fokina GI, et al. Development of antibodies to axonal neurofilaments in the progression of chronic tick-borne encephalitis. *Acta Virol* 1991; **35**: 458–63.

Ford AL, et al. Microglia induce CD4 T lymphocyte final effector function and death. *J Exp Med* 1996; **184**: 1737–45.

Gisslen M, et al. Cerebrospinal fluid antibodies directed against neuron-associated gangliosides in HIV-1 infection. *Infection* 2000; **28**: 143–8.

Glass JD, Wesselingh SL. Microglia in HIV-associated neurological diseases. *Microsc Res Tech* 2001; **15**: 95–105.

Greider FB, Vogel SN. Role of interferon and interferon regulatory factors in early protection against Venezuelan equine encephalitis virus infection. *Virology* 1999; **257**: 106–18.

Griffin DE. Immunoglobulins in the cerebrospinal fluid: Changes during acute viral encephalitis in mice. *J Immunol* 1981; **126**: 27–31.

Griffin DE. Immune responses to RNA-virus infections of the CNS. *Nat Rev Immunol* 2003; **3**: 493–502.

Hailer NP, et al. Astrocytic factors deactivate antigen presenting cells that infiltrate the central nervous system. *Brain Pathol* 1998; **8**: 459–74.

Haring JS, et al. High-magnitude, virus-specific CD4 T cell response in the central nervous system of coronavirus-infected mice. *J Virol* 2001; **75**: 3043–7.

Harrison JK, et al. Role of neuronally derived fractalkine in mediating interactions between neurons and CX3CR1-expressing microglia. *Proc Natl Acad Sci USA* 1998; **95**: 10896–901.

Hassin-Baer S, et al. Stiff-person syndrome following West Nile fever. *Arch Neurol* 2004; **61**: 938–41.

Hatalski CG, et al. Evolution of the immune response in the central nervous system following infection with Borna disease virus. *J Neuroimmunol* 1998; **90**: 137–42.

Hawke S, *et al.* Long-term persistence of activated cytotoxic T lymphocytes after viral infection of the central nervous system. *J Exp Med* 1998; **187**: 1575–82.

Hoek RM, *et al.* Down-regulation of the macrophage lineage through interactions with OX2 (CD200). *Science* 2000; **270**: 1768–71.

Hooper DC, *et al.* Collaboration of antibody and inflammation in clearance of rabies virus from the central nervous system. *J Virol* 1998; **72**: 3711–9.

Irani DN. The susceptibility of mice to immune-mediated neurologic disease correlates with the degree to which their lymphocytes resist the effects of brain-derived gangliosides. *J Immunol* 1998; **161**: 2746–52.

Irani DN, Griffin DE. Isolation of brain parenchymal lymphocytes for flow cytometric analysis. Application to acute viral encephalitis. *J Immunol Meth* 1992; **139**: 223–31.

Irani DN, Griffin DE. Regulation of lymphocyte homing into the brain during viral encephalitis at various stages of infection. *J Immunol* 1996; **156**: 3850–7.

Irani DN, *et al.* Brain-derived gangliosides regulate the cytokine production and proliferation of activated T cells. *J Immunol* 1996; **157**: 4333–40.

Irani DN, *et al.* Regulation of brain-derived T cells during acute central nervous system inflammation. *J Immunol* 1997; **158**: 2318–26.

Jarosinski KW, *et al.* Specific deficiency in nuclear factor-κB activation in neurons of the central nervous system. *Lab Invest* 2001; **81**: 1275–88.

Johnson MD, *et al.* Evidence for transforming growth factor-β expression in human leptomeningeal cells and transforming growth factor-β-like activity in human cerebrospinal fluid. *Lab Invest* 1992; **67**: 360–8.

Johnson RT. *Viral Infections of the Nervous System.* 2nd edn. Philadelphia: Lippincott-Raven, 1998.

Kagi D, *et al.* Cytotoxicity mediated by T cells and natural killer cells is greatly impaired in perforin-deficient mice. *Nature* 1994; **369**: 31–7.

Karpus WJ, *et al.* Inhibition of Theiler's virus-mediated demyelination by peripheral immune tolerance induction. *J Immunol* 1995; **155**: 947–57.

Kimura T, Griffin DE. The role of CD8 + T cells and major histocompatibility complex class I expression in the central nervous system of mice infected with neurovirulent Sindbis virus. *J Virol* 2000; **74**: 6117–25.

Komatsu T, *et al.* Neuronal expression of NOS-1 is required for host recovery from viral encephalitis. *Virology* 1999; **258**: 389–95.

Lane TE, *et al.* Dynamic regulation of α- and β-chemokine expression in the central nervous system during mouse hepatitis virus-induced demyelinating disease. *J Immunol* 1998; **160**: 970–8.

Levine B, Griffin DE. Persistence of viral RNA in mouse brains after recovery from acute alphavirus encephalitis. *J Virol* 1992; **66**: 6429–35.

Levine B, *et al.* Antibody-mediated clearance of alphavirus infection from neurons. *Science* 1991; **254**: 856–60.

Li W, *et al.* Molecular and cellular mechanisms of neuronal death in HIV dementia. *Neurotox Res* 2005; **8**: 119–34.

Liang XH, *et al.* Resistance of interleukin-1β-deficient mice to fatal Sindbis virus encephalitis. *J Virol* 1999; **73**: 2563–7.

Lin MT, *et al.* Mouse hepatitis virus is cleared from the central nervous system of mice lacking perforin-mediated cytolysis. *J Virol* 1997; **71**: 383–91.

Lipton HL, Dal Canto MC. Theiler's virus-induced demyelination: Prevention by immunosuppression. *Science* 1976; **192**: 62–4.

Liu T, *et al.* γ-Interferon can prevent herpes simplex virus type 1 reactivation from latency in sensory neurons. *J Virol* 2001; **75**: 11178–84.

Maciejewski-Lenoir D, *et al.* Characterization of fractalkine in rat brain cells: Migratory and activation signals for CX3CR1-expressing microglia. *J Immunol* 1999; **163**: 1628–35.

Marten NW, *et al.* Role of viral persistence in retaining CD8+ T cells within the central nervous system. *J Virol* 2000; **74**: 7903–10.

Medana I, *et al.* Fas ligand (CD95L) protects neurons against perforin-mediated T lymphocyte cytotoxicity. *J Immunol* 2001; **167**: 674–81.

Miller SD, *et al.* Persistent infection with Theiler's virus leads to CNS autoimmunity via epitope spreading. *Nat Med* 1997; **3**: 1133–6.

Muller U, *et al.* Functional role of type I and type II interferons in antiviral defense. *Science* 1994; **264**: 1918–21.

Murray PD, *et al.* CD4+ and CD8+ T cells make discrete contributions to demyelination and neurologic disease in a viral model of multiple sclerosis. *J Virol* 1998; **72**: 7320–9.

Nargi-Aizenman JL, *et al.* Neural degeneration, paralysis and death due to acute viral encephalomyelitis are prevented by glutamate receptor antagonists. *Ann Neurol* 2004; **55**: 541–9.

Neumann H. Control of glial immune function by neurons. *Glia* 2001; **36**: 191–9.

Njenga MK, *et al.* The immune system preferentially clears Theiler's virus from the grey matter of the central nervous system. *J Virol* 1997; **71**: 8592–601.

Parra B, *et al.* Kinetics of cytokine mRNA expression in the central nervous system following lethal and nonlethal coronavirus-induced acute encephalomyelitis. *Virology* 1997; **233**: 260–70.

Parra B, *et al.* IFN-γ is required for viral clearance from central nervous system oligodendroglia. *J Immunol* 1999; **162**: 1641–7.

Patterson CE, *et al.* Immune-mediated protection from measles virus-induced central nervous system disease is noncytolytic and γ-interferon dependent. *J Virol* 2002; **76**: 4497–506.

Pearce BD, *et al.*. Cytokine induction during T cell-mediated clearance of mouse hepatitis virus from neurons in vivo. *J Virol* 1994; **68**: 5483–95.

Pereira RA, Simmons A. Cell surface expression of H2 antigens on primary sensory neurons in response to acute but not latent herpes simplex virus infection in vivo. *J Virol* 1999; **73**: 6484–9.

Pereira RA, *et al.* Granzyme A, a noncytolytic component of CD8+ cell granules, restricts the spread of herpes simplex virus in the peripheral systems of experimentally infected mice. *J Virol* 2000; **74**: 1029–32.

Pope JG, *et al.* Flow cytometric and functional analysis of central nervous system-infiltrating cells in SJL/J mice with Theiler's virus-induced demyelinating disease. Evidence for a CD4+ T cell-mediated pathology. *J Immunol* 1996; **156**: 4050–8.

Pope JG, *et al.* Characterization of and functional antigen presentation by central nervous system mononuclear cells from mice infected with Theiler's murine encephalomyelitis virus. *J Virol* 1998; **72**: 7762–71.

Ramakrishna C, *et al.* Mechanisms of central nervous system viral persistence: The critical role of antibody and B cells. *J Immunol* 2002; **168**: 1204–11.

Ransohoff RM, *et al.* Three or more routes for leukocyte migration into the central nervous system. *Nat Rev Immunol* 2003; **3**: 569–81.

Robertson B, *et al.* Interferon-γ-responsive neuronal sites in the normal rat brain: Receptor protein distribution and cell activation revealed by Fos induction. *Brain Res Bull* 2000; **52**: 61–74.

Rossi CP, *et al.* Theiler's virus infection of perforin-deficient mice. *J Virol* 1998; **72**: 4515–9.

Rumbaugh JA, Nath A. Developments in HIV neuropathogenesis. *Curr Pharm Des* 2006; **12**: 1023–44.

Sandberg K, *et al.* Expression of α/β interferons (IFN-α/β) and their relationship to IFN-α/β-induced genes in lymphocytic choriomeningitis. *J Virol* 1994; **68**: 7358–66.

Solomon T, *et al.* Interferon alfa-2a in Japanese encephalitis: A randomized double-blinded placebo-controlled trial. *Lancet* 2003; **361**: 821–6.

Stevenson PG, *et al.* The immunogenicity of intracerebral virus infection depends on anatomical site. *J Virol* 1997; **71**: 145–51.

Stohlman SA, *et al.* CTL effector function within the central nervous system requires CD4+ T cells. *J Immunol* 1998; **160**: 2896–904.

Storm P, *et al.* Perforin-deficient CD8+ T cells mediate fatal lymphocytic choriomeningitis despite impaired cytokine production. *J Virol* 2006; **80**: 1222–30.

Sussman MA, *et al.* T cell-mediated clearance of mouse hepatitis virus strain JHM from the central nervous system. *J Virol* 1989; **63**: 3051–6.

Tschen SI, *et al.* Recruitment kinetics and composition of antibody-secreting cells within the central nervous system following viral encephalomyelitis. *J Immunol* 2002; **168**: 2922–9.

Tyor WR, *et al.* Long term intraparenchymal Ig secretion after acute viral encephalitis in mice. *J Immunol* 1992; **149**: 4016–20.

Ubol S, *et al.* Roles of immunoglobulin valency and the heavy-chain constant domain in antibody-mediated downregulation of Sindbis virus replication in persistently infected neurons. *J Virol* 1995; **69**: 1990–3.

van Pesch V, *et al.* The leader protein of Theiler's virus inhibits immediate-early α/β interferon production. *J Virol* 2001; **75**: 7811–7.

Wesselingh SL, *et al.* Intracerebral cytokine mRNA expression during fatal and nonfatal alphavirus encephalitis suggests a predominant type 2 T cell response. *J Immunol* 1994; **152**: 1289–97.

Wesselingh SL, *et al.* Intracerebral cytokine messenger RNA expression in acquired immunodeficiency syndrome dementia. *Ann Neurol* 1993: **33**: 576–82.

Wesselingh SL, Thompson KA. Immunopathogenesis of HIV-associated dementia. *Curr Opin Neurol* 2001; **14**: 375–9.

Williams K, *et al.* Magnetic resonance spectroscopy reveals that activated monocytes contribute to neuronal injury in SIV neuroAIDS. *J Clin Invest* 2005; **115**: 2534–45.

Zink MC, *et al.* Neuroprotective and anti-human immunodeficiency virus activity of minocycline. *J Am Med Assoc* 2005; **293**: 2003–11.

Chronic HIV infection of the CNS: role of the immune system in virological control and the generation of pathology

Carolyn F. Orr and Bruce J. Brew

Introduction

Human immunodeficiency virus (HIV)-associated dementia (HAD) has decreased in incidence since the advent of highly active antiretroviral therapy (HAART), but its prevalence has increased, at least in part due to the life-extending benefit of HAART. It still causes considerable morbidity in HIV-positive individuals. HIV productively infects only macrophages and microglia, but injury and apoptotic death occur in neurons. Macrophages and microglia are the key mediators of the neurodegeneration observed in HAD. Activation of these cells, mediated through either exposure to infection, viral proteins or inflammatory mediators, and their subsequent release of toxins leads to neuronal and astrocytic dysfunction, thereby underpinning the pathogenesis of HAD, although viral proteins also contribute directly to neuronal injury. The precise mechanism of the neuropathogenic process is, nevertheless, still unknown. In this chapter, the potential mechanisms of neurodegeneration and the role of the immune system in HAD are reviewed.

Epidemiology

HIV is a retrovirus that leads to profound CD4 lymphocyte depletion, progressive immunodeficiency and the acquired immune deficiency syndrome (AIDS). HAART has transformed the prognosis of individuals affected with HIV, but it remains a lethal disease. HIV infection can affect any part of the nervous system. In the brain, it leads to cognitive impairment, motor dysfunction and behavioral changes (McArthur et al., 2005). In its severest form, this manifests as a subacute, dementing process known as HIV-associated dementia (HAD), HIV encephalopathy, or the AIDS dementia complex. Prior to HAART, HAD affected 25% of

individuals with advanced HIV with an incidence of 7% per year (MacArthur et al., 1993; Dore et al., 1997). Mean survival after onset of HAD was 6 months (Bouwman et al., 1998; Dore et al., 2003). In developed countries, HAART has increased the survival post onset of HAD to at least 44 months and halved its incidence (Dore et al., 1999, 2003). However, given the increasing life expectancy of HIV-infected individuals, the prevalence of HAD has doubled (Dore et al., 1999, 2003; Maschke et al., 2000), causing a relative increase in HAD as an AIDS-defining illness in the post-HAART era (Persidksy and Gendelman, 2003). HAD is now recognized as the commonest cause of dementia in people under 40 (Kaul et al., 2005). HIV-associated minor cognitive/motor disorder (MCMD) is a milder clinical manifestation of HIV infection of the brain that affects 30% of the HIV-positive population. It is also associated with increased morbidity and mortality and also appears to be increasing (McArthur et al., 2003). Most investigators consider that MCMD is a less severe form of HAD rather than a distinct entity in its own right, but definitive proof is lacking at this stage.

Pathology

HAD is characterized macroscopically by generalized cerebral atrophy particularly in the hippocampus, frontal and temporal cortex (Navia et al., 1986; Ketzler et al., 1990; Everall et al., 1991; Masliah et al., 1992a; Brew et al., 1995a). There is dendritic pruning (Masliah et al., 1997), loss of synapses (Everall et al., 1999) and the accumulation of beta amyloid precursor protein (Giometto et al., 1997). There is loss of large pyramidal neurons and interneurons in the cortex, spiny neurons in the putamen, medium size neurons

Inflammatory Diseases of the Central Nervous System, ed. T. Kilpatrick, R. M. Ransohoff and S. Wesselingh. Published by Cambridge University Press. © Cambridge University Press 2010

in the globus pallidus and interneurons in the hippocampus (Petito and Roberts, 1995; Giometto et al., 1997; Masliah et al., 1997; Thompson et al., 2001). The loss of cortical neurons partly correlates with dementia severity (Asare et al., 1996). There is a marked inflammatory response, with activation of microglia (Glass et al., 1993), perivascular mononuclear cell and lymphocyte infiltration (Glass et al., 1993, 1995), and the formation of microglial nodules and multinucleated giant cells (MNGCs) (Sharer et al., 1985; Dickson, 1986; Wiley et al., 1986). Microglial nodules are collections of lymphocytes and microglia/macrophages (Navia et al., 1986). MNGCs express CD14 and CD45 and are thought to develop through fusion of infected macrophages and microglia (Sharer et al., 1985; Dickson, 1986; Wiley et al., 1986; Michaels et al., 1988; Sharer, 1992; Fischer-Smith et al., 2001; Williams and Hickey, 2002). MNGCs are always present in HAD and are considered the hallmark of HIV neuropathology (Sharer et al., 1985; Dickson, 1986; Wiley et al., 1986; Cherner et al., 2002; Sacktor et al., 2002). HIV encephalitis refers to the combination of infiltrating mononuclear cells and MNGCs. Astrocytosis and diffuse thinning of white matter also occur (Petito and Cash, 1992; Glass et al., 1993; Power et al., 1993; Buttner et al., 1996), and occasionally leptomeningeal fibrosis or vacuolar leukoencephalopathy (Budka, 1991). HAD is clinically a subcortical dementia and these neuropathological changes are most prominent in the basal ganglia (Kure et al., 1991; Brew et al., 1995a; Everall et al., 1995). HIV-related white matter changes, together with neuronal loss and injury are likely to be the pathological substrate of HAD. Decreased synaptic and dendritic density (Masliah et al., 1997; Everall et al., 1999) selective neuronal loss (Masliah et al., 1992a; Fox et al., 1997) and especially increased numbers of activated microglia (Glass et al., 1995) are the pathologic features most closely associated with cognitive impairment.

HIV infection, the brain, and the immune response

The immune system in the CNS

Tropism and viral co-receptors

Upon initial infection, HIV enters helper T lymphocytes and monocytes/macrophages in the blood. HIV enters these cells through interactions between HIV's cell surface glycoprotein receptors gp120 and gp41, and the host cell's CD4 molecule and a chemokine co-receptor: CXCR4 in lymphocytes and CCR5 or occasionally CCR3 in macrophages (Jordan et al., 1991; He et al., 1997; Albright et al., 1999). HIV variants that grow productively in T cell lines but not macrophages are classified as T-tropic, whereas those that grow productively in macrophages but less efficiently in T cell lines are called macrophage-tropic (Kedzierska and Crowe, 2002). Most macrophage-tropic viruses use the CCR5 chemokine receptor, whereas most T-tropic strains use the CXCR4 chemokine receptor (Albright et al., 1999). HIV isolated from the cerebrospinal fluid (CSF) or brain of HIV patients usually displays predominant macrophage tropism (Liu et al., 1990; Ioannidis et al., 1995; Brew et al., 1996). HIV infection of helper T lymphocytes leads to their death, whereas infection of macrophages is less cytopathic and creates a viral reservoir (Nicholson et al., 1986).

Of all the cell types in the brain, only perivascular macrophages and microglia express CD4 antigen, are commonly infected by HIV, and are capable of productive (whole virus producing) infection (Morner et al., 2003). Part of the mononuclear phagocytic system, microglia and perivascular macrophages are bone marrow-derived cells, responsible for phagocytosis, cytokine and chemokine secretion and regulation, antigen presentation, and neurotrophin production (Aloisi et al., 2001). In the absence of dendritic cells, perivascular macrophages and microglia are the resident immunocompetent cells of the brain. They differ in location, morphology, and the presence of specific cell-surface markers (Guillemin and Brew, 2004). Perivascular macrophages are flat, elongated cells located around blood vessels. Microglia are located in the brain parenchyma and morphologically appear as ramified cells in the healthy brain and are amoeboid when activated (Hickey et al., 1992; Lassmann et al., 1993). Perivascular macrophages are replenished throughout life by the migration of circulating monocytes to the brain (Hickey et al., 1992; Lassmann et al., 1993; Hickey, 2001; Ransohoff et al., 2003), a process accelerated under inflammatory conditions (Hickey and Kimura, 1988; Hickey et al., 1992; Lassmann and Hickey, 1993). Microglia appear to turn over much more slowly (Guillemin and Brew, 2004). Most studies assume that perivascular macrophages are CD14+CD45+ and parenchymal microglia CD14–CD45low (Ulvestad et al., 1994a, 1994b), but no marker expression profile reliably differentiates these two cell types (Guillemin and Brew, 2004), complicating reliable evaluation of these studies. Whether parenchymal microglia as well as perivascular macrophages constitute the major reservoir of productive HIV infection in the brain is controversial (Wiley *et al.*, 1986; Takahashi *et al.*, 1996; Williams *et al.*, 2001; Cosenza *et al.*, 2002; Fischer-Smith *et al.*, 2004). It seems likely that perivascular macrophages are the cell type predominantly involved in the early stages of brain infection, with parenchymal microglia infected later, although it remains unclear exactly when (Hughes *et al.*, 1997). Parenchymal microglia express the HIV co-receptor CCR5 (Rottman *et al.*, 1997; Albright *et al.*, 1999; van der Meer *et al.*, 2000; Williams *et al.*, 2001) and can support HIV replication in vitro (Watkins *et al.*, 1990; Albright *et al.*, 2000), but express viral antigens less frequently in vivo than perivascular macrophages. These infected parenchymal cells could, in fact, be monocytes that have entered the brain from the bloodstream and then adopted a microglial phenotype rather than being sourced as a consequence of primary infection of CNS microglia (Wiley *et al.*, 1986; Petito and Cash, 1992; Takahashi *et al.*, 1996; Williams *et al.*, 2001; Cosenza *et al.*, 2002; Fischer-Smith *et al.*, 2004; Gonzalez-Scarano and Martin-Garcia, 2005). In addition to parenchymal microglia and perivascular macrophages, which will be collectively referred to as brain macrophages from here on, the CNS contains other infected macrophage populations, including meningeal and choroid plexus macrophages. Their biology and kinetics of turnover are different and this could influence HIV neuropathogenesis (Harouse *et al.*, 1989; Falangola *et al.*, 1995).

Compared to the rest of the body, the CNS has selective and modified immune reactivity. Virtually all expression of major histocompatibility class II molecules is restricted to reactive microglia and perivascular macrophages (Bo *et al.*, 1994). Few leukocytes are present in the normal CNS, but there is an increased proportion of central memory T cells (CD27 and CD45RO+). There is a relative lack of lymphatic drainage (Ransohoff *et al.*, 2003), and the blood–brain barrier (BBB), a selectively permeable continuous cellular layer of brain microvascular endothelial cells linked to each other by tight junctions, regulates the traffic of cells and substances from the bloodstream to the CNS (Ballabh *et al.*, 2004). Immune surveillance of the brain occurs by trafficking of activated leukocytes from

blood across the choroid plexus into the cerebrospinal fluid, to the subarachnoid space and to the parenchymal perivascular space (Ransohoff *et al.*, 2003). Most leukocyte traffic consists of activated T cells, but monocytes also cross the BBB (Hickey, 2001; Ransohoff *et al.*, 2003). Leukocyte migration to the brain is dependent on activation of the incoming cell, up-regulation of adhesion molecules on the microvascular endothelium, and appropriate cytokine and chemokine stimulation.

Natural history of CNS infection

HIV crosses the blood–brain barrier to enter the brain soon after the peripheral infection of circulating T cells and monocytes (Davis *et al.*, 1992; An *et al.*, 1999), as evidenced by the occasional case of meningoencephalitis at seroconversion (Ho *et al.*, 1985; Johnson *et al.*, 1988; Brew *et al.*, 1989b; Jolles *et al.*, 1996; Melzer *et al.*, 2003), although viral entry into the brain is usually asymptomatic. During acute infection, there is a steep decline in the number of CD4 helper T cells in the blood. HIV-specific CD8 cytotoxic T-lymphocytes and antibodies appear in blood and brain shortly after initial infection and are critical in halting this early phase of HIV infection (Van Wielink, 1990; Jassoy *et al.*, 1992). Patients then enter a presymptomatic phase of varying duration until the onset of clinical disease. This presymptomatic period is characterized by a low fraction of infected CD4 cells, and increased death rates of both CD4 and CD8 cells. HIV antigens and antibodies are found within the CSF during the presymptomatic phase, and it is unclear whether there is no productive infection or whether it occurs at a very low level (Goudsmit *et al.*, 1986; Chiodi *et al.*, 1986, 1992; Resnick *et al.*, 1988; Davis *et al.*, 1992; Bell *et al.*, 1993; Spector *et al.*, 1993; Gosztonyi *et al.*, 1994; Sinclair *et al.*, 1994; An *et al.*, 1996; Gray *et al.*, 1996; Price, 2000). There is also activation of brain macrophages, high levels of MHC class II expression, and low-grade lymphocytic infiltration: mostly CD8+ cytotoxic T cells with fewer B cells (Anthony *et al.*, 2005; McCrossan *et al.*, 2006). Overall, there exists a state of chronic, generalized activation of immune cells both within the brain and in the blood (Derdeyn and Silvestri, 2005).

Control of viral replication, both in the brain and in the periphery, is probably mediated by CD8 cytotoxic T lymphocytes (Sethi *et al.*, 1988; Jassoy *et al.*, 1992; Sopper *et al.*, 1998; Schmitz *et al.*, 1999), which can suppress HIV replication through chemokine-mediated interactions, as well as through direct cell–cell contact (Cocchi et al., 1995; Lusso, 2006). Over time, the peripheral CD4 helper T cell count in the blood decreases, systemic immunosuppression develops and the protective effect of CD8 cytotoxic T lymphocytes declines. There is increased traffic of infected monocytes across the BBB, the number of activated and/or infected monocytes in the brain increases, productive infection of HIV reappears and HAD is clinically manifest (Albright et al., 2003). When HIV reappears in the brain, it is not known whether this represents virus reseeding of the brain from the periphery or if the endogenous control mechanisms that inhibit HIV replication have broken down.

The simian immunodeficiency macaque model recapitulates key features of HIV CNS infection, targeting CD4 lymphocytes and macrophages and producing a late encephalitis with active virus replication in the CNS, neurodegeneration, and psychomotor impairment (Murray et al., 1992; Zink et al., 1999; Sopper et al., 2002; Zink and Clements, 2002). In the SIV model, virus enters the CNS early after infection (Chakrabarti et al., 1991; Davis et al., 1992; Lackner et al., 1994; Smith et al., 1995), but productive infection is observed for only 2 weeks post-infection (Chakrabarti et al., 1991; Davis et al., 1992; Lackner et al., 1994; Smith et al., 1995). CD8 T lymphocytes then enter the brain and a humoral immune response is observed (Sopper et al., 2002). The cellular immune response appears protective, with severe encephalitis developing in animals after CD8 cell depletion (Schmitz et al., 1999; Sopper et al., 2002). Productive CNS infection reappears when the animal develops terminal AIDS (Chakrabarti et al., 1991; Davis et al., 1992; Lackner et al., 1994; Smith et al., 1995) and in SIV represents reactivation of latent infection rather than reinfection from the periphery (Zink and Clements, 2002). Infected perivascular cells are the major reservoir of infection and spread to parenchymal microglia does not occur (Chakrabarti et al., 1991). Although no HIV replication is observed during the presymptomatic phase in the macaque monkey, this may not accurately reflect the situation in human HIV infection, where it is likely that there is variable but low-level HIV replication kept in check by T cell immunity.

HIV probably enters the brain in infected, activated monocytes that migrate across the BBB to replenish the population of perivascular macrophages as part of their normal immune surveillance function

(the "Trojan horse" hypothesis) (Peluso et al., 1985; Haase et al., 1986; Georgsson, 1994; Romero et al., 2000; Gartner, 2000). Monocyte replenishment of brain perivascular macrophages explains the perivascular distribution of the neuropathology of HAD. HIV might also enter the brain in infected CD4 helper T lymphocytes (Hickey et al., 1991; Lassmann et al., 1993; Hickey, 2001), by transcytosis of endothelial cells (Bomsel, 1997; Banks et al., 2001; Liu et al., 2002) or by direct infection (Edinger et al., 1997; Argyris et al., 2003; Bobardt et al., 2004). Significant structural and functional abnormalities in the blood–brain barrier also occur in HIV CNS infection and seem to be reversible with HAART (McArthur et al., 1992; Weis et al., 1996; Giovannoni et al., 1998; Sporer et al., 1998; Dallasta et al., 1999; Persidsky et al., 2000). While the precise contribution of BBB compromise to HIV entry to the CNS and HAD is unknown, it is most likely important.

Inside the CNS, infiltrating macrophages down-regulate their activation markers, adopt a ramified phenotype and enter a resting phase. HIV is sequestered as a latent infection within these macrophages (Finzi et al., 1997; Wong et al., 1997b) and can later reactivate under the appropriate environmental conditions (Albright et al., 2004). Antiretroviral drugs are not effective against resting cells, and have limited penetration into the CSF compared with the rest of the body. This establishes the CNS as a potential sanctuary site for HIV (Pardridge et al., 2002) with possible implications for the development of drug resistance.

Macrophages and microglia are the only host cells that enable productive HIV infection within the brain, but astrocytes can also be infected (Kaul et al., 2001; Anderson et al., 2002). Astrocytes do not express CD4 or the main HIV co-receptors so that the mechanism of viral entry is unclear (Brack-Werner, 1999; Dong and Benveniste, 2001). They can only support restricted infection, where the production of virions stops at the stage of regulatory proteins (Takahashi et al., 1996; Thompson et al., 2004). Endothelial cells are capable of virion production in experimental systems, but most investigators consider infection of this cell to be of limited, if any, significance (Chi et al., 2000). There is no evidence of oligodendrocyte infection in vivo (Codazzi et al., 1995).

Neurons and HIV

Although neurons express chemokine receptors, they do not express the CD4 molecule and are not infected by HIV. There is, nevertheless, significant neuronal cell death in HIV-infected brains, including apoptosis (Adle-Biassette et al., 1995; Gelbard et al., 1995; Petito and Roberts, 1995). Surprisingly, there is little correlation between the number of HIV-infected cells in the brain and cognitive impairment (Glass et al., 1995; Masliah et al., 1997), although there is a relationship between CSF viral load and HAD severity in patients not on HAART (Brew et al., 1997; Ellis et al., 1997; McArthur et al., 1997; Guillemin et al., 2005a). The discordance between productive viral burden in the brain and clinical deficit suggests that HIV infection is not itself directly toxic to neurons. How then are the functionally important neurons injured in HIV-infected brain?

Pathogenesis of HAD

The severity of HAD more closely parallels brain inflammation than productive brain infection. Evidence is mounting that brain macrophages are the key mediators of the neurodegeneration observed in HIV infection. Pathological changes in the brains of patients with HAD correlate better with the presence of activated macrophages than with viral load (Gelman, 1993; Glass et al., 1995; Adle-Biassette et al., 1999; Gartner, 2000; Williams and Hickey, 2002; Fischer-Smith et al., 2004), and the clinical severity of HAD is strongly associated with numbers of activated brain macrophages (Glass et al., 1995). Progression to HAD correlates with increased expression of macrophage activation markers (Glass et al., 1995), macrophage synthesis of quinolinic acid (QA) and arachidonic acid and related metabolites (Achim et al., 1993), increased tumor necrosis factor-α (TNF-α) (Wesselingh et al., 1993, 1997), increased mRNA for inducible nitric oxide synthetase (iNOS) (Bukrinsky et al., 1995; Blond et al., 1998, 2000; Adamson et al., 1999), increased free radical production, and proliferation and apoptosis of astrocytes (Thompson et al., 2001). In patients on HAART, plasma TNF-α and CSF CCL2 are predictive of progression to HAD (Sevigny et al., 2004). The CSF concentrations of β_2 microglobulin (Brew et al., 1989a, 1992), neopterin (a marker of activated macrophages) (Brew et al., 1990) and QA (Heyes et al., 1991) correlate with the severity of HAD in HAART naive patients.

Infected or activated macrophages can contribute to the development of HAD through several mechanisms. There exist two different theories on how HIV infection results in neuronal injury in the brain. In the 'direct injury' hypothesis, viral gene products such as the envelope protein gp120 (Brenneman et al., 1988), gp41 (Adamson et al., 1996), Tat (transcriptional transactivator) (Nath et al., 1996), Nef (van Marle et al., 2004), and viral protein R (Vpr) (Patel et al., 2000) are proposed to injure neurons directly. Although these molecules can exert toxicity on neurons in-vitro, there is currently limited evidence for in vivo toxicity at physiological concentrations (Gonzalez-Scarano and Martin-Garcia, 2005). This could reflect difficulties in quantification of these products in vivo.

In the "indirect or bystander" hypothesis, neuronal injury is chiefly mediated by brain macrophages. Infected brain macrophages produce pro-inflammatory cytokines and chemokines, and potentially neurotoxic chemicals, including eicosanoids, arachidonic acid (Achim et al., 1993), nitric oxide (Adamson et al., 1996), glutamate (Jiang et al., 2001), L-cysteine (Jiang et al., 2001), nitric oxide (Bukrinsky et al., 1995; Blond et al., 1998, 2000; Adamson et al., 1999), platelet activating factor (Gelbard et al., 1994), QA (Achim et al., 1993; Kerr et al., 1998), Ntox (Giulian et al., 1996), and excitatory amino acids (Giulian et al., 1990; Jiang et al., 2001). These can promote activation and recruitment of uninfected brain macrophages, leading to further up-regulation of cytokines, chemokines, and endothelial adhesion molecules, release of other neurotoxic chemicals, matrix metalloproteinases, and complement from brain macrophages, triggering recruitment of other immune cells into the brain. This inflammatory cascade could lead to either the injury or death of bystander neurons. It has been demonstrated in vitro that transient exposure of macrophages to a viral protein (Tat) can activate sustained macrophage production of inflammatory cytokines. This "hit and run phenomenon" suggests that macrophages could be activated by viral products in a single event and once initiated, chronic activation could be self-perpetuating, maintained in an autocrine or paracrine fashion by the continued presence of macrophage-derived molecules (Nath et al., 1999). The direct and indirect theories are not mutually exclusive, and although the available data supports a role for both, the balance of evidence favors the indirect form of neurotoxicity (Gonzalez-Scarano and Martin-Garcia, 2005). Along with loss of neurotrophins and astrocytic dysfunction through infection and as a consequence of macrophage-mediated products, this brain-macrophage inflammatory cascade appears to underlie the pathogenic process.

Molecular response

Matrix metalloproteinases

Increased expression of extracellular matrix degrading proteases is observed in the CSF and brain tissue of HAD patients (Wesselingh et al., 1997; Adamson et al., 1999; Patton et al., 1998; Smith et al., 2001; Heyes et al., 2001; Griffin 1997). These matrix metalloproteinases (MMPs), including MMP-2, MMP-7 and MMP-9, are produced by HIV-infected macrophages (Conant et al., 1999; Johnston et al., 2000) and could compromise the blood brain barrier and contribute directly towards neuronal toxicity (Chapman et al., 2000; Gu et al., 2002).

Adhesion molecules

Adhesion molecules are located on brain microvascular endothelial cells and mediate the migration of activated leukocytes and monocytes into the brain. Macrophage-derived TNF-α and IL-1β induce up-regulation of intercellular adhesion molecule-1 (ICAM-1), vascular cell adhesion molecule-1 (VCAM-1), and E-selectin facilitating cell trafficking, correlating with macrophage infiltration into the brain in HAD (Nottet et al., 1994, 1996). The ICAM-1 is increased in HAD CSF (Heidenreich et al., 1994), and increased expression of VCAM-1 and E-selectin are implicated in monocyte migration into the brain during HIV and SIV infection (Sasseville et al., 1994; Nottet et al., 1996; Persidsky et al., 1997a).

Complement

There is increased production of complement in the brain of HIV-infected patients and activation of the complement cascade could contribute towards HAD pathogenesis (Jongen et al., 2000; Speth et al., 2005). Synthesis of soluble complement proteins by brain macrophages is up-regulated and expression of cellular complement receptors is modulated by HIV (Gasque et al., 1993; Haga et al., 1996; Thomas et al., 2000; Speth et al., 2002a, 2002b). HIV also up-regulates complement expression in astrocytes and neurons (Speth et al., 2001, 2002a) and HIV envelope proteins gp41 and gp120 can activate the complement cascade (Speth et al., 1997). Complement can directly lyse neurons, which express only small amounts of the membrane-bound negative regulator CD59 (Singhrao et al., 2000), which itself is down-regulated by viral gp41 (Chong and Lee, 2000). Complement activation can lead to release of arachidonic acid and its metabolites, and contribute towards oxidative stress through stimulation of respiratory burst activity. Complement opsonization of neurons might also lead to their phagocytosis by brain macrophages, and complement components such as C5a are capable of inducing neuronal apoptosis (Farkas et al., 1998). Complement can also opsonize HIV, resulting in increased monocyte infection which might increase viral entry to the brain (Thieblemont et al., 1995). Complement components C3a and C5a mediate enhanced infiltration of potentially infected monocytes into the brain, and activate signaling cascades in astrocytes and microglia. They might contribute to the reactive astrocytosis and microgliosis observed in the HAD brain.

Cytokines

Cytokines are small polypeptide molecules with pleiotropic activity that form the primary means of communication between neurons, glia and leukocytes (Raivich et al., 1999). Infected or activated macrophages release pro-inflammatory cytokines such as TNF-α and IL-1β, which can activate uninfected macrophages, induce migration of leukocytes into the CNS, exacerbate excitotoxicity and up-regulate the expression of MHC molecules and hence the antigen-presenting capacity of cells (Kaul and Lipton, 2004). The TNF-α, IL-1β, interferon-γ (IFN-γ), IL-1α, IL-6 and CXCL8 (IL-8), which are generally pro-inflammatory, are all increased in the HAD brain (Perrella et al., 1992; Gelbard et al., 1993; Wesselingh et al., 1993, 1997; Glass et al., 1995; Talley et al., 1995; Zhao et al., 2001; Xiong et al., 2003). Activated microglia also increase expression of TNF receptor in HAD (Sippy et al., 1995). Progression to HAD is predicted by high concentrations of TNF-α in plasma (Sevigny et al., 2004), and polymorphisms in the TNF-α promoter are associated with HAD (Quasney et al., 2001), suggesting that pro-inflammatory TNF-α, which induces astrocytosis and is chemotactic for macrophages, is critical for neurotoxicity (Wesselingh et al., 1993).

Cytokines modulate transcription of HIV and production of progenitor virions, and stimulation of CNS cell cultures by pro-inflammatory cytokines induces HIV replication (Swingler et al., 1992; Janabi et al., 1998). Since these cytokines are induced by HIV infection, a vicious circle involving ongoing viral replication and cytokine synthesis could exist in vivo. In contrast, there is reduced IL-4, IL-10, IL-12 and TGF-β, which are considered, in general, to be anti-inflammatory cytokines (Wesselingh *et al.*, 1993; Schuitemaker, 1994; Griffin, 1997; Persidsky *et al.*, 1999; Nunnari *et al.*, 2003). Overall, there exists an activated, dysregulated and generally pro-inflammatory milieu in the HIV-infected brain.

Chemokines

Chemokines are cytokines chemotactic to leukocytes and microglia (Wong and Fish, 2003; Ambrosini and Aloisi, 2004), which modulate the expression of adhesion molecules on brain endothelial cells and mediate leukocyte recruitment into the brain (Dietrich *et al.*, 2002). Chemokine receptors are present on astrocytes and neurons as well as macrophages (Rottman, 1997; Zhang *et al.*, 1998; Zheng *et al.*, 1999b). Chemokine receptors CCR5 and CXCR4 serve as co-receptors for HIV and their endogenous ligands can directly compete with HIV's envelope proteins gp120 and gp41. Altered synthesis of these chemokine co-receptors in vivo could be a mechanism to reduce host cell infectivity. In support of this as a defense mechanism in vivo, it has been observed that a mutation in the CCR5 gene causing loss of the protein confers protection to infection in homozygotes and slows progression to AIDS in heterozygotes (Liu *et al.*, 1996).

Infected and immune-activated brain macrophages produce large amounts of chemokines, including CCL2 (macrophage chemotactic protein-1; MCP-1), CX3CL1 (fractalkine), CCL5 (RANTES; regulated upon activation normal T cell expressed and secreted) and CCL3 (macrophage inflammatory proteins-1α; MIP-1α) and CCL4 (MIP-1β), CXCL12 (SDF-1α; stromal-derived factor-1α) and CXCL10, all of which are found increased in both CSF and brain tissue of patients with HAD (Schmidtmayerova *et al.*, 1996; Cinque *et al.*, 1998; Conant *et al.*, 1998; Hesselgesser *et al.*, 1998b; Kelder *et al.*, 1998; Sanders *et al.*, 1998; Westmoreland *et al.*, 1998; Zhang *et al.*, 1998; Letendre *et al.*, 1999; Zheng *et al.*, 1999a; Lazarini *et al.*, 2000; Persidsky *et al.*, 2000; Wu *et al.*, 2000; Pereira *et al.*, 2001; Langford *et al.*, 2002; Erichsen *et al.*, 2003; Rostasy *et al.*, 2003; Sporer *et al.*, 2003). Increased expression of the chemokine receptors CCR3 and CCR5 is also found in HAD (Klein *et al.*, 1999; Vallat *et al.*, 1998). Chemokines act on their receptors to trigger G-protein-mediated modulation of calcium channels and the inositol triphosphate, adenylate cyclase and mitogen-activated protein kinase pathways (Persidsky and Gendelman, 2003). These signal transduction pathways have important roles in normal neuronal homeostasis and their activation could link inflammation to neuronal apoptosis (Giulian *et al.*, 1990). Microglia and astrocytes produce chemokines in vitro after stimulation with viral proteins, inflammatory cytokines, lipopolysaccharide (LPS) or CD40L (Hurwitz *et al.*, 1995; Conant *et al.*, 1998; McManus *et al.*, 1998; Perry *et al.*, 1998; Cotter *et al.*, 2001). Increased or altered chemokine production could contribute to the HAD pathogenesis through recruitment and activation of macrophages, propagation of inflammation, BBB breakdown, and induction of neuronal apoptosis (Sanders *et al.*, 1998). The roles of chemokines in the HAD brain are, however, complex, with not all necessarily being pathogenic and some possibly even neuroprotective.

The best-characterized chemokines up-regulated in HAD are the β-chemokines CCL2, CCL5, and CX3CL1, and the α-chemokine CXCL12 (Sozzani *et al.*, 1995; Meucci *et al.*, 1998; Wu *et al.*, 2000; Cotter *et al.*, 2002; Erichsen *et al.*, 2003; Gonzalez-Scarano and Martin-Garcia, 2005). The CCL2, believed to be produced by brain macrophages, activated astrocytes, and endothelial cells (Sozzani *et al.*, 1995), is up-regulated by the viral protein Tat (Pu *et al.*, 2003). Levels of CCL2 correlate with the likelihood and severity of dementia (Cinque *et al.*, 1998; Conant *et al.*, 1998; Sevigny *et al.*, 2004). A mutant CXCL2 allele causes increased infiltration of monocytes into tissues and is associated with a 4.5-fold increased risk of HAD (Gonzalez *et al.*, 2002). Mutations of the CXCL2 receptor, CCR2, are also associated with HAD (Singh *et al.*, 2004). The CCL5 is produced by astrocytes and brain macrophages (Gonzalez-Scarano and Martin-Garcia, 2005). It is increased in HIV and SIV infection and its receptors CCR5, CCR1 and CCR 3 are all expressed in the infected brain (Gonzalez-Scarano and Martin-Garcia, 2005). Production of CX3CL1 is increased following incubation with HIV virions or envelope protein gp120 (Erichsen *et al.*, 2003). Gene polymorphisms in CX3CR1 affect the time to development of AIDS (Faure *et al.*, 2000). The CX3CL1 inhibits Fas-mediated apoptosis of microglia (Boehme *et al.*, 2000). Both neurotoxic and neuroprotective effects of β-chemokines have so far been demonstrated in vitro, but no neurotoxic effects of β-chemokines have been so far demonstrated in vivo (Meucci et al., 1998, 2000; Kaul and Lipton, 1999; Tong et al., 2000; Eugenin et al., 2003). The CXCL12 is an α-chemokine and the natural ligand for CXCR4 (Wu et al., 2000). Both CXCL12 and CXCR4 are widely expressed in the brain (Ohtani et al., 1998). Hippocampal neurons express increased CXCR4 and reduced CCR5 in HAD (Petito et al., 2001). The HIV and Tat up-regulate CXCL12 expression both in vitro and in vivo (Hesselgesser et al., 1998a; Zheng et al., 1999b; Langford et al., 2002; Rostasy et al., 2003). Ligation of CXCR4 by either CXCL12 or viral gp120 can initiate signal transduction pathways that ends in neuronal apoptosis (Hesselgesser et al., 1998b; Zheng et al., 1999a, 1999b; Pandey and Bolsover, 2000). In mixed human neuronal/glial culture, both HIV and gp120 activate microglia via CXCR4 leading to toxin production and neuronal apoptosis (Hesselgesser et al., 1998b; Kaul and Lipton, 1999; Zheng et al., 1999b; Kaul et al., 2001). The CXCL12 can be cleaved to a highly neurotoxic truncated fragment which no longer binds CXCR4 by macrophage-derived matrix metalloproteinase-2 (MMP-2) (Zhang et al., 2003). The CXCL12 is neuroprotective against gp120 (Corasaniti et al., 2001), and increased CXCL12 expression might protect neurons from infection by HIV. On the other hand, CXCL12 also induces astrocyte proliferation and could therefore mediate the astrocytosis of HIV encephalitis (Bonavia et al., 2003).

In summary, HIV-1 infection and secondary immune activation induce the production of chemokines from brain macrophages and/or astrocytes. The net effect of the altered chemokine and chemokine receptor profile in HAD brain is still unknown. How and under what circumstances chemokines exert protective or toxic effects are central questions currently under investigation.

Neurotrophins

Microglia express a variety of neurotrophins, including brain-derived neurotrophic factor (BDNF) and nerve growth factor (NGF) (Streit et al., 2002). Neurotrophins can facilitate removal of excitotoxins and dead cells allowing regeneration of damaged neurons, and have anti-inflammatory effects on brain macrophages themselves, causing reduced expression of activation molecules (Wei and Jonakait, 1999). In HAD, activated macrophages overproduce BDNF and

NGF (Soontornniyomkij et al., 1998; Boven et al., 1999; Garaci et al., 1999). Production of neurotrophins in the infected brain could be neuroprotective through limitation of inflammation. This could be relevant to the control of HIV replication and absence of neuronal death in HIV infection before very late disease. Alternatively, NGF can protect brain macrophages from apoptosis and could therefore contribute to the long-term persistence of the viral reservoir in the brain (Garaci et al., 1999; Cosenza et al., 2004).

The role of astrocytes

Astrocytes have important roles in supporting neuronal function via provision of metabolic and tropic factors, aiding repair processes and maintenance of the BBB (Ambrosini and Aloisi, 2004). Dysfunction of astrocytes could result from their restrictive infection with HIV and from dysregulation of their local cytokine/chemokine environment, resulting from infection of brain macrophages. Dysfunctional astrocytes are less able to provide neurons with neurotrophic support or to buffer glutamate, and this could contribute towards neuronal injury. In support of this, the density of apoptotic astrocytes correlates with the rate of progression of HAD (Thompson et al., 2001).

Astrocytes could potentially contribute to HIV neuropathogenesis through dysregulated or excessive production of cytokines, chemokines, adhesion molecules, and complement components. Pro-inflammatory cytokines and QA which are up-regulated in HAD induce chemokine production by astrocytes (Tornatore et al., 1991; Conant et al., 1998; Meucci et al., 1998; Hori et al., 1999; Persidsky et al., 1999; Guillemin et al., 2003c; John et al., 2003; Zhang et al., 2003) Viral proteins such as gp120 or Tat stimulate the expression of ICAM-1 and VCAM-1 in astrocytes (Toneatto et al., 1999; Woodman et al., 1999) and could facilitate infiltration of infected cells into the brain (Woodman et al., 1999). Astrocytes can synthesize complement components either under the influence of pro-inflammatory cytokines or by direct incubation with HIV (Speth et al., 2001, 2002a, 2002b), leading to lysis of virions, immune cell activation and attraction of microglia, peripheral T-cells, and macrophages. Astrocytes also express receptors for complement activation products and HIV modulates astrocyte sensitivity to complement (Kohleisen et al., 1999). Astrocytes directly modulate neuronal survival by regulation of expression of glutamate transporters and NMDA receptor subunits which influence neuronal sensitivity to oxidative stress, and viral Tat and gp120 impair glutamate uptake by astrocytes by inhibiting transcription of the glutamate transporter gene (Wang *et al.*, 2004; Zhou *et al.*, 2004). Astrocytes can up-regulate the production of apoptotic factors such as Fas and Fas ligand (Sabri *et al.*, 2001), and cell cultures from Tat-expressing astrocytes induce neuronal death (Wang *et al.*, 2004; Zhou *et al.*, 2004). Astrocytes could also modulate the immune response. Viral Nef protein decreases astrocytic expression of MHC I and this could protect HIV-infected cells from attack (Schwartz *et al.*, 1996; Yang *et al.*, 2002). Astrocytes also possess limited phagocytic activity and can ingest apoptotic lymphocytes, potentially reducing inflammatory responses (Ren and Savill, 1998; Magnus *et al.*, 2002). Astrocytes can also suppress HIV replication in macrophages (Nottet *et al.*, 1995; Brack-Werner, 1999; Tanaka *et al.*, 1999; Aloisi *et al.*, 2001; Bezzi *et al.*, 2001).

Astrocytes are physiological regulators of microglial and macrophage inflammatory responses, and indirectly modulate neuronal survival through reduction of the macrophage inflammatory response (Min *et al.*, 2006). In co-cultures of activated brain macrophages and astrocytes compared to macrophage-only cultures, macrophages adopt a ramified phenotype and produce significantly lower levels of pro-inflammatory molecules (Nottet *et al.*, 1995; Tanaka and Maeda, 1996; Speth *et al.*, 2005). This anti-inflammatory effect is mediated by astrocytic induction of the antioxidant enzyme hemoxygenase-1 in microglia, which down-regulates microglial activation (Min *et al.*, 2006). Astrocytic dysfunction could release brain macrophages from the dormant state, allowing propagation and amplification of the toxic inflammatory response.

Cytokine/chemokine communications between brain macrophages and astrocytes, and viral proteins produced by brain macrophages, are involved in the balance of protective and destructive actions by these cells. In early HIV infection, astrocytes could down-regulate the inflammatory activity of brain macrophages whereas later, the virus-induced functional impairment of astrocytes might be over-ridden by strong pro-inflammatory signals, resulting in toxic microglial inflammation.

Lessons from animal models of HAD

Neuronal injury and behavioral abnormalities correlate with microglial activation in SIV-infected macaques (Berman *et al.*, 1999). Minocycline, an anti-inflammatory drug which is neuroprotective in animal models of several neurodegenerative disorders (Chen *et al.*, 2000; Van Den Bosch *et al.*, 2002; Wu *et al.*, 2002; Metz *et al.*, 2004), when given to macaques after SIV inoculation suppressed SIV replication in the brain, decreased encephalitis, decreased infiltration and/or activation of macrophages, reduced infiltration of T lymphocytes, reduced axonal degeneration, and decreased expression of MHC class II and MCP-1 (Zink *et al.*, 2005). The expression of MCP-1 directly correlated with macrophage activation and astrocytosis (Zink and Clements, 2002; Zink *et al.*, 2005), whereas MIP-1α, MIP-1β and RANTES did not (Zink and Clements, 2002).

Severe combined immunodeficient (SCID) mice that are stereotaxically inoculated with HIV-infected monocytes into the brain also develop neurodegeneration, brain macrophage and astrocyte activation, leukocyte invasion, neural injury, and cognitive impairment (Persidsky *et al.*, 1997b, 2001; Limoges *et al.*, 2000, 2001; Zink *et al.*, 2002; Anderson *et al.*, 2003). There is increased expression of pro-inflammatory cytokines such as TNF-α and Il-6 and up-regulation of adhesion molecules (Persidsky *et al.*, 1997b). Disease progression in the SCID mouse model relates both to the number of macrophages and the ability of the viral strain to replicate in macrophages (Nukuna *et al.*, 2004). Inhibitors of TNF-α and matrix metalloproteinases are neuroprotective causing reduction in microglial activation and astrogliosis (Persidksy *et al.*, 2001). After the development of an HIV-specific cytotoxic T cell response, viral-infected macrophages were cleared from the brain in a response characterized by ongoing microgliosis and astrocytosis, expression of IL-10, and neurotrophin production (Poluektova *et al.*, 2004).

Why does HAD develop late and why only in some?

HIV enters the brain early after viral infection, but HAD occurs years later and only in some infected people (Meltzer *et al.*, 1990). How does HIV, which reaches the CNS very early in the course of systemic infection and which probably continues to expose the brain throughout its untreated course, remain asymptomatic for years, yet go on to cause the devastating neurological dysfunction of HAD late in the disease course? Why in some patients only? Clinical risk factors for HAD include low CD4 lymphocyte count, increased CSF β_2-microglobulin and increased age

145

(Quasney *et al.*, 2001), suggesting that immunosuppression, inflammation and possibly duration of disease are important. Alterations in the virus itself, as well as alterations in peripheral blood monocytes and enhanced monocyte trafficking into the brain, might be important.

Prior to HAART, HAD usually occurred in advanced disease in association with profound immunosuppression (median CD4 count of 50/µl) (Dore *et al.*, 1999). In late infection in the setting of functionally impaired helper CD4 T lymphocytes, circulating HIV-specific CD8 T cells become partially anergic and unable to eliminate infected cells (Pitcher *et al.*, 1999; Trimble *et al.*, 2000), suggesting that loss of effective T cell immunity enabled resumption of viral production in the brain. In support of this, administration of CD8-depleting monoclonal antibodies to SIV-infected macaque monkeys led to a persistent loss of CD8 T cells, clinical AIDS and SIV encephalitis (Schmitz *et al.*, 1999). However, not all immunosuppressed monkeys develop encephalitis, and not all humans with profound immunodeficiency develop HAD. In patients treated with HAART, the CD4 lymphocyte count can be normal at HAD onset (McArthur, 2004). Immunodeficiency is not, therefore, a prerequisite for HAD, and nadir CD4 cell count and duration of disease could be more important risk factors for HAD than current CD4 count in HAART-treated patients.

The transition of CNS infection from benign to damaging could occur through evolution of the virus to a more neuropathogenic phenotype. Different viral clones have varied ability to infect brain macrophages and prime them for activation. Brain- and CSF-derived viral sequences also differ from the extra-CNS virus (Steuler *et al.*, 1992; Keys *et al.*, 1993; Kuiken *et al.*, 1995; Hughes *et al.*, 1997) and specific neuro-virulent HIV strains could evolve within the CNS (Cheng-Mayer and Levy *et al.*, 1988; Chiodi *et al.*, 1989; Chesebro *et al.*, 1992; Power *et al.*, 1998; Johnston *et al.*, 2001). In macaque monkeys, the strain of virus affects the likelihood of SIV encephalitis, and this difference appears to relate to viral ability to grow in macrophages (Demuth *et al.*, 2000; Sopper *et al.*, 2002). Viral evolution correlates with disease progression in humans and could be important for the development of HAD (Wong *et al.*, 1997a). HIV strains that predominate during the long asymptomatic phase are also usually restricted to CCR5 usage. These macrophage-tropic strains alone may not be sufficient to cause clinical disease. Late in the course of systemic HIV disease, HIV strains could emerge that use CXCR4, and peripheral virus shifts from predominant macrophage tropism to T tropism (Lusso, 2006). This phenotypic switch does not occur in SIV and is not an absolute prerequisite in human HAD, but could be a contributory factor to its pathogenesis (Kimata *et al.*, 1999).

Levels of circulating activated monocytes correlate with the risk of HAD (Pulliam *et al.*, 1997), and enhanced monocyte trafficking during late stage HIV infection could play a role in HAD pathogenesis (Liu *et al.*, 2000). Specific monocyte subsets also emerge in late disease; they express CD14/CD16 and CD14/CD69 surface markers and have enhanced ability to migrate and secrete neurotoxins (Pulliam *et al.*, 1997; Fischer-Smith *et al.*, 2001; Luo *et al.*, 2003). The appearance of these monocytes in blood and brain correlates with the development of HAD (Thieblemont *et al.*, 1995; Pulliam *et al.*, 1997). If increased monocyte entry plays a primary role in initiating a more generalized state of microglial activation, limiting this entry could lead initially to a normalization of perivascular macrophage levels, followed by a return of resident microglia to their resting state. In support of this, imaging studies show that glial activation diminishes after 6–9 months of HAART (Chang *et al.*, 1999a, 1999b). Since most antiretroviral drugs penetrate the brain poorly, but do lead to reduced numbers of circulating monocytes (Amirayan-Chevillard *et al.*, 2000), this delayed reversal of glial activation might be explained by a decreased number and/or activation state of peripheral monocytes and reduced trafficking into the brain, rather than a direct effect on brain macrophages, with the delayed response corresponding to an alteration in the turnover rate of perivascular macrophages (Hickey *et al.*, 1992; Chang *et al.*, 1999b; Bechmann *et al.*, 2001).

The kynurenine pathway and immune tolerance

Quinolinic acid is produced by the oxidative catabolism of tryptophan through the kynurenine pathway. The QA is a neurotoxin both with acute and chronic low-level exposure. Activation of the kynurenine pathway causes increased production of this and other potentially neurotoxic metabolites. Toxicity is mediated by activation of NMDA receptors, leading to influx of calcium, triggering of proteases, formation of free radicals, induction of mitochondrial dysfunction, inhibition of glutamate uptake and lipid peroxidation (Guillemin *et al.*, 2005a). Under normal conditions there is very little QA in the brain, and only small amounts are required to cause neuronal injury (Stone *et al.*, 2003). Quinolinic acid is involved in the pathogenesis of several inflammatory brain disorders, including Huntington's disease and certain viral infections (Stone *et al.*, 2003).

Within the CNS, QA is produced primarily by macrophages after up-regulation of its synthetic enzymes including indoleamine-2,3-dioxygenase (IDO), the first enzyme in the kynurenine pathway and its rate-limiting step (Heyes *et al.*, 1997; Pemberton *et al.*, 1997; Kohler *et al.*, 1988; Smith *et al.*, 2001). Pro-inflammatory cytokines such as IFN-γ increase IDO expression, whereas the anti-inflammatory IL-4 reduces it (Musso *et al.*, 1994; Pemberton *et al.*, 1997; Smith *et al.*, 2001; Guillemin *et al.*, 2005a). HIV and its proteins Nef and Tat induce IDO in human macrophages through induction of pro-inflammatory cytokines (Grant *et al.*, 2000; Smith *et al.*, 2001).

The activity of IDO is significantly increased in HAD brains compared to both controls and patients with AIDS but with no cognitive impairment (Sardar *et al.*, 1995), and QA is considerably elevated to levels that are neurotoxic in vitro (Heyes *et al.*, 1991, 2001; Brouwers *et al.*, 1993). Levels of QA within the CSF correlate with the likelihood and severity of cognitive dysfunction (Heyes *et al.*, 1991; Kaul *et al.*, 2001), and is directly related to viral load (Brew *et al.*, 1995a, 1995b). Antiviral treatment reduces CSF QA levels (Valle *et al.*, 2004). Most QA in the HAD brain is produced by cytokine-activated but non-infected macrophages, favoring the indirect theory of macrophage-mediated toxicity (Nuovo and Alfieri, 1996). QA at brain concentrations found in HAD can also increase chemokine production and induce apoptosis in astrocytes (Guillemin *et al.*, 2003c, 2005a, 2005b). In SIV-infected macaques there is also increased QA (Depboylu *et al.*, 2004), and the severity of neurological symptoms correlates with brain QA levels (Heyes *et al.*, 1992). Suppression of IDO expression reduces viral burden and macrophage activation (Depboylu *et al.*, 2004).

In addition to producing neurotoxic metabolites, the kynurenine pathway is a major regulator of the immune response leading to immune tolerance (Fallarino *et al.*, 2002; Grohmann *et al.*, 2003; Mellor *et al.*, 2003) and is critical in preventing fetal rejection (Munn *et al.*, 1998). Quinolinic acid inhibits T cell proliferation through local tryptophan depletion, causing lymphocyte anergy and apoptosis (Munn *et al.*, 1999; Hwu *et al.*, 2000). In SCID mice, inhibition of IDO activity during HIV brain infection enhances CD8 T lymphocyte-mediated clearance of HIV-infected macrophages (Potula *et al.*, 2005), and IDO expression by brain macrophages might in vivo allow HIV to escape cytotoxic T cell-mediated clearance. Activation of the kynurenine pathway in HIV-infected macrophages could thus be a critical mechanism in the maintenance of immune tolerance to the virus and allowing viral persistence.

Host and viral factors relating to QA production could be relevant to the fact that only a subset of patients develop HAD, with significant interindividual differences in QA production in response to HIV infection (Kerr *et al.*, 1997). Not all strains of HIV can induce the kynurenine pathway in macrophages (Grant *et al.*, 2000), and the degree of viral macrophage tropism correlates with the level of QA production (Brew *et al.*, 1995b). This variability could reflect differences in virulence, as inhibition of QA production by HIV-infected macrophages is neuroprotective (Kerr *et al.*, 1997).

Effect of HAART upon HAD

To what extent does HAART control brain infection? HAART reduces viral load, increases circulating T cells and at least partially restores immune competence. Not all HAD patients improve on HAART, possibly reflecting irreversible neuronal loss, and HAART does not eradicate HIV or completely stop viral replication. Despite excellent compliance and an undetectable viral load, HIV persists in cellular reservoirs such as macrophages and in sanctuary sites such as the brain and lymphoid tissue. Cognitively normal patients with AIDS treated with HAART showed ongoing microglial activation comparable with that seen in AIDS and HIVE in the absence of astrogliosis or lymphocytic invasion (Petito *et al.*, 2001; Anthony *et al.*, 2005). This ongoing macrophage inflammation could be due to productive brain infection below the limits of detection in CSF, or could be secondary to previous damage (Brew, 2004). Dysregulation or loss of astrocytes, which normally down-regulate microglial inflammation, could also contribute. The increased pro-inflammatory and reduced anti-inflammatory cytokine milieu in the brain might be a third contributor to unchecked immune activation.

There is evidence for a change in the neuropathology of HAD in HAART-treated patients. Most patients show an attenuation of the inflammatory response. There is more involvement of the hippocampus and increased cerebral atherosclerosis (Morgello *et al.*, 2002; Anthony *et al.*, 2005). Occasionally a fulminant inflammatory leukoencephalopathy occurs that may be triggered by HAART-induced immune reconstitution (Gray *et al.*, 2003). The longer survival of HAART-treated patients makes them more likely to be exposed to confounding conditions. Testosterone deficiency can cause cognitive deficits and occurs in roughly 30% of late-stage HIV (Gouchie and Kimura, 1991), and hepatitis C infection superimposed on HIV can also worsen cognitive deficits (Valcour *et al.*, 2004). Of interest, however, is that there is evidence that neuropsychological impairment could be shifting from a subcortical to a cortical basis in HAART-treated patients, reminiscent of Alzheimer's pathology (Brew, 2004; Cysique *et al.*, 2004a). A study of asymptomatic HIV-positive patients showed increased verbal memory impairment on neuropsychological testing (Cysique *et al.*, 2004b). In addition, PET studies show less prominent basal ganglia hypermetabolism, with new mesial temporal lobe abnormalities post-HAART (Brew, 2004). It is suggested that HAART-treated HAD could predispose to an Alzheimer's-like form of the disease.

Alzheimer's pathology

In the HIV-infected brain, there are significant pathological changes reminiscent of Alzheimer's disease (Andreasen *et al.*, 2001). There is increased expression of amyloid precursor protein (APP) (Nebuloni *et al.*, 2001), and the occurrence of APP-rich lesions coincides with the presence of HAD (Adle-Biassette *et al.*, 1995). Accumulation of beta amyloid (Aβ) fragments of APP occurs more commonly in HIV-infected patients (Green *et al.*, 2005), and more so in HAART-treated and older patients (Esiri *et al.*, 1998; Green *et al.*, 2005; Rempel and Pulliam, 2005), and there is increased ubiquitin staining in the white matter (Gelman and Schuenke, 2004). There is premature deposition of hyperphosphorylated Tau in HIV-infected brains (Anthony *et al.*, 2004, 2006).The CSF total and phosphorylated tau concentrations are elevated in HAD patients, whereas the neurotoxic, amyloidogenic Aβ42 proteolytic fragment of APP is significantly lower in HAD patients (Brew *et al.*, 2005). Increased CSF Tau reflects neuronal and axonal

injury, whereas a reduction of CSF Aβ42 could reflect the deposition of Aβ into senile plaques. HIV-infected patients with the ApoE4 allele, a genetic risk factor for AD, are more likely to be demented and to have more severe dementia than those without it (Corder *et al.*, 1998). Overall, these changes suggest accelerated neuro-aging, and HIV infection could increase the risk of Alzheimer's disease or accelerate its expression in those who are otherwise destined to develop it. The mechanisms underlying these changes are unknown, but the inflammatory response in the brain to HIV infection could promote the production and accumulation of APP and favor formation of amyloid plaques (An *et al.*, 1997; Esiri *et al.*, 1998). The pro-inflammatory cytokines increased in the HIV brain increase the activity of the γ-secretase enzyme, which degrades APP to amyloid beta (Aβ) fragments, including the toxic Aβ42 molecule (Liao *et al.*, 2004), and viral Tat inhibits the degradation of Aβ by its enzyme neprilysin (Rempel and Pulliam, 2005). Amyloidogenic APP proteolytic fragments such as the neurotoxic Aβ42 increase target cell infectivity by HIV and could increase the vulnerability of the brain to HIV infection (Wojtowicz *et al.*, 2002). The Aβ42 fibrils can also induce brain macrophage QA synthesis (Guillemin *et al.*, 2003a, 2003b).

There appears to be increased neuro-aging in the HAART group. Neuro-inflammation, rather than viral burden, could be a potential factor in the pathogenesis of these Alzheimer's-like changes, as HAART-treated brains have a low viral burden but ongoing brain macrophage inflammation, particularly in the hippocampus (Anthony *et al.*, 2005). Given the increased life expectancy of HAART-treated HIV-infected individuals, premature neurodegeneration could become an increasing problem over time.

Conclusion

Sustained brain inflammation is an essential factor in many neurodegenerative disorders, and HIV infection leads to dysregulation of immune control and induction of inappropriate immune tolerance. The immune response within the CNS to HIV infection could be a double-edged sword. In early disease, microglia and other brain macrophages might be protective and counteract the negative effects of infection, through direct control of HIV replication, secretion of neurotrophins and elimination of debris and apoptotic cells (Verani *et al.*, 2005). Later on in HIV infection, perhaps in the context of loss of regulation from astrocytes and peripheral immune dysregulation, macrophage activation and inflammation become toxic to neurons via unregulated production of pro-inflammatory cytokines, chemokines, and oxidative products (Schwartz *et al.*, 2006). Precisely which factors are responsible for this switch from protective to neuro-degenerative macrophage inflammation are unknown. Further knowledge of the mechanisms underlying macrophage activation and pathogenesis could lead to novel therapeutic and preventive strategies for the control of HIV disease.

References

Achim CL, *et al.* Quantitation of human immunodeficiency virus, immune activation factors, and quinolinic acid in AIDS brains. *J Clin Invest* 1993; **91**(6): 2769–75.

Adamson DC, *et al.* Immunologic NO synthase: elevation in severe AIDS dementia and induction by HIV-1 gp41. *Science* 1996; **274**(5294): 1917–21.

Adamson DC, *et al.* Rate and severity of HIV-associated dementia (HAD): correlations with Gp41 and iNOS. *Mol Med* 1999; **5**(2): 98–109.

Adle-Biassette H, *et al.* Neuronal apoptosis in HIV infection in adults. *Neuropathol Appl Neurobiol* 1995; **21**(3): 218–27.

Adle-Biassette H, *et al.* Neuronal apoptosis does not correlate with dementia in HIV infection but is related to microglial activation and axonal damage. *Neuropathol Appl Neurobiol* 1999; **25**(2): 123–33.

Albright AV, *et al.* Microglia express CCR5, CXCR4, and CCR3, but of these, CCR5 is the principal coreceptor for human immunodeficiency virus type 1 dementia isolates. *J Virol* 1999; **73**(1): 205–13.

Albright AV, *et al.* Characterization of cultured microglia that can be infected by HIV-1. *J Neurovirol* 2000; **6** (Suppl 1): S53–60.

Albright AV, *et al.* Pathogenesis of human immunodeficiency virus-induced neurological disease. *J Neurovirol* 2003; **9**(2): 222–7.

Albright AV, *et al.* Low-level HIV replication in mixed glial cultures is associated with alterations in the processing of p55(Gag). *Virology* 2004; **325**(2): 328–39.

Aloisi F, *et al.* Intracerebral regulation of immune responses. *Ann Med* 2001; **33**(8): 510–5.

Ambrosini E, Aloisi F. Chemokines and glial cells: A complex network in the central nervous system. *Neurochem Res* 2004; **29**(5): 1017–38.

Amirayan-Chevillard N, *et al.* Impact of highly active anti-retroviral therapy (HAART) on cytokine production and monocyte subsets in HIV-infected patients. *Clin Exp Immunol* 2000; **120**(1): 107–12.

An SF, *et al.* Axonal damage revealed by accumulation of beta-APP in HIV-positive individuals without AIDS. *J Neuropathol Exp Neurol* 1997; **56**(11): 1262–8.

An SF, *et al.* Early entry and widespread cellular involvement of HIV-1 DNA in brains of HIV-1 positive asymptomatic individuals. *J Neuropathol Exp Neurol* 1999; **58**(11): 1156–62.

Anderson E, *et al.* HIV-1-associated dementia: a metabolic encephalopathy perpetrated by virus-infected and immune-competent mononuclear phagocytes. *J Acquir Immune Defic Syndr* 2002; **31**(Suppl 2): S43–54.

Anderson ER, *et al.* Hippocampal synaptic dysfunction in a murine model of human immunodeficiency virus type 1 encephalitis. *Neuroscience* 2003; **118**(2): 359–69.

Andreasen N, *et al.* Evaluation of CSF-tau and CSF-Abeta42 as diagnostic markers for Alzheimer disease in clinical practice. *Arch Neurol* 2001; **58**(3): 373–9.

Anthony IC, *et al.* Effects of human immunodeficiency virus encephalitis and drug abuse on the B lymphocyte population of the brain. *J Neurovirol* 2004; **10**(3): 181–8.

Anthony IC, *et al.* Influence of HAART on HIV-related CNS disease and neuroinflammation. *J Neuropathol Exp Neurol* 2005; **64**(6): 529–36.

Anthony IC, *et al.* Accelerated Tau deposition in the brains of individuals infected with human immunodeficiency virus-1 before and after the advent of highly active anti-retroviral therapy. *Acta Neuropathol (Berl)* 2006; **111**(6): 529–38.

Argyris EG, *et al.* Human immunodeficiency virus type 1 enters primary human brain microvascular endothelial cells by a mechanism involving cell surface proteoglycans independent of lipid rafts. *J Virol* 2003; **77**(22): 12140–51.

Asare E, *et al.* Neuronal pattern correlates with the severity of human immunodeficiency virus-associated dementia complex. Usefulness of spatial pattern analysis in clinicopathological studies. *Am J Pathol* 1996; **148**(1): 31–8.

Ballabh P, *et al.* The blood–brain barrier: an overview. Structure, regulation, and clinical implications. *Neurobiol Dis* 2004; **16**(1): 1–13.

Bechmann I, *et al.* Turnover of rat brain perivascular cells. *Exp Neurol* 2001; **168**(2): 242–9.

Berman NE, *et al.* Microglial activation and neurological symptoms in the SIV model of NeuroAIDS: association of MHC-II and MMP-9 expression with behavioral deficits and evoked potential changes. *Neurobiol Dis* 1999; **6**(6): 486–98.

Bezzi P, *et al.* CXCR4-activated astrocyte glutamate release via TNFalpha: Amplification by microglia triggers neurotoxicity. *Nat Neurosci* 2001; **4**(7): 702–10.

Blond D, *et al.* Nitric oxide synthesis enhances human immunodeficiency virus replication in primary human macrophages. *J Virol* 2000; **74**(19): 8904–12.

Bo L, *et al.* Detection of MHC class II-antigens on macrophages and microglia, but not on astrocytes and endothelia in active multiple sclerosis lesions. *J Neuroimmunol* 1994; **51**(2): 135–46.

Boehme SA, *et al.* The chemokine fractalkine inhibits Fas-mediated cell death of brain microglia. *J Immunol* 2000; **165**(1): 397–403.

Bomsel M. Transcytosis of infectious human immunodeficiency virus across a tight human epithelial cell line barrier. *Nat Med* 1997; **3**(1): 42–7.

Bonavia R, *et al.* Chemokines and their receptors in the CNS: Expression of CXCL12/SDF-1 and CXCR4 and their role in astrocyte proliferation. *Toxicol Lett* 2003; **139**(2–3): 181–9.

Bouwman FH, *et al.* Variable progression of HIV-associated dementia. *Neurology* 1998; **50**(6): 1814–20.

Brack-Werner R. Astrocytes: HIV cellular reservoirs and important participants in neuropathogenesis. *AIDS* 1999; **13**(1): 1–22.

Brenneman DE, *et al.* Neuronal cell killing by the envelope protein of HIV and its prevention by vasoactive intestinal peptide. *Nature* 1988; **335**(6191): 639–42.

Brew BJ. Evidence for a change in AIDS dementia complex in the era of highly active antiretroviral therapy and the possibility of new forms of AIDS dementia complex. *AIDS* 2004; **18**(Suppl 1): S75–8.

Brew BJ, *et al.* Cerebrospinal fluid beta 2 microglobulin in patients infected with human immunodeficiency virus. *Neurology* 1989; **39**(6): 830–4.

Brew BJ, *et al.* Cerebrospinal fluid neopterin in human immunodeficiency virus type 1 infection. *Ann Neurol* 1990; **28**(4): 556–60.

Brew BJ, *et al.* Cerebrospinal fluid beta 2-microglobulin in patients with AIDS dementia complex: An expanded series including response to zidovudine treatment. *AIDS* 1992; **6**(5): 461–5.

Brew BJ, *et al.* AIDS dementia complex and HIV-1 brain infection: Clinical–virological correlations. *Ann Neurol* 1995a; **38**(4): 563–70.

Brew BJ, *et al.* Quinolinic acid production is related to macrophage tropic isolates of HIV-1. *J Neurovirol* 1995b; **1**(5–6): 369–74.

Brew BJ, *et al.* The relationship between AIDS dementia complex and the presence of macrophage tropic and non-syncytium inducing isolates of human immunodeficiency virus type 1 in the cerebrospinal fluid. *J Neurovirol* 1996; **2**(3): 152–7.

Brew BJ, *et al.* Levels of human immunodeficiency virus type 1 RNA in cerebrospinal fluid correlate with AIDS dementia stage. *J Infect Dis* 1997; **175**(4): 963–6.

Brew BJ, *et al.* CSF amyloid beta42 and tau levels correlate with AIDS dementia complex. *Neurology* 2005; **65**(9): 1490–2.

Brouwers P, *et al.* Quinolinic acid in the cerebrospinal fluid of children with symptomatic human immunodeficiency virus type 1 disease: Relationships to clinical status and therapeutic response. *J Infect Dis* 1993; **168**(6): 1380–6.

Budka H. The definition of HIV-specific neuropathology. *Acta Pathol Jpn* 1991; **41**(3): 182–91.

Buttner A, *et al.* Vascular changes in the cerebral cortex in HIV-1 infection. II. An immunohistochemical and lectinhistochemical investigation. *Acta Neuropathol (Berl)* 1996; **92**(1): 35–41.

Chakrabarti L, *et al.* Early viral replication in the brain of SIV-infected rhesus monkeys. *Am J Pathol* 1991; **139**(6): 1273–80.

Chang L, *et al.* Cerebral metabolite abnormalities correlate with clinical severity of HIV-1 cognitive motor complex. *Neurology* 1999a; **52**(1): 100–8.

Chang L, *et al.* Highly active antiretroviral therapy reverses brain metabolite abnormalities in mild HIV dementia. *Neurology* 1999b; **53**(4): 782–9.

Chapman GA, *et al.* Fractalkine cleavage from neuronal membranes represents an acute event in the inflammatory response to excitotoxic brain damage. *J Neurosci* 2000; **20**(15): RC87.

Chen M, *et al.* Minocycline inhibits caspase-1 and caspase-3 expression and delays mortality in a transgenic mouse model of Huntington disease. *Nat Med* 2000; **6**(7): 797–801.

Cheng-Mayer C, Levy JA. Distinct biological and serological properties of human immunodeficiency viruses from the brain. *Ann Neurol* 1988; **23**(Suppl): S58–61.

Cherner M, *et al.* Neurocognitive dysfunction predicts postmortem findings of HIV encephalitis. *Neurology* 2002; **59**(10): 1563–7.

Chi D, *et al.* The effects of HIV infection on endothelial function. *Endothelium* 2000; **7**(4): 223–42.

Chong YH, Lee MJ. *Expression of complement inhibitor protein CD59 in human neuronal and glial cell lines treated with HIV-1 gp41 peptides. J Neurovirol* 2000; **6**(1): 51–60.

Cinque P, *et al.* Cerebrospinal fluid HIV-1 RNA levels: Correlation with HIV encephalitis. *AIDS* 1998; **12**(4): 389–94.

Cocchi F, *et al.* Identification of RANTES, MIP-1 alpha, and MIP-1 beta as the major HIV-suppressive factors produced by CD8+ T cells. *Science* 1995; **270**(5243): 1811–5.

Codazzi F, *et al.* HIV-1 gp120 glycoprotein induces {Ca2+}i responses not only in type-2 but also type-1 astrocytes and oligodendrocytes of the rat cerebellum. *Eur J Neurosci* 1995; **7**(6): 1333–41.

Conant K, *et al.* Induction of monocyte chemoattractant protein-1 in HIV-1 Tat-stimulated astrocytes and elevation in AIDS dementia. *Proc Natl Acad Sci USA* 1998; **95**(6): 3117–21.

Conant K, *et al.* Cerebrospinal fluid levels of MMP-2, 7, and 9 are elevated in association with human immunodeficiency virus dementia. *Ann Neurol* 1999; **46**(3): 391–8.

Corasaniti MT, *et al.* Evidence that the HIV-1 coat protein gp120 causes neuronal apoptosis in the neocortex of rat via a mechanism involving CXCR4 chemokine receptor. *Neurosci Lett* 2001; **312**(2): 67–70.

Corder EH, *et al.* HIV-infected subjects with the E4 allele for APOE have excess dementia and peripheral neuropathy. *Nat Med* 1998; **4**(10): 1182–4.

Cosenza MA, *et al.* HIV-1 expression protects macrophages and microglia from apoptotic death. *Neuropathol Appl Neurobiol* 2004; **30**(5): 478–90.

Cotter R, *et al.* Fractalkine (CX3CL1) and brain inflammation: Implications for HIV-1-associated dementia. *J Neurovirol* 2002; **8**(6): 585–98.

Cysique LA, *et al.* Antiretroviral therapy in HIV infection: are neurologically active drugs important? *Arch Neurol* 2004a; **61**(11): 1699–704.

Cysique LA, *et al.* Prevalence and pattern of neuropsychological impairment in human immunodeficiency virus-infected/

acquired immunodeficiency syndrome (HIV/AIDS) patients across pre- and post-highly active antiretroviral therapy eras: A combined study of two cohorts. *J Neurovirol* 2004b; **10**(6): 350–7.

Dallasta LM, *et al.* Blood–brain barrier tight junction disruption in human immunodeficiency virus-1 encephalitis. *Am J Pathol* 1999; **155**(6): 1915–27.

Davis LE, *et al.* Early viral brain invasion in iatrogenic human immunodeficiency virus infection. *Neurology* 1992; **42**(9): 1736–9.

Demuth M, *et al.* Relationship between viral load in blood, cerebrospinal fluid, brain tissue and isolated microglia with neurological disease in macaques infected with different strains of SIV. *J Neurovirol* 2000; **6**(3): 187–201.

Depboylu C, *et al.* Brain virus burden and indoleamine-2,3-dioxygenase expression during lentiviral infection of rhesus monkey are concomitantly lowered by 6-chloro-2′,3′-dideoxyguanosine. *Eur J Neurosci* 2004; **19**(11): 2997–3005.

Derdeyn CA, Silvestri G. Viral and host factors in the pathogenesis of HIV infection. *Curr Opin Immunol* 2005; **17**(4): 366–73.

Dickson DW. Multinucleated giant cells in acquired immunodeficiency syndrome encephalopathy. Origin from endogenous microglia? *Arch Pathol Lab Med* 1986; **110**(10): 967–8.

Dietrich JB. The adhesion molecule ICAM-1 and its regulation in relation with the blood–brain barrier. *J Neuroimmunol* 2002; **128**(1–2): 58–68.

Dong Y, Benveniste EN. Immune function of astrocytes. *Glia* 2001; **36**(2): 180–90.

Dore GJ, *et al.* Trends in incidence of AIDS illnesses in Australia from 1983 to 1994: The Australian AIDS cohort. *J Acquir Immune Defic Syndr Hum Retrovirol* 1997; **16**(1): 39–43.

Dore GJ, *et al.* Changes to AIDS dementia complex in the era of highly active antiretroviral therapy. *AIDS* 1999; **13**(10): 1249–53.

Dore GJ, *et al.* Marked improvement in survival following AIDS dementia complex in the era of highly active antiretroviral therapy. *AIDS* 2003; **17**(10): 1539–45.

Edinger AL, *et al.* CD4-independent, CCR5-dependent infection of brain capillary endothelial cells by a neurovirulent simian immunodeficiency virus strain. *Proc Natl Acad Sci USA* 1997; **94**(26): 14742–7.

Erichsen D, *et al.* Neuronal injury regulates fractalkine: Relevance for HIV-1 associated dementia. *J Neuroimmunol* 2003; **138**(1–2): 144–55.

Esiri MM, *et al.* Prevalence of Alzheimer plaques in AIDS. *J Neurol Neurosurg Psychiatry* 1998; **65**(1): 29–33.

Eugenin EA, *et al.* MCP-1 (CCL2) protects human neurons and astrocytes from NMDA or HIV-tat-induced apoptosis. *J Neurochem* 2003; **85**(5): 1299–311.

Everall I, *et al.* Assessment of neuronal density in the putamen in human immunodeficiency virus (HIV) infection. Application of stereology and spatial analysis of quadrats. *J Neurovirol* 1995; **1**(1): 126–9.

Everall IP, *et al.* Cortical synaptic density is reduced in mild to moderate human immunodeficiency virus neurocognitive disorder. HNRC Group. HIV Neurobehavioral Research Center. *Brain Pathol* 1999; **9**(2): 209–17.

Falangola MF, *et al.* HIV infection of human choroid plexus: a possible mechanism of viral entry into the CNS. *J Neuropathol Exp Neurol* 1995; **54**(4): 497–503.

Fallarino F, *et al.* T cell apoptosis by tryptophan catabolism. *Cell Death Differ* 2002; **9**(10): 1069–77.

Farkas I, *et al.* A neuronal C5a receptor and an associated apoptotic signal transduction pathway. *J Physiol* 1998; **507**(Pt 3): 679–87.

Faure S, *et al.* Rapid progression to AIDS in HIV+ individuals with a structural variant of the chemokine receptor CX3CR1. *Science* 2000; **287**(5461): 2274–7.

Finzi D, *et al.* Identification of a reservoir for HIV-1 in patients on highly active antiretroviral therapy. *Science* 1997; **278**(5341): 1295–300.

Fischer-Smith T, *et al.* CNS invasion by CD14+/CD16+ peripheral blood-derived monocytes in HIV dementia: Perivascular accumulation and reservoir of HIV infection. *J Neurovirol* 2001; **7**(6):528–41.

Fischer-Smith T, *et al.* Macrophage/ microglial accumulation and proliferating cell nuclear antigen expression in the central nervous system in human immunodeficiency virus encephalopathy. *Am J Pathol* 2004; **164**(6): 2089–99.

Fox L, *et al.* Neurodegeneration of somatostatin-immunoreactive neurons in HIV encephalitis. *J Neuropathol Exp Neurol* 1997; **56**(4): 360–8.

Garaci E, *et al.* Nerve growth factor is an autocrine factor essential for the survival of macrophages infected with HIV. *Proc Natl Acad Sci USA* 1999; **96**(24): 14013–8.

Garaci E, *et al.* Anti-nerve growth factor Ab abrogates macrophage-mediated HIV-1 infection and depletion of CD4+ T lymphocytes in hu-SCID mice. *Proc Natl Acad Sci USA* 2003; **100**(15): 8927–32.

Gartner S. HIV infection and dementia. *Science* 2000; **287**(5453): 602–4.

Gelbard HA, *et al.* Platelet-activating factor: A candidate human immunodeficiency virus type 1-induced neurotoxin. *J Virol* 1994; **68**(7): 4628–35.

Gelbard HA, *et al.* Apoptotic neurons in brains from paediatric patients with HIV-1 encephalitis and progressive encephalopathy. *Neuropathol Appl Neurobiol* 1995; **21**(3): 208–17.

Gelman BB. Diffuse microgliosis associated with cerebral atrophy in the acquired immunodeficiency syndrome. *Ann Neurol* 1993; **34**(1): 65–70.

Gelman BB, Schuenke K. Brain aging in acquired immunodeficiency syndrome: Increased ubiquitin-protein conjugate is correlated with decreased synaptic protein but not amyloid plaque accumulation. *J Neurovirol* 2004; **10**(2): 98–108.

Giometto B, *et al.* Accumulation of beta-amyloid precursor protein in HIV encephalitis: Relationship with neuropsychological abnormalities. *Ann Neurol* 1997; **42**(1): 34–40.

Giulian D, *et al.* Secretion of neurotoxins by mononuclear phagocytes infected with HIV-1. *Science* 1990; **250**(4987): 1593–6.

Giulian D, *et al.* Study of receptor-mediated neurotoxins released by HIV-1-infected mononuclear phagocytes found in human brain. *J Neurosci* 1996; **16**(10): 3139–53.

Glass JD, *et al.* Clinical-neuropathologic correlation in HIV-associated dementia. *Neurology* 1993; **43**(11): 2230–7.

Glass JD, *et al.* Immunocytochemical quantitation of human immunodeficiency virus in the brain: correlations with dementia. *Ann Neurol* 1995; **38**(5): 755–62.

Gonzalez E, *et al.* HIV-1 infection and AIDS dementia are influenced by a mutant MCP-1 allele linked to increased monocyte infiltration of tissues and MCP-1 levels. *Proc Natl Acad Sci USA* 2002; **99**(21): 13795–800.

Gonzalez-Scarano F, Martin-Garcia J. The neuropathogenesis of AIDS. *Nat Rev Immunol* 2005; **5**(1): 69–81.

Gosztonyi G, *et al.* Human immunodeficiency virus (HIV) distribution in HIV encephalitis: Study of 19 cases with combined use of in situ hybridization and immunocytochemistry. *J Neuropathol Exp Neurol* 1994; **53**(5): 521–34.

Gouchie C, Kimura D. The relationship between testosterone levels and cognitive ability patterns. *Psychoneuroendocrinology* 1991; **16**(4): 323–34.

Goudsmit J, *et al.* Intrathecal synthesis of antibodies to HTLV-III in patients without AIDS or AIDS related complex. *Br Med J (Clin Res Ed)* 1986; **292**(6530): 1231–4.

Grant RS, *et al.* Induction of indolamine 2,3-dioxygenase in primary human macrophages by human immunodeficiency virus type 1 is strain dependent. *J Virol* 2000; **74**(9): 4110–5.

Gray F, *et al.* The changing pattern of HIV neuropathology in the HAART era. *J Neuropathol Exp Neurol* 2003; **62**(5): 429–40.

Green DA, *et al.* Brain deposition of beta-amyloid is a common pathologic feature in HIV positive patients. *AIDS* 2005; **19**(4): 407–11.

Griffin DE. Cytokines in the brain during viral infection: clues to HIV-associated dementia. *J Clin Invest* 1997; **100**(12): 2948–51.

Grohmann U, *et al.* Tolerance, DCs and tryptophan: Much ado about IDO. *Trends Immunol* 2003; **24**(5): 242–8.

Gu Z, *et al.* S-nitrosylation of matrix metalloproteinases: Signaling pathway to neuronal cell death. *Science* 2002; **297**(5584): 1186–90.

Guillemin GJ, Brew BJ. Microglia, macrophages, perivascular macrophages, and pericytes: A review of function and identification. *J Leukoc Biol* 2004; **75**(3): 388–97.

Guillemin GJ, *et al.* A beta 1–42 induces production of quinolinic acid by human macrophages and microglia. *Neuroreport* 2003a; **14**(18): 2311–5.

Guillemin GJ, *et al.* Quinolinic acid in the pathogenesis of Alzheimer's disease. *Adv Exp Med Biol* 2003b; **527**: 167–76.

Guillemin GJ, *et al.* Quinolinic acid upregulates chemokine production and chemokine receptor expression in astrocytes. *Glia* 2003c; **41**(4): 371–81.

Guillemin GJ, *et al.* Involvement of quinolinic acid in AIDS dementia complex. *Neurotox Res* 2005a; **7**(1–2): 103–23.

Guillemin GJ, *et al.* Quinolinic acid selectively induces apoptosis of human astrocytes: Potential role in AIDS dementia complex. *J Neuroinflam* 2005b; **2**: 16.

Harouse JM, *et al.* Human choroid plexus cells can be latently infected with human immunodeficiency virus. *Ann Neurol* 1989; **25**(4): 406–11.

He J, *et al.* CCR3 and CCR5 are co-receptors for HIV-1 infection of microglia. *Nature* 1997; **385**(6617): 645–9.

Heidenreich F, *et al.* Serum and cerebrospinal fluid levels of soluble intercellular adhesion molecule 1 (sICAM-1) in patients with HIV-1 associated neurological diseases. *J Neuroimmunol* 1994; **52**(2): 117–26.

Hesselgesser J, *et al.* Identification and characterization of the CXCR4 chemokine receptor in human T cell lines: Ligand binding, biological activity, and HIV-1 infectivity. *J Immunol* 1998a; **160**(2): 877–83.

Hesselgesser J, *et al.* Neuronal apoptosis induced by HIV-1 gp120 and the chemokine SDF-1 alpha is mediated by the chemokine receptor CXCR4. *Curr Biol* 1998b; **8**(10): 595–8.

Heyes MP, *et al.* Quinolinic acid in cerebrospinal fluid and serum in HIV-1 infection: Relationship to clinical and neurological status. *Ann Neurol* 1991; **29**(2): 202–9.

Heyes MP, *et al.* Relationship of neurologic status in macaques infected with the simian immunodeficiency virus to cerebrospinal fluid quinolinic acid and kynurenic acid. *Brain Res* 1992; **570**(1–2): 237–50.

Heyes MP, *et al.* Elevated cerebrospinal fluid quinolinic acid levels are associated with region-specific cerebral volume loss in HIV infection. *Brain* 2001; **124**(Pt 5): 1033–42.

Hickey WF. Basic principles of immunological surveillance of the normal central nervous system. *Glia* 2001; **36**(2): 118–24.

Hickey WF, Kimura H. Perivascular microglial cells of the CNS are bone marrow-derived and present antigen in vivo. *Science* 1988; **239**(4837): 290–2.

Hickey WF, *et al.* T-lymphocyte entry into the central nervous system. *J Neurosci Res* 1991; **28**(2): 254–60.

Hickey WF, *et al.* Bone marrow-derived elements in the central nervous system: An immunohistochemical and ultrastructural survey of rat chimeras. *J Neuropathol Exp Neurol* 1992; **51**(3): 246–56.

Ho DD, *et al.* Isolation of HTLV-III from cerebrospinal fluid and neural tissues of patients with neurologic syndromes related to the acquired immunodeficiency syndrome. *N Engl J Med* 1985; **313**(24): 1493–7.

Hughes ES, *et al.* Investigation of the dynamics of the spread of human immunodeficiency virus to brain and other tissues by evolutionary analysis of sequences from the p17gag and env genes. *J Virol* 1997; **71**(2): 1272–80.

Hwu P, *et al.* Indoleamine 2,3-dioxygenase production by human dendritic cells results in the inhibition of T cell proliferation. *J Immunol* 2000; **164**(7): 3596–9.

Ioannidis JP, *et al.* Long-term productive human immunodeficiency virus-1 infection in human infant microglia. *Am J Pathol* 1995; **147**(5): 1200–6.

Janabi N, *et al.* Induction of human immunodeficiency virus type 1 replication in human glial cells after pro-inflammatory cytokines stimulation: Effect of IFNgamma, IL1beta, and TNFalpha on differentiation and chemokine production in glial cells. *Glia* 1998; **23**(4): 304–15.

Jassoy C, *et al.* Detection of a vigorous HIV-1-specific cytotoxic T lymphocyte response in cerebrospinal fluid from infected persons with AIDS dementia complex. *J Immunol* 1992; **149**(9): 3113–9.

Jiang ZG, *et al.* Glutamate is a mediator of neurotoxicity in secretions of activated HIV-1-infected macrophages. *J Neuroimmunol* 2001; **117**(1–2): 97–107.

John GR, *et al.* Cytokines: Powerful regulators of glial cell activation. *Neuroscientist* 2003; **9**(1): 10–22.

Johnston JB, *et al.* Lentivirus infection in the brain induces matrix metalloproteinase expression: Role of envelope diversity. *J Virol* 2000; **74**(16): 7211–20.

Johnston JB, *et al.* HIV-1 Tat neurotoxicity is prevented by matrix metalloproteinase

inhibitors. *Ann Neurol* 2001; **49**(2): 230–41.

Jongen PJ, *et al.* Cerebrospinal fluid C3 and C4 indexes in immunological disorders of the central nervous system. *Acta Neurol Scand* 2000; **101**(2): 116–21.

Jordan CA, *et al.* Infection of brain microglial cells by human immunodeficiency virus type 1 is CD4 dependent. *J Virol* 1991; **65**(2): 736–42.

Kaul M, Lipton SA. Chemokines and activated macrophages in HIV gp120-induced neuronal apoptosis. *Proc Natl Acad Sci USA* 1999; **96**(14): 8212–16.

Kaul M, Lipton SA. Signaling pathways to neuronal damage and apoptosis in human immunodeficiency virus type 1-associated dementia: Chemokine receptors, excitotoxicity, and beyond. *J Neurovirol* 2004; **10**(Suppl 1): 97–101.

Kaul M, *et al.* Pathways to neuronal injury and apoptosis in HIV-associated dementia. *Nature* 2001; **410**(6831): 988–94.

Kaul M, *et al.* HIV-1 infection and AIDS: Consequences for the central nervous system. *Cell Death Differ*, 2005; **12**(Suppl 1): 878–92.

Kedzierska K, Crowe SM. The role of monocytes and macrophages in the pathogenesis of HIV-1 infection. *Curr Med Chem* 2002; **9**(21): 1893–903.

Kerr SJ, *et al.* Kynurenine pathway inhibition reduces neurotoxicity of HIV-1-infected macrophages. *Neurology* 1997; **49**(6): 1671–81.

Kerr SJ, *et al.* Chronic exposure of human neurons to quinolinic acid results in neuronal changes consistent with AIDS dementia complex. *AIDS* 1998; **12**(4): 355–63.

Kimata JT, *et al.* Coreceptor specificity of temporal variants of simian immunodeficiency virus Mne. *J Virol* 1999; **73**(2): 1655–60.

Klein RS, *et al.* Chemokine receptor expression and signaling in macaque and human fetal neurons and astrocytes: Implications for the neuropathogenesis of AIDS. *J Immunol* 1999; **163**(3): 1636–46.

Kohleisen B, *et al.* Stable expression of HIV-1 Nef induces changes in growth properties and activation state of human astrocytes. *AIDS* 1999; **13**(17): 2331–41.

Kohler C, *et al.* Localization of quinolinic acid metabolizing enzymes in the rat brain. Immunohistochemical studies using antibodies to 3-hydroxyanthranilic acid oxygenase and quinolinic acid phosphoribosyltransferase. *Neuroscience* 1988; **27**(1): 49–76.

Kuiken CL, *et al.* Differences in human immunodeficiency virus type 1 V3 sequences from patients with and without AIDS dementia complex. *J Gen Virol* 1995; **76**(Pt 1): 175–80.

Kure K, *et al.* Human immunodeficiency virus-1 infection of the nervous system: An autopsy study of 268 adult, pediatric, and fetal brains. *Hum Pathol* 1991; **22**(7): 700–10.

Langford D, *et al.* Expression of stromal cell-derived factor 1alpha protein in HIV encephalitis. *J Neuroimmunol* 2002; **127**(1–2): 115–26.

Lassmann H, Hickey WF. Radiation bone marrow chimeras as a tool to study microglia turnover in normal brain and inflammation. *Clin Neuropathol* 1993; **12**(5): 284–5.

Lassmann H, *et al.* Bone marrow derived elements and resident microglia in brain inflammation. *Glia* 1993; **7**(1): 19–24.

Liao YF, *et al.* Tumor necrosis factor-alpha, interleukin-1beta, and interferon-gamma stimulate gamma-secretase-mediated cleavage of amyloid precursor protein through a JNK-dependent MAPK pathway. *J Biol Chem* 2004; **279**(47): 49523–32.

Liu NQ, *et al.* Human immunodeficiency virus type 1 enters brain microvascular endothelia by macropinocytosis dependent on lipid rafts and the mitogen-activated protein kinase signaling pathway. *J Virol* 2002; **76**(13): 6689–700.

Liu R, *et al.* Homozygous defect in HIV-1 coreceptor accounts for resistance of some multiply-exposed individuals to HIV-1 infection. *Cell* 1996; **86**(3): 367–77.

Liu Y, *et al.* Analysis of human immunodeficiency virus type 1 gp160 sequences from a patient with HIV dementia: Evidence for monocyte trafficking into brain. *J Neurovirol* 2000; **6**(Suppl 1): S70–81.

Luo X, *et al.* Macrophage proteomic fingerprinting predicts HIV-1-associated cognitive impairment. *Neurology* 2003; **60**(12): 1931–7.

Lusso P. HIV and the chemokine system: 10 years later. *Embo J* 2006; **25**(3): 447–56.

Magnus T, *et al.* Astrocytes are less efficient in the removal of apoptotic lymphocytes than microglia cells: Implications for the role of glial cells in the inflamed central nervous system. *J Neuropathol Exp Neurol* 2002; **61**(9): 760–6.

Maschke M, *et al.* Incidence and prevalence of neurological disorders associated with HIV since the introduction of highly active antiretroviral therapy (HAART). *J Neurol Neurosurg Psychiatry* 2000; **69**(3): 376–80.

Masliah E, *et al.* Selective neuronal vulnerability in HIV encephalitis. *J Neuropathol Exp Neurol* 1992a; **51**(6): 585–93.

Masliah E, *et al.* Dendritic injury is a pathological substrate for human immunodeficiency virus-related cognitive disorders. HNRC Group. The HIV Neurobehavioral Research Center. *Ann Neurol* 1997; **42**(6): 963–72.

McArthur JC. HIV dementia: An evolving disease. *J Neuroimmunol* 2004; **157**(1–2): 3–10.

McArthur JC, *et al.* The diagnostic utility of elevation in cerebrospinal fluid beta 2-microglobulin in HIV-1 dementia. Multicenter AIDS Cohort Study. *Neurology* 1992; **42**(9): 1707–12.

McArthur JC, *et al.* Dementia in AIDS patients: incidence and risk factors. Multicenter AIDS Cohort Study. *Neurology* 1993; **43**(11): 2245–52.

McArthur JC, *et al.* Human immunodeficiency virus-associated dementia: an evolving disease. *J Neurovirol* 2003; **9**(2): 205–21.

McArthur JC, *et al.* Neurological complications of HIV infection. *Lancet Neurol* 2005; **4**(9): 543–55.

McCrossan M, *et al.* An immune control model for viral replication in the CNS during presymptomatic HIV infection. *Brain* 2006; **129**(Pt 2): 503–16.

McManus CM, *et al.* Cytokine induction of MIP-1 alpha and MIP-1 beta in human fetal microglia. *J Immunol* 1998; **160**(3): 1449–55.

Melzer MS, *et al.* Meningoencephalitis due to primary HIV infection. HIV infection may also cause rash or glandular fever type illness. *Br Med J* 2003; **326**(7388): 552.

Meltzer MS, *et al.* Role of mononuclear phagocytes in the pathogenesis of human immunodeficiency virus infection. *Annu Rev Immunol* 1990; **8**: 169–94.

Metz LM, *et al.* Minocycline reduces gadolinium-enhancing magnetic resonance imaging lesions in multiple sclerosis. *Ann Neurol* 2004; **55**(5): 756.

Meucci O, *et al.* Chemokines regulate hippocampal neuronal signaling and gp120 neurotoxicity. *Proc Natl Acad Sci USA* 1998; **95**(24): 14500–5.

Meucci O, *et al.* Expression of CX3CR1 chemokine receptors on neurons and their role in neuronal survival. *Proc Natl Acad Sci USA* 2000; **97**(14): 8075–80.

Michaels J, *et al.* Microglia in the giant cell encephalitis of acquired immune deficiency syndrome: Proliferation, infection and fusion. *Acta Neuropathol (Berl)* 1988; **76**(4): 373–9.

Min KJ, *et al.* Astrocytes induce hemeoxygenase-1 expression in microglia: A feasible mechanism for preventing excessive brain inflammation. *J Neurosci* 2006; **26**(6): 1880–7.

Morgello S, *et al.* Autopsy findings in a human immunodeficiency virus-infected population over 2 decades: Influences of gender, ethnicity, risk factors, and time. *Arch Pathol Lab Med* 2002; **126**(2): 182–90.

Morner A, *et al.* Productive HIV-2 infection in the brain is restricted to macrophages/microglia. *AIDS* 2003; **17**(10): 1451–5.

Munn DH, *et al.* Prevention of allogeneic fetal rejection by tryptophan catabolism. *Science* 1998; **281**(5380): 1191–3.

Munn DH, *et al.* Inhibition of T cell proliferation by macrophage tryptophan catabolism. *J Exp Med* 1999; **189**(9): 1363–72.

Murray EA, *et al.* Cognitive and motor impairments associated with SIV infection in rhesus monkeys. *Science* 1992; **255**(5049): 1246–9.

Musso T, *et al.* Interleukin-4 inhibits indoleamine 2,3-dioxygenase expression in human monocytes. *Blood* 1994; **83**(5): 1408–11.

Nath A, *et al.* Identification of a human immunodeficiency virus type 1 Tat epitope that is neuroexcitatory and neurotoxic. *J Virol* 1996; **70**(3): 1475–80.

Nath A, *et al.* Transient exposure to HIV-1 Tat protein results in cytokine production in macrophages and astrocytes. A hit and run phenomenon. *J Biol Chem* 1999; **274**(24): 17098–102.

Navia BA, *et al.* The AIDS dementia complex: II. Neuropathology. *Ann Neurol* 1986; **19**(6): 525–35.

Nebuloni M, *et al.* Beta amyloid precursor protein and patterns of HIV p24 immunohistochemistry in different brain areas of AIDS patients. *AIDS* 2001; **15**(5): 571–5.

Nicholson JK, *et al.* In vitro infection of human monocytes with human T lymphotropic virus type III/ lymphadenopathy-associated virus (HTLV-III/LAV). *J Immunol* 1986; **137**(1): 323–9.

Nottet HS, *et al.* Role for oxygen radicals in self-sustained HIV-1 replication in monocyte-derived macrophages: Enhanced HIV-1 replication by N-acetyl-L-cysteine. *J Leukoc Biol* 1994; **56**(6): 702–7.

Nottet HS, *et al.* A regulatory role for astrocytes in HIV-1 encephalitis. An overexpression of eicosanoids, platelet-activating factor, and tumor necrosis factor-alpha by activated HIV-1-infected monocytes is attenuated by primary human astrocytes. *J Immunol* 1995; **154**(7): 3567–81.

155

Nottet HS, *et al.* Mechanisms for the transendothelial migration of HIV-1-infected monocytes into brain. *J Immunol* 1996; **156**(3): 1284–95.

Nukuna A, *et al.* Levels of human immunodeficiency virus type 1 (HIV-1) replication in macrophages determines the severity of murine HIV-1 encephalitis. *J Neurovirol* 2004; **10**(Suppl 1): 82–90.

Nuovo GJ, Alfieri ML. AIDS dementia is associated with massive, activated HIV-1 infection and concomitant expression of several cytokines. *Mol Med* 1996; **2**(3): 358–66.

Ohtani Y, *et al.* Expression of stromal cell-derived factor-1 and CXCR4 chemokine receptor mRNAs in cultured rat glial and neuronal cells. *Neurosci Lett* 1998; **249**(2–3): 163–6.

Pandey V, Bolsover SR. Immediate and neurotoxic effects of HIV protein gp120 act through CXCR4 receptor. *Biochem Biophys Res Commun* 2000; **274**(1): 212–5.

Pardridge WM. Targeting neurotherapeutic agents through the blood–brain barrier. *Arch Neurol* 2002; **59**(1): 35–40.

Patel CA, *et al.* Human immunodeficiency virus type 1 Vpr induces apoptosis in human neuronal cells. *J Virol* 2000; **74**(20): 9717–26.

Patton BL, *et al.* Synaptic laminin prevents glial entry into the synaptic cleft. *Nature* 1998; **393**(6686): 698–701.

Peluso R, *et al.* A Trojan Horse mechanism for the spread of visna virus in monocytes. *Virology* 1985; **147**(1): 231–6.

Pemberton LA, *et al.* Quinolinic acid production by macrophages stimulated with IFN-gamma, TNF-alpha, and IFN-alpha. *J Interferon Cytokine Res* 1997; **17**(10): 589–95.

Pereira CF, *et al.* Enhanced expression of fractalkine in HIV-1 associated dementia. *J Neuroimmunol* 2001; **115**(1–2): 168–75.

Perrella O, *et al.* Cerebrospinal fluid cytokines in AIDS dementia complex. *J Neurol* 1992; **239**(7): 387–8.

Perry SW, *et al.* Platelet-activating factor receptor activation. An initiator step in HIV-1 neuropathogenesis. *J Biol Chem* 1998; **273**(28): 17660–4.

Persidsky Y, Gendelman HE. Mononuclear phagocyte immunity and the neuropathogenesis of HIV-1 infection. *J Leukoc Biol* 2003; **74**(5): 691–701.

Persidsky Y, *et al.* A model for monocyte migration through the blood-brain barrier during HIV-1 encephalitis. *J Immunol* 1997a; **158**(7): 3499–510.

Persidsky Y, *et al.* An analysis of HIV-1-associated inflammatory products in brain tissue of humans and SCID mice with HIV-1 encephalitis. *J Neurovirol* 1997b; **3**(6): 401–16.

Persidsky Y, *et al.* Microglial and astrocyte chemokines regulate monocyte migration through the blood–brain barrier in human immunodeficiency virus-1 encephalitis. *Am J Pathol* 1999; **155**(5): 1599–611.

Persidsky Y, *et al.* Mononuclear phagocytes mediate blood–brain barrier compromise and neuronal injury during HIV-1-associated dementia. *J Leukoc Biol* 2000; **68**(3): 413–22.

Persidsky Y, *et al.* Reduction in glial immunity and neuropathology by a PAF antagonist and an MMP and TNFalpha inhibitor in SCID mice with HIV-1 encephalitis. *J Neuroimmunol* 2001; **114**(1–2): 57–68.

Petito CK, Cash KS. Blood–brain barrier abnormalities in the acquired immunodeficiency syndrome: Immunohistochemical localization of serum proteins in postmortem brain. *Ann Neurol* 1992; **32**(5): 658–66.

Petito CK, Roberts B. Evidence of apoptotic cell death in HIV encephalitis. *Am J Pathol* 1995; **146**(5): 1121–30.

Petito CK, *et al.* Hippocampal injury and alterations in neuronal chemokine co-receptor expression in patients with AIDS. *J Neuropathol Exp Neurol* 2001; **60**(4): 377–85.

Pitcher CJ, *et al.* HIV-1-specific CD4+ T cells are detectable in most individuals with active HIV-1 infection, but decline with prolonged viral suppression. *Nat Med* 1999; **5**(5): 518–25.

Poluektova L, *et al.* Neuroregulatory events follow adaptive immune-mediated elimination of HIV-1-infected macrophages: Studies in a murine model of viral encephalitis. *J Immunol* 2004; **172**(12): 7610–7.

Potula R, *et al.* Inhibition of indoleamine 2,3-dioxygenase (IDO) enhances elimination of virus-infected macrophages in an animal model of HIV-1 encephalitis. *Blood* 2005; **106**(7): 2382–90.

Power C, *et al.* Cerebral white matter changes in acquired immunodeficiency syndrome dementia: alterations of the blood–brain barrier. *Ann Neurol* 1993; **34**(3): 339–50.

Pu H, *et al.* HIV-1 Tat protein upregulates inflammatory mediators and induces monocyte invasion into the brain. *Mol Cell Neurosci* 2003; **24**(1): 224–37.

Pulliam L, *et al.* Unique monocyte subset in patients with AIDS dementia. *Lancet* 1997; **349**(9053): 692–5.

Quasney MW, *et al.* Increased frequency of the tumor necrosis factor-alpha-308 A allele in adults with human immunodeficiency virus dementia. *Ann Neurol* 2001; **50**(2): 157–62.

Raivich G, *et al.* Neuroglial activation repertoire in the injured brain: graded response, molecular mechanisms and cues to physiological function. *Brain Res Brain Res Rev* 1999; **30**(1): 77–105.

Ransohoff RM, *et al.* Three or more routes for leukocyte migration into the central nervous system. *Nat Rev Immunol* 2003; **3**(7): 569–81.

Rempel HC, Pulliam L. HIV-1 Tat inhibits neprilysin and elevates amyloid beta. *AIDS* 2005; **19**(2): 127–35.

Ren Y, Savill J. Apoptosis: The importance of being eaten. *Cell Death Differ* 1998; **5**(7): 563–8.

Rostasy K, *et al.* SDF-1alpha is expressed in astrocytes and neurons in the AIDS dementia complex: An in vivo and in vitro study. *J Neuropathol Exp Neurol* 2003; **62**(6): 617–26.

Rottman JB, *et al.* Cellular localization of the chemokine receptor CCR5. Correlation to cellular targets of HIV-1 infection. *Am J Pathol* 1997; **151**(5): 1341–51.

Sabri F, *et al.* Elevated levels of soluble Fas and Fas ligand in cerebrospinal fluid of patients with AIDS dementia complex. *J Neuroimmunol* 2001; **114**(1–2): 197–206.

Sacktor N, *et al.* HIV-associated cognitive impairment before and after the advent of combination therapy. *J Neurovirol* 2002; **8**(2): 136–42.

Sanders VJ, *et al.* Chemokines and receptors in HIV encephalitis. *AIDS* 1998; **12**(9): 1021–6.

Sardar AM, *et al.* Increased concentrations of the neurotoxin 3-hydroxykynurenine in the frontal cortex of HIV-1-positive patients. *J Neurochem* 1995; **64**(2): 932–5.

Sasseville VG, *et al.* Monocyte adhesion to endothelium in simian immunodeficiency virus-induced AIDS encephalitis is mediated by vascular cell adhesion molecule-1/ alpha 4 beta 1 integrin interactions. *Am J Pathol* 1994; **144**(1): 27–40.

Schmitz JE, *et al.* Control of viremia in simian immunodeficiency virus infection by CD8+ lymphocytes. *Science* 1999; **283**(5403): 857–60.

Schuitemaker H. IL4 and IL10 as potent inhibitors of HIV1 replication in macrophages in vitro: A role for cytokines in the in vivo virus host range? *Res Immunol* 1994; **145**(8–9): 588–92.

Schwartz M, *et al.* Microglial phenotype: Is the commitment reversible? *Trends Neurosci* 2006; **29**(2): 68–74.

Schwartz O, *et al.* Endocytosis of major histocompatibility complex class I molecules is induced by the HIV-1 Nef protein. *Nat Med* 1996; **2**(3): 338–42.

Sevigny JJ, *et al.* Evaluation of HIV RNA and markers of immune activation as predictors of HIV-associated dementia. *Neurology* 2004; **63**(11): 2084–90.

Sharer LR, *et al.* Multinucleated giant cells and HTLV-III in AIDS encephalopathy. *Hum Pathol* 1985; **16**(8): 760.

Singh KK, *et al.* CCR2 polymorphisms affect neuropsychological impairment in HIV-1-infected adults. *J Neuroimmunol* 2004; **157**(1–2): 185–92.

Singhrao SK, *et al.* Spontaneous classical pathway activation and deficiency of membrane regulators render human neurons susceptible to complement lysis. *Am J Pathol* 2000; **157**(3): 905–18.

Sippy BD, *et al.* Increased expression of tumor necrosis factor-alpha receptors in the brains of patients with AIDS. *J Acquir Immune Defic Syndr Hum Retrovirol* 1995; **10**(5): 511–21.

Smith DG, *et al.* Quinolinic acid is produced by macrophages stimulated by platelet activating factor, Nef and Tat. *J Neurovirol* 2001; **7**(1): 56–60.

Smith MO, *et al.* Early intrathecal events in rhesus macaques (*Macaca mulatta*) infected with pathogenic or nonpathogenic molecular clones of simian immunodeficiency virus. *Lab Invest* 1995; **72**(5): 547–58.

Soontornniyomkij V, *et al.* Expression of brain-derived neurotrophic factor protein in activated microglia of human immunodeficiency virus type 1 encephalitis. *Neuropathol Appl Neurobiol* 1998; **24**(6): 453–60.

Sopper S, *et al.* Protective role of the virus-specific immune response for development of severe neurologic signs in simian immunodeficiency virus-infected macaques. *J Virol* 1998; **72**(12): 9940–7.

Sopper S, *et al.* Macaque animal model for HIV-induced neurological disease. *J Neural Transm* 2002; **109**(5–6): 747–66.

Sozzani S, *et al.* Receptors, signal transduction, and spectrum of action of monocyte chemotactic protein-1 and related chemokines. *J Leukoc Biol* 1995; **57**(5): 788–94.

Speth C, *et al.* Complement receptors in HIV infection. *Immunol Rev* 1997; **159**: 49–67.

Speth C, *et al.* Human immunodeficiency virus type 1 induces expression of complement factors in human astrocytes. *J Virol* 2001; **75**(6): 2604–15.

Speth C, *et al.* Mechanism of human immunodeficiency virus-induced complement expression in astrocytes and neurons. *J Virol* 2002a; **76**(7): 3179–88.

Speth C, *et al.* Neuroinvasion by pathogens: A key role of the complement system. *Mol Immunol* 2002b; **38**(9): 669–79.

Speth C, *et al.* HIV-infection of the central nervous system: The tightrope walk of innate immunity. *Mol Immunol* 2005; **42**(2): 213–28.

Steuler H, *et al.* Distinct populations of human immunodeficiency virus type 1 in blood and cerebrospinal fluid. *AIDS Res Hum Retrovir* 1992; **8**(1): 53–9.

Stone TW, *et al.* Tryptophan metabolites and brain disorders. *Clin Chem Lab Med* 2003; **41**(7): 852–9.

Streit WJ. Microglia as neuroprotective, immunocompetent cells of the CNS. *Glia* 2002; **40**(2): 133–9.

Swingler S, *et al.* Cytokine augmentation of HIV-1 LTR-driven gene expression in neural cells. *AIDS Res Hum Retrovir* 1992; **8**(4): 487–93.

Takahashi K, *et al.* Localization of HIV-1 in human brain using polymerase chain reaction/in situ hybridization and immunocytochemistry. *Ann Neurol* 1996; **39**(6): 705–11.

Talley AK, *et al.* Tumor necrosis factor alpha-induced apoptosis in human neuronal cells: Protection by the antioxidant N-acetylcysteine and the genes bcl-2 and crmA. *Mol Cell Biol* 1995; **15**(5): 2359–66.

Tanaka J, Maeda N. Microglial ramification requires nondiffusible factors derived from astrocytes. *Exp Neurol* 1996; **137**(2): 367–75.

Tanaka J, *et al.* Morphological differentiation of microglial cells in culture: Involvement of insoluble factors derived from astrocytes. *Neurosci Res* 1999; **34**(4): 207–15.

157

Thieblemont N, *et al.* CD14lowCD16high: A cytokine-producing monocyte subset which expands during human immunodeficiency virus infection. *Eur J Immunol* 1995; **25**(12): 3418–24.

Thompson KA, *et al.* Correlation between neurological progression and astrocyte apoptosis in HIV-associated dementia. *Ann Neurol* 2001; **49**(6): 745–52.

Thompson KA, *et al.* Astrocyte specific viral strains in HIV dementia. *Ann Neurol* 2004; **56**(6): 873–7.

Toneatto S, *et al.* Evidence of blood-brain barrier alteration and activation in HIV-1 gp120 transgenic mice. *AIDS* 1999; **13**(17): 2343–8.

Tornatore C, *et al.* Persistent human immunodeficiency virus type 1 infection in human fetal glial cells reactivated by T-cell factor(s) or by the cytokines tumor necrosis factor alpha and interleukin-1 beta. *J Virol* 1991; **65**(11): 6094–100.

Trimble LA, *et al.* Human immunodeficiency virus-specific circulating CD8 T lymphocytes have down-modulated CD3zeta and CD28, key signaling molecules for T-cell activation. *J Virol* 2000; **74**(16): 7320–30.

Ulvestad E, *et al.* Human microglial cells have phenotypic and functional characteristics in common with both macrophages and dendritic antigen-presenting cells. *J Leukoc Biol* 1994a; **56**(6): 732–40.

Ulvestad E, *et al.* Phenotypic differences between human monocytes/macrophages and microglial cells studied in situ and in vitro. *J Neuropathol Exp Neurol* 1994b; **53**(5): 492–501.

Valcour VG, *et al.* Cognitive impairment in older HIV-1-seropositive individuals: Prevalence and potential mechanisms. *AIDS* 2004; **18**(Suppl 1): S79–86.

Vallat AV, *et al.* Localization of HIV-1 co-receptors CCR5 and CXCR4 in the brain of children with AIDS. *Am J Pathol* 1998; **152**(1): 167–78.

Valle M, *et al.* CSF quinolinic acid levels are determined by local HIV infection: Cross-sectional analysis and modeling of dynamics following antiretroviral therapy. *Brain* 2004; **127**(Pt 5): 1047–60.

van der Meer P, *et al.* Immunohistochemical analysis of CCR2, CCR3, CCR5, and CXCR4 in the human brain: potential mechanisms for HIV dementia. *Exp Mol Pathol* 2000; **69**(3): 192–201.

van Marle G, *et al.* Human immunodeficiency virus type 1 Nef protein mediates neural cell death: A neurotoxic role for IP-10. *Virol* 2004; **329**(2): 302–18.

Van Wielink G, *et al.* Intrathecal synthesis of anti-HIV IgG: Correlation with increasing duration of HIV-1 infection. *Neurology* 1990; **40**(5): 816–19.

Verani A, *et al.* Macrophages and HIV-1: Dangerous liaisons. *Mol Immunol* 2005; **42**(2): 195–212.

Wang Z, *et al.* Effects of human immunodeficiency virus type 1 on astrocyte gene expression and function: Potential role in neuropathogenesis. *J Neurovirol* 2004; **10**(Suppl 1): 25–32.

Watkins BA, *et al.* Specific tropism of HIV-1 for microglial cells in primary human brain cultures. *Science* 1990; **249**(4968): 549–53.

Wei R, Jonakait GM. Neurotrophins and the anti-inflammatory agents interleukin-4 (IL-4), IL-10, IL-11 and transforming growth factor-beta1 (TGF-beta1) down-regulate T cell costimulatory molecules B7 and CD40 on cultured rat microglia. *J Neuroimmunol* 1999; **95**(1–2): 8–18.

Wesselingh SL, *et al.* Intracerebral cytokine messenger RNA expression in acquired immunodeficiency syndrome dementia. *Ann Neurol* 1993; **33**(6): 576–82.

Wesselingh SL, *et al.* Cellular localization of tumor necrosis factor mRNA in neurological tissue from HIV-infected patients by combined reverse transcriptase/polymerase chain reaction in situ hybridization and immunohistochemistry. *J Neuroimmunol* 1997; **74**(1–2): 1–8.

Wiley CA, *et al.* Cellular localization of human immunodeficiency virus infection within the brains of acquired immune deficiency syndrome patients. *Proc Natl Acad Sci USA* 1986; **83**(18): 7089–93.

Williams KC, Hickey WF. Central nervous system damage, monocytes and macrophages, and neurological disorders in AIDS. *Annu Rev Neurosci* 2002; **25**: 537–62.

Williams KC, *et al.* Perivascular macrophages are the primary cell type productively infected by simian immunodeficiency virus in the brains of macaques: Implications for the neuropathogenesis of AIDS. *J Exp Med* 2001; **193**(8): 905–15.

Wojtowicz WM, *et al.* Stimulation of enveloped virus infection by beta-amyloid fibrils. *J Biol Chem* 2002; **277**(38): 35019–24.

Wong JK, *et al.* In vivo compartmentalization of human immunodeficiency virus: Evidence from the examination of pol sequences from autopsy tissues. *J Virol* 1997a; **71**(3): 2059–71.

Wong JK, *et al.* Recovery of replication-competent HIV despite prolonged suppression of plasma viremia. *Science* 1997b; **278**(5341): 1291–5.

Wong MM, Fish EN. Chemokines: Attractive mediators of the immune response. *Semin Immunol* 2003; **15**(1): 5–14.

Woodman SE, *et al.* Human immunodeficiency virus type 1 TAT protein induces adhesion molecule expression in astrocytes. *J Neurovirol* 1999; **5**(6): 678–84.

Wu DT, *et al.* Mechanisms of leukocyte trafficking into the CNS. *J Neurovirol* 2000; **6**(Suppl 1): S82–5.

Yang OO, *et al.* Nef-mediated resistance of human immunodeficiency virus type 1 to antiviral cytotoxic T lymphocytes. *J Virol* 2002; **76**(4): 1626–31.

Zhang K, *et al.* HIV-induced metalloproteinase processing of the chemokine stromal cell derived factor-1 causes neurodegeneration. *Nat Neurosci* 2003; **6**(10): 1064–71.

Zhang L, *et al.* In vivo distribution of the human immunodeficiency virus/simian immunodeficiency virus coreceptors: CXCR4, CCR3, and CCR5. *J Virol* 1998; **72**(6): 5035–45.

Zheng J, *et al.* Intracellular CXCR4 signaling, neuronal apoptosis and neuropathogenic mechanisms of HIV-1-associated dementia. *J Neuroimmunol* 1999a; **98**(2): 185–200.

Zheng J, *et al.* Lymphotropic virions affect chemokine receptor-mediated neural signaling and apoptosis: Implications for human immunodeficiency virus type 1-associated dementia. *J Virol* 1999b; **73**(10): 8256–67.

Zhou BY, *et al.* Astrocyte activation and dysfunction and neuron death by HIV-1 Tat expression in astrocytes. *Mol Cell Neurosci* 2004; **27**(3): 296–305.

Zink MC, Clements JE. A novel simian immunodeficiency virus model that provides insight into mechanisms of human immunodeficiency virus central nervous system disease. *J Neuroviro* 2002; **8**(Suppl 2): 42–8.

Zink MC, *et al.* Neuroprotective and anti-human immunodeficiency virus activity of minocycline. *J Am Med Assoc* 2005; **293**(16): 2003–11.

Chapter 2

Brain inflammation during bacterial meningitis

Trine H. Mogensen and Lars Østergaard

Introduction

Bacterial meningitis – inflammation of the meninges, subarachnoid space, and brain ventricles – remains a devastating infectious disease and an important cause of mortality and morbidity worldwide. In developed countries, the estimated annual incidence of bacterial meningitis is 4–6 cases per 100,000 adults, with *Streptococcus pneumoniae* and *Neisseria meningitidis* being responsible for 80% of cases (van de Beek *et al.*, 2006a). In contrast, group B streptococcus, *Escherichia coli*, and *Listeria monocytogenes* are the main causes of neonatal meningitis (Kim, 2003). Mortality from bacterial meningitis remains unacceptably high, with a rate of 20–30%, despite advances in anti-microbial therapy. Furthermore, as many as 30–50% of survivors sustain neurological sequelae, such as hearing impairment, seizure disorders, learning disabilities, and behavioral problems (Kim, 2003; van de Beek *et al.*, 2006a; Zwijnenburg *et al.*, 2006). Bacterial meningitis can develop when bacteria invade the central nervous system (CNS) either by the hematogenous route whereby they traverse the blood–brain barrier (BBB) or via spread from a focal infection in the vicinity of the CNS. Bacterial multiplication in the CNS subsequently triggers an inflammatory response, including cytokine- and chemokine-production, as well as leukocyte recruitment, resulting in meningeal inflammation and pleocytosis of the cerebrospinal fluid. Classical signs and symptoms are fever, headache, nuchal rigidity, and altered level of consciousness (van de Beek *et al.*, 2004). Although the generation of an inflammatory response is of crucial importance for the elimination of the invading pathogen, exaggerated inflammation can be harmful to the host. Therefore, CNS inflammation, if not tightly regulated, can cause cerebral ischemia and edema, increased intracranial pressure, and neuronal injury (Koedel *et al.*, 2002a). It has long been recognized that the inflammatory reaction to the pathogen, rather than the pathogen itself, plays a major role in the neuropathology during bacterial meningitis. Accordingly, anti-inflammatory adjunctive treatment of bacterial meningitis with glucocorticoids is a promising approach, and large clinical trials have demonstrated significant benefit from such treatment (de Gans *et al.*, 2002).

This chapter describes some important aspects of brain inflammation during bacterial meningitis, including mechanisms of bacterial invasion and spread through the BBB, activation of the inflammatory response, and some of the mechanisms by which Toll-like receptors (TLRs), cytokines, leukocyte recruitment, and leukocyte activation contribute to resolution and immunopathology. We also consider the importance of host genetic factors and bacterial pathogenic factors for the development of inflammation and disease. Finally, molecular targets of anti-inflammatory treatment are discussed together with clinical management of the disease.

Bacterial entry into the CNS

Mucosal colonization, invasion, and spread

Almost all human pathogenic bacteria have the potential to cause meningitis, and it is currently unknown why only a minor group of pathogens account for most cases of meningitis. The first prerequisite is the ability to gain access into the CNS. Pathogens can enter the CNS to cause meningitis via different routes, including:

(i) hematogenous spread and crossing of the BBB;

(ii) invasion from a contiguous source of infection (e.g. during sinusitis/mastoiditis); and

(iii) less commonly by direct inoculation into the CSF in cases of meningeal laceration during skull fracture or in the presence of ventricular shunts (Kim, 2003).

Inflammatory Diseases of the Central Nervous System, ed. T. Kilpatrick, R. M. Ransohoff and S. Wesselingh. Published by Cambridge University Press. © Cambridge University Press 2010

Hematogenous spread is considered the most important, and several sequential steps of host–pathogen interaction are involved. First, bacterial colonization of mucosal surfaces of the upper respiratory or gastrointestinal tract sometimes results in bacterial invasion of the bloodstream, causing bacteremia. Predisposing factors to invasive disease are viral infection, which is thought to create a milieu favorable to pathogen adherence and invasion through the exposure and up-regulation of cell adhesion molecules and receptors, and by suppressing the local immune response and decreasing phagocytosis (Abramson et al., 1982; O'Brien et al., 2000).

Another important factor seems to be a threshold level of bacteremia, since several studies in humans and experimental animals indicate a correlation between the magnitude of bacteremia and the development of meningitis (Koedel et al., 2002a). A sufficiently large amount of bacteria needs to be present in the bloodstream for an appropriate amount of time in order to sustain intravascular survival and facilitate penetration into the subarachnoid space. Of note, all fresh bacterial isolates from patients with pneumococcal meningitis are encapsulated (Austrian, 1981), and the polysaccharide capsule is considered an important virulence factor. Besides acting as a shield to prevent complement activation, the capsule is also endowed with anti-phagocytic properties, enabling the pneumococcus to survive in the bloodstream (Koedel et al., 2002a).

Bacterial invasion through the BBB

For most bacteria, a sustained high-grade bacteremia is necessary but not sufficient for the development of meningitis. A crucial step is the ability of bacteria to cross the BBB. This physiological and anatomical barrier is characterized by several specific cellular components, which regulate the passage of molecules, ions, toxins, and pathogens into and out of the brain. The BBB is composed of brain microvascular endothelial cells (BMEC) characterized by specific tight junctions, limited pinocytic activity, and specific carrier and transport systems that all contribute to its highly specialized functions (Koedel et al., 2002a). The blood–cerebrospinal fluid (CSF) barrier, on the other hand, is composed of epithelial-like cells in continuity with the ependymal lining of the brain ventricles, and is located at the choroid plexuses, which constitute the largest interface between the blood and the CSF (Koedel et al.,

2002a). Whether meningitis-causing pathogens enter the CNS through the BBB or the blood–CSF barrier remains an unresolved question. However, results from experimental animal models have suggested that most bacteria, including S. pneumoniae, enter through the BBB, whereas others, such as Haemophilus influenzae, seem to enter through the blood–CSF barrier (Sylvester et al., 1992; Tan et al., 1995). In principle, passage through the BBB or blood–CSF barrier could occur by several different mechanisms, of which transcellular passage seems to be the preferred route, at least for S. pneumoniae and E. coli (Tuomanen, 1996). For example, pneumococci utilize the platelet-activating factor receptor and invade endothelial cells in a vacuole, thereby gaining access to the CNS as live bacteria by transcytosis (Cundell et al., 1995). Such passage involves cytoskeletal rearrangements and several different signaling pathways, which may, however, vary between different meningitis-causing bacteria (Kim, 2003). During bacterial meningitis, the BBB is partially disrupted, but this increase in BBB permeability only seems to occur secondary to bacterial entry and inflammation. It has been suggested that the primary bacterial entry into the CNS takes place without any change in BBB permeability, and that even the resultant pleocytosis is relatively independent of BBB disruption (Kim, 2003).

Bacterial survival and multiplication in the subarachnoid space

The CNS is considered a relatively immune-privileged organ. In the absence of pathogens, the CSF is almost devoid of polymorphonuclear leukocytes, complement components and immunoglobulins (Koedel et al., 2002a), which represent essential components of the immune response. Therefore, local host defences are rather inefficient in eliminating invading pathogens, especially encapsulated bacteria such as S. pneumoniae and N. meningitidis. However, when these bacteria start multiplying, they undergo autolysis during transition from exponential growth to the stationary phase or due to exposure to antibiotics (Moore et al., 2005). In this process, bacterial cell wall components, toxins, enzymes, and bacterial DNA are liberated, and these components alert the organism as to the presence of an invading pathogen and synergistically activate the immune response.

Activation of the innate immune response by pattern recognition receptors

Toll-like receptors (TLRs)

One of the key components of the innate immune system is the family of TLRs. These pattern recognition receptors (PRR) recognize evolutionarily conserved pathogen-associated molecular patterns (PAMPs) present on most types of microorganisms (Iwasaki and Medzhitov, 2004). Once TLRs are activated, they signal to the host the presence of invading pathogens and trigger signaling cascades leading to anti-microbial and inflammatory responses involving both innate and adaptive immunity (Iwasaki and Medzhitov, 2004). To date, 10 TLRs have been identified in humans, and they each recognize different microbial structures. Located on the cell surface, TLR1, 2, 4, 5, 6, and 10 mainly recognize bacterial products unique to the invading organism; TLR2 recognizes bacterial lipoproteins, such as peptidoglycan, and lipoteichoic acids, TLR4 mainly recognizes lipopolysaccharide (LPS), and TLR5 detects bacterial flagellin (Akira et al., 2006). In contrast, TLR3, 7, and 8, which together with TLR9 are located within endosomal compartments, are specialized primarily in viral detection and more generally in recognition of RNA (Mogensen and Paludan, 2005; Akira et al., 2006) with dsRNA being recognized by TLR3 and ssRNA by TLR7 and 8 (Mogensen and Paludan, 2005). Finally, TLR9 recognizes unmethylated bacterial and viral CpG DNA (Mogensen et al., 2003; Akira et al., 2006). Studies have demonstrated broad expression of TLRs in the human CNS. Whereas microglia cells were found to express a wide range of different TLRs, astrocytes and oligodendrocytes primarily expressed TLR2 and TLR3. Importantly, TLR expression was up-regulated in the CNS during inflammation as a means of enhancing the response (Bsibsi et al., 2002).

Engagement of a TLR ligand results in intracellular signal transduction mediated by downstream adaptor molecules, kinases, and transcription factors. The pathways leading to activation of the transcription factor nuclear factor (NF)-κB and mitogen-activated protein kinases (MAPKs) are considered key components of this response (Akira and Takeda, 2004). The TLR-activated signaling pathways responsible for activating NF-κB proceed through (i) an adaptor protein (most importantly MyD88), (ii) members of the interleukin (IL)-1 receptor-associated kinase family, (iii) tumor necrosis factor (TNF) receptor-associated factor 6, and (iv) transforming growth factor (TGF)-β-activated protein kinase-1, which activates (v) the inhibitory protein κB kinase (IKK) complex. Finally, IKK phosphorylates the inhibitory κB (IκB) protein and targets it for degradation, hence liberating NF-κB, which migrates to the nucleus and activates transcription of target genes (Dunne and O'Neill, 2003; Akira and Takeda, 2004). It appears that NF-κB plays a pivotal role in TLR-induced pro-inflammatory signaling by up-regulating the expression of a wide range of cytokines, chemokines, cell adhesion molecules, and receptors involved in the generation of an inflammatory response (Ghosh et al., 1998; Karin and Ben-Neriah, 2000).

TLR activation by pathogenetic factors of *N. meningitidis* and *S. pneumoniae*

During recent years, the involvement and function of TLRs in the pathogenesis of bacterial meningitis has been studied extensively (Koedel et al., 2003, 2004; Smirnova et al., 2003), and knowledge about the ability of individual bacterial pathogenesis factors to activate different TLRs has increased substantially (Akira et al., 2006; Mogensen et al., 2006). As described above, the basic paradigm states that Gram-positive bacteria activate TLR2 via lipoteicoic acid and peptidoglycans, whereas LPS of Gram-negative bacteria activates TLR4 (Poltorak et al., 1998; Hirschfeld et al., 1999; Schwandner et al., 1999). Given the fact that a microorganism contains several PAMPs and hence may activate several individual TLRs simultaneously, the emerging picture is more complex than initially anticipated.

The ability of peptidoglycan and lipoteichoic acid from *S. pneumoniae* to activate TLR2 is well described (Moore et al., 2003), whereas controversy remains as to the contribution from TLR4 activated by the pneumococcal toxin pneumolysin (Yoshimura et al., 1999; Malley et al., 2003). Furthermore, TLR9 has been implicated in generation of the inflammatory response during pneumococcal infection, possibly via activation mediated by bacterial DNA (Mogensen et al., 2006; Albiger et al., 2007). Intriguingly, in a model of pneumococcal meningitis, TLR2-deficient mice were found to respond to live pathogens to almost the same extent as wild-type mice (Koedel et al., 2002a). This phenomenon may be explained by redundancy, i.e. even if TLR2 plays a major role in the inflammatory response triggered by pneumococci, alternative TLRs can substitute in the absence of TLR2. This is in agreement with the finding that MyD88, an adaptor common to most TLR-activated signaling pathways, has been demonstrated to be required for mounting an immune response to *S. pneumoniae* in the CNS (Koedel *et al.*, 2004).

With regards to *N. meningitidis*, several studies have confirmed the essential role of TLR4 in the recognition of meningococcal lipooligosaccharide (LOS) (Zughaier *et al.*, 2004). This notion is further supported by an association between an increased susceptibility to meningococcal disease in humans and rare TLR4 mutations (Smirnova *et al.*, 2003). Additionally, porins (outer membrane proteins of menigococci) trigger TLR2 signaling (Ingalls *et al.*, 2000; Massari *et al.*, 2002), suggesting that TLR2 contributes to the activation of inflammation during meningococcal infection.

In studies of TLR- and NF-κB activation by whole live bacteria in vitro, it was demonstrated that *S. pneumoniae* activated TLR2 and TLR9, whereas *N. meningitidis* was able to activate TLR2, TLR4, and TLR9 (Mogensen *et al.*, 2006). Thus, distinct, yet overlapping, sets of TLRs are used to mount the inflammatory response. This phenomenon could be favorable to the host in several ways, for instance by allowing the host to activate several different cell types expressing different TLRs, to fine-tune the immune response by utilizing different TLRs in synergy or in a sequential manner, and finally to avoid immune evasion (Mogensen *et al.*, 2006).

NOD proteins and the inflammasome

In addition to the TLRs, another family of PRRs has recently been identified (Martinon and Tschopp, 2005). This family of proteins named nucleotide-binding oligomerization domain (NOD)-like receptor (NLR)s are involved in detecting intracellular pathogens and danger signals in general (Agostini *et al.*, 2004; Martinon and Tschopp, 2005; Mariathasan *et al.*, 2006). Among the NLRs, the NOD proteins detect the bacterial degradation products myramyl di- and tri-peptides, thereby leading to activation of the NF-κB and MAPK signaling pathways and inflammatory gene expression (Martinon and Tschopp, 2005). Although no direct evidence of a role for NOD proteins in meningitis exists, it has been demonstrated that *S. pneumoniae* is recognized by NOD2 (Opitz *et al.*, 2004), and that this PRR is expressed by astrocytes (Sterka *et al.*, 2006). Another important

function of NLRs is to sense intracellular pathogens and activate caspase-1, which, in turn, converts pro-IL-1β to IL-1β (Martinon and Tschopp, 2005; Akira *et al.*, 2006). In cells exposed to an appropriate stimulus (e.g. LPS), inactive IL-1β precursor accumulates in the cytosol. Conversion of pro-IL-1β to active IL-1β requires assembly of a protein scaffold termed the inflammasome, which is composed of an NLR family member, such as NAcht leucine-rich-repeat protein (NALP) 1 or 3, an adaptor protein called ASC, and pro-caspase-1. Oligomerization of these proteins results in activation of caspase-1, which subsequently cleaves and activates the accumulated IL-1β precursor, ultimately resulting in secretion of biologically active IL-1β (Agostini *et al.*, 2004; Martinon and Tschopp, 2005). Mutations in NALPs and other components of the inflammasome have been linked to relatively rare hereditary periodic fever syndromes (Kastner, 2005). However, evidence on their important role in the first line of defense against bacteria, including pneumococci, is accumulating (Koedel *et al.*, 2002b), and as described below, experimental animal models of pneumococcal meningitis strongly indicate a crucial role of caspase-1 signaling and IL-1β secretion in the pathogenesis of bacterial meningitis (Koedel *et al.*, 2002a). Therefore, it appears likely that more information on the inflammasome will provide additional insight into the pathogenesis of infectious diseases, including bacterial meningitis.

The inflammatory response during bacterial meningitis

Due to the fact that the brain is encapsulated in the skull with only limited capacity for swelling and edema to occur, before severe brain injury may take place, the early innate immune response aimed at eliminating invading pathogens soon after their entry into the CNS is of special relevance and importance. Early containment of the infection and recruitment of leukocytes into the subarachnoid space is mediated by cytokines, chemokines, and complement and through up-regulation of cell adhesion molecules.

Cytokines

Cytokines play an important regulatory role in the initiation, maintenance, and termination of inflammatory reactions. Interleukins-1 and -6 and tumor necrosis factor-α (TNF-α) are regarded as prominent early-phase cytokines, which are all up-regulated in the CSF from patients with bacterial meningitis.

Importantly, these cytokines have been demonstrated to be produced by macrophage-equivalent brain cells, including astrocytes and microglia, as well as cerebral BMECs (Saez-Llorens and McCracken, 2003; Fowler et al., 2004). In CSF samples from patients with bacterial meningitis, concentrations of IL-1 correlated with severity of disease (van Furth et al., 1996), and high CSF concentrations of IL-1β, IL-6, TNF-α, and TGF-β have been associated with poor clinical outcome in children with bacterial meningitis (Paul et al., 2003).

In addition to these cytokines, several factors involved in their production are of interest. For instance, caspase 1, which is involved in generating mature, biologically active IL-1, is up-regulated in the brain during experimental pneumococcal meningitis, and depletion of the caspase 1 gene or pharmacological inhibition of caspase1 was followed by a significantly reduced inflammatory host response to pneumococci (Koedel et al., 2002b). Similarly, TNF-α converting enzyme (TACE), which produces the active soluble form of TNF-α by proteolytic cleavage, might contribute to CNS inflammation, since treatment with the TACE inhibitor BB-1101 attenuated neuronal injury in a rat model of pneumococcal meningitis (Leib et al., 2001). However, in murine pneumococcal CNS infection, deficiency of neither TNF-α nor the TNF-α receptor had any significant impact on bacterial titres in the brain or leukocyte recruitment into the subarachnoid space (Wellmer et al., 2001).

In contrast to IL-1 and TNF-α, which are particularly effective in inducing the expression of chemokines and cell adhesion molecules, IL-6 seems to be one of the factors responsible for controlling the extent of the inflammatory response by down-regulating these mediators of inflammation (Koedel et al., 2002a). This is supported by findings in IL-6-deficient mice, where pneumococcal inoculation in the CNS caused an increase in CSF pleocytosis and chemokine concentrations compared with wild-type mice (Paul et al., 2003).

Chemotactic factors: complement and chemokines

The role of chemotactic factors in the CSF during bacterial meningitis is an area of interest, because it is largely responsible for the development of pleocytosis, a hallmark of meningitis.

Complement activation significantly contributes to innate immunity by complementing antibodies in the killing of bacteria and by exhibiting strong chemotactic activity (Emonts et al., 2003; Zwijnenburg et al., 2006). Three different pathways of complement activation, including the classical pathway, the alternative pathway, and the mannose-binding lectin (MBL) pathway all converge on a common final pathway, which generates the membrane attack complex and the potent inflammatory molecules and chemotaxins C3a and C5a (Koedel et al., 2002a; Zwijnenburg et al., 2006). The brain appears to represent a major site of complement activation, and local complement activation has been demonstrated in experimental animal studies, as well as in CSF from patients with bacterial meningitis (Ernst et al., 1984; Stahel et al., 1997).

Chemokines contribute to leukocyte recruitment by activating integrins necessary for leukocyte attachment and by inducing leukocyte migration across the endothelium and through the extracellular matrix. Additionally, chemokines stimulate leukocyte activation by enhancing superoxide generation, granule release, and phagocytosis (Zwijnenburg et al., 2006). Chemokines are induced during inflammation by cytokines like IL-1 and TNF-α, and by bacterial products such as LPS (Zwijnenburg et al., 2006). Several chemokines, belonging to both the CXC and CC families of chemokines, have been implicated in bacterial meningitis, with CXCL8, CXCL1, CCL2, CCL3, and CCL4 all being present in the CSF from patients with bacterial meningitis, although with varying capacity to exert chemotactic activity in vivo and in vitro (Zwijnenburg et al., 2006). Furthermore, the murine CXCR2 ligand and neutrophil/monocyte chemoattractant CXCL2/MIP-2 displayed increased expression in a mouse model of pneumococcal meningitis, and the release of these two chemokines was dependent on the integrity of IL-1 signaling (Koedel et al., 2002a; Zwijnenburg et al., 2006).

Leukocyte recruitment

Leukocyte migration into the CNS is an intricate process that involves the up-regulation and interaction between adhesion receptors and their ligands on both leukocytes and host endothelial cells. The process involves (i) tethering mediated by selectins, (ii) triggering induced by cytokines, chemokines, complement products, and bacterial cell wall components, adhesion between integrins, such as CD11b/CD18 on leukocytes, and their integrin ligands/receptors, including intercellular adhesion molecule (ICAM)1, (iii) firm adhesion, and (iv) emigration along a chemotactic gradient (Koedel et al., 2002a).

Although leukocyte recruitment is acknowledged to represent a key aspect of the protective response during bacterial meningitis, leukocytes at the same time are believed to play a major role in the exaggerated inflammatory response that can ultimately lead to tissue damage in the brain. In experimental animal models involving mice deficient in selectins as well as in experiments with neutralizing antibodies against ICAM, leukocyte recruitment was severely attenuated as was meningitis-induced intracranial complications (Tuomanen et al., 1989; Tang et al., 1996).

Mediators of brain damage

An entire plethora of mediators contribute to the pleocytosis and increased BBB permeability during bacterial meningitis. In addition to the effects of pro-inflammatory cytokines and chemokines, which synergistically support further inflammation by enhancing cytokine gene expression in a self-perpetuating cycle, a massive leukocyte influx occurs through up-regulation of selectins and integrins. Activated leukocytes release several potentially cytotoxic and tissue-destructive agents, including reactive oxygen species (ROS) and proteolytic enzymes, and a substantial amount of evidence suggests a central role of these mediators in the pathogenesis of bacterial meningitis (Koedel et al., 2002a; Scheld et al., 2002). First, oxidants, particularly peroxynitrite, can cause brain damage by inducing lipid peroxidation, ultimately leading to loss of membrane function and integrity. Alternatively, peroxynitrite can induce DNA damage and subsequent poly-(ADP ribose) polymerase activation, energy depletion, and cell injury (Beckman and Koppenol, 1996; Kastenbauer et al., 2002). Second, leukocytes release proteolytic enzymes, such as matrix metalloproteinases (MMPs) 8 and 9 with the capacity to degrade extracellular matrix proteins like collagen IV and laminin, thereby contributing to tissue destruction and BBB disruption (Yong et al., 2001). Increased levels of MMP8 and 9 have been detected in the CSF of patients with bacterial meningitis, and high concentrations of MMP9 have been considered a marker for the development of neurological sequelae after bacterial meningitis (Leppert et al., 2000). Finally, experimental studies with pharmacological inhibitors have suggested that excitatory amino acids contribute to the neuropathology during bacterial meningitis (Leib et al., 1996), and increased levels of glutamate in the CSF have been associated with poor clinical outcome in patients with meningitis (Spranger et al., 1996).

Taken together, endothelial cell injury and dysfunction impairs cerebrovascular autoregulation and integrity of the BBB, subsequently leading to vasogenic cerebral edema, which together with cytotoxic and interstitial edema caused by inflammation and ischemia, ultimately results in cerebral ischemia and increased intracranial pressure with the potential risk of cerebral herniation (Koedel et al., 2002a).

Neuropathology

Examinations of histopathological material from experimental animals and of fatal human cases of bacterial meningitis have revealed that necrotic cortical injury and apoptotic hippocampal injury are the most prominent pathological findings (Nau et al., 1999; Kim, 2003). However, during post-mortem examination of severe cases of bacterial meningitis in humans, several other types of neuropathology have been documented, including vasculitis, focal necrosis of cortical neurons, apoptotic neuronal cell death in the dentate gyrus, and loss of myelinated fibers in the subcortical white matter, cerebellum, and brain stem (Rorke and Pitts, 1963; Koedel et al., 2002a). Intriguingly, dexamethasone, now widely used as adjunctive treatment of bacterial meningitis (see below), seems to aggravate hippocampal injury in experimental models of pneumococcal meningitis (Zysk et al., 1996).

Molecular targets of anti-inflammatory adjunctive treatment

For decades, it has been recognized that immunopathology – that is, the exaggerated activation of the host's immune response induced by either bacteria or their products – plays a major role in the pathogenesis of bacterial infection in the CNS (Chaudhuri and Behan, 2004). Therefore, besides being of fundamental biological interest, understanding the molecular mechanisms underlying brain inflammation during bacterial meningitis could be of clinical relevance, since all these inducers, mediators, and effectors are potential targets of therapeutic intervention. As described above, a large number of components, including TLRs, NF-κB, cytokines, chemokines, complement, reactive oxygen species, nitric oxide, matrix metalloproteinases (MMPs), arachidonic acid metabolites, neuropeptides, and caspases are recognized potential targets of anti-inflammatory treatment of bacterial meningitis. However, these approaches, whether they are directed to the modulation of leukocyte influx, to the blockade of reactive oxygen species or to the inhibition of NF-κB, caspase, MMP, or cytokine (particularly TNF-α and IL-1) activity are all presently at the experimental stage, with the exception of the glucorticoid dexamethasone, which remains the only currently accepted adjunctive therapy for the treatment of bacterial meningitis (van de Beek et al., 2006b). Given that glucocorticoids are known to interfere with many signaling pathways and molecules triggered by TLR activation, it has been hypothesized that TLR signaling pathways could be important targets for glucocorticoid action (Moynagh, 2003). Therefore, TLR antagonists could represent a rational target for future anti-inflammatory therapy in the treatment of bacterial meningitis (Kanzler et al., 2007). The great challenge is to inhibit the detrimental components of the immune response while leaving untouched an appropriate and necessary immune response, essential for the resolution of infection and elimination of the invading pathogen.

Clinical management with anti-inflammatory adjunctive treatment

In contrast to all other organ systems, the CNS is encompassed by bone (the skull and the spine). It is therefore not possible for the inflamed meninges to expand outward, and an increased pressure is thus applied inwards. This pressure contributes to CNS ischemia and necrosis. Optimal clinical management therefore aims at balancing strategies to kill the invading bacteria, with control of the magnitude of the inflammatory response caused by the pathogen. An attempt to kill the bacteria should be initiated as soon as possible using bacteriocidal antibiotics covering all potential pathogens. The inflammatory response can be modified by several agents, but only one, dexamethasone, is used in clinical practice.

Glucocorticoids: mechanism of action

While the introduction of glucocorticoids as adjunctive therapy of bacterial meningitis is relatively recent, these agents have been widely used for many years for the treatment of other diseases, where their potent anti-inflammatory and immunosuppressive effects may be desirable. The molecular mechanisms behind these effects are of great complexity and are only partly understood. Briefly, glucocorticoids bind to the intracellular glucocorticoid receptor and through subsequent binding to glucocorticoid response elements activate expression of genes with anti-inflammatory

effects (such as the IL-1 receptor antagonist, IL-10, lipocortin and IκBα). Alternatively, glucocorticoids inhibit the production of pro-inflammatory molecules, including cytokines, chemokines, and cell adhesion molecules by binding and inhibition of the transcription factors NF-κB and AP-1, upstream signal transduction pathways, or by direct interference with the transcriptional machinery (Moynagh, 2003).

Glucocorticoids: clinical trials

In a systematic review on glucocorticoid use in acute bacterial meningitis, van de Beek and coworkers identified 32 clinical trials of which 20 fulfilled the quality criteria outlined by the Cochrane Library (van de Beek et al., 2007). Dexamethasone was used in 17 studies, and most clinical data thus concern the use of this specific glucocorticoid.

Effect of glucocorticoids on mortality

In adults, adjuvant therapy with glucocorticoids resulted in a reduction in death from 21.9% in the placebo group to 11.7% in the intervention group – a statistically and clinically highly significant reduction by 43% (Bennett et al., 1963; Girgis et al., 1989; Bhaumik and Behari, 1998; Thomas et al., 1999; de Gans et al., 2002). In contrast to the beneficial effect on mortality seen in adults, no difference between glucocorticoid therapy and placebo could be found in children (Belsey et al., 1969; DeLemos and Haggerty, 1969; Lebel et al., 1988, 1989; Girgis et al., 1989; Odio et al., 1991; Schaad et al., 1993; King et al., 1994; Ciana et al., 1995; Kanra et al., 1995; Kilpi et al., 1995; Wald et al., 1995; Qazi et al., 1996; Molyneux et al., 2002). One of the explanations of this difference between adults and children could be the various responsible organisms. Thus, Haemophilus influenzae is the predominant organism in children, and the effect of glucocorticoids in terms of mortality on this organism is not shown. Glucocorticoids had a beneficial effect in both pneumococcal meningitis, with a reduction of 41% and in meningitis caused by other bacteria except H. influenzae, with a reduction in mortality of 23% (Belsey et al., 1969; DeLemos and Haggerty, 1969; Lebel et al., 1988, 1989; Girgis et al., 1989; Odio et al., 1991; Schaad et al., 1993; King et al., 1994; Ciana et al., 1995; Kanra et al., 1995; Kilpi et al., 1995; Wald et al., 1995; Qazi et al., 1996; Molyneux et al., 2002).

Effect of glucocorticoids on complications

Severe hearing loss, defined as bilateral hearing loss for less than 60 dB or the need for bilateral hearing aids, is one of the most common complications in children with meningitis caused by *H. influenzae*. Although glucocorticoids do not reduce mortality in children, there is a marked reduction in severe hearing loss of 63% by the use of these agents. This beneficial effect, however, is only found in studies performed in high-income countries.

Neurological sequelae are defined as focal neurological deficits (other than hearing loss) including epilepsy, severe ataxia, and severe memory or concentration disturbance. The risk of these complications can be reduced from 9 to 6% by the use of glucocorticoids when assessed between 6 and 12 months after discharge (Lebel *et al.*, 1988; Girgis *et al.*, 1989; Odio *et al.*, 1991; Schaad *et al.*, 1993; King *et al.*, 1994; Kanra *et al.*, 1995; Kilpi *et al.*, 1995; Wald *et al.*, 1995; Qazi *et al.*, 1996). However, when assessing the complications between discharge and 6 weeks after hospital discharge, only a small but non-significant benefit is found in children (Lebel *et al.*, 1988, 1989; Ciana *et al.*, 1995; Kanra *et al.*, 1995; Kilpi *et al.*, 1995; Bhaumik and Behari, 1998; Thomas *et al.*, 1999; de Gans *et al.*, 2002; Molyneux *et al.*, 2002).

Sequence of administration

In nine studies, glucocorticoids have been given with or before the first dose of antibiotic, and in seven studies glucocorticoids have been given after the first doses of antibiotic. No statistically significant difference could be found between the results of these two groups of studies. However, in terms of mortality, the beneficial effect was higher by giving the glucocorticoid before or with the first dose of antibiotics, whereas in terms of severe hearing loss, late administration of glucocorticoids seems to perform better.

Side effects of glucocorticoid use

The risk of side-effects is generally low using a short course of glucocorticoids. Accordingly, there was no difference in side-effects between patients receiving and not receiving glucocorticoids (Bennet *et al.*, 1963; Belsey *et al.*, 1969; Lebel *et al.*, 1988, 1989; Odio *et al.*, 1991; Schaad *et al.*, 1993; King *et al.*, 1994; Kanra *et al.*, 1995; Kilpi *et al.*, 1995; Wald *et al.*, 1995; Qazi *et al.*, 1996; Bhaumik and Behari, 1998; de Gans *et al.*, 2002; Molyneux *et al.*, 2002). This included the risk of gastrointestinal tract bleeding.

State of the art

At the present time, a 4-day regimen of dexamethasone (0.6 mg/kg daily) preferably given before or with the first dose of antibiotics should be used in adults and children with acute bacterial meningitis. Since antibiotics are often given before a definite diagnosis of acute bacterial meningitis is established, it may be reasonable to administer dexamethasone with the antibiotics and then cease the dexamethasone again if examination of the CSF does not reveal a diagnosis of meningitis or the suspicion of a bacterial cause.

Conclusion

Bacterial meningitis remains a serious condition with considerable mortality and morbidity despite appropriate treatment with antibiotics. It is well-established that immunopathology plays a major role in the pathogenesis of bacterial meningitis. Central nervous system inflammation, if not tightly regulated, can cause cerebral ischemia and edema, increased intracranial pressure, and neuronal injury. Understanding the molecular mechanisms underlying brain inflammation during bacterial meningitis is therefore of fundamental biological interest and not least of clinical importance. Although several potential targets of therapeutic intervention have been identified, specific pharmacological inhibition of these mediators is presently at the experimental stage, with the exception of the glucocorticoid dexamethasone, which remains the only currently accepted adjunctive therapy for the treatment of patients with bacterial meningitis (van de Beek *et al.*, 2006b). Future clinical trials should be designed to further clarify the timing of dexamethasone administration and the diverse effects of dexamethasone observed depending on the microbiological etiology (de Gans *et al.*, 2002; Nguyen *et al.*, 2007; Scarborough *et al.*, 2007). In addition, it will be important to define the populations that will benefit most from dexamethasone treatment and identify subpopulations that may not benefit from such treatment, including certain populations in the developing world with extensive co-morbidity of tuberculosis and chronic HIV infection (de Gans *et al.*, 2002; Nguyen *et al.*, 2007; Scarborough *et al.*, 2007). Finally, TLR antagonists could represent a rational target for future anti-inflammatory therapy in the treatment of bacterial meningitis (Kanzler *et al.*, 2007). The great challenge remains to inhibit the detrimental components of the immune response while leaving untouched an appropriate and necessary immune response, essential for the resolution of infection and elimination of invading pathogens.

References

Abramson JS, *et al.* Inhibition of neutrophil lysosome-phagosome fusion associated with influenza virus infection in vitro. Role in depressed bactericidal activity. *J Clin Invest* 1982; **69**: 1393–7.

Agostini L, *et al.* NALP3 forms an IL-1β-processing inflammasome with increased activity in Muckle–Wells autoinflammatory disorder. *Immunity* 2004; **20**: 319–25.

Akira S, Takeda K. Toll-like receptor signalling. *Nat Rev Immunol* 2004; **4**: 499–511.

Akira S, *et al.* Pathogen recognition and innate immunity. *Cell* 2006; **124**: 783–801.

Albiger B, *et al.* Toll-like receptor 9 acts at an early stage in host defence against pneumococcal infection. *Cell Microbiol* 2007; **9**: 633–44.

Austrian R. Some observations on the pneumococcus and on the current status of pneumococcal disease and its prevention. *Rev Infect Dis* 1981; 3(Suppl): S1–17.

Beckman JS, Koppenol WH. Nitric oxide, superoxide, and peroxynitrite: the good, the bad, and the ugly. *Am J Physiol* 1996; **271**: C1424–37.

Belsey MA, *et al.* Dexamethasone in the treatment of acute bacterial meningitis: The effect of study design on the interpretation of results. *Pediatrics* 1969; **44**: 503–13.

Bennett IL, *et al.* The effectiveness of hydrocortisone in the management of severe infections. *J Am Med Assoc* 1963; **183**: 462–5.

Bhaumik S, Behari M. Role of dexamethasone as adjunctive therapy in acute bacterial meningitis in adults. *Neurol India* 1998; **46**: 2258.

Bsibsi M, *et al.* Broad expression of Toll-like receptors in the human central nervous system. *J Neuropathol Exp Neurol* 2002; **61**: 1013–21.

Chaudhuri A, Behan PO. Fatigue in neurological disorders. *Lancet* 2004; **363**: 978–88.

Ciana G, *et al.* Effectiveness of adjunctive treatment with steroids in reducing short-term mortality in a high-risk population of children with bacterial meningitis. *J Trop Pediatr* 1995; **41**: 164–8.

Cundell DR, *et al.* Streptococcus pneumoniae anchor to activated human cells by the receptor for platelet-activating factor. *Nature* 1995; **377**: 435–8.

de Gans J, *et al.* Dexamethasone in adults with bacterial meningitis. *N Engl J Med* 2002; **347**: 1549–56.

DeLemos RA, Haggerty RJ. Corticosteroids as an adjunct to treatment in bacterial meningitis. A controlled clinical trial. *Pediatrics* 1969; **44**: 30–4.

Dunne A, O'Neill LA. The interleukin-1 receptor/Toll-like receptor superfamily: Signal transduction during inflammation and host defense. *Sci STKE* 2003; re3.

Emonts M, *et al.* Host genetic determinants of *Neisseria meningitidis* infections. *Lancet Infect Dis* 2003; **3**: 565–77.

Ernst JD, *et al.* Complement (C5)-derived chemotactic activity accounts for accumulation of polymorphonuclear leukocytes in cerebrospinal fluid of rabbits with pneumococcal meningitis. *Infect Immun* 1984; **46**: 81–6.

Fowler MI, *et al.* Different meningitis-causing bacteria induce distinct inflammatory responses on interaction with cells of the human meninges. *Cell Microbiol* 2004; **6**: 555–67.

Ghosh S, *et al.* NF-κB and Rel proteins: Evolutionarily conserved mediators of immune responses. *Annu Rev Immunol* 1998; **16**: 225–60.

Girgis NI, *et al.* Dexamethasone treatment for bacterial meningitis in children and adults. *Pediatr Infect Dis J* 1989; **8**: 848–51.

Hirschfeld M, *et al.* Cutting edge: Inflammatory signaling by *Borrelia burgdorferi* lipoproteins is mediated by toll-like receptor 2. *J Immunol* 1999; **163**: 2382–6.

Ingalls RR, *et al.* Differential roles of TLR2 and TLR4 in the host response to Gram-negative bacteria: Lessons from a lipopolysaccharide-deficient mutant of *Neisseria meningitidis. J Endotoxin Res* 2000; **6**: 411–5.

Iwasaki A, Medzhitov R. Toll-like receptor control of the adaptive immune responses. *Nat Immunol* 2004; **5**: 987–95.

Kanra GY, *et al.* Beneficial effects of dexamethasone in children with pneumococcal meningitis. *Pediatr Infect Dis J* 1995; **14**: 490–4.

Kanzler H, *et al.* Therapeutic targeting of innate immunity with Toll-like receptor agonists and antagonists. *Nat Med* 2007; **13**: 552–9.

Karin M, Ben-Neriah Y. Phosphorylation meets ubiquitination: The control of NF-κB activity. *Annu Rev Immunol* 2000; **18**: 621–63.

Kastenbauer S, *et al.* Oxidative stress in bacterial meningitis in humans. *Neurology* 2002; **58**: 186–91.

Kastner DL. Hereditary periodic fever syndromes. *Hematology Am Soc Hematol Educ Program* 2005; 74–81.

Kilpi T, *et al.* Oral glycerol and intravenous dexamethasone in preventing neurologic and audiologic sequelae of childhood bacterial meningitis. The Finnish Study Group. *Pediatr Infect Dis J* 1995; **14**: 270–8.

Kim KS. Pathogenesis of bacterial meningitis: From bacteraemia to neuronal injury. *Nat Rev Neurosci* 2003; **4**: 376–85.

King SM, *et al.* Dexamethasone therapy for bacterial meningitis: Better never than late? *Can J Infect Dis* 1994; **5**: 210–15.

Koedel U, *et al.* Pathogenesis and pathophysiology of pneumococcal meningitis. *Lancet Infect Dis* 2002a; **2**: 721–36.

Koedel U, *et al.* Role of Caspase-1 in experimental pneumococcal meningitis: Evidence from pharmacologic Caspase inhibition and Caspase-1-deficient mice. *Ann Neurol* 2002b; **51**: 319–29.

Koedel U, *et al.* Toll-like receptor 2 participates in mediation of immune response in experimental pneumococcal meningitis. *J Immunol* 2003; **170**: 438–44.

Koedel U, et al. MyD88 is required for mounting a robust host immune response to Streptococcus pneumoniae in the CNS. Brain 2004; 127: 1437–45.

Lebel MH, et al. Dexamethasone therapy for bacterial meningitis. Results of two double-blind, placebo-controlled trials. N Engl J Med 1988; 319: 964–71.

Lebel MH, et al. Magnetic resonance imaging and dexamethasone therapy for bacterial meningitis. Am J Dis Child 1989; 143: 301–6.

Leib SL, et al. Neuroprotective effect of excitatory amino acid antagonist kynurenic acid in experimental bacterial meningitis. J Infect Dis 1996; 173: 166–71.

Leib SL, et al. Inhibition of matrix metalloproteinases and tumour necrosis factor α converting enzyme as adjuvant therapy in pneumococcal meningitis. Brain 2001; 124: 1734–42.

Leppert D, et al. Matrix metalloproteinase (MMP)-8 and MMP-9 in cerebrospinal fluid during bacterial meningitis: Aassociation with blood–brain barrier damage and neurological sequelae. Clin Infect Dis 2000; 31: 80–4.

Malley R, et al. Recognition of pneumolysin by Toll-like receptor 4 confers resistance to pneumococcal infection. Proc Natl Acad Sci USA 2003; 100: 1966–71.

Mariathasan S, et al. Cryopyrin activates the inflammasome in response to toxins and ATP. Nature 2006; 440: 228–32.

Martinon F, Tschopp J. NLRs join TLRs as innate sensors of pathogens. Trends Immunol 2005; 26: 447–54.

Massari P, et al. Cutting edge: Immune stimulation by neisserial porins is toll-like receptor 2 and MyD88 dependent. J Immunol 2002; 168: 1533–7.

Mogensen TH, Paludan SR. Reading the viral signature by Toll-like receptors and other pattern recognition receptors. J Mol Med 2005; 83: 180–92.

Mogensen TH, et al. Activation of NF-κB in virus-infected macrophages is dependent on mitochondrial oxidative stress and intracellular calcium: Downstream involvement of the kinases TGF-β-activated kinase 1, mitogen-activated kinase/extracellular signal-regulated kinase kinase 1, and IκB kinase. J Immunol 2003; 170: 6224–33.

Mogensen TH, et al. Live Streptococcus pneumoniae, Haemophilus influenzae, and Neisseria meningitidis activate the inflammatory response through Toll-like receptors 2, 4, and 9 in species-specific patterns. J Leukoc Biol 2006; 80: 267–77.

Molyneux EM, et al. Dexamethasone treatment in childhood bacterial meningitis in Malawi: A randomised controlled trial. Lancet 2002; 360: 211–8.

Moore LJ, et al. Penicillin enhances the toll-like receptor 2-mediated proinflammatory activity of Streptococcus pneumoniae. J Infect Dis 2003; 188: 1040–8.

Moore LJ, et al. Induction of pro-inflammatory cytokine release by human macrophages during exposure of Streptococcus pneumoniae to penicillin is influenced by minimum inhibitory concentration ratio. Int J Antimicrob Agents 2005; 26: 188–96.

Moynagh PN. Toll-like receptor signalling pathways as key targets for mediating the anti-inflammatory and immunosuppressive effects of glucocorticoids. J Endocrinol 2003; 179: 139–44.

Nau R, et al. Apoptosis of neurons in the dentate gyrus in humans suffering from bacterial meningitis. J Neuropathol Exp Neurol 1999; 58: 265–74.

Nguyen TH, et al. Dexamethasone in Vietnamese adolescents and adults with bacterial meningitis. N Engl J Med 2007; 357: 2431–40.

O'Brien KL, et al. Severe pneumococcal pneumonia in previously healthy children: The role of preceding influenza infection. Clin Infect Dis 2000; 30: 784–9.

Odio CM, et al. The beneficial effects of early dexamethasone administration in infants and children with bacterial meningitis. N Engl J Med 1991; 324: 1525–31.

Opitz B, et al. Nucleotide-binding oligomerization domain proteins are innate immune receptors for internalized Streptococcus pneumoniae. J Biol Chem 2004; 279: 36426–32.

Paul R, et al. Lack of IL-6 augments inflammatory response but decreases vascular permeability in bacterial meningitis. Brain 2003; 126: 1873–82.

Poltorak M. et al. Defective LPS signaling in C3H/HeJ and C57BL/10ScCr mice: Mutations in Tlr4 gene. Science 1998; 282: 2085–8.

Qazi SA, et al. Dexamethasone and bacterial meningitis in Pakistan. Arch Dis Child 1996; 75: 482–8.

Rorke LB, Pitts FW. Purulent meningitis: The pathologic basis of clinical manifestations. Clin Pediatr (Phil) 1963; 2: 64–71.

Saez-Llorens X, McCracken GH, Jr. Bacterial meningitis in children. Lancet 2003; 361: 2139–48.

Scarborough M, et al. Corticosteroids for bacterial meningitis in adults in sub-Saharan Africa. N Engl J Med 2007; 357: 2441–50.

Schaad UB, et al. Dexamethasone therapy for bacterial meningitis in children. Swiss Meningitis Study Group. Lancet 1993; 342: 457–61.

Scheld WM, et al. Pathophysiology of bacterial meningitis: Mechanism(s) of neuronal injury. J Infect Dis 2002; 186(Suppl 2): S225–33.

Schwandner R, et al. Peptidoglycan- and lipoteichoic acid-induced cell activation is mediated by toll-like receptor 2. J Biol Chem 1999; 274: 17406–9.

Smirnova I, et al. Assay of locus-specific genetic load implicates rare Toll-like receptor 4 mutations in meningococcal susceptibility. Proc Natl Acad Sci USA 2003; 100: 6075–80.

Spranger M, et al. Excess glutamate levels in the cerebrospinal fluid predict clinical outcome of bacterial meningitis. Arch Neurol 1996; 53: 992–6.

Stahel PF, et al. Complement C3 and factor B cerebrospinal fluid concentrations in bacterial and aseptic meningitis. *Lancet* 1997; **349**: 1886–7.

Sterka D, Jr, *et al.* Functional expression of NOD2, a novel pattern recognition receptor for bacterial motifs, in primary murine astrocytes. *Glia* 2006; **53**: 322–30.

Sylvester I, *et al.* Neutrophil attractant protein-1-immunoglobulin G immune complexes and free anti-NAP-1 antibody in normal human serum. *J Clin Invest* 1992; **90**: 471–81.

Tan TQ, *et al.* Hematogenous bacterial meningitis in an intercellular adhesion molecule-1-deficient infant mouse model. *J Infect Dis* 1995; **171**: 342–9.

Tang T, *et al.* Cytokine-induced meningitis is dramatically attenuated in mice deficient in endothelial selectins. *J Clin Invest* 1996; **97**: 2485–90.

Thomas R, *et al.* Trial of dexamethasone treatment for severe bacterial meningitis in adults. Adult Meningitis Steroid Group. *Intens Care Med* 1999; **25**: 475–80.

Tuomanen E. Entry of pathogens into the central nervous system. *FEMS Microbiol Rev* 1996; **18**: 289–99.

Tuomanen EI, *et al.* Reduction of inflammation, tissue damage, and mortality in bacterial meningitis in rabbits treated with monoclonal antibodies against adhesion-promoting receptors of leukocytes. *J Exp Med* 1989; **170**: 959–69.

van de Beek D, *et al.* Clinical features and prognostic factors in adults with bacterial meningitis. *N Engl J Med* 2004; **351**: 1849–59.

van de Beek D, *et al.* Community-acquired bacterial meningitis in adults. *N Engl J Med* 2006a; **354**: 44–53.

van de Beek D, *et al.* Drug Insight: Adjunctive therapies in adults with bacterial meningitis. *Nat Clin Pract Neurol* 2006b; **2**: 504–16.

van de Beek D, *et al.* Corticosteroids for acute bacterial meningitis. Cochrane Database Syst Rev 2007; CD004405.

van Furth AM, *et al.* Roles of pro-inflammatory and anti-inflammatory cytokines in pathophysiology of bacterial meningitis and effect of adjunctive therapy. *Infect Immun* 1996; **64**: 4883–90.

Wald ER, *et al.* Dexamethasone therapy for children with bacterial meningitis. Meningitis Study Group. *Pediatrics* 1995; **95**: 21–8.

Wellmer A, *et al.* Effect of deficiency of tumor necrosis factor α or both of its receptors on *Streptococcus pneumoniae* central nervous system infection and peritonitis. *Infect Immun* 2001; **69**: 6881–6.

Yong VW, *et al.* Metalloproteinases in biology and pathology of the nervous system. *Nat Rev Neurosci* 2001; **2**: 502–11.

Yoshimura A, *et al.* Cutting edge: recognition of Gram-positive bacterial cell wall components by the innate immune system occurs via Toll-like receptor 2. *J Immunol* 1999; **163**: 1–5.

Zughaier SM, *et al. Neisseria meningitidis* lipooligosaccharide structure-dependent activation of the macrophage CD14/Toll-like receptor 4 pathway. *Infect Immun* 2004; **72**: 371–80.

Zwijnenburg PJ, *et al.* Chemotactic factors in cerebrospinal fluid during bacterial meningitis. *Infect Immun* 2006; **74**: 1445–51.

Zysk G, *et al.* Anti-inflammatory treatment influences neuronal apoptotic cell death in the dentate gyrus in experimental pneumococcal meningitis. *J Neuropathol Exp Neurol* 1996; **55**: 722–8.

Parasitic infections of the brain: malaria and beyond

Stephen J. Rogerson and Danny A. Milner Jr

Introduction

Despite successful public health initiatives, the number of people actually infected with parasitic disease is increasing, due to population growth in many disease-endemic areas. Parasitic diseases cause an enormous burden of neurological disease, although human central nervous system (CNS) involvement is not an obligatory phase in the life cycle of any common human parasite. Therefore, the study of parasitic CNS disease, and, logically, neuro-inflammatory reactions, is one of abnormalities in either the parasite's natural life cycle or the human host's immune response. The inflammatory milieu in parasitic CNS infections, although classically labelled as largely eosinophilic, is highly variable and not conserved across classes or even species (Table 13.1). This chapter will focus on *Plasmodium falciparum*, the most common parasitic cause of neurological symptoms.

Malaria: epidemiology, burden and immunity

Malaria causes over 500 million disease episodes and upwards of a million deaths each year (Murphy and Breman, 2001; Snow *et al.*, 2005). In malaria-endemic areas, exposed individuals acquire immunity to clinical disease, but frequently still carry infection (Bottius *et al.*, 1996). Severe illness and mortality are largely restricted to preschool children in Africa (the great majority) and to non-immune adults in Asia. Cerebral malaria (CM), severe malarial anemia (SMA) and respiratory distress are the most common manifestations of severe, life-threatening disease (Marsh *et al.*, 1995). Although four species of *Plasmodium* can infect man (*P. malariae*, *P. vivax*, *P. ovale*, and *P. falciparum*), almost all CM is due to *P. falciparum*, for two reasons. First, parasitized red blood cells (PRBC) sequester and become concentrated in the microcirculation of the brain and other vital organs because they adhere to host endothelial receptors, facilitating their evasion of splenic clearance. Second, *P. falciparum* efficiently invades erythrocytes of all stages, unlike *P. vivax* (which invades reticulocytes). Together, these factors allow the development of extremely high parasite burdens, and lead to the targeting of large numbers of metabolically active mature-stage parasites to the cerebral vasculature.

Clinical features and complications of cerebral malaria

Cerebral malaria is a diffuse, reversible encephalopathy, defined clinically as Blantyre coma score ≤ 2 (Molyneux *et al.*, 1989) for ≥ 4 h in the presence of malarial parasitemia, without other identifiable cause, and after controlling for hypoglycemia and seizures (World Health Organization, 2000). This clinical syndrome encompasses multiple disease processes, and may lack specificity for malaria. In an autopsy study from Malawi, 7 of 31 children with clinical CM had no sequestration, and other diagnoses could be made (Taylor *et al.*, 2004). Importantly, 95% of children with pathological CM had malaria-associated findings in the optic fundus, while 90% of children with other pathological diagnoses had no such changes (Taylor *et al.*, 2004). These changes have prognostic significance in life (Beare *et al.*, 2004), and fundoscopy is increasingly recognized as a critical clinical tool in diagnostic and interventional studies of CM.

Mortality rates from CM are 10–20% despite treatment, and over 10% of survivors have major residual neurological defects, such as hemiparesis, blindness, ataxia, and aphasia (Molyneux *et al.*, 1989; Brewster *et al.*, 1990; Marsh *et al.*, 1995). Neurocognitive impairments are common and are often persistent (Carter *et al.*, 2005). Malaria is estimated to be the eighth most common cause of disability-adjusted life years globally (Lopez *et al.*, 2006).

Inflammatory Diseases of the Central Nervous System, ed. T. Kilpatrick, R. M. Ransohoff and S. Wesselingh. Published by Cambridge University Press. © Cambridge University Press 2010

Table 13.1 Selected examples of patterns of neuro-inflammatory injury in parasitic diseases.

Organism	Inflammatory cells	CNS cells	Cytokines	Pathological findings in the CNS
Acanthamoeba castellani in granulomatous amebic encephalitis	Macrophages, T lymphocytes (primary source of IFN-γ)	Microglia (activation), endothelium (induced apoptosis)	TNF-α, INF-γ, IL-1β, IL-6 (important for prevention of infection in the immunocompetent)	Direct cytotoxicity and apoptosis of tissue with granulomatous encephalitis (in the immunosuppressed)
Angiostrongylus cantonensis in eosinophilic meningitis	Eosinophils	N/A	N/A	Third stage larvae, after ingestion, die after migration to the meninges, releasing antigen; eosinophils enter CSF in abundance in response to antigen
Taenia solium in neurocysticercosis	None in live larval stage; B lymphocytes, T lymphocytes, natural killer cells, monocyte/macrophages at death of larvae	None in live larval stage; astrocytes at death of larvae	Minimal in live larval stage; TNF-α, IL-5, IL-6, IL-10 at death of larvae	Immunologically silent cysts (1 to hundreds) in the white and gray matter causing "mass effect" with focal neurological signs; granulomatous inflammation at death of larvae and/or calcifications
Toxoplasma gondii in reactivation toxoplasmosis	Neutrophils, CD11c and CD11b + cells (transmigration of parasite across blood–brain barrier), CD4+ and CD8+ lymphocytes (primary source of IFN-γ), dendritic cells, B cells	Endothelium (↑ ICAM-1), microglia, astrocytes, neurons	↑TNF-α, INF-γ, IL-1, IL-12 (acutely protective Th1 response); ↑IL-10 with decreased Th1 response (chronic protection)	Immunosuppression, especially HIV, decreases T cells, allowing reactivation without control leading to tissue necrosis, abundant tissue tachyzoites, neutrophils, and macrophages
Trypanosoma brucei in African trypanosomiasis (i.e. African sleeping sickness)	CD8+ T lymphocytes	Astrocytes (gliosis), microglia (activation), endothelium (↑ ICAM-1, VCAM-1, and E-selectin)	↑TNF-α, INF-γ, IL-1β; ↓IL-10, IL-6	Blood–brain barrier breakdown with leakage, perivascular cuffing with lymphocytes, gliosis, "Mott" cells (i.e. plasma cells with immunoglobulin), parasites in the CSF

Neuropathology in cerebral malaria

Marchifava and Bignami were the first to describe sequestration (Marchiafava and Bignami, 1892). Young children constituted 87% of individuals who died of malaria in Panama (Kean and Smith, 1944; Arieti, 1946; Kean and Taylor, 1946), and in Ghana different patterns of cerebral pathology were all considered compatible with CM (Edington, 1954). Despite this diversity of pathology, the dogma remains; sequestration of the parasitized erythrocyte is a primary cause of mortality in adults and children.

The pathologic findings associated with the clinical syndrome of CM include a swollen edematous brain with or without frank herniation; a slate gray cerebral and cerebellar cortex; petechial hemorrhages on the cerebellar surface and in the white matter of the cerebellar and cerebral cortex; sequestered parasites within the blood vessels; macrophages containing

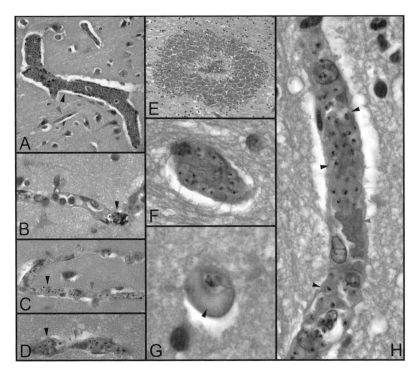

Figure 13.1 Cerebral sequestration within brain tissue obtained from pediatric patients in Africa. Sequestration can be extremely variable, being dense in some blood vessels (Panel A, black arrow) but sparse in others (Panel A, red arrow). Pigment-laden macrophages are important in the removal of *P. falciparum* from sequestered sites in the body but can become greatly enlarged with masses of pigment (Panel B, black arrow). Within a single segment of vessel (Panels C, D, black arrow) sequestration can be focal and adjacent to segments that are apparently unaffected (Panels C, D, red arrow). Ring hemorrhages are a classic finding (Panel E) that usually include fibrin thrombi within the core in and around the damaged vessel. Larger vessels with sequestration appear to maintain blood flow through the center (Panel F). Fibrin thrombi are occasionally seen without ring hemorrhages (Panel G, black arrow). In a given specimen, a mixture of PRBC with pathogens at different stages of development and with different levels of hemoglobin loss (Panel H, black arrows) can be identified when compared to unaffected cells (Panel H, red arrow).

numerous parasite pigment granules (i.e. hemozoin); and ring hemorrhages (grossly visible petechial hemorrhages, primarily located around small capillaries). These findings are illustrated in Figure 13.1. In Malawi, whereas most children meeting the clinical case definition of CM had these pathological changes at autopsy (Taylor *et al.*, 2004), 6 of 31 children had sequestration without intravascular inflammation (and no other cause of death), while 7 lacked cerebral pathology, and had another anatomic cause of death discernable outside of the CNS. In South East Asian adults, predominant sequestration was the most common finding (MacPherson *et al.*, 1985). The processes leading to death in either "pure" cerebral sequestration or cases with intravascular inflammatory changes remain poorly understood.

Parasite sequestration is tissue-specific. For example, PRBC sequester in the neurohypophysis (an extension of the brain) but not in the endocrine tissue of the adenohypophysis. The retina is another extension of the brain's vascular network, and can be examined during life; as discussed above, retinal changes associated with malaria correlate with histological findings (Lewallen *et al.*, 1993; Beare *et al.*, 2004). Comparing outcomes in relation to retinal pathology could shed light on the pathogenesis of fatal disease.

Mechanisms of development of cerebral malaria

It is now generally accepted that sequestration is necessary, but not always sufficient, for the development of CM (although debate has been extensive), and that in many instances a dysregulated host inflammatory response is a key factor in development of CM. The intensity of sequestration was significantly greater in children with confirmed CM than in children with clinical CM and another cause of death (Seydel *et al.*, 2006). Most fatal cases have intravascular inflammation (Taylor *et al.*, 2004), suggesting the host response is fundamental to disease pathology and outcome. True "neuroinflammation", with cerebral infiltrates of immune cells, is not a feature of CM, but activation of perivascular macrophages and microglia occurs (reviewed below).

Clinical CM can also develop in some instances through severe systemic illness due to malaria, associated with acidosis and other metabolic upsets (Clark *et al.*, 2006).

The basis for sequestration

Cerebral capillaries and post-capillary venules can be packed with trophozoite and schizont-infected cells, collectively representing sequestered PRBC. Interactions

Table 13.2 Receptors implicated in sequestration of *P. falciparum*-infected erythrocytes and first description.

CD36 (Barnwell *et al.*, 1985)
Intercellular adhesion molecule-1 (Berendt *et al.*, 1989)*
Thrombospondin (Roberts *et al.*, 1985)
Heparin† (Carlson *et al.*, 1992)
E-selectin (Ockenhouse *et al.*, 1992)
Vascular cell adhesion molecule 1 (Ockenhouse *et al.*, 1992)
P-selectin (Udomsangpetch *et al.*, 1997)
CD31 (Treutiger *et al.*, 1997)
αVβ3 integrin (Siano *et al.*, 1998)
Complement receptor 1† (Rowe *et al.*, 1997)
Chondroitin sulphate A* (Rogerson *et al.*, 1995)
Hyaluronic acid* (Beeson *et al.*, 2000)
Non-immune IgG* (Flick *et al.*, 2001)

* Implicated in placental malaria. Role in EC adhesion unknown.
† Involved in adhesion of PRBC to uninfected RBC; role in EC adhesion unknown.

between parasite ligands such as the *Plasmodium falciparum* erythrocyte membrane protein 1 (PfEMP1) family of proteins and host endothelial cell receptors such as CD36, ICAM-1, and (in the case of placental malaria) chondroitin sulphate A (CSA) are implicated in PRBC adhesion (Table 13.2). Platelets expressing CD36 can play ancillary roles in bridging between PRBC and the endothelium, and the facilitation of "clumping" of PRBC (Pain *et al.*, 2001; Wassmer *et al.*, 2004).

Multiple host receptors have been associated with in-vitro cytoadherence of PRBC. Two larger studies examining the adhesion properties of PRBC from infected hosts both reported higher adhesion to CD36 by isolates from children with less severe malaria (Newbold *et al.*, 1997; Rogerson *et al.*, 1999). This inverse relationship could be relevant to immunomodulation of dendritic cells by PRBC adhesion through CD36 (Urban *et al.*, 1999), or to involvement of CD36 in non-opsonic clearance of PRBC by phagocytes (McGilvray *et al.*, 2000), which are postulated to be potentially protective interactions. On the other hand, endothelial activation and up-regulation of surface receptors such as ICAM-1 and E-selectin can be induced by cytokines such as TNF-α, and by the parasite toxin glycosylphosphatidylinositol (GPI) (Schofield *et al.*, 1996): in adults, ICAM-1 expression co-localized with PRBCs (Turner *et al.*, 1994).

The parasite protein PfEMP1 is the most important ligand for sequestration of PRBC, and is the dominant variant surface antigen (VSA) expressed on the PRBC surface. The PfEMP1 is encoded by the *var* gene family, which is comprised of about 60 members per genome (Gardner *et al.*, 2002). A single *var* gene is expressed at one time, but PRBC switch *var* expression at a rate of 2% per generation (Roberts *et al.*, 1992). Different PfEMP1s can adhere to different receptors, and adhesion is mediated by specific domains within these proteins. The extracellular portion of PfEMP1 comprises a variable number of Duffy binding like domains, or DBLs, and one or more cysteine-rich interdomain regions (or CIDR). Domains are classified as α to ε, based on sequence homology, and DBLα and CIDR1 form a relatively conserved head structure. A unique exception to this is the PfEMP1 encoded by the *var2csa* gene, which lacks DBLα and CIDR domains (Salanti *et al.*, 2003; Duffy *et al.*, 2005): interestingly, this gene is highly conserved among isolates causing placental malaria (Tuikue Ndam *et al.*, 2005; Duffy *et al.*, 2006).

An enduring question has been whether particular parasites are especially prone to cause CM. Laboratory studies suggest certain "common" variants or VSA types to be particularly associated with severe disease, and with disease in young children (Bull *et al.*, 2000; Nielsen *et al.*, 2002). Recently, attempts have begun to characterize PfEMP1 sequences associated with severe malaria and CM, although clear answers are yet to emerge (Jensen *et al.*, 2004; Bull *et al.*, 2005; Kaestli *et al.*, 2006; Rottmann *et al.*, 2006).

We do not know why some parasites sequester in the brain, and others in the gut, subcutaneous tissue, or elsewhere. Although most children are infected with multiple parasite clones, different clones do not sequester in different tissues (Montgomery *et al.*, 2006; Dobano *et al.*, 2007). Whether *var* gene and PfEMP1 expression differ between different tissues is an important but presently unresolved question.

Bioactive parasite products and disease

Sequestered parasites release various products that interact primarily with the innate immune system. Innate immune cells frequently respond to infectious disease by recognizing pathogen-associated molecular patterns (PAMPs). At least two PAMPs have been described in malaria. The GPI molecule of *P. falciparum* activates macrophages to release pro-inflammatory molecules, and endothelial cells (ECs) to up-regulate receptor expression (Schofield *et al.*, 1996; Tachado *et al.*, 1996), potentially increasing sequestration of PRBC (as discussed below). The glycan moiety causes many of the symptoms of severe malaria in mice, which can be protected by immunization with conjugated GPI glycan (Schofield *et al.*, 2002).

Hemozoin is another *P. falciparum*-derived PAMP, reported to interact with Toll-like receptor (TLR) 9 (Coban *et al.*, 2005). It reportedly has both activating (Coban *et al.*, 2005) and immunosuppressive (Schwarzer *et al.*, 1992) effects on macrophages.

Microvascular obstruction

The clinical course of CM is not like that of stroke or of cerebral hypoxia, in which focal or generalized neurological deficits persist, often indefinitely. Total cerebral blood flow is within normal limits in adults with CM (Warrell *et al.*, 1988), and middle cerebral artery blood flow was increased in a proportion of children with CM (Newton *et al.*, 1996). However, the heterogeneous nature of sequestration (with some venules being packed with PRBC, but with others empty) is beyond the resolution of these technologies. Capillary obstruction by adherent, rigid PRBC may be exacerbated by adhesion of uninfected RBC to PRBC (Pongponratn *et al.*, 1991) (termed rosetting in vitro) or by clumping of PRBC, perhaps bridged by platelets (Pain *et al.*, 2001), which co-localize with PRBC in autopsy samples (Grau *et al.*, 2003). Moreover, uninfected RBC are more rigid in severe malaria, due to oxidative damage to the RBC membrane (Dondorp *et al.*, 2004). In affected vessels, these factors could severely restrict flow, while vasoactive mediators released could result in increased flow in nearby, unparasitised vessels.

Endothelial cell changes and blood–brain barrier alterations in cerebral malaria

Cerebral malaria is associated with changes in endothelial cell (EC) receptor expression, altered expression of EC junctional proteins, and with EC damage, resulting in impaired blood–brain barrier (BBB) function. Although evidence for a general increase in vascular permeability is conflicting (Medana and Turner, 2006), several pathways are suggested to lead to BBB alteration in malaria, including reduced microcirculatory flow due to sequestration (resulting in local hypoxia), the effects of PRBC adhesion on EC receptor expression,

cytokine release, and induction of EC apoptosis by PRBC (reviewed in Pino *et al.*, 2005; Hunt and Grau, 2006; Medana and Turner, 2006). Platelets can potentiate the effects of malaria and cytokines on ECs (Wassmer *et al.*, 2006a), perhaps by releasing transforming growth factor-beta (TGFβ) which increases EC apoptosis (Wassmer *et al.*, 2006b). Systemic consequences of malaria illness could also affect BBB function through metabolic disturbance, such as accumulation of quinolinic acid (Medana *et al.*, 2005).

Increased BBB permeability was seen in African children but not Thai adults with CM (Brown *et al.*, 2001). In autopsy cases, PRBC sequestration is associated with decreased expression of cell junctional protein expression and with activation of perivascular macrophages (Brown *et al.*, 1999, 2001). Intracranial hypertension can develop late in the disease and has a poor prognosis (Newton *et al.*, 1997). In mice, cerebral edema, due to BBB breakdown, develops in terminal CM (Penet *et al.*, 2005).

Animal models of cerebral malaria

Mouse and monkey models of CM reproduce certain features of the human disease, but both have the shortcoming that cerebral sequestration of PRBC is minimal (De Souza and Riley, 2002). This caveat notwithstanding, important insights into immunopathogenesis of CM, and especially the roles of innate and acquired immune cells, have emerged from animal studies (reviewed by Schofield and Grau, 2005). Mouse strains differ in their susceptibility to CM, and most work on pathogenesis has been done in strains that demonstrate a marked pro-inflammatory immune response to disease, not seen in CM-resistant mouse strains.

The most widely used parasite species is *P. berghei* ANKA (PbA), which sequesters in deep organs. The pathology is characterized by plugging of cerebral vessels with leukocytes, accompanied by petechial hemorrhages. Clinically, mice develop fitting and coma, analogous to human CM. Survivors, and CM-resistant mice, succumb to severe anaemia at about D21 post-infection. The natural history of CM is divided into induction and effector phases, and identifying the key players in the former process is critical to understanding the subsequent immunopathology. T cell induction probably occurs in the spleen, with subsequent migration to the brain (Renia *et al.*, 2006): migration is directed by molecules such as chemokines and their receptors. Chemokine receptor 5 (CCR5) and CCR2 are expressed by CD8+ T cells (Belnoue *et al.*, 2002), and CCR5-deficient mice are partially protected from CM (Belnoue *et al.*, 2003). Trafficking is then facilitated by up-regulation of endothelial cell adhesion molecules, such as ICAM-1, VCAM-1 and E-selectin (as seen in human CM: Turner *et al.*, 1994), although the key receptors for leukocyte recruitment in murine CM are not known.

Cytokines and other inflammatory mediators

Tumor necrosis factor-α (TNF-α)

Injection of TNF-α drastically increased the severity of malaria in mice, and anti-TNF antibody blocked the development of CM in mice infected with *P. berghei* ANKA (Clark *et al.*, 1987; Grau *et al.*, 1987). Subsequent human studies showed that TNF-α levels are increased in CM compared to non-CM patients (Grau *et al.*, 1989b), and are highest in children with fatal CM (Kwiatkowski *et al.*, 1990). Release of TNF-α in response to malarial toxin appears to be mediated by MAP Kinase pathways, with a central role for JNK2 (Lu *et al.*, 2006), suggesting a potential therapeutic target. However, attempts to block TNF-α activity in malaria have not been successful (van Hensbroek *et al.*, 1996).

Interferon-γ (IFN-γ)

Levels of IFN-γ are increased in symptomatic malaria, and the level of in-vitro production of IFN-γ by CD4+ T cells stimulated with malaria antigen correlates with protection from infection (Luty *et al.*, 1999). In patients, strong early IFN-γ responses (De Souza *et al.*, 1997) appear to be protective. On the other hand, blockade of IFN-γ can abrogate CM in the *P. berghei* ANKA model; moreover, this blockade abrogates the increase in TNF-α levels that is normally seen, implying that activation of IFNγ-producing cells could occur upstream of TNF-α induction (Grau *et al.*, 1989a). In humans, NK cells and γδ T cells are key sources of IFN-γ (Hensmann and Kwiatkowski, 2001; Artavanis-Tsakonas and Riley, 2002). Heterogeneity in NK cell IFNγ responses, based on the expression profile of genes encoding the killer cell immunoglobulin-like receptors (Kir), has been observed in humans, and is a determinant of disease outcome in mice (Hansen *et al.*, 2005).

Lymphotoxin α

This cytokine shows similar induction in inflammatory processes to that exhibited by TNF-α, and acts through an overlapping series of receptors. However, in PbA-infected mice, LTα$^{-/-}$ knockout mice were protected from CM, unlike TNF-α$^{-/-}$ mice (Engwerda *et al.*, 2002). The role of LTα in human CM is not presently known.

Other cytokines and mediators

Interleukin-10 (IL10) is an "anti-inflammatory" cytokine. Levels are elevated in children with CM (Lyke *et al.*, 2004), but levels of IL10 in the plasma were lower in adults with CM than in those with hyperparasitemia, shock, and jaundice. In the same study, IL10 levels fell as disease progressed in adults with fatal CM (Day *et al.*, 1999). Knockout mice deficient in IL10 develop increased sequestration and cerebral edema in response to *P. chabaudi* infection (Sanni *et al.*, 2004), and susceptible mice were protected against CM by recombinant IL10 (Kossodo *et al.*, 1997). Together, these data suggest IL10 plays an important protective role in CM.

Interleukin 12 (IL12) is released from macrophages, B cells and other cells early in malaria infection, stimulating the release of IFN-γ from NK and T cells. The levels of IL12 have not been associated specifically with CM (Lyke *et al.*, 2004). Nevertheless, in mice, IL12 is important in protection from severe anemia (Stevenson *et al.*, 2001).

Reactive oxygen species (ROS) and nitric oxide (NO) probably do not have causative roles in CM pathogenesis, although the expression of inducible NO synthase expression is a common event in CM (Maneerat *et al.*, 2000; Clark *et al.*, 2003) and NO could actually be protective (Anstey *et al.*, 1996; Sanni *et al.*, 1999; Lopansri *et al.*, 2003).

Cellular involvement

T cells and T cell subsets

In mice, the onset of symptoms coincides with sequestration of leukocytes, including T cells and mice lacking T cells do not develop CM (reviewed in Renia *et al.*, 2006).

Depletion of CD4+ T cells in mice abrogated CM development, and reconstitution by adoptive transfer restored disease pathogenesis (Grau *et al.*, 1986; Yanez *et al.*, 1996). These cells could be primarily involved in the induction of CM, or in the effector phase.

More recently, it was identified that depletion of CD8+ T cells, but not CD4+ T cells, abrogated CM pathology in 129Sv/ev × C57BL/6 mice (Belnoue *et al.*, 2002). The CD8+ T cells produce perforin, which can cause apoptosis of brain ECs (Potter *et al.*, 2006a), suggesting that CD8+ T cells could be important effectors of CM. The Fas/FasL system could be important in mediating CD8+ T cell-mediated axonal damage (Potter *et al.*, 2006b).

Depletion of γδ T cells early during infection abrogated the development of CM in C57BL/6 mice, but mice genetically incapable of making γδ T cells still developed disease (Yanez *et al.*, 1999). These cells could therefore have a helper or facilitatory role in disease pathogenesis.

Role of CNS in induction of pathology

Evidence is accumulating to suggest that cells within the CNS participate actively in the immunological reactions to malaria. Altered BBB function (reviewed above) leads to microglial activation and redistribution, and to astrocyte damage, possibly due to local cytokine release (Hunt *et al.*, 2006). Studies in murine CM using retinal whole mount preparations (Chang-Ling *et al.*, 1992) have allowed *in-situ* study of the effects of malaria on the distribution and morphology of astrocytes (Medana *et al.*, 1996) and microglia (Medana *et al.*, 2001). Astrocytes normally contribute to tight junctions and regulate the neuronal environment, ensheathing cerebral and retinal vessels. In fatal murine CM, ensheathment is disrupted, the arrangement of astrocytes is distorted and gliosis occurs (Medana *et al.*, 1996).

Seizures, both clinical and subclinical, are common in CM, and contribute to sequelae. Interferon-γ controls tryptophan metabolism through the indoleamine 2,3-dioxygenase (IDO) pathway, and imbalances in the production of neuroprotective kynurenine and neurotoxic quinolinic acid can lead to neuronal damage, both in vitro and in vivo (reviewed in Hunt *et al.*, 2006). Interferon-γ induces IDO, and a resultant increase in quinolinic acid levels in the brain and CSF has been reported in human and murine CM (Hunt *et al.*, 2006).

Conclusion

Cerebral malaria, the most important parasitic disease affecting the CNS, is associated with inflammatory immune responses, including intravascular macrophage accumulation and cytokine release, and (in late disease) with activation of microglia and other neural cells. Despite detailed human and animal studies of its pathogenesis, there remain many uncertainties, particularly regarding the fundamental steps in pathogenesis that lead to a fatal outcome. Identification of these steps could pave the way for adjunctive immunomodulatory therapy for this devastating condition.

References

Anstey NM, et al. Nitric oxide in Tanzanian children with malaria: Inverse relationship between malaria severity and nitric oxide production/nitric oxide synthase type 2 expression. *J Exp Med* 1996; **184**: 557–67.

Arieti S. Histopathologic changes in cerebral malaria and their relation to psychotic sequels. *Arch Neurol Psychiatry* 1946; **56**: 79–104.

Artavanis-Tsakonas K, Riley EM. Innate immune response to malaria: Rapid induction of IFN-gamma from human NK cells by live *Plasmodium falciparum*-infected erythrocytes. *J Immunol* 2002; **169**(6): 2956–63.

Barnwell JW, et al. Monoclonal antibody OKM5 inhibits the in vitro binding of *Plasmodium falciparum*-infected erythrocytes to monocytes, endothelial, and C32 melanoma cells. *J Immunol* 1985; **135**: 3494–7.

Beare NA, et al. Prognostic significance and course of retinopathy in children with severe malaria. *Arch Ophthalmol* 2004; **122**(8): 1141–7.

Beeson JG, et al. Adhesion of *Plasmodium falciparum*-infected erythrocytes to hyaluronic acid in placental malaria. *Nat Med* 2000; **6**: 86–90.

Belnoue E, et al. CCR5 deficiency decreases susceptibility to experimental cerebral malaria. *Blood* 2003; **101**(11): 4253–9.

Belnoue E, et al. On the pathogenic role of brain-sequestered alphabeta CD8+ T cells in experimental cerebral malaria. *J Immunol* 2002; **169**(11): 6369–75.

Berendt AR, et al. Intercellular adhesion molecule-1 is an endothelial cell adhesion molecule for *Plasmodium falciparum*. *Nature* 1989; **341**: 57–9.

Bottius E, et al. Malaria: Even more chronic in nature than previously thought; evidence for subpatent parasitaemia detectable by the polymerase chain reaction. *Trans R Soc Trop Med Hyg* 1996; **90**: 15–9.

Brewster DR, et al. Neurological sequelae of cerebral malaria in children. *Lancet* 1990; **336**: 1039–43.

Brown H, et al. Evidence of blood–brain barrier dysfunction in human cerebral malaria. *Neuropathol Appl Neurobiol* 1999; **25**(4): 331–40.

Brown H, et al. Blood–brain barrier function in cerebral malaria in Malawian children. *Am J Trop Med Hyg* 2001; **64**(3–4): 207–13.

Bull PC, et al. *Plasmodium falciparum* variant surface antigen expression patterns during malaria. *PLoS Pathogens* 2005; **1**(3): e26.

Bull PC, et al. *Plasmodium falciparum*-infected erythrocytes: Agglutination by diverse Kenyan plasma is associated with severe disease and young host age. *J Infect Dis* 2000; **182**(1): 252–9.

Carlson J, et al. Disruption of *Plasmodium-falciparum* erythrocyte rosettes by standard heparin and heparin devoid of anticoagulant activity. *Am J Trop Med Hyg* 1992; **46**(5): 595–602.

Carter JA, et al. Persistent neurocognitive impairments associated with severe falciparum malaria in Kenyan children. *J Neurol Neurosurg Psychiatry* 2005; **76**(4): 476–81.

Chang-Ling T, et al. Early microvascular changes in murine cerebral malaria detected in retinal wholemounts. *Am J Pathol* 1992; **140**(5): 1121–30.

Clark IA, et al. Possible roles of tumor necrosis factor in the pathology of malaria. *Am J Pathol* 1987; **129**: 192–9.

Clark IA, et al. Tissue distribution of migration inhibitory factor and inducible nitric oxide synthase in falciparum malaria and sepsis in African children. *Malaria J* 2003; **2**(1): 6.

Clark IA, et al. Human malarial disease: A consequence of inflammatory cytokine release. *Malaria J* 2006; **5**(1): 85.

Coban C, et al. Toll-like receptor 9 mediates innate immune activation by the malaria pigment hemozoin. *J Exp Med* 2005; **201**(1): 19–25.

Day NP, et al. The prognostic and pathophysiologic role of pro- and antiinflammatory cytokines in severe malaria. *J Infect Dis* 1999; **180**(4): 1288–97.

De Souza JB, et al. Early gamma interferon responses in lethal and nonlethal murine blood-stage malaria. *Infect Immun* 1997; **65**(5): 1593–8.

De Souza JB, Riley EM. Cerebral malaria: The contribution of studies in animal models to our understanding of immunopathogenesis. *Microbes Infect* 2002; **4**(3): 291–300.

Dobano C, et al. Expression of merozoite surface protein markers by *Plasmodium falciparum* infected erythrocytes in peripheral blood and tissues of children with fatal malaria. *Infect Immun* 2007; **75**(2): 643–52.

Dondorp AM, et al. Reduced microcirculatory flow in severe falciparum malaria: Pathophysiology and electron-microscopic pathology. *Acta Trop* 2004; **89**(3): 309–17.

Duffy MF, et al. Broad analysis reveals a consistent pattern of *var* gene transcription in *Plasmodium falciparum* repeatedly selected for a defined adhesion phenotype. *Mol Microbiol* 2005; **56**(3): 774–88.

Duffy MF, et al. Transcribed var genes associated with placental malaria in Malawian women. *Infect Immun* 2006; **74**(8): 4875–83.

Edington GM. Cerebral malaria in the Gold Coast African: Four autopsy reports. *Ann Trop Med Parasitol* 1954; **48**(3): 300–6.

Engwerda CR, et al. Locally up-regulated lymphotoxin alpha, not systemic tumor necrosis factor alpha, is the principle mediator of murine cerebral malaria. *J Exp Med* 2002; **195**(10): 1371–7.

Flick K, et al. Role of nonimmune IgG bound to PfEMP1 in placental malaria. *Science* 2001; **293**(5537): 2098–100.

Gardner MJ, et al. Genome sequence of the human malaria parasite *Plasmodium falciparum*. *Nature* 2002; **419**: 498–511.

Grau GE, et al. L3T4+ T lymphocytes play a major role in the pathogenesis of murine cerebral malaria. *J Immunol* 1986; **137**: 2348–54.

Grau GE, *et al.* Tumor necrosis factor (cachectin) as an essential mediator in murine cerebral malaria. *Science* 1987; **237**: 1210–2.

Grau GE, *et al.* Monoclonal antibody against interferon g can prevent experimental cerebral malaria and its associated overproduction of tumor necrosis factor. *Proc Natl Acad Sci USA* 1989a; **86**: 5572–4.

Grau GE, *et al.* Tumor necrosis factor and disease severity in children with *falciparum* malaria. *N Engl J Med* 1989b; **320**: 1586–91.

Grau GE, *et al.* Platelet accumulation in brain microvessels in fatal pediatric cerebral malaria. *J Infect Dis* 2003; **187**(3): 461–6.

Hansen DS, *et al.* The natural killer complex regulates severe malarial pathogenesis and influences acquired immune responses to *Plasmodium berghei* ANKA. *Infect Immun* 2005; **73**(4): 2288–97.

Hensmann M, Kwiatkowski D. Cellular basis of early cytokine response to *Plasmodium falciparum*. *Infect Immun* 2001; **69**(4): 2364–71.

Hunt N, Grau G. Blood–brain barrier in parasitic disease. *Int J Parasitol* 2006; **36**(5): 503–4.

Hunt NH, *et al.* Immunopathogenesis of cerebral malaria. *Int J Parasitol* 2006; **36**(5): 569–82.

Jensen AT, *et al. Plasmodium falciparum* associated with severe childhood malaria preferentially expresses PfEMP1 encoded by group A *var* genes. *J Exp Med* 2004; **199**(9): 1179–90.

Kaestli M, *et al.* Virulence of malaria is associated with differential expression of *Plasmodium falciparum* var gene subgroups in a case-control study. *J Infect Dis* 2006; **193**(11): 1567–74.

Kean BH, Smith JA. Death due to estivo-autumnal malaria. *Am J Trop Med Hyg* 1944; **34**: 317–22.

Kean BH, Taylor CE. Medical shock in the pathogenesis of algid malaria. *Am J Trop Med Hyg* 1946; **35**: 209–19.

Kossodo S, *et al.* Interleukin-10 modulates susceptibility in experimental cerebral malaria. *Immunology* 1997; **91**: 536 40.

Kwiatkowski DA *et al.* TNF concentration in fatal cerebral, non-fatal cerebral, and uncomplicated *Plasmodium falciparum* malaria. *Lancet* 1990; **336**(8725): 1201–4.

Lewallen S, *et al.* Ocular fundus findings in Malawian children with cerebral malaria. *Ophthalmology* 1993; **100**(6): 857–61.

Lopansri BK, *et al.* Low plasma arginine concentrations in children with cerebral malaria and decreased nitric oxide production. *Lancet* 2003; **361**(9358): 676–8.

Lopez AD, *et al.* Global and regional burden of disease and risk factors, 2001: Systematic analysis of population health data. *Lancet* 2006; **367**(9524): 1747–57.

Lu Z, *et al.* Disruption of JNK2 decreases the cytokine response to *Plasmodium falciparum* glycosylphosphatidylinositol in vitro and confers protection in a cerebral malaria model. *J Immunol* 2006; **177**(9): 6344–52.

Luty AJ., *et al.* Interferon-gamma responses are associated with resistance to reinfection with *Plasmodium falciparum* in young African children. *J Infect Dis* 1999; **179**(4): 980–8.

Lyke KE, *et al.* Serum levels of the proinflammatory cytokines interleukin-1 beta (IL-1beta), IL-6, IL-8, IL-10, tumor necrosis factor alpha, and IL-12(p70) in Malian children with severe *Plasmodium falciparum* malaria and matched uncomplicated malaria or healthy controls. *Infect Immun* 2004; **72**(10): 5630–7.

MacPherson GG, *et al.* "Human cerebral malaria. A quantitative ultrastructural analysis of parasitized erythrocyte sequestration. *Am J Pathol* 1985; **119**: 385–401.

Maneerat Y, *et al.* Inducible nitric oxide synthase expression is increased in the brain in fatal cerebral malaria. *Histopathology* 2000; **37**: 269–77.

Marchiafava E, Bignami A. Sulle febbre malariche estivo-autumnali. *Bull del R Acad Med di Roma* 1892; **297**(18).

Marsh K, *et al.* Indicators of life-threatening malaria in African children. *N Engl J Med* 1995; **332**: 1399–404.

McGilvray ID, *et al.* Nonopsonic monocyte/macrophage phagocytosis of *Plasmodium falciparum*-parasitized erythrocytes: A role for CD36 in malarial clearance. *Blood* 2000; **96**(9): 3231–40.

Medana IM, *et al.* Redistribution and degeneration of retinal astrocytes in experimental murine cerebral malaria: Relationship to disruption of the blood–retinal barrier. *Glia* 1996; **16**(1): 51–64.

Medana IM, *et al.* Central nervous system in cerebral malaria: 'Innocent bystander' or active participant in the induction of immunopathology? *Immunol Cell Biol* 2001; **79**(2): 101–20.

Medana IM, *et al.* Cerebrospinal fluid levels of markers of brain parenchymal damage in Vietnamese adults with severe malaria. *Trans R Soc Trop Med Hyg* 2005; **99**(8): 610–7.

Medana IM, Turner GD. Human cerebral malaria and the blood–brain barrier. *Int J Parasitol* 2006; **36**(5): 555–68.

Molyneux ME, *et al.* Clinical features and prognostic indicators in paediatric cerebral malaria: A study of 131 comatose Malawian children. *Q J Med* 1989; **71**: 441–59.

Montgomery J, *et al.* Genetic analysis of circulating and sequestered populations of *Plasmodium falciparum* in fatal pediatric malaria. *J Infect Dis* 2006; **194**(1): 115–22.

Murphy SC, Breman JG. Gaps in the childhood malaria burden in Africa: Cerebral malaria, neurological sequelae, anemia, respiratory distress, hypoglycemia, and complications of pregnancy. *Am J Trop Med Hyg* 2001; **64**(Suppl): 57–67.

Newbold C, *et al.* Receptor-specific adhesion and clinical disease in *Plasmodium falciparum*. *Am J Trop Med Hyg* 1997; **57**: 389–98.

Newton CR, *et al.* Intracranial hypertension in Africans with cerebral malaria. *Arch Dis Child* 1997; **76**(3): 219–26.

Newton CR, *et al*. Perturbations of cerebral hemodynamics in Kenyans with cerebral malaria. *Pediatr Neurol* 1996; **15**(1): 41–9.

Nielsen MA, *et al*. *Plasmodium falciparum* variant surface antigen expression varies between isolates causing severe and nonsevere malaria and is modified by acquired immunity. *J Immunol* 2002; **168**(7): 3444–50.

Ockenhouse CF, *et al*. Human vascular endothelial cell adhesion receptors for *Plasmodium falciparum*-infected erythrocytes: Roles for endothelial leukocyte adhesion molecule 1 and vascular cell adhesion molecule 1. *J Exp Med* 1992; **176**: 1183–9.

Pain A, *et al*. Platelet-mediated clumping of *Plasmodium falciparum*-infected erythrocytes is a common adhesive phenotype and is associated with severe malaria. *Proc Natl Acad Sci USA* 2001; **98**(4): 1805–10.

Penet MF, *et al*. Imaging experimental cerebral malaria in vivo: Significant role of ischemic brain edema. *J Neurosci* 2005; **25**(32): 7352–8.

Pino P, *et al*. Blood–brain barrier breakdown during cerebral malaria: Suicide or murder? *Thromb Haemost* 2005; **94**(2): 336–40.

Pongponratn E, *et al*. Microvascular sequestration of parasitized erythrocytes in human falciparum malaria: A pathological study. *Am J Trop Med Hyg* 1991; **44**(2): 168–75.

Potter S, *et al*. Perforin mediated apoptosis of cerebral microvascular endothelial cells during experimental cerebral malaria. *Int J Parasitol* 2006a; **36**(4): 485–96.

Potter SM, *et al*. A role for Fas–Fas ligand interactions during the late-stage neuropathological processes of experimental cerebral malaria. *J Neuroimmunol* 2006b; **173**(1–2): 96–107.

Renia L, *et al*. Pathogenic T cells in cerebral malaria. *Int J Parasitol* 2006; **36**(5): 547–54.

Roberts DD, *et al*. Thrombospondin binds falciparum malaria

parasitized erythrocytes and may mediate cytoadherence. *Nature* 1985; **318**: 64–6.

Roberts DJ, *et al*. Rapid switching to multiple antigenic and adhesive phenotypes in malaria. *Nature* 1992; **357**: 689–92.

Rogerson SJ, *et al*. Chondroitin sulfate A is a cell surface receptor for *Plasmodium falciparum*-infected erythrocytes. *J Exp Med* 1995; **182**: 15–20.

Rogerson SJ, *et al*. Cytoadherence characteristics of *Plasmodium falciparum*-infected erythrocytes from Malawian children with severe and uncomplicated malaria. *Am J Trop Med Hyg* 1999; **61**: 467–72.

Rottmann M, *et al*. Differential expression of var gene groups is associated with morbidity caused by *Plasmodium falciparum* infection in Tanzanian children. *Infect Immun* 2006; **74**(7): 3904–11.

Rowe JA, *et al*. *P. falciparum* rosetting mediated by a parasite-variant erythrocyte membrane protein and complement-receptor 1. *Nature* 1997; **388**(6639): 292–5.

Salanti A, *et al*. Selective upregulation of a single distinctly structured *var* gene in chondroitin sulphate A-adhering *Plasmodium falciparum* involved in pregnancy-associated malaria. *Mol Microbiol* 2003; **49**(1): 179–91.

Sanni LA, *et al*. Are reactive oxygen species involved in the pathogenesis of murine cerebral malaria? *J Infect Dis* 1999; **179**(1): 217–22.

Sanni LA, *et al*. Cerebral edema and cerebral hemorrhages in interleukin-10-deficient mice infected with *Plasmodium chabaudi*. *Infect Immun* 2004; **72**(5): 3054–8.

Schofield L, Grau GE. Immunological processes in malaria pathogenesis. *Nat Rev Immunol* 2005; **5**(9): 722–35.

Schofield L, *et al*. Synthetic GPI as a candidate anti-toxic vaccine in a model of malaria. *Nature* 2002; **418**(6899): 785–9.

Schofield L, *et al*. Glycosylphosphatidylinositol toxin

of *Plasmodium* upregulates intercellular adhesion molecule-1, vascular cell adhesion molecule-1, and E-selectin expression in vascular endothelial cells and increases leukocyte and parasite cytoadherence via tyrosine kinase-dependent signal transduction. *J Immunol* 1996; **156**: 1886–96.

Schwarzer E, *et al*. Impairment of macrophage functions after ingestion of *Plasmodium falciparum*-infected erythrocytes or isolated malarial pigment. *J Exp Med* 1992; **176**(4): 1033–41.

Seydel KB, *et al*. The distribution and intensity of parasite sequestration in comatose Malawian children. *J Infect Dis* 2006; **194**(2): 208–15.

Siano JP, *et al*. *Plasmodium falciparum*: Cytoadherence to $a_v b_3$ on human microvascular endothelial cells. *Am J Trop Med Hyg* 1998; **59**: 77–9.

Snow RW, *et al*. The global distribution of clinical episodes of *Plasmodium falciparum* malaria. *Nature* 2005; **434**(7030): 214–17.

Stevenson MM, *et al*. Modulation of host responses to blood-stage malaria by interleukin-12: From therapy to adjuvant activity. *Microbes Infect* 2001; **3**: 49–59.

Tachado SD, *et al*. Glycosylphosphatidylinositol toxin of *Plasmodium* induces nitric oxide synthase expression in macrophages and vascular endothelial cells by a protein tyrosine kinase-dependent and protein kinase C-dependent signaling pathway. *J Immunol* 1996; **156**: 1897–907.

Taylor TE, *et al*. Differentiating the pathologies of cerebral malaria by postmortem parasite counts. *Nat Med* 2004; **10**(2): 143–5.

Treutiger CJ, *et al*. PECAM-1/CD31, an endothelial receptor for binding *Plasmodium falciparum*-infected erythrocytes. *Nature Med* 1997; **2**(12): 1405–08.

Tuikue Ndam NG, *et al*. High level of var2csa transcription by *Plasmodium falciparum* isolated from the placenta. *J Infect Dis* 2005; **192**(2): 331–5.

Turner GDH, *et al*. An immunohistochemical study of the

pathology of fatal malaria. Evidence for widespread endothelial activation and a potential role for intercellular adhesion molecule-1 in cerebral sequestration. *Am J Pathol* 1994; **145**: 1057–69.

Udomsangpetch R, *et al.* Promiscuity of clinical *Plasmodium faciparum* isolates for multiple adhesion molecules under flow conditions. *J Immunol* 1997; **158**: 4358–64.

Urban B, *et al. Plasmodium falciparum*-infected erythrocytes modulate the maturation of dendritic cells. *Nature* 1999; **400**(6739): 73–7.

van Hensbroek MB, *et al.* The effect of a monoclonal antibody to tumor necrosis factor on survival from childhood cerebral malaria. *J Infect Dis* 1996; **174**(5): 1091–7.

Warrell DA, *et al.* Cerebral anaerobic glycolysis and reduced cerebral oxygen transport in human cerebral malaria. *Lancet* 1988; **2**(8610): 534–8.

Wassmer SC, *et al.* Platelets potentiate brain endothelial alterations induced by *Plasmodium falciparum. Infect Immun* 2006a; **74**(1): 645–53.

Wassmer SC, *et al.* TGF-{beta}1 released from activated platelets can induce TNF-stimulated human brain endothelium apoptosis: A new mechanism for microvascular lesion during cerebral malaria. *J Immunol* 2006b; **176**(2): 1180–4.

Wassmer SC, *et al.* Platelets reorientate *Plasmodium falciparum*-infected erythrocyte cytoadhesion to activated endothelial cells. *J Infect Dis* 2004; **189**(2): 180–9.

World Health Organization. Severe falciparum malaria. *Trans R Soc Trop Med Hyg* 2000; **94**(Suppl 1): S1–90.

Yanez DM, *et al.* Gamma delta T-cell function in pathogenesis of cerebral malaria in mice infected with *Plasmodium berghei* ANKA. *Infect Immun* 1999; **67**(1): 446–8.

Yanez DM, *et al.* Participation of lymphocyte subpopulations in the pathogenesis of experimental murine cerebral malaria. *J Immunol* 1996; **157**(4): 1620–4.

Role of the inflammatory process in traumatic brain damage

Cristina Morganti-Kossmann, Laveniya Satgunaseelan, Nicole Bye, Phuong Nguyen, and Thomas Kossmann

Introduction

Still a hidden epidemic, traumatic brain injury (TBI) remains the major cause of death of young people under the age of 45 in industrialized countries. Despite the fact that prevention is a fundamental key to reduce morbidity and mortality in patients with severe TBI, much effort in clinical and fundamental research aims to improve the therapeutic options both from the medical and the surgical perspective. The pathophysiology of traumatic injury to the brain is complex. Most of the improvement in survival rate and enhanced neurological recovery following TBI has been obtained through advances in critical care management. Many reasons have been proffered for the failure of pharmacological trials in TBI patients, ranging from inappropriate inclusion criteria, heterogeneity of injury types, lack of suitable outcome measures, a too rapid transition from preclinical to clinical studies, and statistical aspects for data analysis. In conclusion, it is clear that intensive clinical and basic research is required to more fully understand the pathogenesis of TBI. In addition, putative therapies require validation in multiple animal models that reproduce various types of brain damage before being submitted to clinical trial.

Classification of brain injury

Generally, the severity of TBI is clinically assessed using the Glasgow coma scale (GCS 1–14), which is a neurological scale reflecting severe (3–8), moderate (9–12) and mild head injury (13–14) (Teasdale and Jennett, 1974). In general terms, the damage caused to the brain in response to trauma can be distinguished qualitatively into patterns based on both distribution of the insult and its tempo (focal versus diffuse) (immediate or primary and delayed or secondary) (Figure 14.1). The heterogeneity of these types of

damage is also reflected in differences in their pathophysiology, which renders TBI a complex process. Focal closed brain damage consists of single or multiple localized lesions such as contusions or acute epidural, subdural, or intracerebral hematomas that may arise from deformations of the skull generating damage to the underlying tissue, often accompanied by lesions to the opposite aspect of the brain termed *contre-coup* injuries. Consequently, a contusion with a necrotic core, together with damage of the surrounding vessels, is observed (Marion, 1999; Graham *et al.*, 2002).

Diffuse axonal injury in humans can be of various degrees (1–4) and does not necessarily require contact with the skull, but rather is caused by acceleration/deceleration forces. In diffuse axonal injury, the initial damage to the axonal membrane results in changes in ionic concentrations, which progress to dysfunction of axonal transport, loss of microtubular ultrastructure, mitochondrial impairment, and deposition of amyloid precursor protein (APP), which is currently the best early histological marker of axonal damage. Ultimately, grading is best achieved by counting the number of damaged axons using macroscopic and microscopic examination, which reveals the classical hallmark of axonal swelling and retraction balls, as well as petechial hemorrhages (Adams *et al.*, 1989; Sahuquillo *et al.*, 1989; Povlishock and Christman, 1995).

It is therefore apparent that focal and diffuse brain injuries involve distinct mechanical dynamics and physiological and morphological abnormalities which, in turn, trigger selective cascades with variable outcomes determining the extent and type of secondary brain damage. By definition, secondary brain damage begins at the time of injury and progresses over the ensuing hours, days, and weeks, leading to delayed loss of neuronal cells and worsening of the neurological outcome. Neuronal cell death has traditionally been

Inflammatory Diseases of the Central Nervous System, ed. T. Kilpatrick, R. M. Ransohoff and S. Wesselingh. Published by Cambridge University Press. © Cambridge University Press 2010

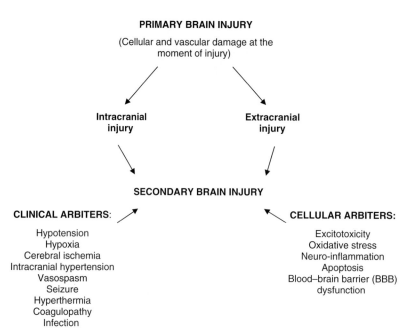

Figure 14.1 The damage caused to the brain in response to trauma.

thought to take place in two phases, encompassing an early necrotic and a long-term apoptotic phase. Cell death via necrosis appears to occur immediately after the mechanical impact associated with the primary injury, consequent to sudden changes to the cell membrane and metabolic constitution of the cell. However, axonal disconnection after TBI, which progresses from "retraction balls" in the days following injury to Wallerian degeneration by 3 months post-injury, is an example of the protracted course of necrosis that can occur in TBI. Furthermore (Colicos and Dash, 1996; Hausmann *et al.*, 2004), apoptotic cell death has been observed as acutely as one day post-TBI and as long-term as 22 weeks after injury (Marciano *et al.*, 2004).

Physiological consequences involved in secondary brain damage

Subsequent to severe TBI, patients can experience respiratory impairment leading to hypoxia and hypertension, further compromising cerebral perfusion pressure. This can directly exacerbate the neurotoxic insults induced by the traumatic injury and, in the case of ischemia, also predispose to delayed reperfusion injuries once cerebral perfusion is restored. These systemic changes can also contribute to cerebral edema by augmenting the blood–brain barrier permeability (BBB; vasogenic edema) and/or by causing cell swelling (cytotoxic edema). The increase in brain mass elevates

the intracranial pressure which in concert with edema, BBB dysfunction, and regional ischemic damage compounds the neural degeneration (Marmarou, 2003; Unterberg *et al.*, 2004; Beaumont *et al.*, 2006).

Biochemistry of TBI

There is a wide number of molecular cascades that become activated following TBI which collectively contribute to secondary neuronal cell death. In principle, this cytotoxicity can be induced by either excitotoxicity, oxidative stress, or inflammation (see below). The concentration of excitatory neurotransmitters such as glutamate is increased immediately after TBI via both excessive release from dying neurons and reduced uptake by astrocytes. High glutamate concentrations activate the NMDA receptors causing intracellular Ca^{2+} influx, free radical production, cellular swelling and ultimately cell death (Furukawa *et al.*, 2003). Dysfunction of cerebral blood flow can lead to ischemic injury associated with hypoxia which, when followed by a sudden reperfusion, can lead to liberation of damaging oxygen free radicals. These radicals cause the peroxidation of lipids, proteins, and DNA, thus contributing to cell membrane damage (Lewen *et al.*, 2000). Mitochondrial dysfunction with impaired oxidative phosphorylation can lead to the release of cytochrome c and activation of the intrinsic pathway of cell apoptosis (Hausmann *et al.*, 2004).

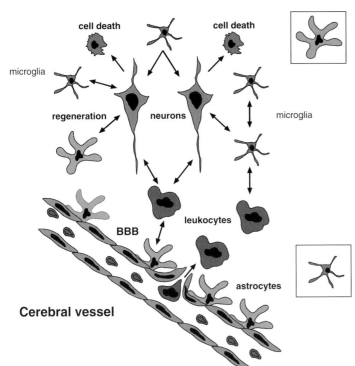

Activated astrocytes

Anisomorphic:
Localized at the glial scar
Release of neurotoxic molecules:
TNF, NO, oxygen radicals.
Killing of neurons, oligodendrocytes

Isomorphic:
Distant from the injury site
glutamate uptake
release of energy substrates,
neurotrophic factors, anti-oxidants,
extracellular matrix, anti-
inflammatory cytokines.
BBB restoration and tissue repair

Activated microglia

M1: stimulated by TNF, LPS or
IFN$_\gamma$ = cytotoxicity

M2: stimulated by IL-4, IL-13,
IL-10 = immune suppression and
tissue remodeling

Figure.14.2 Modes of activation of astrocytes and microglia.

Cerebral inflammation induced by TBI

We and others have proposed that two competing cerebral inflammatory effects are elicited in the context of neuropathological diseases (Morganti-Kossmann et al., 1992). These opposite and complex properties are not only displayed by the whole inflammatory cascade, but are also fundamental features of individual immune mediators. Although the intrinsic characteristics of the central nervous system (CNS) render it refractory to immune activation, studies of various neuropathologies have clearly shown that it can mount significant inflammatory responses. This role is specifically played by glial cells, namely microglia and astrocytes, which become rapidly activated in response to a pathological challenge.

A classical model for neuro-inflammation is based upon the injection of the endotoxin lipopolysaccharide (LPS) directly into the parenchyma, which results in both humoral and cellular activation (Hauss-Wegrzyniak et al., 2000). Resident glial cells have the ability to express a variety of immunological antigens on the cell membrane, to secrete a large number of cytokines and chemokines, as well as to up-regulate cell adhesion molecules (Thibeault et al., 2001). Despite the abundant use of the LPS model, some have expressed concern regarding its suitability to understand the cellular and molecular changes induced by traumatic injury. It is conceivable that similar to what has been proposed for T cells, microglia could become polarized in terms of the repertoire of cytokines and chemokines induced, depending on the stimulus used for challenge (Figure 14.2). It has already been reported that the response of macrophages can be dichotomous; for example, when stimulated by either LPS, interferon-gamma (IFNγ) or tumor necrosis factor-alpha (TNF-α), these cells exhibit a so-called M1 polarization or type 1 immunological response characterized by cytotoxic and anti-tumoral properties (Mantovani et al., 2004). On the other hand, M2 responses are multifaceted and they can be induced by either interleukin (IL) 4 or 13 cytokines known to be involved in allergy and the killing of parasites (M2a response); by either toll-like receptor (TLR) or IL-1 receptor agonists mediating immunoregulation (M2b response); and by IL-10 leading to immune suppression and tissue remodeling (M2c response). Thus, the cellular function of macrophages, and potentially that of microglia, is likely to be contextual.

Astrocytes also appear to be distinguished by two phenotypes: the reactive or anisomorphic astrocytes which form the glial scar and which release neurotoxic molecules thereby killing neurons and oligodendrocytes, and isomorphic astrocytes which are only transiently activated and release trophic factors that enhance neuronal survival and tissue repair (Figure14.2) (Liberto et al., 2004). Following the early release of cytokines by activated microglia, astrocytes can exert several functions. Reactive gliosis is overt in TBI and has been shown to impair neurite outgrowth and potentially to contribute to tissue damage by secreting cytokines such as TNF-α, arachidonic acid, nitric oxide (NO), and reactive oxygen species. Alternatively, astrocytes represent a valuable source of energy provided by storage of glycogen that can rapidly be made available to neurons when energy is scarce. They can also convert excessive concentrations of the cytotoxic agent glutamate into glutamine and promote angiogenesis and induce neurovascularization via the release of epidermal growth factor (EGF), fibroblast growth factor (FGF), insulin-like growth factor (IGF) and vascular endothelial growth factor (VEGF), as well as contribute to the reformation of the integrity of the BBB. Furthermore, through the synthesis of neurotrophic factors induced by TNF-α, IL-1 and IL-6, astrocytes support neuronal survival, neurite outgrowth, and neurogenesis by increasing the proliferation of progenitor cells and the differentiation of newly formed neurons (Dong and Benveniste, 2001; Nakajima and Kohsaka, 2004).

In comparison to other tissues, the inflammatory response elicited in the brain tends to be of a lesser magnitude than in peripheral tissues, as exhibited by lower concentrations of inflammatory cytokines. This could be either due to relative sequestration based on the BBB or the properties of intrinsic neural cells such as microglia, which when cultured in vitro have been shown to secrete anti-inflammatory cytokines spontaneously.

Studies aimed at defining the inflammatory response following brain trauma began in the early 1990s focusing both on animal models of TBI, and the characterization of cerebrospinal fluid (CSF) collected from head trauma patients. Both approaches have yielded similar results, revealing that several cytokines are released soon after injury in brain homogenates of animals subjected to TBI and that these same cytokines are detected in CSF samples from patients but not from controls. However, we also demonstrated a fundamental difference between humans and animals: the up-regulation of cytokines in humans is identifiable for days to weeks post-injury (Kossmann et al., 1995; Hans et al., 1999a), whereas in animals subjected to TBI they are no longer detectable at these time points, even though the activation of astrocytes and microglia persists for weeks.

In addition to the activation of resident cells of the CNS, the injured brain attracts the migration of neutrophils and, to a lesser extent, lymphocytes, especially within focal lesion. These cells secrete a variety of cytokines and free radicals that generate a state of oxidative stress, which contribute to tissue damage. Over time, these cells are cleared from the lesion either through apoptosis or via migration towards the meningeal structures. In several animal models, neutrophils have been shown to be recruited early after injury with their infiltration peaking at around 24 h, whereas macrophages/microglia are found in abundance by 2–7 days (Aihara et al., 1995). Many of these cells are found to localize within the penumbra, the tissue surrounding the primary injury, which is most vulnerable to secondary damage (Beer et al., 2000). These data suggest that the nature of the inflammatory responses exerted by the cytokines and the relevant immune cells is likely to be a key determinant of the extent of secondary brain damage and the ultimate neurological outcome.

Interestingly, important differences have been identified in the nature of the cellular response to focal TBI (as detailed above) as opposed to diffuse axonal injury (DAI). In DAI, whilst resident CNS cells are activated, there is generally a paucity of infiltrating leukocytes (Csuka et al., 2000).

The role of cytokines in the post-traumatic inflammatory response

Cytokines were originally referred to as "lymphokines" and "monokines" (generated by activated lymphocytes, monocytes, and macrophages, respectively), but their production by other cell types has altered this notion. Under physiological conditions, cytokines typically exist in near undetectable concentrations within the CNS; however, in several neurological diseases, including multiple sclerosis, stroke, and HIV dementia, elevated concentrations of several cytokines have been documented (Merrill and Benveniste, 1996; Griffin, 1997; Feuerstein et al., 1998). Traumatic brain injury is no different – the immune mediators are up-regulated within the CNS by resident cells that adopt an immunological function and by infiltrating leukocytes that enter subsequent to BBB disruption. A positive feedback loop is then established whereby both glia and infiltrating hematogenous cells secrete cytokines, and the cytokines themselves in turn activate further glia and recruit additional leukocytes from the periphery, acting largely in an autocrine and paracrine fashion.

In comparison to focal TBI, there is currently a paucity of data concerning the cytokine response in either experimental or clinical DAI.

Interleukin 1 – the archetypal pro-inflammatory mediator

The role of IL-1 has been extensively characterized in focal injury models. Well known as a major player in the hypothalamic–pituitary axis, IL-1 is thought to be the primary pro-inflammatory cytokine responsible for initiating the "cytokine cycle" (Gentleman et al., 2004). Interleukin-1 exists in two forms: IL-1α, the membrane-bound form, and IL-1β, the secreted form which is the main agonist induced in the brain in response to injury (Rothwell, 1991). Interestingly, the main source of IL-1 in the CNS are activated microglia, an acknowledged exacerbator of neuro-inflammation, which also express the IL-1 receptor (IL-1R1) (Pinteaux et al., 2002). Once bound to its receptor, IL-1 activates various signal transduction pathways, including the ubiquitous transcription factor nuclear factor κB (NF-κB), and p38 mitogen-activated protein kinases (O'Neill and Greene, 1998). Such activation results in the transcription of other inflammatory factors (e.g. prostaglandin-E2 (PGE2) and IL-6) (Norris et al., 1994; Caggiano and Kraig, 1999). Therefore, it is not surprising that the neurotoxicity of IL-1 is thought to arise indirectly from its propensity to induce other pro-inflammatory cytokines (Chung and Benveniste, 1990; Aloisi et al., 1992), as well as its capacity to stimulate the production of inflammatory mediators such as cyclo-oxygenase-2 (COX-2), phospholipase A2 (PLA$_2$) and prostaglandins (Molina-Holgado et al., 2000). It is important to note that IL-1 does not cause neuronal damage of its own accord – rather, it has a synergistic effect with other injurious factors, especially in the context of either ischemia or excitotoxicity (Rothwell, 1999, 2003; Allan, 2002).

Focal models of TBI were the first to demonstrate alterations of IL-1 expression in the brain. A fluid percussion model in the rat showed a rapid increase in IL-1β mRNA (Fan et al., 1995), whilst in our laboratory IL-18 (a recently identified member of the IL-1 family known for its interferon-γ inducing properties) has also been found to be elevated in a murine closed head injury model and in severe TBI patients (Yatsiv et al., 2002). Other studies of TBI patients, both adult and pediatric, showed strong correlations of IL-1 with poor functional outcome (Tasci et al., 2003; Chiaretti et al., 2005) and high expression, by in-situ hybridization, in contused human brain tissue excised from victims, 3–5 days after trauma (Holmin and Hojeberg, 2004).

Open head injury models, which reproduce stab wound and gunshot injury in the human, have illustrated the deleterious effects of IL-1, using IL-1R1 knockout mice. In the absence of IL-1R, not only was endogenous microglial activation and recruitment of macrophages from the periphery abrogated, but the production of a variety of inflammatory mediators, including COX-2, other pro-inflammatory cytokines (TNF-α and IL-6) and chemotactic molecules (VCAM-1 and ICAM-1) were also reduced (Basu et al., 2002). There are many other examples of IL-1 inhibition yielding improved outcomes in experimental TBI: for example, IL-1 receptor antagonist (IL-1 RA) administered in both a fluid percussion model and aseptic cryogenic injury reduced neuronal damage (Toulmond and Rothwell, 1995; Jones et al., 2005), whilst corroborative results supporting a negative role of IL-1 were shown in transgenic mice over-expressing endogenous IL-1 RA in which improved neurological outcome and decreased expression of pro-inflammatory cytokines after closed focal head injury were identified (Tehranian et al., 2002). Neutralization of the most recently identified isoform of IL-1, IL-18, using a binding protein (IL-18 BP), also improved neurological recovery in mice post TBI (Yatsiv et al., 2002).

The role of IL-1 in diffuse brain injury has only begun to be characterized, with Marmarou's well-known impact-acceleration model. As with focal injury, intrathecal levels of both IL-1α and IL-1β mRNA have been found to be elevated in rodent brains within 12 h of diffuse axonal injury (Lu et al., 2005a, 2005b; Kamm et al., 2006). Similarly, antibodies to IL-1α and IL-1β reduced neuronal injury, particularly in the hippocampus (Lu et al., 2005a, 2005b). In these circumstances, IL-1 α has been found to be expressed by astrocytes and IL-1β by neurons, as opposed to predominant expression by macrophages/microglia in contusion-type damage (Holmin et al., 1997;

Lu *et al.*, 2005b). This is in keeping with the observation that reactive astrocytosis is a key component of the neural response to diffuse axonal injury (Csuka *et al.*, 2000).

The role of astrocytes in the IL-1-mediated immune response is an important one – the homotypic response of astrocytes to all CNS injury (that is, to proliferate and hypertrophy), is known to be modulated by IL-1 (Balasingam *et al.*, 1994; Lin *et al.*, 2006). However, another dimension to the reactive astroglial response (which eventuates in the formation of the glial scar) is the fact that IL-1 induces the expression of nerve growth factor (NGF) in astrocytes (DeKosky *et al.*, 1996). This is one of several potential neuroprotective responses that IL-1 can induce, which possibly includes inhibition of both calcium influx into neurons (Plata-Salaman and Ffrench-Mullen, 1992) and of *N*-methyl-D-aspartate (NMDA) receptor-mediated neuronal excitation (Coogan and O'Connor, 1997). Thus the cytokine IL-1 can exert both pro- and anti-inflammatory effects.

Tumor necrosis factor-α – breaking from the pro-inflammatory stereotype

Tumor necrosis factor-alpha was initially portrayed as a purveyor of a diverse range of injurious functions. Its deleterious effects in the brain are widespread, ranging from recruitment of leukocytes to the CNS (Pober and Cotran, 1990), induction of BBB damage through activation of proteolytic enzymes (Rosenberg *et al.*, 1995), regulation of the expression of the potent inflammatory mediator, anaphylatoxin C5a (Stahel *et al.*, 2000a), and blockade of migration of astrocytes to the site of injury (Faber-Elman *et al.*, 1995). In the case of diffuse axonal injury, TNF-α contributes indirectly to secondary damage and regeneration failure through a variety of mechanisms, including the inhibition of astrocytic repopulation, induction of oligodendrocyte death and myelin destruction (Tchelingerian *et al.*, 1995). An important determinant of outcome, namely cerebral edema, is also affected by TNF-α: this influence is possibly mediated via damage to the microvasculature, as demonstrated in the percussion injury model (Kita *et al.*, 1997). However, the best characterized role of TNF-α is in the activation, increased production and hypertrophy of microglia (Kita *et al.*, 1997; Rostworowski *et al.*, 1997; Knoblach *et al.*, 1999), although it is also thought to contribute to

astrogliosis (Chung and Benveniste, 1990; Benveniste, *et al.*, 1995; Hua *et al.*, 2002).

Increased TNF-α expression has been identified in various animal models in the acute phase of TBI including fluid percussion, stab wound, closed head, and closed cortical injury. The temporal profile of release of TNF-α is consistent between experiments, with detectable levels present at 1 h, peaking at 3–8 h and decreasing within 24 h. This short latency suggests that endogenous production of TNF-α within the CNS is involved and, consistent with this, TNF-α mRNA can be detected within 1 h of trauma in the contused cerebral hemisphere of the injured rat (Taupin *et al.*, 1993; Shohami *et al.*, 1994; Fan *et al.*, 1996; Kita *et al.*, 1997; Rostworowski *et al.*, 1997; Stover *et al.*, 2000). Interestingly, findings in the contralateral hemisphere in models of focal injury demonstrate the global nature of the cerebral inflammatory response, with increases in TNF-α mRNA and protein after fluid percussion injury in both the contralateral cortex and hippocampus of injured mice (Taupin *et al.*, 1993; Fan *et al.*, 1996). The only diffuse injury model published to date showed significant increases of TNF-α in serum within 24 h, but not in cerebral tissue. This, once again, indicates the need to consider diffuse injury separately (Kamm *et al.*, 2006).

Involvement of TNF-α in damage has also been supported by experiments using various methods of inhibition. First, low molecular weight substances that suppress the synthesis of TNF-α, including a phosphodiesterase inhibitor which blocks TNF-α mRNA expression (pentoxifylline) (Shohami *et al.*, 1996) and dexanabinol, a post-transcriptional inhibitor of TNF-α and NMDA receptor antagonist (Shohami *et al.*, 1997), attenuated cerebral edema and improved functional outcome in mice subjected to closed focal head injury. Second, soluble TNF-α receptors and binding protein (TNF-α BP), representing macromolecules that bind to TNF-α to inhibit its function, resulted in improved neurological outcomes when they were applied either peripherally (intravenous administration), or centrally (intraventricular administration) (Shohami *et al.*, 1996; Knoblach *et al.*, 1999).

Outcomes in transgenic and knockout mice have, however, also played a pivotal role in demonstrating that TNF-α is not necessarily solely "pro-inflammatory". Whilst one murine model demonstrated that over-expression of the cytokine causes a chronic inflammatory and degenerative state (Probert *et al.*, 1997), we showed that deficiency of the TNF-α gene as a TNF/lymphotoxin-α double knockout yielded increased post-traumatic mortality (Stahel *et al.*, 2000b). Those TNF-α-deficient mice which survived displayed an improved neurological recovery in the days following trauma, with no significant difference in either the degree of BBB dysfunction, cell death, or neutrophil infiltration as compared to wild-type mice. This finding has been supported by another closed cortical injury model, whereby deficits in memory and motor function in the acute post-traumatic period were less in TNF-α knockout mice, whereas their recovery from injury was prolonged and cortical tissue loss at 4 weeks was greater (Scherbel *et al.*, 1999). Co-injection of TNF-α with the excitotoxin α-amino-3-hydroxy-5-methyl-4-isoxazole propionic acid (AMPA) into the striatum of the rodent brain significantly reduced AMPA-mediated striatal tissue loss, whereas co-injection with IL-1β caused considerable cell death (Allan, 2002). Collectively, these results suggest that TNF-α exerts both early deleterious and late neuroprotective effects.

It is now well recognized that TNF-α signals through two receptors, namely TNFR1 and TNFR2, and that their individual signaling pathways contribute to the bimodal function of this cytokine. Binding to TNFR1, which leads to activation of the p55 signaling pathway, activates apoptosis via FADD (Fas-associated death domain) or FLICE (FADD-like IL-1 converting enzyme), which in turn instigates caspase activity. Binding to TNFR1 or TNFR2 could also cause the activation of NF-κB via TRADD (TNF-α receptor-associated death domain) and TNF-α-associated factors (TRAF1 and TRAF2) (Shohami *et al.*, 1999; Sullivan *et al.*, 1999). The NF-κB is known to mediate the pro-inflammatory effects of IL-1 (O'Neill and Greene, 1998), via the induction of COX-2, PLA2, intracellular adhesion molecular-1 (ICAM-1, discussed below) and pro-inflammatory cytokines (Lee and Burckart, 1998). However, NF-κB is also capable of inducing "protective" genes via the production of antioxidants (manganese superoxide dismutase), a calcium binding protein and inhibitor of apoptosis (calbindin) as well as anti-inflammatory cytokines (Mattson *et al.*, 2000). Thus, duality of function is not a feature exclusive to cytokines, but appears to characterize all stages of the neuro-inflammatory process following TBI.

We and others have reported that TNF-α is elevated in both the serum and CSF of TBI patients (Goodman *et al.*, 1990; Ross *et al.*, 1994). The potentiality for duality

of function of TNF-α in human TBI has also been demonstrated, via its association with both the pro-inflammatory IL-18 and the anti-inflammatory IL-10 (Csuka *et al.*, 1999; Schmidt *et al.*, 2004). More specifically, we have identified that in 28 TBI patients monitored over a 3-week period, the mean CSF TNF-α level was elevated above the mean serum level, lending credence to the findings in animal models that TNF-α is endogenously produced within the CNS (Csuka *et al.*, 1999). The converse was found in a separate study of 29 patients over 10 days post-injury, whereby soluble TNF receptors (which have anti-inflammatory properties due to their ability to bind circulating TNF-α) were found to be more readily detected in plasma than in CSF (Maier *et al.*, 2006).

Such findings signify a shift in the view of inflammatory cytokines from a clinical perspective. For instance, early therapeutic intervention is likely to treat the deleterious effects of TNF-α, whilst ongoing inhibition could prevent its protective properties. Marklund and colleagues (2005) demonstrated that ongoing treatment of rats subjected to fluid percussion injury with monoclonal antibodies targeting TNF-α showed no effect on either neurological outcome or brain swelling 1 week post-injury. In a recent study by Browne *et al.* (2006) on fluid percussion-injured rats, prolonged administration of the non-steroidal anti-inflammatory drug ibuprofen worsened cognitive ability but had no effect on eventual hippocampal tissue loss, as evaluated at 4 months post-injury. Such findings support the view that there is a complexity to treating the neuro-inflammatory response in the patient, and provide insight into why many clinical trials in the head-injured have been negative (Narayan *et al.*, 2002) – a failure to recognize the duality of cytokine activity after head injury.

Interleukin-6 – the original Janus cytokine

Interleukin-6 (IL-6) provides a typical example of the dual functions that cytokines can exert during ischemia, hypoxia, or TBI (Singhal *et al.*, 2002). The IL-6 is also responsible for protection against glutamate excitotoxicity and oxidative stress (Penkowa *et al.*, 2000), the induction of NGF (Kossmann *et al.*, 1996), the inhibition of TNF-α, and the induction of IL-1-RA (Benveniste *et al.*, 1995). However, its role as a pro-inflammatory cytokine is well known, inducing up-regulation of chemokine production, adhesion molecule expression, and enhancement of leukocyte recruitment (Modur *et al.*, 1997; Romano *et al.*, 1997). The IL-6 also plays a major role in acute phase reactions, both in the periphery and CNS, as shown earlier in our clinical research (Kossmann *et al.*, 1995), and is produced by a wide range of cells, from B lymphocytes to microglia. The actions of IL-6 are propagated through its receptor (IL-6-R), which is made up of two membrane glycoproteins: an 80-kDa binding receptor protein and a signal transducing protein (gp130). When bound, the substrate–receptor complex induces homodimerization of gp130, which leads to activation of signaling cascades within the cytoplasm (Benveniste, 1998). The receptor also exists in a soluble form (s-IL-6-R), which when associated with gp130 can act autonomously to activate IL-6-mediated pathways and was found elevated in the CSF of TBI patients, together with IL-6 (Hans *et al.*, 1999a).

In many different animal models, IL-6 has been shown to exhibit the same time-line of release whether the traumatic phenomenon is focal or diffuse, generally commencing at 1 h and peaking between 2 and 8 h in the rat (Woodroofe *et al.*, 1991; Taupin *et al.*, 1993; Shohami *et al.*, 1994; Hans *et al.*, 1999b). A similar pattern, with an early peak of IL-6 at 3–6 days, has also been identified in human studies (Kossmann *et al.*, 1996). The IL-6 also appears to be synthesized within the brain, which is supported by the presence of IL-6 mRNA within the cortex, thalamus, hippocampus, and dentate gyrus, and high concentrations of IL-6 within the CSF of rats subjected to diffuse injury (Hans *et al.*, 1999b; Rhodes *et al.*, 2002). Studies of focal injury models have demonstrated that astrocytes are unlikely producers of IL-6, with microglia, neurons, and peripherally recruited macrophages the probable cellular sites of synthesis (Woodroofe *et al.*, 1991; Hans *et al.*, 1999b). However, astrocytes rely on IL-6 for activation (Swartz *et al.*, 2001).

The role of astrogliosis in pathogenesis after CNS injury is uncertain, as it could either exacerbate scar formation and thereby inhibit repair or aid in re-establishing the integrity of the BBB (Rostworowski *et al.*, 1997). Astroglial reactivity is defined by increased expression of either glial fibrillary acidic protein (GFAP) or of its mRNA within these cells which, in turn, corresponds with increases in pro-inflammatory cytokine gene transcription, including that of TNF-α (Rostworowski *et al.*, 1997; Herx and Yong, 2001). It is in this post-injury context that IL-6 exerts its many protective effects upon resident cells of

the CNS. It has been found that transgenic mice in which IL-6 is expressed behind the GFAP promoter show improved revascularization after aseptic cerebral injury, with IL-6 providing an indirect angiogenic signal (Swartz *et al.*, 2001). Focal cerebral injury in IL-6 knockout mice not only resulted in increased numbers of apoptotic neurons and worsened BBB breakdown, but also decreased gliosis and astrocyte activation (Penkowa *et al.*, 1999, 2000; Swartz *et al.*, 2001). In contrast, in diffuse injury models, GFAP-positive cells did not express IL-6 which was, instead, mainly localized on neurons (Hans *et al.*, 1999a; Rhodes *et al.*, 2002). This pattern was observed despite the fact that reactive astrocytes can be identified within hours and up to 2 weeks post-injury in this model (Csuka *et al.*, 2000). This, once again, highlights the need to recognize the very different inflammatory responses mounted in focal and diffuse injury.

The IL-6 has also been found to influence neurotrophin production by astrocytes in human studies, such that astrocyte cultures exposed to the CSF of TBI patients, known to contain IL-6, demonstrated elevated production of NGF, whereas astrocytes exposed to control CSF did not generate the neurotrophin (Kossmann *et al.*, 1996). Production of NGF was also attenuated with the incubation of CSF with an anti-IL-6 antibody. This raises the distinct possibility that neuroregeneration can be driven by cytokines that are endogenously produced within the CNS. It is also important to note that IL-6 levels have been observed to be higher in the CSF than in serum after TBI: it has also been postulated that IL-6 of cerebral origin can influence the peripheral acute phase response (Kossmann *et al.*, 1995).

The complexity of IL-6 induced activity has shown itself in the contradictory findings in patient outcome studies. The study by Winter *et al.* (2004) performed on brain microdialysis measurements in 14 TBI patients showed increased levels of IL-6 in survivors, and a correlation between increasing levels of IL-6 and positive Glasgow Outcome Scale (GOS) at 6 months. Singhal *et al.* (2002) quantified IL-6 in the CSF of 36 patients and found similar associations. In direct contrast, two studies, with sample sizes of 62 and 84 patients, identified serum IL-6 to be a marker of poor prognosis post-TBI (Arand *et al.*, 2001; Minambres *et al.*, 2003). These conflicting results once again support the notion that TBI is a complex process with cytokines playing multiple roles in different settings, both within the CNS and in the periphery.

The anti-inflammatory cytokines – interleukin-10 and transforming growth factor-beta

The most commonly studied anti-inflammatory cytokines include IL-10 and transforming growth factor beta (TGF-β), both of which possess immunosuppressive properties within the CNS (Morganti-Kossmann et al., 2001). Both cytokines are produced by glia and lymphopoietic cells (Aloisi et al., 1992; Xiao et al., 1996), with IL-10 production postulated to be a result of sympathetic activation (Woiciechowsky et al., 1998). The primary method through which anti-inflammatory cytokines exert their effects is via the inhibition of a variety of pro-inflammatory cytokines, including IL-1 and IFN-γ (Benveniste et al., 1995; Knoblach et al., 1999; Kremlev and Palmer, 2005): they also serve to attenuate MHC II expression, microglial activation and leukocyte adhesion (Balasingam and Yong, 1996; Benveniste, 1998).

Experimental studies have illustrated the neuroprotective benefit conferred by IL-10. Elevated levels of IL-10 in the brain have been observed in models of diffuse cerebral injury within 24 h of trauma (Kamm et al., 2006), whereas exogenous administration of IL-10 has been observed to improve neurological recovery and to significantly reduce levels of the pro-inflammatory cytokine, TNF-α, in the injured cortex of rodents subjected to focal injury (Knoblach and Faden, 1998). Similarly, in patients with TBI, increases in CSF concentrations of IL-10 have been detected in the 24 h following trauma (Hayakata et al., 2004), and have been found to correlate with decreased levels of TNF-α in the CSF (Csuka et al., 1999). The TGF-β has been shown to be elevated in the CSF of sufferers of TBI, with a lesser increase identified in the serum at 3 weeks post-injury. A correlation between TGF-β levels and BBB dysfunction was found, as demonstrated by the CSF–serum albumin quotient (Q_A ratio); this was highly indicative of a leakage of the cytokine from serum to the CSF, although the high levels of TGF-β in the CSF could suggest intrathecal production (Morganti-Kossmann et al., 1999). Elevations of IL-10 in the serum of severely head injured patients have also been observed (Shimonkevitz et al., 1999; Maier et al., 2001), but have been found to be non-specific to TBI in the multi-trauma setting (Hensler et al., 2000). Furthermore, the beneficial role of IL-10 is not consistently replicated in human studies, as it has been associated with higher mortality in children (Bell et al., 1997) and severe septic complications in multi-trauma patients (Neidhardt et al., 1997). Thus, IL-10 could confer benefit centrally in decreasing pro-inflammatory damage within the CNS, but could also have detrimental effects by contributing to systemic immunosuppression in the multi-trauma patient. Therefore the dichotomy between central (or intracerebral) and peripheral events needs to be considered. This is particularly important in the context of both intracerebral and systemic production of cytokines, and the fact that patients often suffer both multi-trauma and TBI.

Chemokines – the importance of cellular communication

In addition to cytokines, chemokines are required for the induction of the infiltration of peripheral leukocytes into the CNS after TBI. These small, soluble molecules, which play a role in the developing CNS, are grouped into two families: the CXC or α chemokines, of which IL-8 is a prime example, and the CC or β chemokines, which includes monocyte chemoattractant protein-1, or MCP-1. These molecules are largely produced by peripheral leukocytes, although evidence now exists for their production within the brain (Ransohoff and Tani, 1998; Morganti-Kossmann et al., 2001).

The IL-8, also named in rodents as macrophage inflammatory protein-2 (MIP-2), has powerful chemotactic and activating properties for neutrophils, known to be propagators of proteolytic-mediated secondary brain injury (Sherwood and Prough, 2000; Morganti-Kossmann et al., 2001). Whalen et al. (2000) demonstrated an association between increased mortality and higher CSF IL-8 levels in children with severe head injury, illustrating its reputation as a contributor to pro-inflammatory damage. Evidence of high production of IL-8 in the CSF of patients with severe TBI has been found within 6 h of injury (Kossmann et al., 1997; Maier et al., 2001; Kushi et al., 2003; Hayakata et al., 2004). This has led to speculation that IL-8 could have other functions within the CNS, including the induction of BBB dysfunction. On the other hand, recombinant IL-8 has also been shown to stimulate the production of NGF by cultured mouse astrocytes (Kossmann et al., 1997; Morganti-Kossmann et al., 1997). Given the potent neutrophil chemotactic properties of IL-8, concomitant elevation of adhesion molecules, such as E-selectin and intracellular adhesion molecule-1 (ICAM-1), would be expected. Although we demonstrated that ICAM-1 correlated with the index of BBB disruption in TBI patients (Pleines *et al.*, 1998), experimental studies show maximal elevation of ICAM-1 at 7 days, well after peak neutrophil accumulation, which occurs at 24 h (Clark *et al.*, 1994; Rancan *et al.*, 2001). However, MIP-2 is abundantly produced by murine astrocytes and microvascular endothelial cells when stimulated by either ICAM-1 or TNF-α (Otto *et al.*, 2000), and since its kinetics differ depending on the stimulus, two separate signaling pathways are hypothesized to be operative. Clearly, further study of the interactions between MIP2/IL-8, ICAM-1, and neutrophil recruitment is required.

The role of MCP-1 in TBI is also yet to be fully elucidated, but it is known to play an important role in blood-borne monocyte recruitment (Stamatovic *et al.*, 2005). Although there have not been any patient studies to date on MCP-1, a variety of experimental models have demonstrated up-regulation of this chemokine. In our laboratory, brain MCP-1 protein levels have recently been shown to peak by 4 h following closed focal head injury in mice (Bye *et al.*, 2006). Furthermore, MCP-1 mRNA expression was significantly increased after focal brain injury, and was consistently associated with the presence of infiltrating leukocytes (Glabinski *et al.*, 1996). Diffuse injury proved no different, with elevation of MCP-1 detectable in the rodent brain (Rancan *et al.*, 2001), correlating with perivascular localization of monocytes/macrophages. On the other hand, as previously reported by Csuka and colleagues (2000), neutrophil infiltration was not detected, and there was a commensurate lack of IL-8 expression. It can thus be concluded that the pattern of chemokine release is an aspect of neuro-inflammation that, in all likelihood, modulates the cellular response and probably in a contextual way, dependent on the nature of the primary brain injury.

Microdialysis – a new horizon of cytokine detection

The studies discussed so far used a variety of techniques to ascertain levels of inflammatory mediators. In experimental studies, this often involves immunohistochemistry or ELISA techniques utilizing brain homogenates of animals sacrificed at various timepoints post-injury. On the other hand, human studies have involved analysis of CSF and serum collected at set intervals. Using these methods, the neuroscientist can only gain an indirect insight into the extracellular

events that occur within the brain parenchyma. Microdialysis, by contrast, provides us with an antemortem temporal measure of the extracellular environment. A microdialysis system comprises a probe or catheter that is implanted in the brain, which is perfused at low flow rates in order to mimic a blood capillary, allowing the diffusion of molecules from the extracellular fluid, across a semipermeable membrane to be collected in vials every 10–60 min (Robinson and Justice Jr, 1991; Hillered *et al.*, 2005). To date, there have been few studies detailing cytokine detection using microdialysis. This is mainly due to the fact that cytokines are large molecules that are difficult to recover using a microdialysis probe. However, the availability of 100 kDa plus pore-sized probes has led to improved recovery of cytokines at reasonable time intervals, thus allowing for adequate temporal resolution of the secretion profiles of these molecules. Winter and colleagues (2002, 2004) were the first to measure cytokines in humans using microdialysis and focused on the kinetics of IL-6 expression. The pore size was 3000 kDa, inserted away from focal injury into the uninjured frontal region to detect damage secondary to diffuse injury. Previously, Woodroofe *et al.* (1991) had assessed the neuro-inflammatory response following probe insertion, finding no increase in the acute period post-TBI in the rat: in contrast, IL-1β was found to be elevated within 60 min of insertion in a more recent study (Fassbender *et al.*, 2000).

Conclusion

Historically, research devoted to elucidating the function of cerebral inflammation following trauma has lagged behind similar work directed to other neurological diseases such as stroke, multiple sclerosis, and spinal cord injury. Therefore, in spite of the progress achieved in the last decade in understanding the various components of the immune responses in TBI models and in patients, more needs to be done to clarify many of the contradictory results concerning the role of humoral and cellular immune activation. Much can be learnt from the study of the aforementioned diseases, which can then be applied to the model systems used in TBI research. Overall, the factors that seem more likely to influence whether any given cytokine exerts either beneficial or detrimental effects include the kinetics of its expression and the expression patterns of its receptor subunits. Compared to infectious diseases, the concentration of cytokines in the injured brain is much lower, suggesting that, in this context, they are more likely to exert a reparative role by inducing neurotrophic factors and extracellular matrix proteins that are involved in augmenting the survival of compromised neural cells. The most compelling evidence to support a protective role for cytokines derives from studies of cytokine-deficient mice in which in the majority of cases display either more severe injury or no obvious effect after TBI. In those instances in which cytokines have proven to be deleterious, it is also quite likely that total inhibition of activity will prove to be counterproductive. This has been well demonstrated in transgenic mice overexpressing the inhibitory molecule IL-1 RA at either the homozygous or heterozygous level, and secondly through the administration of anti-inflammatory compounds using alternative therapeutic regimens, either of short or prolonged duration. In the first instance, Tehranian et al. (2002) showed that the best outcome following TBI was seen in animals in which IL-1β was only partially inhibited, namely in the IL-1RA heterozygous mice,

as compared to the homozygous transgenic lineage. On the other hand, anti-inflammatory treatment with IL-10, in a model of spinal cord injury, revealed that a single injection was beneficial, whereas protracted treatment resulted in only transient protection, suggesting that attenuation of the early inflammatory response could be neuroprotective, while a later inflammatory response could be essential for tissue recovery (Bethea et al., 1999). In line with these experimental data, our group has recently shown transient benefit when the anti-inflammatory tetracycline, minocycline, was administered over 4 days post-TBI; minocycline decreased lesion volume and improved neurological outcome at 1 day post-trauma, but this response was not maintained at 4 days (Bethea et al., 1999).

Clearly, given the complexity of the inflammatory cascade, together with the multiple and redundant roles displayed by cytokines and the distinct phases of the cellular elements involved, it will be necessary for any successful therapeutic strategy in TBI to selectively target specific aspects of the inflammatory response.

References

Adams JH, *et al.* Diffuse axonal injury in head injury: Definition, diagnosis and grading. *Histopathology* 1989; **15**: 49–59.

Aihara N, *et al.* Altered immunoexpression of microglia and macrophages after mild head injury. *J Neurotrauma* 1995; **12**: 53–63.

Allan SM. Varied actions of proinflammatory cytokines on excitotoxic cell death in the rat central nervous system. *J Neurosci Res* 2002; **67**: 428–34.

Aloisi F, *et al.* Production of hemolymphopoietic cytokines (IL-6, IL-8, colony-stimulating factors) by normal human astrocytes in response to IL-1 beta and tumor necrosis factor-alpha. *J Immunol* 1992; **149**: 2358–66.

Arand M, *et al.* Early inflammatory mediator response following isolated traumatic brain injury and other major trauma in humans. *Langenbecks Arch Surg* 2001; **386**: 241–8.

Balasingam V, *et al.* Reactive astrogliosis in the neonatal mouse brain and its modulation by cytokines. *J Neurosci* 1994; **14**: 846–56.

Balasingam V, Yong VW. Attenuation of astroglial reactivity by interleukin-10. *J Neurosci* 1996; **16**: 2945–55.

Basu A, *et al.* The type 1 interleukin-1 receptor is essential for the efficient activation of microglia and the induction of multiple proinflammatory mediators in response to brain injury. *J Neurosci* 2002; **22**: 6071–82.

Beaumont A, *et al.* Bolus tracer delivery measured by MRI confirms edema without blood–brain barrier permeability in diffuse traumatic brain injury. *Acta Neurochir Suppl* 2006; **96**: 171–4.

Beer R, *et al.* Expression of Fas and Fas ligand after experimental traumatic brain injury in the rat. *J Cereb Blood Flow Metab* 2000; **20**: 669–77.

Bell MJ, *et al.* Interleukin-6 and interleukin-10 in cerebrospinal fluid after severe traumatic brain injury in children. *J Neurotrauma* 1997; **14**: 451–7.

Benveniste EN. Cytokine actions in the central nervous system. *Cytokine Growth Factor Rev* 1998; **9**: 259–75.

Benveniste EN, *et al.* Differential regulation of astrocyte TNF-alpha expression by the cytokines TGF-beta, IL-6 and IL-10. *Int J Dev Neurosci* 1995; **13**: 341–9.

Bethea JR, *et al.* Systemically administered interleukin-10 reduces tumor necrosis factor-alpha production and significantly improves functional recovery following traumatic spinal cord injury in rats. *J Neurotrauma* 1999; **16**: 851–63.

Browne KD, *et al.* Chronic ibuprofen administration worsens cognitive outcome following traumatic brain injury in rats. *Exp Neurol* 2006; **201**: 301–7.

Bye N, *et al.* The chemokine MCP-1 modulates post-traumatic inflammation following closed head injury in the mouse (Oral). In *8th International Neurotrauma Symposium*, Rotterdam; 2006.

Caggiano A, Kraig RP. Prostaglandin E receptor subtypes in cultured rat microglia and their role in reducing lipopolysaccharide-induced interleukin-1 α production. *J Neurochem* 1999; **72**: 565–75.

Chiaretti A, *et al.* Interleukin 1beta and interleukin 6 relationship with paediatric head trauma severity and outcome. *Childs Nerv Syst* 2005; **21**: 185–93.

Chung IY, Benveniste EN. Tumor necrosis factor-alpha production by astrocytes. Induction by lipopolysaccharide, IFN-gamma, and IL-1 beta. *J Immunol* 1990; **144**: 2999–3007.

Clark RS, *et al.* Neutrophil accumulation after traumatic brain injury in rats: Comparison of weight drop and controlled cortical impact models. *J Neurotrauma* 1994; **11**: 499–506.

Colicos MA, Dash PK. Apoptotic morphology of dentate gyrus granule cells following experimental cortical impact injury in rats: Possible role in spatial memory deficits. *Brain Res* 1996; **739**: 120–31.

Coogan A, O'Connor JJ. Inhibition of NMDA receptor-mediated synaptic transmission in the rat dentate gyrus in vitro by IL-1 beta. *Neuroreport* 1997; **8**: 2107–10.

Csuka E, *et al.* Cell activation and inflammatory response following traumatic axonal injury in the rat. *Neuroreport* 2000; **11**: 2587–90.

Csuka E, *et al.* IL-10 levels in cerebrospinal fluid and serum of patients with severe traumatic brain injury: Relationship to IL-6, TNF-alpha, TGF-beta1 and blood–brain barrier function. *J Neuroimmunol* 1999; **101**: 211–21.

DeKosky ST, *et al.* Interleukin-1 receptor antagonist suppresses neurotrophin response in injured rat brain. *Ann Neurol* 1996; **39**: 123–7.

Dong Y, Benveniste EN. Immune function of astrocytes. *Glia* 2001; **36**: 180–90.

Faber-Elman A, *et al.* Vitronectin overrides a negative effect of TNF-alpha on astrocyte migration. *FASEB J* 1995; **9**: 1605–13.

Fan L, *et al.* Experimental brain injury induces expression of interleukin-1 beta mRNA in the rat brain. *Brain Res Mol Brain Res* 1995; **30**: 125–30.

Fan L, *et al.* Experimental brain injury induces differential expression of tumor necrosis factor-alpha mRNA in the CNS. *Brain Res Mol Brain Res* 1996; **36**: 287–91.

Fassbender K, *et al.* Temporal profile of release of interleukin-1beta in neurotrauma. *Neurosci Lett* 2000; **284**: 135–8.

Feuerstein GZ, *et al.* The role of cytokines in the neuropathology of stroke and neurotrauma. *Neuroimmunomodulation* 1998; **5**: 143–59.

Furukawa T, *et al.* The glutamate AMPA receptor antagonist, YM872, attenuates cortical tissue loss, regional cerebral edema, and neurological motor deficits after experimental brain injury in rats. *J Neurotrauma* 2003; **20**: 269–78.

Gentleman SM, *et al.* Long-term intracerebral inflammatory

response after traumatic brain injury. *Forensic Sci Int* 2004; **146**: 97–104.

Glabinski AR, *et al.* Chemokine monocyte chemoattractant protein-1 is expressed by astrocytes after mechanical injury to the brain. *J Immunol* 1996; **156**: 4363–8.

Goodman JC, *et al.* Elevation of tumor necrosis factor in head injury. *J Neuroimmunol* 1990; **30**: 213–7.

Graham DI, *et al.* Trauma. In Graham DI, Lantos PL (Eds.) *Greenfield's Neuropathology*, vol. 2. London: Arnold, 2002; pp. 823–98.

Griffin DE. Cytokines in the brain during viral infection: Clues to HIV-associated dementia. *J Clin Invest* 1997; **100**: 2948–51.

Hans VH, *et al.* Interleukin-6 and its soluble receptor in serum and cerebrospinal fluid after cerebral trauma. *Neuroreport* 1999a; **10**: 409–12.

Hans VH, *et al.* Experimental axonal injury triggers interleukin-6 mRNA, protein synthesis and release into cerebrospinal fluid. *J Cereb Blood Flow Metab* 1999b; **19**: 184–94.

Hausmann R, *et al.* Neuronal apoptosis following human brain injury. *Int J Legal Med* 2004; **118**: 32–6.

Hauss-Wegrzyniak B, *et al.* Behavioral and ultrastructural changes induced by chronic neuroinflammation in young rats. *Brain Res* 2000; **859**: 157–66.

Hayakata T, *et al.* Changes in CSF S100B and cytokine concentrations in early-phase severe traumatic brain injury. *Shock* 2004; **22**: 102–7.

Hensler T, *et al.* The effect of additional brain injury on systemic interleukin (IL)-10 and IL-13 levels in trauma patients. *Inflamm Res* 2000; **49**: 524–8.

Herx LM, Yong VW. Interleukin-1 beta is required for the early evolution of reactive astrogliosis following CNS lesion. *J Neuropathol Exp Neurol* 2001; **60**: 961–71.

Hillered L, *et al.* Translational neurochemical research in acute human brain injury: The current status and potential future for cerebral microdialysis. *J Neurotrauma* 2005; **22**: 3–41.

Holmin S, Hojeberg B. In situ detection of intracerebral cytokine expression after human brain contusion. *Neurosci Lett* 2004; **369**: 108–14.

Holmin S, *et al.* Delayed cytokine expression in rat brain following experimental contusion. *J Neurosurg* 1997; **86**: 493–504.

Hua LL, *et al.* Modulation of astrocyte inducible nitric oxide synthase and cytokine expression by interferon beta is associated with induction and inhibition of interferon gamma-activated sequence binding activity. *J Neurochem* 2002; **83**: 1120–8.

Jones NC, *et al.* Antagonism of the interleukin-1 receptor following traumatic brain injury in the mouse reduces the number of nitric oxide synthase-2-positive cells and improves anatomical and functional outcomes. *Eur J Neurosci* 2005; **22**: 72–8.

Kamm K, *et al.* The effect of traumatic brain injury upon the concentration and expression of interleukin-1beta and interleukin-10 in the rat. *J Trauma* 2006; **60**: 152–7.

Kita T, *et al.* The expression of tumor necrosis factor-alpha in the rat brain after fluid percussive injury. *Int J Legal Med* 1997; **110**: 305–11.

Knoblach SM, Faden AI. Interleukin-10 improves outcome and alters proinflammatory cytokine expression after experimental traumatic brain injury. *Exp Neurol* 1998; **153**: 143–51.

Knoblach SM, *et al.* Early neuronal expression of tumor necrosis factor-alpha after experimental brain injury contributes to neurological impairment. *J Neuroimmunol* 1999; **95**: 115–25.

Kossmann T, *et al.* Intrathecal and serum interleukin-6 and the acute-phase response in patients with severe traumatic brain injuries. *Shock* 1995; **4**: 311–7.

Kossmann T, *et al.* Interleukin-6 released in human cerebrospinal fluid following traumatic brain injury may trigger nerve growth factor production in astrocytes. *Brain Res* 1996; **713**: 143–52.

Kossmann T, *et al.* Interleukin-8 released into the cerebrospinal fluid after brain injury is associated with blood–brain barrier dysfunction and nerve growth factor production. *J Cereb Blood Flow Metab* 1997; **17**: 280–9.

Kremlev SG, Palmer C. Interleukin-10 inhibits endotoxin-induced pro-inflammatory cytokines in microglial cell cultures. *J Neuroimmunol* 2005; **162**: 71–80.

Kushi H, *et al.* IL-8 is a key mediator of neuroinflammation in severe traumatic brain injuries. *Acta Neurochir Suppl* 2003; **86**: 347–50.

Lee JI, Burckart GJ. Nuclear factor kappa B: Important transcription factor and therapeutic target. *J Clin Pharmacol* 1998; **38**: 981–93.

Lewen A, *et al.* Free radical pathways in CNS injury. *J Neurotrauma* 2000; **17**: 871–90.

Liberto CM, *et al.* Pro-regenerative properties of cytokine-activated astrocytes. *J Neurochem* 2004; **89**: 1092–100.

Lin HW, *et al.* Astrogliosis is delayed in type 1 interleukin-1 receptor-null mice following a penetrating brain injury. *J Neuroinflammation* 2006; **3**: 15.

Lu KT, *et al.* Extracellular signal-regulated kinase-mediated IL-1-induced cortical neuron damage during traumatic brain injury. *Neurosci Lett* 2005a; **386**: 40–5.

Lu KT, *et al.* Effect of interleukin-1 on traumatic brain injury-induced damage to hippocampal neurons. *J Neurotrauma* 2005b; **22**: 885–95.

Maier B, *et al.* Delayed elevation of soluble tumor necrosis factor receptors p75 and p55 in cerebrospinal fluid and plasma after traumatic brain injury. *Shock* 2006; **26**: 122–7.

Maier B, *et al.* Differential release of interleukins 6, 8, and 10 in cerebrospinal fluid and plasma after traumatic brain injury. *Shock* 2001; **15**: 421–6.

Mantovani A, *et al.* The chemokine system in diverse forms of macrophage activation and polarization. *Trends Immunol* 2004; **25**: 677–86.

Marciano PG, *et al*. Neuron-specific mRNA complexity responses during hippocampal apoptosis after traumatic brain injury. *J Neurosci* 2004; **24**: 2866–76.

Marion DW. *Traumatic Brain Injury*. New York: Thieme, 1999.

Marklund N, *et al*. Administration of monoclonal antibodies neutralizing the inflammatory mediators tumor necrosis factor alpha and interleukin-6 does not attenuate acute behavioral deficits following experimental traumatic brain injury in the rat. *Restor Neurol Neurosci* 2005; **23**: 31–42.

Marmarou A. Pathophysiology of traumatic brain edema: Current concepts. *Acta Neurochir Suppl* 2003; **86**: 7–10.

Mattson MP, *et al*. Roles of nuclear factor kappaB in neuronal survival and plasticity. *J Neurochem* 2000; **74**: 443–56.

Merrill JE, Benveniste EN. Cytokines in inflammatory brain lesions: Helpful and harmful. *Glia* 1996; **19**: 331–8.

Minambres E, *et al*. Correlation between transcranial interleukin-6 gradient and outcome in patients with acute brain injury. *Crit Care Med* 2003; **31**: 933–8.

Modur V, *et al*. Retrograde inflammatory signaling from neutrophils to endothelial cells by soluble interleukin-6 receptor alpha. *J Clin Invest* 1997; **100**: 2752–6.

Molina-Holgado E, *et al*. Induction of COX-2 and PGE(2) biosynthesis by IL-1beta is mediated by PKC and mitogen-activated protein kinases in murine astrocytes. *Br J Pharmacol* 2000; **131**: 152–9.

Morganti-Kossmann CM, *et al*. Production of cytokines following brain injury: Beneficial and deleterious for the damaged tissue. *Mol Psychiat* 1997; **2**: 133–6.

Morganti-Kossmann CM, *et al*. TGF-beta is elevated in the CSF of patients with severe traumatic brain injuries and parallels blood–brain barrier function. *J Neurotrauma* 1999; **16**: 617–28.

Morganti-Kossmann MC, *et al*. Cytokines and neuropathology. *Trends Pharmacol Sci* 1992; **13**: 286–91.

Morganti-Kossmann MC, *et al*. Role of cerebral inflammation after traumatic brain injury: A revisited concept. *Shock* 2001; **16**: 165–77.

Nakajima K, Kohsaka S. Microglia: Neuroprotective and neurotrophic cells in the central nervous system. *Curr Drug Targets Cardiovasc Haematol Disord* 2004; **4**: 65–84.

Narayan RK, *et al*. Clinical trials in head injury. *J Neurotrauma* 2002; **19**: 503–57.

Neidhardt R, *et al*. Relationship of interleukin-10 plasma levels to severity of injury and clinical outcome in injured patients. *J Trauma* 1997; **42**: 863–70.

Norris JG, *et al*. Signal transduction pathways mediating astrocyte IL-6 induction by IL-1 beta and tumor necrosis factor-alpha. *J Immunol* 1994; **152**: 841–50.

O'Neill LAJ, Greene C. Signal transduction pathways activated by the IL-1 receptor family: Ancient signaling machinery in mammals, animals and plants. *J Leukoc Biol* 1998; **63**: 650–7.

Otto VI, *et al*. sICAM-1 and TNF-alpha induce MIP-2 with distinct kinetics in astrocytes and brain microvascular endothelial cells. *J Neurosci Res* 2000; **60**: 733–42.

Penkowa M, *et al*. Impaired inflammatory response and increased oxidative stress and neurodegeneration after brain injury in interleukin-6-deficient mice. *Glia* 2000; **32**: 271–85.

Penkowa M, *et al*. Strongly compromised inflammatory response to brain injury in interleukin-6-deficient mice. *Glia* 1999; **25**: 343–57.

Pinteaux E, *et al*. Expression of interleukin-1 receptors and their role in interleukin-1 actions in murine microglial cells. *J Neurochem* 2002; **83**: 754–63.

Plata-Salaman CR, Ffrench-Mullen JM. Interleukin-1 beta depresses calcium currents in CA1 hippocampal neurons at pathophysiological concentrations. *Brain Res Bull* 1992; **29**: 221–3.

Pleines UE, *et al*. Soluble ICAM-1 in CSF coincides with the extent of cerebral damage in patients with severe traumatic brain injury. *J Neurotrauma* 1998; **15**: 399–409.

Pober JS, Cotran RS. Cytokines and endothelial cell biology. *Physiol Rev* 1990; **70**: 427–51.

Povlishock JT, Christman CW. The pathobiology of traumatically induced axonal injury in animals and humans: A review of current thoughts. *J Neurotrauma* 1995; **12**: 555–64.

Probert L, *et al*. TNF-alpha transgenic and knockout models of CNS inflammation and degeneration. *J Neuroimmunol* 1997; **72**: 137–41.

Rancan M, *et al*. Upregulation of ICAM-1 and MCP-1 but not of MIP-2 and sensorimotor deficit in response to traumatic axonal injury in rats. *J Neurosci Res* 2001; **63**: 438–46.

Ransohoff RM, Tani M. Do chemokines mediate leukocyte recruitment in post-traumatic CNS inflammation? *Trends Neurosci* 1998; **21**: 154–9.

Rhodes JK, *et al*. Expression of interleukin-6 messenger RNA in a rat model of diffuse axonal injury. *Neurosci Lett* 2002; **335**: 1–4.

Robinson TE, Justice JB Jr. *Microdialysis in the Neurosciences*. Amsterdam: Elsevier, 1991.

Romano M, *et al*. Role of IL-6 and its soluble receptor in induction of chemokines and leukocyte recruitment. *Immunity* 1997; **6**: 315–25.

Rosenberg GA, *et al*. Tumor necrosis factor-alpha-induced gelatinase B causes delayed opening of the blood–brain barrier: An expanded therapeutic window. *Brain Res* 1995; **703**: 151–5.

Ross SA, *et al*. The presence of tumor necrosis factor in CSF and plasma after severe head injury. *Br J Neurosurg* 1994; **8**: 419–25.

Rostworowski M, *et al*. Astrogliosis in the neonatal and adult murine brain post-trauma: elevation of inflammatory cytokines and the lack of requirement for endogenous interferon-gamma. *J Neurosci* 1997; **17**: 3664–74.

Rothwell N. Interleukin-1 and neuronal injury: Mechanisms, modification, and therapeutic potential. *Brain Behav Immun* 2003; **17**: 152–7.

Rothwell NJ. Functions and mechanisms of interleukin 1 in the brain. *Trends Pharmacol Sci* 1991; **12**: 430–6.

Rothwell NJ. Cytokines – killers in the brain? *J Physiol* 1999; **514**: 3–17.

Sahuquillo J, et al. Diffuse axonal injury after severe head trauma. A clinico-pathological study. *Acta Neurochir (Wien)* 1989; **101**: 149–58.

Scherbel U, et al. Differential acute and chronic responses of tumor necrosis factor-deficient mice to experimental brain injury. *Proc Natl Acad Sci USA* 1999; **96**: 8721–6.

Schmidt OI, et al. Tumor necrosis factor-mediated inhibition of interleukin-18 in the brain: A clinical and experimental study in head-injured patients and in a murine model of closed head injury. *J Neuroinflam* 2004; **1**: 13.

Sherwood ER, Prough DS. Interleukin-8, neuroinflammation, and secondary brain injury. *Crit Care Med* 2000; **28**: 1221–3.

Shimonkevitz R, et al. Transient monocyte release of interleukin-10 in response to traumatic brain injury. *Shock* 1999; **12**: 10–6.

Shohami E, et al. Inhibition of tumor necrosis factor alpha (TNFalpha) activity in rat brain is associated with cerebroprotection after closed head injury. *J Cereb Blood Flow Metab* 1996; **16**: 378–84.

Shohami E, et al. Cytokine production in the brain following closed head injury: Dexanabinol (HU-211) is a novel TNF-alpha inhibitor and an effective neuroprotectant. *J Neuroimmunol* 1997; **72**: 169–77.

Shohami E, et al. Dual role of tumor necrosis factor alpha in brain injury. *Cytokine Growth Factor Rev* 1999; **10**: 119–30.

Shohami E, et al. Closed head injury triggers early production of TNF alpha and IL-6 by brain tissue. *J Cereb Blood Flow Metab* 1994; **14**: 615–9.

Singhal A, et al. Association between cerebrospinal fluid interleukin-6 concentrations and outcome after severe human traumatic brain injury. *J Neurotrauma* 2002; **19**: 929–37.

Stahel PF, et al. Intracerebral complement C5a receptor (CD88) expression is regulated by TNF and lymphotoxin-alpha following closed head injury in mice. *J Neuroimmunol* 2000a; **109**: 164–72.

Stahel PF, et al. Experimental closed head injury: Analysis of neurological outcome, blood–brain barrier dysfunction, intracranial neutrophil infiltration, and neuronal cell death in mice deficient in genes for pro-inflammatory cytokines. *J Cereb Blood Flow Metab* 2000b; **20**: 369–80.

Stamatovic SM, et al. Monocyte chemoattractant protein-1 regulation of blood–brain barrier permeability. *J Cereb Blood Flow Metab* 2005; **25**: 593–606.

Stover JF, et al. Temporal profile of cerebrospinal fluid glutamate, interleukin-6, and tumor necrosis factor-alpha in relation to brain edema and contusion following controlled cortical impact injury in rats. *Neurosci Lett* 2000; **288**: 25–8.

Sullivan PG, et al. Exacerbation of damage and altered NF-kappaB activation in mice lacking tumor necrosis factor receptors after traumatic brain injury. *J Neurosci* 1999; **19**: 6248–56.

Swartz KR, et al. Interleukin-6 promotes post-traumatic healing in the central nervous system. *Brain Res* 2001; **896**: 86–95.

Tasci A, et al. Prognostic value of interleukin-1 beta levels after acute brain injury. *Neurol Res* 2003; **25**: 871–4.

Taupin V, et al. Increase in IL-6, IL-1 and TNF levels in rat brain following traumatic lesion. Influence of pre- and post-traumatic treatment with Ro5 4864, a peripheral-type (p site) benzodiazepine ligand. *J Neuroimmunol* 1993; **42**: 177–85.

Tchelingerian JL, et al. Differential oligodendroglial expression of the tumor necrosis factor receptors in vivo and in vitro. *J Neurochem* 1995; **65**: 2377–80.

Teasdale G, Jennett B. Assessment of coma and impaired consciousness. A practical scale. *Lancet* 1974; **2**: 81–4.

Tehranian R, et al. Improved recovery and delayed cytokine induction after closed head injury in mice with central overexpression of the secreted isoform of the interleukin-1 receptor antagonist. *J Neurotrauma* 2002; **19**: 939–51.

Thibeault I, et al. Regulation of the gene encoding the monocyte chemoattractant protein 1 (MCP-1) in the mouse and rat brain in response to circulating LPS and proinflammatory cytokines. *J Comp Neurol* 2001; **434**: 461–77.

Toulmond S, Rothwell NJ. Interleukin-1 receptor antagonist inhibits neuronal damage caused by fluid percussion injury in the rat. *Brain Res* 1995; **671**: 261–6.

Unterberg AW, et al. Edema and brain trauma. *Neuroscience* 2004; **129**: 1021–9.

Whalen MJ, et al. Interleukin-8 is increased in cerebrospinal fluid of children with severe head injury. *Crit Care Med* 2000; **28**: 929–34.

Winter CD, et al. A microdialysis method for the recovery of IL-1beta, IL-6 and nerve growth factor from human brain in vivo. *J Neurosci Meth* 2002; **119**: 45–50.

Winter CD, et al. Raised parenchymal interleukin-6 levels correlate with improved outcome after traumatic brain injury. *Brain* 2004; **127**: 315–20.

Woiciechowsky C, et al. Sympathetic activation triggers systemic interleukin-10 release in immunodepression induced by brain injury. *Nat Med* 1998; **4**: 808–13.

Woodroofe MN, et al. Detection of interleukin-1 and interleukin-6 in adult rat brain, following mechanical injury, by in vivo microdialysis: Evidence of a role for microglia in cytokine production. *J Neuroimmunol* 1991; **33**: 227–36.

Xiao BG, *et al*. Shift from anti- to proinflammatory cytokine profiles in microglia through LPS-

or IFN-gamma-mediated pathways. *Neuroreport* 1996; **7**: 1893–8.

Yatsiv I, *et al*. Elevated intracranial IL-18 in humans and mice after traumatic brain injury and

evidence of neuroprotective effects of IL-18-binding protein after experimental closed head injury. *J Cereb Blood Flow Metab* 2002; **22**: 971–8.

HIV-associated neurocognitive disorders: clinical features and therapeutic challenges

Nicoline Schiess and Justin C. McArthur

Introduction

This chapter focuses on the evolution, clinical features and treatment of HIV-associated neurocognitive disorders (HAND) from the pre-treatment era to the present. The definition of HIV-dementia (HIV-D) has now been expanded to include less severe forms, such as minor cognitive motor disorder (MCMD) and asymptomatic neurocognitive impairment (ANI) (Antinori *et al.*, 2007). Recently revised diagnostic criteria and the utility of neuro-imaging and laboratory tests are discussed. Medical treatment, including central nervous system (CNS) penetration and completed treatment trials are summarized.

Evolution and prevalence of HAND

Since it first came to the world's attention in the early 1980s, the spectrum of the medical conditions associated with HIV/AIDS has expanded dramatically. This is particularly apparent in relation to the cognitive changes accompanying the disease. In 1987, this was emphasized when HIV dementia (HIV-D) was acknowledged as an AIDS indicator illness. Also called HIV encephalopathy and AIDS dementia complex, HIV-D was characterized then by a subcortical dementia which progresses over weeks to months that includes cognitive and behavioral changes such as short-term memory loss, apathy, and mental slowing. In addition, motor symptoms are often present in the form of tremor, fine motor-movement difficulties, and gait dysfunction (Navia *et al.*, 1986). Minor cognitive motor disorder (MCMD, or recently renamed MND) represents a milder form of HIV-D, and indeed with highly active antiretroviral therapy (HAART) the more severe forms of HIV-D are much less common. One particular point to emphasize is the continued high prevalence of measurable cognitive abnormalities even in medically asymptomatic HIV+ individuals receiving HAART. In one cohort of 46 individuals who had advanced HIV infection, the majority had undetectable plasma HIV RNA levels, but 19 had asymptomatic neurocognitive impairment. This suggests that HAART has not succeeded in eliminating HAND. Before HAART was introduced, HIV-D had an annual incidence of 7% among patients with AIDS, and it was estimated that 20–30% of all AIDS patients would ultimately develop HIV-D (McArthur *et al.*, 1993). With the advent of HAART, the incidence of HIV-D decreased, but, as those with HIV infection live longer, the overall number of people infected expands, and the prevalence of the disease has actually doubled since the early 1990s (McArthur *et al.*, 2003). The HIV-associated neurocognitive disorders have been recognized in most countries, including resource-limited countries, and comparable cross-sectional prevalence rates have been reported. For example, the Asia–Pacific NeuroAIDS Consortium surveyed 8 countries and found an overall rate of 12% in a cohort where two-thirds were using HAART (Wright *et al.*, 2008). In Australia, the proportion of AIDS patients diagnosed with HIV-D actually increased from 5.2% in 1993 to 6.8% in 2000 (Sacktor, 2002). A recent preliminary study from China reported that the proportion of patients with HIV-D was 17%, higher than seen in developed countries (Wu *et al.*, 2007) and in Kampala, Uganda, the cross-sectional frequency in an untreated outpatient setting was an alarming 31% (Wong *et al.*, 2007). New screening tests such as the International HIV Dementia Scale (IHDS) could make the diagnosis of HIV-D easier in cross-cultural studies (Sacktor *et al.*, 2005a, 2005b).

The onset of either HIV-D or MCMD is usually insidious and can be overlooked in cursory examinations of patients. Although it can initially appear only subtly, it can have deleterious effects for the patient in regard to medication compliance, employability, driving skills, and other everyday functions in work or the

Inflammatory Diseases of the Central Nervous System, ed. T. Kilpatrick, R. M. Ransohoff and S. Wesselingh. Published by Cambridge University Press. © Cambridge University Press 2010

complex activities of daily living (van Gorp *et al.*, 1999; Wilkie *et al.*, 1998; Heaton *et al.*, 2004; Marcotte *et al.*, 2004). The prognosis is about 3.5 years in HAART-treated individuals (Dore *et al.*, 2003), but was less than 6 months before HAART (McArthur *et al.*, 1993, 2003). As awareness and knowledge of this disorder increases, the definition of HAND is expanding. The National Institute of Mental Health (NIMH) recently added "asymptomatic neurocognitive impairment" (ANI) to the definition of HAND in an effort to recognize the subtle asymptomatic, yet clinically significant, cognitive impairment that often heralds the more severe forms of HAND, and is predictive of HIV encephalitis (Cherner *et al.*, 2002; Antinori *et al.*, 2007). In many ways, ANI and MCMD are analogous to the minor cognitive impairment that can eventually transform into Alzheimer's disease.

There are several identified risk-factors for HIV-D, including anemia, low CD4 counts (Childs *et al.*, 1999), intravenous and non-intravenous drug abuse (Woody *et al.*, 1999), systemic HIV symptoms (McArthur *et al.*, 1993), and increased age. Recently, declining platelet counts and hemoglobin levels were noted to be predictive of HIV-D in a cohort with advanced HIV disease (Wachtmann *et al.*, 2006), suggesting that changes within the bone marrow could "drive" the subsequent development of neurological disease. Highly active antiretroviral therapy can produce significant improvements in the neurocognitive deficits that characterize HIV-D or MCMD, and usually parallel immune system reconstitution (Figure 15.1).

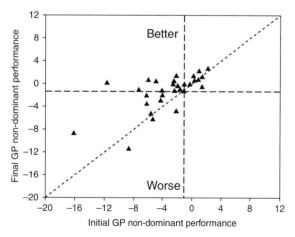

Figure 15.1 Neurocognitive improvement on the grooved-pegboard (GP) test following initiation of HAART therapy. Movement up and to the left indicates improvement, and as can be seen, most individuals respond. (From McArthur JC, with permission. Davis *et al.*, 2002.)

In HAART-treated individuals, as CD4 counts and plasma HIV RNA levels respond, so have the characteristics of HIV-related dementia changed substantially. As patients' life expectancies increase with successful HAART, cortical aspects of dementia have begun to surface (Cysique *et al.*, 2006a, 2006b) superimposed on the well-known subcortical deficits of HIV-D; in particular, retrograde amnesia and loss of remote memories are indicative of the diffuse cortical changes that can occur (Sadek *et al.*, 2004). In addition, pathological studies have confirmed that it is not just subcortical areas that are damaged during HAND. For example, brains from individuals dying with AIDS showed neuronal loss in the frontal cortex (Wiley *et al.*, 1986; Everall *et al.*, 1999), which correlated with the severity of HIV-D prior to death. In fact, in one study, cortical neuronal changes in the hippocampus represented the strongest predictor of HIV-D (Moore *et al.*, 2006).

Clinical features of HIV-D and MCMD

Features before HAART

Without HAART, HIV-D generally presents as the subacute or chronic onset of a subcortical dementia. It begins to manifest only with the advanced immunosuppression of late-stage HIV/AIDS with CD4 counts <200, and is generally rare in patients with well-controlled viral loads and high/normal CD4 counts. It was particularly unusual to encounter HIV-D among so-called "long-term non-progressors", and indeed, studies from homosexual or bisexual men in the Multicenter AIDS Cohort study, and men and women in the AIDS Link to Intravenous Drug Use in the 1980s, defined no significant neurocognitive decline in medically asymptomatic HIV+ individuals (Egan *et al.*, 1990; Selnes *et al.*, 1990).

In the pre-HAART era, HIV-D initially presented subtly, with the earliest and most frequent symptoms being forgetfulness, gait difficulty, difficulty with concentration, depressive symptoms, and delayed thought processing. Behavioral symptoms of apathy and social withdrawal were common. Leg weakness, loss of balance, and changes in handwriting were motor symptoms that also appeared early in the disease (Navia *et al.*, 1986).

Although neurocognitive deficits were found to usually occur in conjunction with constitutional symptoms of AIDS (Miller *et al.*, 1990), the "real-world" impact of neurocognitive impairment, of itself, can have a profound effect on everyday functioning (Heaton *et al.*, 2004). Furthermore, HIV-D appears to have an independent negative effect on survival, above and beyond the systemic features (Mayeux *et al.*, 1993). In some cases, HIV-D can be the presenting symptom of HIV/AIDS (Navia and Price, 1987). Depression can also be a serious aspect of HIV and can confound performances on neurocognitive testing. Depression, like HIV-D, has shown improvement secondary to initiation of HAART (Gibbie *et al.*, 2006). Revised research criteria for HAND, classified as either HIV-associated asymptomatic neurocognitive impairment, mild neurocognitive disorder, or dementia, are available.

Today with HAART as the standard of care, three subtypes of HIV-D, defined by their temporal course have emerged:

1. "subacute progressive" dementia very similar to the above description of HIV-D in the pre-HAART era;
2. "chronic active" dementia in patients who are either non-compliant with medication or who have viral resistance to HAART; and
3. "chronic inactive" dementia in patients who are stable and compliant with their treatment regimens (McArthur *et al.*, 2003).

Recently, an NIMH consensus conference has revised and expanded these terms (Table 15.1) (Antinori *et al.*, 2007).

The importance of recognizing and treating the early onset of HAND cannot be over-emphasized. Even mild neuropsychological impairment should be taken seriously because of the functional importance of the deficit, including poorer medication compliance and higher rates of mortality (Hinkin *et al.*, 2002). Lifestyle impacts such as unemployment, increasing need for help with activities of daily living and depression are often underappreciated impacts of HIV-D or MND (Heaton *et al.*, 2004). There are multiple, practical aids to offer patients to help with their daily activities. For example, medication adherence difficulties can frequently be circumvented with verbal prompting devices, which have been shown to be effective in neurocognitively impaired individuals (Andrade *et al.*, 2005). To date, no medication regimen other than HAART has been shown to halt or reverse the onset of HIV-associated neurocognitive decline and while severe HIV-D has declined secondary to HAART, mild cognitive impairment is still prevalent and a source of morbidity and mortality (Neuenburg *et al.*, 2002; Cysique *et al.*, 2006a).

Confounding illnesses

One of the challenges in making an initial diagnosis of HIV-D is the multitude of confounding factors that can mimic the neuropsychiatric features of HAND (Table 15.2). Some of these illnesses, such as trauma, tuberculosis, syphilis, drug abuse, and cerebrovascular disease, can be ruled out with imaging and laboratory methods. Other disorders like acute HIV leukoencephalitis, depression, immune reconstitution syndrome (IRIS), CNS escape, some opportunistic infections, and neurodegenerative diseases such as Alzheimer's are more challenging to diagnose (Wojna *et al.*, 2007). An important caveat is that these conditions often exist simultaneously and a patient who tests positive for one of the above confounding illnesses can still have HIV-D.

Immune reconstitution inflammatory syndrome (IRIS)

When assessing cognitive changes in the context of HIV and HAART, it is important to include in the differential the possibility of immune reconstitution inflammatory syndrome (IRIS). Also known as immune reconstitution syndrome (IRS) and immune reconstitution disease (IRD), IRIS is yet another new disease entity associated with HIV. The IRIS consists

Table 15.1 Theoretical temporal features of HAND with HAART (NIMH)

Active HIV disease	Poorly controlled HIV replication and no/incomplete immunological recovery
Inactive HIV disease	Well controlled HIV replication and immunological recovery
Progressive HAND	Equivalent to "subacute" or "chronic active" in previous classifications
Stable HAND	Fixed neurological deficits; previously called "chronic inactive"
Improving HAND	Improving or regressing neurological or neurocognitive deficits
Fluctuating HAND	Fluctuating neurological or neurocognitive deficits

Table 15.2 Confounding illnesses for HAND and distinguishing features

Confounding illness	Diagnosis
Trauma	History/imaging
Cerebrovascular disease	MRI with DWI and perfusion imaging
Opportunistic infections: Toxoplasmosis, Primary CNS lymphoma, Cryptococcus-PML	Imaging; ring-enhancing mass lesions; large contrast enhancing lesion(s) with edema; non-enhancing mass lesions in basal ganglia with meningitis; patchy, multifocal subcortical white matter changes on MRI
Anxiety, depression	Psychiatric evaluation
Alcohol consumption	History/urinary toxicology screen
Drug abuse	History/urinary toxicology screen
Syphilis/tuberculosis	Laboratory tests/history/CSF and imaging
Metabolic encephalopathy	Laboratory tests (electrolytes, thyroid function tests, ammonia, urine analysis)
Vitamin B_{12} deficiency	Plasma B_{12}, methylmalonic acid, homocysteine, MCV
IRIS	1. Worsening neurological status. 2. New/worsening neuroradiological findings. 3. A decrease in plasma viral load of >1 log 10. 4. Presence of symptoms not explained by a newly acquired disease or by the usual course of a previously acquired illness. 5. Histopathology demonstrating T cell infiltration (Riedel *et al.*, 2006).
CNS escape	CSF HIV RNA levels >> plasma HIV RNA levels (Wendel *et al.*, 2003)
Alzheimer's	Neurocognitive testing should reveal clear cortical dementia vs. subcortical. Imaging shows atrophy or is normal. FDG-PET imaging shows frontotemporal hypometabolism. PIB-PET scans show amyloid.

of an unforeseen clinical deterioration after the initiation of HAART that is attributable to recovery of the immune system. Inclusive criteria include:

1. diagnosis of AIDS;
2. treatment with HAART;
3. infectious or inflammatory (autoimmune) symptoms appearing after the initiation of HAART; and
4. new symptoms unexplainable by new infection or side effects of HAART (Shelburne *et al.*, 2002).

The IRIS can affect multiple parts of the body and has a variable presentation according to the infectious agent to which the exuberant inflammatory response is directed. Infectious agents seen with IRIS include *Mycobacterium avium* complex, cryptococcus, cytomegalovirus, herpes zoster, *Pneumocystis carinii* and JC virus, which causes progressive multifocal leukoencephalopathy (PML) (Shelburne *et al.*, 2002). In some series approximately 15–25% of HAART patients will develop some form of IRIS, and this risk increases to 45% in the setting of an already present opportunistic infection (Shelburne *et al.*,

2006). Recently, it has been identified that HIV encephalitis can manifest as a part of IRIS (Venkataramana *et al.*, 2006), with neurological worsening that may respond to steroids. The frequency of this entity is uncertain.

The diagnosis of CNS IRIS is a difficult challenge, as cases can mistakenly be attributed to worsening of already extant HIV-D or CNS opportunistic infections. Thus, in addition to the initial systemic criteria proposed for IRIS, new guidelines have been added specifically for the CNS and include:

1. worsening neurological status;
2. new or worsening neuroradiological findings;
3. a decrease in plasma viral load of >1 log 10;
4. presence of symptoms not explained by a newly acquired disease or by the usual course of a previously acquired illness;
5. histopathology demonstrating T cell infiltration (Riedel *et al.*, 2006).

Treatment for IRIS currently consists of corticosteroids and possible changes in HAART, with variable results (Venkataramana *et al.*, 2006).

CNS escape

The HIV virus enters the brain very early in the course of infection and then becomes latent within the relative sanctuary of the brain. An important question that arises when patients are on HAART is the idea of viral CNS escape (Wendel *et al.*, 2003). With viral load well controlled in the systemic circulation, can the hidden virus in the brain escape through the blood–brain barrier (BBB) back into the circulation and re-infect the patient? The penetration of HAART through the BBB is a challenge, as the tight junctions on blood vessel endothelium provide a significant barrier. Also, drugs that are highly bound to proteins are less able to cross the BBB (Ellis *et al.*, 2007) and the physical characteristics of the drugs themselves, such as molecular size, charge, and lipophilic characteristics, can affect penetration. The CNS escape phenomenon appears, however, to be a rare event as most of the antiretroviral agents in use have relatively strong CNS penetration, which leads to decreased CNS HIV replication, as measured by CSF HIV RNA levels (McArthur *et al.*, 2006).

Disease co-factors

A host genetic susceptibility for HAND has been proposed for some time, focusing on various immune response genes, including tumor necrosis factor-alpha (Quasney *et al.*, 2001), the monocyte chemoattractant protein-1 (MCP-1/CCL-2) (Gonzales *et al.*, 2002), and others. To date, these putative associations have not influenced clinical practice (McArthur *et al.*, 2005). The HIV infection often co-exists with other diseases or conditions that can pose a significant confound in evaluation, or independently add to the neurocognitive effects of HIV. For example, chemical dependencies with alcohol and drugs are very common, as well as co-infection with other infectious agents. Hepatitis C, in particular, has been shown to have a significant correlation with HIV and occurs in 50–80% of patients who acquire HIV through intravenous drug abuse (Sulkowski *et al.*, 2000). The hepatitis C virus can impact on neurocognitive performance either indirectly through hepatic effects, or directly through pathological changes in the brain itself. The liver damage associated with co-infection of hepatitis C and HIV is a common and challenging clinical problem. Hepatic fibrosis that accompanies hepatitis C is more aggressive when there is co-infection with HIV (Benhamou *et al.*, 1999). Compounding the duel insult of HIV/hepatitis C

infection on the liver is the added hepatotoxicity of antiretroviral compounds. Antiretroviral therapy increases hepatotoxicity: however, this varies between different types of medications. For example, patients taking ritonavir have a fivefold higher chance of developing severe hepatotoxicity when compared with other antiretroviral drugs. It is important to note that this is usually reversible and withholding antiretroviral therapy on the basis of hepatotoxicity is not recommended (Sulkowski *et al.*, 2000).

To date, hepatitis C has not been identified within the brain, but imaging studies using PET have shown changes in brain function. Neuropsychologically, hepatitis C positive patients are more likely to meet criteria for HIV-D than hepatitis C negative patients and they have worse performances on the Digit Symbol test (Morgello *et al.*, 2005). Hepatits C-positive patients also have more depressive symptoms when compared to patients infected with HIV alone (Clifford *et al.*, 2005). Hepatitis C can therefore be an important co-morbidity for HIV with regard to neurocognitive function.

Drug abuse and dependency have a strong association with HIV either because of concomitant lifestyle choices or because their administration provides a portal for infection. Common drugs in order of frequency include alcohol, marijuana, nitrite inhalants, amphetamines, cocaine, and hallucinogens (Woody *et al.*, 1999). Substance abuse disorders can interfere with the treatment of HIV through direct effects on the brain and cognitive function of patients, as well as with psychosocial aspects that have influence upon compliance with medication and medical follow-up (Ferrando and Batki, 2000). The addition of frequent accompanying psychiatric and behavioral issues further complicates attempts to treat these patients. Drug abuse alone has been associated with macrophage and microglial upregulation into the brain, and HIV-positive drug abusers have increased lymphocytic infiltration in the brain compared to HIV-positive non-drug abusers and HIV-negative drug abusers (Tomlinson *et al.*, 1999).

Of the non-injectable drugs of abuse, methamphetamine is frequently associated with HIV and is often accompanied by high-risk sexual activity in homosexual men (Woody *et al.*, 1999). It is known that methamphetamines alone can cause vascular injury, ischemia, and neuronal death from excitotoxic injury caused by increased dopaminergic and glutaminergic activity (Stephans and Yamamoto, 1994). When combined with HIV, there are additive effects on brain metabolites that can be seen with MR spectroscopy imaging (Taylor *et al.*, 2000) and also neuropathologically. The frontal cortices of patients with combined methamphetamine abuse and HIV have been found to contain a smaller number of calbindin positive interneurons, as well as microgliosis (Langford *et al.*, 2003). These interneurons also had neuritic processes that were suggestive of aberrant sprouting. While the exact mechanism by which methamphetamine and HIV have additive effects is, as yet, undetermined, there is increasing evidence that methamphetamine-mediated damage on neuronal function in the dopaminergic pathways is a result of mitochondrial dysfunction and oxidative stress (Nath *et al.*, 2002). Clinically, this translates into a higher risk of neuropsychological impairment in methamphetamine-abusing HIV patients (Rippeth *et al.*, 2004; Carey *et al.*, 2006).

CSF changes in HIV-D

In both clinical research and clinical practice, the establishment of a definitive diagnosis of HIV-D or MND and the monitoring of the activity of the neurological disease is largely a clinical judgment by the physician and is reliant upon neuropsychological testing. There are currently no biomarkers available that can either make a non-subjective diagnosis or accurately predict the course of the illness. Laboratory analyses are used to rule out confounding illnesses that often accompany the spectrum of HIV/AIDS, but are not helpful in establishing a concrete diagnosis in and of themselves. The cerebrospinal fluid (CSF) is the logical specimen to use for HAND analysis, as it is the closest fluid to the brain and is readily accessible. In the pre-HAART era, HIV RNA was consistently found in the CSF of patients with HIV-D, and could predict progression to HIV-D (Ellis *et al.*, 1997, 2002). The situation is very different for those on HAART, however, and CSF HIV RNA levels do not correlate with the degree of dementia in patients on HAART (McArthur *et al.*, 2004; Sevigny *et al.*, 2004). The AIDS Clinical Trials Group (ACTG) 736 study team recently showed that CSF RNA was rarely detectable when plasma HIV RNA was <1000 copies/mL and that for those with plasma HIV RNA >1000 copies/ml, recipients of an antiretroviral regimen with good CNS penetration were 5 times more likely to achieve CSF suppression. Furthermore, achieving undetectable HIV RNA in both CSF and plasma was 2.6 times more likely when the HAART regimen had good CNS penetration.

These results suggest that an antiretroviral regimen with good CNS penetration is important in achieving suppression of HIV RNA in both CSF and plasma (Marra *et al.*, 2006).

Considering the lack of any validated individual CSF biomarkers, it could prove more useful eventually to employ a combined panel of CSF markers instead (Antinori *et al.*, 2005). In addition to viral markers such as CSF HIV RNA, immunological markers such as beta-2-microglobulin, CCL-2, neopterin, and quinolinic acid could have utility. In the pre-HAART era, CSF levels of the macrophage activation marker, neopterin, were higher in patients with HAND (Fuchs *et al.*, 1989; Brew *et al.*, 1990). Levels of beta-2-microglobulin within the CSF of greater than 3.8 mg/l were found to be a useful marker for HIV-D (McArthur *et al.*, 1992). The CCL-2, a monocyte chemoattractant, has been associated with CNS HIV replication through its effects on monocyte attraction (Monteiro de Almeida *et al.*, 2005). Further potential CSF biomarkers to include in a putative combined panel are brain-specific markers such as dopamine, 14–3–3 nitrosylated proteins (Li *et al.*, personal communication), S-100 (Pemberton *et al.*, 2001), tau proteins (Berger *et al.*, 1994; Green *et al.*, 2000; Miller *et al.*, 2000), neurofilament proteins (Abdulle *et al.*, 2007) and markers of oxidative stress (Bandaru *et al.*, 2007). These latter markers could potentially differentiate active, progressive HAND from inactive disease. Proteomic and metabolic assays are also under active exploration (Ciborowski *et al.*, 2007). The hope is that over the next few years, biomarker development will succeed such that validated and reliable CSF markers can be brought into widespread use either for diagnosis, or for the early recognition of progressive HAND.

Radiological features of HIV-D

Concomitant with the search for a laboratory biomarker of HAND has been the use of neuro-imaging for diagnosis and monitoring of neurocognitive impairment. Thus far, the most advantageous use of neuro-imaging has been in excluding opportunistic CNS infections and lymphomas in HIV patients who show cognitive changes. However, certain characteristics of HIV-D have increasingly been identified as imaging has become more sophisticated. In both pre- and post-HAART patients, cerebral atrophy and, particularly, caudate atrophy have been shown to be key radiographic characteristics of HIV-D (Jakobsen *et al.*, 1989; Dal Pan *et al.*, 1992; Stout *et al.*, 1998). In addition, thinning of the cerebral cortex in certain regions has a strong association with cognitive impairment. For example, demented HIV patients had cortical thinning in the frontal lobes in comparison to non-demented patients who showed thinning in the striatum, white matter, and posterior cortex, instead (Thompson *et al.*, 2005). As the frontal lobe controls attention, working memory, and executive functioning, atrophy of this critical area correlates well with the clinical features of HIV-D. Patients with HIV-D can also show areas of diffuse demyelination and vacuolation in the periventricular regions that eventually fuse to form a diffuse hyperintensity on FLAIR images (Bakshi, 2004) (Figure 15.2).

Diffusion tensor imaging (DTI) is a special type of MRI that measures the restricted diffusion of water in brain tissues, particularly white matter tracts where the diffusion of water molecules occurs more easily because of the architecture of the parallel bundles of myelinated axons. It has detected abnormalities in the white matter of patients with HIV that correlate with disease severity and inversely with HAART usage (Filippi *et al.*, 2001). Other studies have shown that DTI is also a useful tool to link HIV pathology in neuroanatomic areas with specific cognitive characteristics in HIV-infected patients (Ragin *et al.*, 2005).

Magnetization transfer imaging (MTR) is based on the interaction between water free protons and macromolecular protons in restricted environments. The MTR has been useful in distinguishing the brains of HIV-D patients from controls and findings were associated with the severity of neurocognitive function in the HIV patients (Ragin *et al.*, 2004).

Magnetic resonance spectroscopy (MRS) combines the benefit of anatomical location of MRI with the spectroscopic information provided by nuclear magnetic resonance (NMR). It enables a regional analysis of the profile of key metabolites within the brain. Asymptomatic HIV patients show reductions in *N*-acetyl-aspartate (NAA), with corresponding increases in myo-inositol (MI) and choline (Cho)/creatine (Cr) (Tarasow *et al.*, 2003). These changes have been shown to increase with progressive neuropsychological impairment (Sacktor *et al.*, 2005a, 2005b) and to respond to HAART therapy (Tarasow *et al.*, 2004).

Functional MRI (fMRI) records changing oxygen levels in the blood while it traverses cerebral tissues. These changes are an indicator of the relative metabolic activity of neurons. The greatest advantage of fMRI is the ability to measure brain activity during cognitive tasks undertaken whilst in the scanner. In studying HIV-associated changes with fMRI, it was found that there were differences in the deep gray matter of patients with HIV-associated cognitive dysfunction when compared with normal controls (Tracey *et al.*, 1998).

Single-photon emission computed tomography (SPECT) assesses cerebral blood flow. Using SPECT scans it is possible to detect changes in cerebral blood flow in HIV-infected patients when compared to HIV-negative controls (Costa *et al.*, 1988; Sacktor *et al.*, 1995b) and reduced global cerebral uptake has been associated with impairments in motor speed performance (Sacktor *et al.*, 1995a). The SPECT scans enable the identification of HIV-associated abnormalities prior to the development of changes on CT or MRI scans and thus provide a valuable tool to identify and monitor patients at risk for HIV dementia (Tatsch *et al.*, 1990).

Positron emission tomography (PET) scanning uses radioactive tracers to monitor glucose metabolism in specific areas of the brain. Abnormalities on PET have been found in the pre-frontal and pre-motor regions specifically in HIV seropositive patients (Pascal *et al.*, 1991), and could be even more sensitive to neurocognitive changes than traditional neuropsychological testing (Hinkin *et al.*, 1995). In addition to the decreased metabolism in the frontal

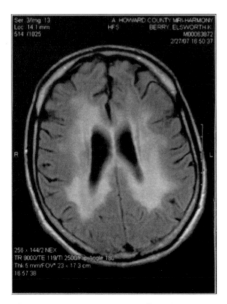

Figure 15.2 FLAIR MRI image of HIV-D. Lesions are symmetric, diffuse and loosely circumscribed, sparing the U-fibers.

and motor regions, hypermetabolism has been found in the basal ganglia and the parietal lobe in HIV-infected patients in some studies (Hinkin et al., 1995); the basal ganglia changes did, however, evolve to hypometabolism with progressive disease (Tucker et al., 2004). Temporal lobe changes identified with PET also appear to be more prevalent in the post-HAART era (Brew, 2004). Newer ligands targeting the peripheral benzodiazepine receptor could be useful in detecting inflammation within the brain (Hammoud et al., 2005).

To date, with the exception of "conventional" MRI, these techniques have only been used for research purposes.

Pathology

The HIV enters the CNS early after the onset of infection and often prior to the appearance of any cognitive or neurological abnormalities (Resnick et al., 1988). However, we believe that after this early entry, the virus is controlled and does not replicate until immunosuppression has developed. Once the virus enters the body it is internalized into host cells via the CD4 receptor, with CXCR4 or CCR5 serving as co-receptors.

Ingress into the brain is probably through circulating activated monocytes, and changes in the bone marrow could allow for the release of greater numbers of activated cells into the circulation (Figure 15.3) (Gartner, 2000). Neuropathologically, the infection results in microglial nodules, astrocytosis, formation of multinucleated giant cells and, indirectly, neuronal loss (Navia et al., 1986). The primary cells infected in the brain are perivascular macrophages. Although astrocytes are known to be infected and to produce viral proteins, the viral genome is not replicated in these cells as it is in monocyte/macrophages (Saito et al., 1994). Neurons themselves are seldom infected by HIV; however, neuronal loss and atrophy is a common finding. Neuronal damage and subsequent death is thought to be mediated via an indirect effect of toxic viral proteins or host cell molecules such as platelet activating factor (PAF), nitric oxide or cytokines (Merrill et al., 1992; Jassoy et al., 1993; Gelbard et al., 1994). The HIV viral proteins tat, nef and rev are thought to play a particularly deleterious role in the dysfunction and ultimate death of neurons (Tornatore et al., 1994; Ranki et al., 1995; Rumbaugh et al., 2006). Neuronal loss is predominantly prevalent in the basal

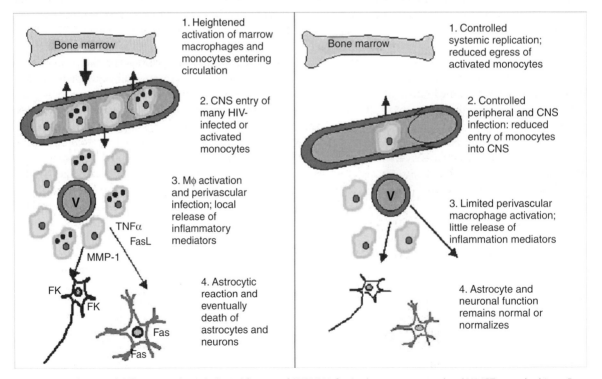

Figure 15.3 Theoretical differences in the pathological features of CNS HIV infection between untreated and HAART-treated subjects. From McArthur JC, with permission. (MØ= macrophages, TNF-α= Tumor necrosis factor α, FasL = Fas Ligand, MMP-1 = matrix metalloproteinase-1, FK = Fractalkine/ CX3CL1.

ganglia and hippocampus (Fox *et al.*, 1997; Maragos *et al.*, 2003; Masliah *et al.*, 1992) and non-NMDA excitatory amino acid receptors on neurons are principally susceptible to toxic viral proteins (Everall *et al.*, 1995; Magnuson *et al.*, 1995).

Synaptodendritic injury is another mechanism that is thought to parallel the severity of cognitive dysfunction in HIV-demented patients (Ellis *et al.*, 2007). Neurons communicate with each other at the synapse connecting the dendrite of one cell with the axonal end of the other. If this crucial connection is disrupted, the communication between the cells is impaired. Ultimately, this can show itself clinically in impaired cognitive functioning. Pathological findings that are indicative of synaptodendritic injury are dendritic beading, atypical sprouting, and retraction of dendritic spines (Ellis *et al.*, 2007). These changes lead to a decreased facility for long-term potentiation, which is crucial for memory formation and consolidation. One important difference between synaptodendritic injury and neuronal loss is the potential reversibility of synaptic changes, and the lack of reversibility of neuronal loss. This could explain how the milder pathology evident in HAART-treated patients (see Figure 15.3) could underlie more fluctuations in cognitive status than was apparent in the pre-HAART era.

Tat

As mentioned previously, a significant component of the damage to neurons of the brain could be mediated through the HIV viral proteins tat and gp120. The HIV protein tat is composed of 101 basic amino acids (Ruben *et al.*, 1989; Robert-Guroff *et al.*, 1990) and is produced in the first segment of viral transcription (Stauber and Pavlakis, 1998). It promotes transcription of the HIV genome (Rosen *et al.*, 1988), regulates the level of gene expression, and is required for effective HIV-1 reverse transcription (Harrich *et al.*, 1997). It is found within the nucleus and nucleolus of HIV-infected cells (Stauber and Pavlakis, 1998) and is excreted by glial cells (Tardieu *et al.*, 1992; Chauhan *et al.*, 2003) and monocytes (Johnston *et al.*, 2001) into surrounding tissue, where it could harm neighbouring cells such as neurons. Tat has been shown unequivocally to be present in the brains of patients with HIV encephalitis (Hofman *et al.*, 1994; Hudson *et al.*, 2000; Valle *et al.*, 2000). Levels of tat mRNA are also elevated in the brains of patients with HIV-D (Wesselingh *et al.*, 1993; Hudson *et al.*, 2000). Strains

of HIV from demented patients may have a glutamate substitution in the second exon of the tat gene. This substitution may decrease tat intracellular uptake, thus increasing the concentrations in the extracellular matrix (Bratanich *et al.*, 1998), leading to enhanced neurovirulence.

While tat neurotoxicity has been convincingly demonstrated in vitro (Rumbaugh *et al.*, 2006), it has also been demonstrated in transgenic mouse models in which tat expression was regulated by GFAP in astrocytes with a doxycycline-inducible promoter to turn the gene on and off (Kim *et al.*, 2003). These mice had behavioral abnormalities that were similar to those observed in human patients with HIV dementia. This study was significant, as it showed that the tat protein itself is sufficient to cause neurobehavioral changes without HIV infection. Another avenue of research that could be relevant is the work suggesting that tat interferes with critical synaptic proteins such as SNAP-25 (Eletto *et al.*, 2008).

Gp120

Gp160 is a glycoprotein on the surface of the HIV virion that is composed of two parts, gp120 and gp 41. It enables the virus to attach to the CD4 receptor and to enter the host cell. Like tat, immunostaining has localized gp120 in brain tissues of HIV-D patients in microglial cells and monocytes (Jones *et al.*, 2000). Gp120 was also found primarily in the basal ganglia and near blood vessels. Along with microglial cells and monocytes it is neurotoxic to astrocytes (Su *et al.*, 2003) and also to neurons (Lipton *et al.*, 1991; Vignoli *et al.*, 2000; Galey *et al.*, 2003). Dopaminergic neurons are the most susceptible to the toxic effects of gp120 (Diop *et al.*, 1995). In addition to direct toxic effects on neurons and other cells of the CNS, gp120 induces the release of inflammatory cytokines and chemokines from monocytes and macrophages (Yi *et al.*, 2004). These can cause direct and indirect oxidative damage to the monocytes. A particularly important aspect of gp120's effect on the brain is the activation of a sodium/proton exchanger on astrocytes. Glutamate accumulation in the extracellular matrix is regulated by astrocytes and this exchanger is important in that regulation. Gp120 stimulates this proton pump, which ultimately depolarizes the membrane (Benos *et al.*, 1994) and inhibits glutamate clearance by astrocytes (Patton *et al.*, 2000). It also decreases glutamate clearance by down-regulating the glutamate transporter gene which, in turn, leads to excitotoxicity and cell damage. Finally, gp120-mediated apoptosis is caspase-activated via multiple pathways (Garden *et al.*, 2004). Any of the above mechanisms and actions makes gp120 an attractive target for possible therapeutic intervention.

Clinical studies of antiretroviral agents for HIV-D

Probably the most difficult aspect of assessing improvement in neuropsychological performances in clinical studies is the determination of which neuropsychiatric tests to use and their reliability and reproducibility. Multiple criteria should be included and test results on at least two domains should be affected in order to categorize the patient as having a neuropsychological impairment. Domains included in the testing should include:

- executive functioning,
- verbal and visual learning,
- fluency,
- speed of information processing,
- delayed recall of verbal and visual material,
- attention and working memory,
- motor skills.

The effects of HAART on HAND

The introduction of HAART therapy in the mid-1990s has decreased the incidence of HIV-associated cognitive decline through virological suppression (Sacktor *et al.*, 2001, 2003). Among the different potential entry points into the brain, the two commonest are through the BBB, and possibly through the blood–CSF barrier, via the choroid plexus. While the BBB is meant to be a protective feature of the brain it can also limit the penetration of antiretrovirals into the brain parenchyma. The virus "uses" this relative sanctuary to reproduce within the brain, protected from a number of the poorly-penetrant antivirals. Completion of a recent study showed that patients on a HAART drug regimen with strong CNS penetration had a fivefold higher chance of having undetectable CSF HIV RNA when plasma HIV RNA was 1000 c/ml or higher (Marra *et al.*, 2006).

The HAART combines multiple drug mechanisms for limiting the replication of HIV. Nucleoside reverse transcriptase inhibitors were the first drugs developed. These drugs inhibit the reverse transcriptase enzyme, which facilitates DNA chain elongation. Subsequently, the non-nucleoside reverse transcriptase inhibitors were developed. These drugs affect reverse transcriptase via non-competitive mechanisms. Protease inhibitors were then introduced to the market and work by impairing viral assembly (Kandanearatchi *et al.*, 2003). Of the nucleoside reverse transcriptase inhibitors, zidovudine (AZT), abacavir (ABC) and stavudine (D4T) show the most CNS penetration (Arendt *et al.*, 2001; Lanier *et al.*, 2001). Of the non-nucleoside reverse transcriptase inhibitors, nevirapine and efavirenz have shown the most promise for CNS efficacy (Price *et al.*, 1999). Indinavir, a protease inhibitor, has also shown promise with high CNS penetration and antiretroviral activity (Martin *et al.*, 1999; Haas *et al.*, 2000). The role of the newer classes of antiretrovirals, fusion inhibitors, integrase inhibitors or CCR5 antagonists is unstudied. The life-saving properties of HAART are truly astounding, yet there is great concern that side effects of pancreatitis, lactic acidosis, impaired glucose tolerance, hypertriglyceridemia, accelerated atherosclerosis, bone density changes, peripheral neuropathy, and lipodystrophy could be limitations for the long-term use of current antiretroviral therapy (ART) regimens.

There have been multiple clinical studies of antiretroviral agents for HAND, and the results have been simultaneously informative and confounding. Initially, the introduction of HAART therapy produced a striking decrease in the incidence of HIV-D. With the addition of HAART, however, the characteristics of HAND have undoubtedly undergone a change. Additionally, HIV dementia has shown itself to be a challenging disease entity to quantify and measure. Often the associations between changes in cognition and the actual functional levels of the patient are weak (Schifitto *et al.*, 2001). Clinical trials studying HIV-D are difficult and expensive to conduct, and comparison between studies is compounded by the fact that the battery of neuropsychological tests used and the analytic techniques employed often differ between studies (Turchan *et al.*, 2003). We will comment here on two illustrative trials of ARTs for HAND which produced contradictory results.

Zidovudine (ZDV) monotherapy for HAD

In this ground-breaking trial, which was the first placebo-controlled trial of ART for HAND, zidovudine was given at an oral dose of 400 mg five times daily or 200 mg five times daily, which is much higher than currently used doses. Neuropsychological performance of both treated groups in the battery was better in comparison to the placebo group (Sidtis *et al.*, 1993).

Abacavir (ABC) as add-on therapy for HAD

The abacavir "ABC" trial serves to illustrate the changing features of HAND in the era of HAART, and has influenced how trials for HAND are designed (Lanier *et al.*, 2001). In essence, the addition of abacavir, a reverse transcriptase inhibitor, to HIV-infected patients with HAD who were already on HAART treatment produced no additional improvement on neurocognitive impairments compared to background antiretrovirals and placebo. This was a discordant result compared to earlier studies of high-dose AZT in the pre-HAART era (Sidtis *et al.*, 1993). A possible explanation for this inconsistency is that some of the patients in the ABC trial had a "burnt out" or inactive form of HIV-D, accounting for their apparent lack of response to abacavir. Alternatively, the patients could have had RT resistance mutations attenuating any response to the drug (Brew *et al.*, 2004, 2007).

A summary of the major clinical HAART trials is given in Table 15.3.

On the basis of the studies to date, we would recommend that established HAD or MCMD be treated with ARTs that are selected with CNS penetration in mind. Letendre *et al.* have proposed a classification of agents based on the level of CNS access, utilizing both theoretical and empirical data, including CSF levels (Langford *et al.*, 2006). In addition, it is also now apparent that the paradigm of treatment interruption for HAART that was tested in the past few years has been unsuccessful; some attempts (e.g. as reported by the Strategies for Management of Antiviral Therapy Study Group [SMART]) have actually been associated with accelerated disease progression (Abdool Karim, 2006). In the opinion of this author, there is currently no place for treatment interruptions in the treatment of HAD. Similarly, current recommendations for the initiation of HAART worldwide do not take into account the presence of HAND (which should probably warrant HAART initiation, no matter what the CD4 count is).

Clinical trials of adjunctive agents for HIV-D

Several adjunctive trials for HAND have been inspired by the results of pathogenic studies that have identified elevated levels of oxidative stress or aberrant immunological mechanisms as potential drivers of the condition. Despite numerous controlled trials, none of the adjunctive agents trialled to date have garnered any clear therapeutic efficacy in neuropsychological performance, and thus not a single phase 3 trial has been conducted. However, a number of significant compounds have been tested in phase II trials, with varying results.

Nimodipine

Nimodipine, a dihydropyridine calcium channel antagonist, was the first non-antiretroviral drug to be tested in a clinical trial. As gp120 from HIV-1 causes cellular damage in central neurons via increased intracellular calcium, blocking these calcium channels might prevent excitotoxicity and subsequent cell death (Dreyer *et al.*, 1990). In a phase I/II trial of nimodipine in 41 patients, no significant toxicity was observed: however, the drug did not generate any obvious improvement on neuropsychological performance. It was an important trial from two perspectives, given that it established a baseline for further clinical trials in HIV and provided a means to evaluate the effectiveness of the NPZ-8 neuropsychological scoring system (Navia *et al.*, 1998; Turchan *et al.*, 2003).

Selegiline

The MAO-B inhibitor selegiline is an antioxidant that has shown promise in recent years in the prevention and treatment of HIV-D (Koutsilieri *et al.*, 2004). Selegiline increases dopamine at the neural synapse by preventing dopamine reuptake and by promoting its release from presynaptic neurons (Kieburtz *et al.*, 1991; Mintz *et al.*, 1996). This is relevant to HIV-infected patients, as it has been shown that a significant amount of damage inflicted by the virus occurs in the basal ganglia (Itoh *et al.*, 2000) and that the basal ganglia of HIV-infected patients have less dopamine and dopa metabolites than do normal controls (Sardar *et al.*, 1996). There have been three clinical trials using selegiline for HAND. In 1998, the Dana Consortium used selegiline orally in 36 pre-HAART patients while another arm of the study received thioctic acid, an antioxidant. The use of selegiline was associated with improvements in verbal memory while thioctic acid did not improve neurocognitive function (Dana Consortium, 1998). A second study by the same group used a transdermal selegiline patch in order to obtain consistently higher therapeutic levels and this

Table 15.3 Summary of the major clinical HAART trials and the outcome on neuropsychological (NP) impairments. (ddI= 2'3'-dideoxyinosine, ddC= 2'3'-dideoxycytosine, NVP= Nevirapine.)

Agent	Mechanism	Outcome	Comments
Zidovudine (ZDV)	Reverse transcriptase inhibitor	Positive NP effect	400 mg five times daily, 200 mg five times daily, placebo five times daily. High-dose ZDV showed greatest improvement (Sidtis *et al.*, 1993)
Abacavir (ABC) – added onto concurrent antiretroviral therapy	Reverse transcriptase inhibitor	No efficacy	600 mg bid, placebo bid. Possible explanation: majority had RT resistance mutations and/or burnt-out disease (Lanier *et al.*, 2001; Brew, 2007).
Zidovudine (ZDV) – alternating ddI versus ZDV+ddI versus ZDV+ddC versus ZDV+ddI+NVP	Reverse transcriptase inhibitor	Triple therapy or ZDV/ddI improved NP	Not solely a trial of HIV-D; no protease inhibitors; all had CD4 <50 (Price *et al.*, 1999).
HAART in Uganda	Reverse transcriptase, protease inhibitor	Positive effect on NP	First demonstration of reversal of HIV-D in resource limited country (RLC) (Sacktor *et al.*, 2006).

was well tolerated. The selegiline treated group also showed improvement on verbal memory and motor/psychomotor performances (Sacktor *et al.*, 2000).

OPC-14117

OPC-14117 is another antioxidant that was initially found to be neuroprotective by prolonging the survival of mice in hypoxic conditions (Oshiro *et al.*, 1991). The agent has a lipophilic structure similar to vitamin E and it acts as an antioxidant by scavenging superoxide anion radicals. The OPC-14117 was also found to decrease edema formation and behavioral deficits after cortical contusion in rats (Kawamata *et al.*, 1997). In an initial clinical trial of OPC-14117 in patients with Huntington's disease, four patients were found to have asymptomatic elevations of liver transaminases (The Huntington Study Group, 1998). Subsequently, a double-blind, placebo-controlled, randomized clinical trial of 30 patients with HIV and cognitive impairment showed it to be safe and well-tolerated and patients taking the drug had better scores on a clinical global impression scale.

Memantine

Memantine is a glutamate ionotropic NMDA receptor antagonist, approved for use in Alzheimer's dementia. Concomitant activation of NMDA receptors by gp120 is required for excitotoxicity and subsequent neuronal damage (Lipton *et al.*, 1991). The in-vitro neurotoxic effects resulting from the simultaneous application of gp120 and tat are blocked by memantine (Nath *et al.*, 2000). These studies suggest that memantine might be useful in the clinical setting of HAND.

Peptide T

Peptide T, otherwise known as DAPTA (D-Ala-peptide T-amide), is an octapeptide contained within the core HIV envelope sequence necessary to bind to CD4 receptors (Pert *et al.*, 1986). By binding to the CD4 receptor, peptide T blocks gp120 binding and subsequent neurotoxicity in vitro. In 1998, a randomized double-blind placebo-controlled trial using intranasal peptide T was conducted and failed to show any statistical difference compared with placebo (Heseltine *et al.*, 1998). A follow-up retrospective analysis of the same patients found that peripheral viral load (plasma and serum) was significantly reduced in the patients treated with peptide T, but no differences were seen in the CSF viral load (Goodkin *et al.*, 2006).

Platelet-activating factor (PAF) antagonists

The PAF antagonists represent another group of potential anti-neurotoxic drugs that have been studied in clinical trials. Initially, large quantities of PAF, a lipid membrane derivative, were found to be present when human glial cells were cultured with monocytes infected with the monocyte-tropic HIV-1 isolate, ADA (Genis *et al.*, 1992). Platelet-activating factor was then found to be present in the CSF of patients infected with HIV-1. When PAF was inoculated into primary neurons, it was found to be a potent neurotoxin (Gelbard *et al.*, 1994). With this in mind, a randomized, double-blind, placebo-controlled clinical trial was conducted with the PAF inhibitor, lexipafant. Results showed that it was well tolerated and safe with a positive trend in verbal memory neuropsychological performance (Schifitto *et al.*, 1999).

CPI-1189

CPI-1189 is a tumor necrosis factor-alpha (TNF-α) inhibitor. The chemical mediators that the immune system produces can be used by HIV to enhance its own viral replication. This has been shown with mediators such as TNF-α and free radicals (Wilt *et al.*, 1995; Richard *et al.*, 1997). Levels of TNF-α mRNA are higher in the brains of HIV-D affected patients compared to patients with AIDS but without dementia (Wesselingh *et al.*, 1993). The CPI-1189 was tested in a double-blind placebo-controlled trial from 1998 to 2000 and was generally well tolerated, but patients treated with the agent did not show any significant improvement in neuropsychometric measures other than on the Grooved Pegboard Test (Clifford *et al.*, 2002).

Valproic acid

Recently, a pilot 10-week placebo-controlled study was conducted using valproic acid as adjunctive therapy for HIV-D. The study was based on previous findings that valproic acid inhibits the apoptosis induced by PAF-activated glycogen synthase kinase (Maggirwar *et al.*, 1999). The results of the study showed that the oral dose of 250 mg twice a day was well tolerated, but there was no significant change in the cognitive performance between the placebo group and the valproic acid treated group after 10 weeks (Schifitto *et al.*, 2006). Conversely, valproate, carbamazepine, and phenytoin were found to activate HIV replication in latently infected monocytes (Robinson *et al.*, 2006). This caveat is important, as HIV-infected macrophages are important players in the development of HIV-D.

Ongoing experimental strategies

As HIV infects CNS cells other than neurons and the by-products of viral infection of these cells ultimately injure neurons, it stands to reason that interfering with or blocking that pathway should protect against neuronal injury and ultimately prevent HAND. This concept, that is the potentiation of neuroprotection, has been a vigorous area of research (Gelbard, 1999). In addition to attempting to neutralize the soluble mediators of viral infection, it has also been shown that macrophage cytokine production and oxidative burst are significantly increased in infected tissues. While these reactions are considered part of a normal immune defense mechanism toward viral infection, they themselves can have neurotoxic effects on the multiple cells in the surrounding tissues.

Glutathione

Glutathione is an antioxidant that occurs naturally in the body and which protects cells from free radicals or toxins that can otherwise cause cell damage and death. By utilizing its sulfhydryl groups, glutathione clears free radicals and maintains mitochondrial function. Glutathione levels are decreased by tat and gp41, whilst glutathione has been found to have protective effects against HIV-1-induced cell death in patients with HIV-D (Sung *et al.*, 2001). Capitalizing on these findings, *N*-acetyl cysteine (NAC) is being studied as a possible drug to stimulate glutathione synthesis. A precursor of glutathione, NAC is currently used as a mucolytic agent for pulmonary disease and for hepatic damage after acetaminophen overdose. By providing a source of sulfhydryl groups, NAC can enhance glutathione-*S*-transferase activity which, by stimulating glutathione synthesis, aids detoxification and scavenges damaging free radicals (Kelly, 1998). The NAC was also shown to decrease serum TNF-α levels and to slow the decrease of CD4 cell counts in HIV-infected patients in a double-blind placebo-controlled trial (Akerlund *et al.*, 2004).

Selenium

Selenium is an essential micronutrient and antioxidant that is necessary for the activity and function of glutathione in preventing oxidative stress and could be beneficial as adjunctive therapy for HIV patients. Selenium concentrations are decreased with HIV disease progression (Cirelli *et al.*, 1991) and by regulating the levels of IL-2, IL-8, and TNF-α, selenium affects T lymphocyte proliferation, differentiation, and cytokine-induced HIV-1 replication (Baum *et al.*, 2000).

Anti-glutaminergic agents

Although memantine is the only anti-glutaminergic drug tested in clinical trials thus far, other similar compounds are putative candidates for neuroprotection. Riluzole has been tested in multiple clinical trials for amyotrophic lateral sclerosis and has been found to have a satisfactory tolerability profile (Lacomblez *et al.*, 2002). Other anti-glutaminergic drugs such as lamotrigine (Yuen, 1994) and pentamidine (Reynolds *et al.*, 1992) are also viable candidates.

Matrix metalloproteinases (MMPs) and minocycline

A factor thought to contribute to HIV infection of the brain and HIV-D is the breakdown of the blood–brain barrier (BBB), followed by trafficking of infected monocytes and macrophages. The basal lamina of endothelial cells is a component part of the BBB and is composed of extracellular matrix proteins, including collagen type IV. The extracellular matrix is continuously being formed and degraded as it is remodeled. Matrix metalloproteinases (MMPs) are members of zinc-containing endopeptidases that target components of the BBB and extracellular matrix. Importantly, it has been shown in animal models that MMP inhibitors decrease damage to the BBB (Rosenberg *et al.*, 1997). Specific subtypes of MMPs (MMP-2, MMP-7, and MMP-9) are particularly proficient in proteolysis of the BBB and have been shown to be elevated in association with HIV-D (Conant *et al.*, 1999). Multiple MMP inhibitors, including BAY12–9566, batismastat, marimastat, AG-3340, OPB-3206, KBR-7785, KBR-8301, and neovastat are currently under study (Wojtowicz-Praga, 1999). Other drugs including statins and minocyline have possible therapeutic potential in this arena as they are known to inhibit the production of MMPs by macrophages (Koh *et al.*, 2001). Minocycline is now entering human trials in the USA (ACTG 5235) on the basis of very positive effects in a macaque model of SIV encephalitis (Zink *et al.*, 2005). This drug has the advantage of a very long safety record, and is widely available and cheap.

Estrogen

Women are increasingly becoming susceptible to HIV-D as they become a significant proportion of the HIV-positive population. For example, of the heterosexually acquired HIV cases between 1999 and 2004 in the United States, 64% were women (Espinoza *et al.*, 2006). In a study of Puerto Rican Hispanic women with HIV, 77.6% of the women had some degree of cognitive impairment (Wojna *et al.*, 2006). Estrogens have been found to be neuroprotective by acting directly on neurons as well as by possessing anti-inflammatory, neuroprotective characteristics (Wilson *et al.*, 2006). Studies are currently ongoing, assessing the possible use of this hormone in HIV-D (Turchan *et al.*, 2003); however, the side effects of breast and uterine cancer risks, as well as possible cognitive impairment in post-menopausal women (Rapp *et al.*, 2003), make this an unlikely hormone for long-term therapy.

While estrogens might themselves have unacceptable side effects, plant extracts known as flavinoids with a combination of weak estrogen receptor affinity, as well as antioxidant and neuroprotective properties (Turchan *et al.*, 2003), remain viable therapeutic candidates.

Conclusion

The impact of HAART on the course, co-morbidities, and mortality of HIV patients has been unprecedented. In consequence, the incidence of HIV-D has decreased, concordant with a reduction in HIV viral load. However, cognitive difficulties in these patients remain a major source of daily morbidity and suffering and should not be understated or overlooked. It is also striking that the prevalence of HAND remains very high even in HAART-treated populations. While none of the experimental therapies outlined in this chapter have, as yet, translated into clinical treatment options for HIV-D, some do warrant further investigation, utilizing more appropriate and sensitive outcome measures. In addition, access to medication regimens that are already available in developed countries needs to be increased on a global scale in order to more effectively combat the international HIV/AIDS pandemic.

References

Abdool Karim SS. Report from the XVI International AIDS Conference. SMART and DART: Intermittent antiretroviral treatment is suboptimal and should be avoided. *AIDS Clin Care* 2006; **18**: 100.

Akerlund B, *et al.* Effect of *N*-acetylcysteine (NAC) treatment on HIV-1 infection: a double-blind placebo-controlled trial. *Eur J Clin Pharmacol* 2004; **50**: 457–61.

Abdulle S, *et al.* CSF neurofilament protein (NFL) – a marker of active HIV-related neurodegeneration. *J Neurol* 2007; **254**: 1026–32.

Andrade AS, *et al.* A programmable prompting device improves adherence to highly active antiretroviral therapy in HIV-infected subjects with memory impairment. *Clin Infect Dis* 2005; **41**: 875–82.

Antinori A, *et al.* Biomarkers of HIV-associated neurocognitive disorders. Report from the Conference: HIV infection and the Central Nervous System: Developed and resource limited settings; 2005.

Antinori A, *et al.* Updated research nosology for HIV-associated neurocognitive disorders. *Neurology* 2007; **69**(18): 1788–99.

Arendt G, *et al.* Therapeutic effects of nucleoside analogues on psychomotor slowing in HIV infection. *AIDS* 2001; **15**: 493–500.

Bandaru VVR, *et al.* Associative and predictive biomarkers of dementia in HIV-1 – infected patients. *Neurology* 2007; **68**: 1481–7.

Baum MD, *et al.* Selenium and interleukins in persons infected with human immunodeficiency virus type I. *J Infect Dis* 2000; **182**(Suppl 1): S69–73.

Benhamou Y, *et al.* Liver fibrosis progression in human immunodeficiency virus and hepatitis C virus coinfected patients. *Hepatology* 1999; **30**: 1054–8.

Benos DJ, *et al.* Cytokines and HIV envelope glycoprotein gp120 stimulate Na+/H exchange in astrocytes. *J Biol Chem* 1994; **269**: 13811–6.

Berger JR, *et al.* Cerebrospinal fluid dopamine in HIV-1 infection. *AIDS* 1994; **8**: 67–71.

Bratanich AC, *et al.* Brain-derived HIV-1 tat sequences from AIDS patients with dementia show increased molecular heterogeneity. *J Neurovirol* 1998; **4**: 387–93.

Brew BJ, *et al.* Cerebrospinal fluid neopterin in human immunodeficiency virus type 1 infection. *Ann Neurol* 1990; **28**: 556–60.

Brew BJ. Evidence for a change in AIDS dementia complex in the era of highly active antiretroviral therapy and the possibility of new forms of AIDS dementia complex. *AIDS* 2004; **18**(Suppl 1): S75–8.

Brew BJ, *et al.* Factors in AIDS dementia complex trial design: results and lessons from the abacavir trial. *PLoS Clin Trials* 2007; **2**(3): e13.

Carey CL, *et al.* Additive deleterious effects of methamphetamine dependence and immunosuppression on neuropsychological functioning in HIV infection. *AIDS Behav* 2006; **10**: 185–90.

Chauhan A, *et al.* Intracellular human immunodeficiency virus Tat expression in astrocytes promotes astrocyte survival but induces potent neurotoxicity at distant sites *via* axonal transport. *J Biol Chem* 2003; **278**: 13512–9.

Cherner M, *et al.* Neurocognitive dysfunction predicts postmortem findings of HIV encephalitis. *Neurology* 2002; **59**: 1563–7.

Childs EA, *et al.* Plasma viral load and CD4 lymphocytes predict HIV-associated dementia and sensory neuropathy. *Neurology* 1999; **52**: 607–13.

Ciborowski P, *et al.* Investigating the human immunodeficiency virus type 1-infected monocyte-derived macrophage secretome. *Virology* 2007; **363**: 198–209.

Cirelli A, *et al.* Serum selenium concentration and disease progress in patients with HIV infection. *Clin Biochem* 1991; **24**: 211–4.

Clifford DB, *et al.* A randomized clinical trial of CPI-1189 for HIV-associated cognitive-motor impairment. *Neurology* 2002; **59**: 1568–73.

Clifford DB, *et al.* The neuropsychological and neurological impact of hepatitis C virus co-infection in HIV-infected subjects. *AIDS* 2005; **19**(Suppl 3): S64–S71.

Conant K, *et al.* Cerebrospinal fluid levels of MMP-2, 7, and 9 are elevated in association with human immunodeficiency virus dementia. *Ann Neurol* 1999; **46**: 391–8.

Costa DC, *et al.* CBF tomograms with 99mTc-HM-PAO in patients with dementia (Alzheimer type and HIV) and Parkinson's disease-initial results. *J Cereb Blood Flow Metab* 1988; **8**: S109–15.

Cysique LA, *et al.* Variable benefit in neuropsychological function in HIV-infected HAART-treated patients. *Neurology* 2006a; **66**: 1447–50.

Cysique LA, *et al.* The neuropsychological profile of symptomatic AIDS and ADC patients in the pre-HAART era: A meta-analysis. *J Int Neuropsychol Soc* 2006b; **12**: 368–82.

Dal Pan GJ, *et al.* Patterns of cerebral atrophy in HIV-1-infected individuals: Results of a quantitative MRI analysis. *Neurology* 1992; **42**: 2125–30.

Dana Consortium on the Therapy of HIV Dementia and Related Cognitive Disorders. Safety and tolerability of the antioxidant OPC-14117 in HIV-associated cognitive impairment. *Neurology* 1997; **49**: 142–6.

Dana Consortium on the Therapy of HIV Dementia and Related Cognitive Disorders. A randomized, double-blind, placebo-controlled trial of deprenyl and thioctic acid in human immunodeficiency virus-associated cognitive impairment. *Neurology* 1998; **50**: 645–51.

Davis HF, *et al.* Assessing HIV-associated dementia: Modified HIV dementia scale versus the Grooved

Pegboard. *AIDS Reader* 2002; **12**: 32–3.

Diop AG, *et al.* Calbindin D28K-containing neurons and not HSP70-expressing neurons, are more resistant to HIV-1 envelope (gp120) toxicity in cortical cell cultures. *J Neurosci Res* 1995; **42**: 252–8.

Dore GJ, *et al.* Marked improvement in survival following AIDS dementia complex in the era of highly active antiretroviral therapy. *AIDS* 2003; **17**: 1539–45.

Dreyer EB, *et al.* HIV-1 coat protein neurotoxicity prevented by calcium channel antagonists. *Science* 1990; **248**: 364–7.

Egan VG, *et al.* The Edinburgh cohort of HIV-positive drug users: Current intellectual function is impaired, but not due to early AIDS dementia complex. *AIDS* 1990; **4**: 651–6.

Eletto D, *et al.* Inhibition of SNAP25 expression by HIV-1 Tat involves the activity of mir-128a. *J Cell Physiol* 2008; **216**: 764–70.

Ellis RJ, *et al.* Cerebrospinal fluid human immunodeficiency virus type 1 RNA levels are elevated in neurocognitively impaired individuals with acquired immunodeficiency syndrome. *Ann Neurol* 1997; **42**: 679–88.

Ellis RJ, *et al.* Progression to neuropsychological impairment in human immunodeficiency virus infection predicted by elevated cerebrospinal fluid levels of human immunodeficiency virus RNA. *Arch Neurol* 2002; **59**: 923–8.

Ellis R, *et al.* HIV and antiretroviral therapy in the brain: Neuronal injury and repair. *Nat Rev Neurosci* 2007; **8**: 33–44.

Espinoza L, *et al.* Characteristics of persons with heterosexually acquired HIV infection, United States 1999–2004. *Am J Public Hlth* 2007; **97**: 1–6.

Everall I, *et al.* Decreased expression of aMPA receptor messenger RNA and protein in AIDS: A model for HIV-associated neurotoxicity. *Nature Med* 1995; **1**: 1174–8.

Everall IP, *et al.* Cortical synaptic density is reduced in mild to moderate human immunodeficiency virus neurocognitive disorder. *Brain Pathol* 1999; **9**: 209–17.

Ferrando SJ, Batki SL. Substance abuse and HIV infection. *New Dir Ment Hlth Serv* 2000; **87**: 57–67.

Filippi CG, *et al.* Diffusion tensor imaging of patients with HIV and normal-appearing white matter on MR images of the brain. *Am J Neuroradiol* 2001; **22**: 277–83.

Fox L, *et al.* Neurodegeneration of somatostatin-immunoreactive neurons in HIV encephalitis. *J Neuropathol Exp Neurol* 1997; **56**(4): 360–8.

Fuchs D, *et al.* Neopterin concentrations in cerebrospinal fluid and serum of individuals infected with HIV-1. *AIDS* 1989; **3**: 285–8.

Galey D, *et al.* Differential transcriptional regulation by human immunodeficiency virus type 1 and gp120 in human astrocytes. *J Neurovirol* 2003; **9**: 358–71.

Garden GA, *et al.* HIV associated neurodegeneration requires p53 in neurons and microglia. *FASEB J* 2004; **18**: 1141–3.

Gartner S. HIV infection and dementia. *Science* 2000; **287**: 602–4.

Gelbard HA. Neuroprotective strategies for HIV-1-associated neurologic disease. *Ann NY Acad Sci* 1999; **890**: 312–13.

Gelbard HA, *et al.* Platelet-activating factor: A candidate human immunodeficiency virus type 1-induced neurotoxin. *J Virol* 1994; **68**: 4628–35.

Genis P, *et al.* Cytokines and arachidonic metabolites produced during human immunodeficiency virus (HIV)-infected macrophage–astroglia interactions: Implications for the neuropathogenesis of HIV disease. *J Exp Med* 1992; **176**: 1703–18.

Gibbie T, *et al.* Depression and neurocognitive performance in individuals with HIV/AIDS: 2-year follow-up. *HIV Med* 2006; 7: 112–21.

Gonzales E, *et al.* HIV-1 infection and AIDS dementia are influenced by a mutant MCP-1 allele linked to increased monocyte infiltration of tissues and MCP-1 levels. *Proc Natl Acad Sci USA* 2002; **99**: 13795–800.

Goodkin K, *et al.* Cerebrospinal and peripheral human immunodeficiency virus type 1 load in a multisite, randomized, double-blind, placebo-controlled trial of D-Ala-peptide T-amide for HIV-1 associated cognitive-motor impairment. *J NeuroVirol* 2006; **12**: 178–89.

van Gorp WG, *et al.* The relationship between employment and neuropsychological impairment in HIV infection. *J Int Neuropsychol Soc* 1999; **5**: 534–9.

Green AJ, *et al.* Cerebrospinal fluid tau concentrations in HIV infected patients with suspected neurological disease. *Sex Transm Infect* 2000; **76**: 443–6.

Haas D, *et al.* Comparative studies of two-times-daily versus three-times-daily indinavir in combination with zidovudine and lamivudine. *AIDS* 2000; **14**: 1973–8.

Hammoud DA, *et al.* Imaging glial cell activation with (11C)-R-PK11195 in patients with AIDS. *J Neurovirol* 2005; **11**: 346–55.

Harrich D, Ulich C, Garcia-Martinez LF, Gaynor RB. Tat is required for efficient HIV-1 reverse transcription. *EMBO J* 1997; **16**: 1224–35.

Heaton RK, *et al.* The impact of HIV-associated neuropsychological impairment on everyday functioning. *J Int Neuropsychol Soc* 2004; **10**: 317–31.

Heseltine PNR, *et al.* Randomized double-blind placebo-controlled trial of peptide T for HIV-associated cognitive impairment. *Arch Neurol* 1998; **55**: 41–51.

Heyes MP, *et al.* Quinolinic acid in cerebrospinal fluid and serum in HIV-1 infection: relationship to clinical and neurological status. *Ann Neurol* 1991; **29**: 202–9.

Hinkin CH, *et al.* Cerebral metabolic change in patients with AIDS: Report of a six-month follow-up using positron-emission tomography. *J Neuropsychiatry Clin Neurosci* 1995; **7**: 180–7.

Hinkin CH, *et al.* Medication adherence among HIV+ adults. *Neurology* 2002; **59**: 1944–50.

Hofman FM, *et al.* Exogenous tat protein activates central nervous system-derived endothelial cells. *J Neuroimmunol* 1994; **54**: 19–28.

Hudson L, *et al.* Detection of the human immunodeficiency virus regulatory protein tat in CNS tissues. *J Neurovirol* 2000; **6**: 145–55.

Huntington Study Group. Safety and tolerability of the free-radical scavenger OPC-14117 in Huntington's disease. *Neurology* 1998; **50**: 1366–73.

Itoh K, *et al.* Neuronal damage of the substantia nigra in HIV-1 infected brains. *Acta Neuropathol (Berl)* 2000; **99**: 376–84.

Jakobsen J, *et al.* Cerebral ventricular enlargement relates to neuropsychological measures in unselected AIDS patients. *Acta Neurol Scand* 1989; **79**: 59–62.

Jassoy C, *et al.* Human immunodeficiency virus type 1-specific cytotoxic T lymphocytes release gamma interferon, tumor necrosis factor-alpha (TNF-alpha) and TNF-beta when they encounter their target antigens. *J Virol* 1993; **67**: 2844–52.

Johnston JB, *et al.* HIV-1 tat neurotoxicity is prevented by matrix metalloproteinase inhibitors. *Ann Neurol* 2001; **49**: 230–41.

Jones MV, *et al.* Immunolocalization of HIV envelope gp120 in HIV encephalitis with dementia. *AIDS* 2000; **14**: 2709–13.

Kandanearatchi A, *et al.* Assessing the efficacy of highly active antiretroviral therapy in the brain. *Brain Pathol* 2003; **13**: 104–10.

Kawamata T, *et al.* Antioxidant, OPC-14117, attenuates edema formation and behavioral deficits following cortical contusion in rats. *Acta Neurochir Suppl* 1997; **70**: 191–3.

Kelly GS. Clinical applications of *N*-acetylcysteine. *Alt Med Rev* 1998; **3**: 114–27.

Kieburtz KD, *et al.* Excitotoxicity and dopaminergic dysfunction in the acquired immunodeficiency syndrome dementia complex. Therapeutic implications. *Arch Neurol* 1991; **48**: 1281–4.

Kim BO, *et al.* Neuropathologies in transgenic mice expressing human immunodeficiency virus type 1 Tat protein under the regulation of the astrocyte-specific glial fibrillary acidic protein promoter and doxycycline. *Am J Pathol* 2003; **162**: 1693–3403.

Koh KK, *et al.* Non-lipid effects of statin on hypercholesterolemic patients established to have coronary artery disease who remained hypercholesterolemic while eating a step-II diet. *Coron Artery Dis* 2001; **12**: 305–11.

Koutsilieri E, *et al.* Monoamine oxidase inhibition and CNS immunodeficiency infection. *NeuroToxicology* 2004; **25**: 267–270.

Lacomblez L, *et al.* Tolerance of riluzole in a phase IIIb clinical trial. *Therapie* 2002; **57**: 65–71.

Langford D, *et al.* Patterns of selective neuronal damage in methamphetamine-user AIDS patients. *J Acquir Immune Defic Syndr* 2003; **34**: 467–74.

Langford D, *et al.* Relationship of antiretroviral treatment to postmortem brain tissue viral load in human immunodeficiency virus-infected patients. *J Neurovirol* 2006; **12**:100–7.

Lanier ER, *et al.* HIV-1 reverse transcriptase sequence in plasma and cerebrospinal fluid of patients with AIDS dementia complex treated with Abacavir. *AIDS* 2001; **15**: 747–51.

Lipton SA, *et al.* Synergistic effects of HIV coat protein and NMDA receptor-mediated neurotoxicity. *Neuron* 1991; **7**: 111–8.

Maggirwar SB, *et al.* HIV-1 tat-mediated activation of glycogen synthase kinase-3B contributes to tat-mediated neurotoxicity. *J Neurochem* 1999; **73**: 578–86.

Magnuson D, *et al.* Human immunodeficiency virus type 1 Tat activates non-*N*-methyl-D-aspartate excitatory amino acid receptors and causes neurotoxicity. *Ann Neurol* 1995; **37**: 373–80.

Maragos WF, *et al.* Neuronal injury in hippocampus with human immunodeficiency virus transactivating protein, TAT. *Neuroscience* 2003; **117**: 43–53.

Marcotte TD, *et al.* A multimodal assessment of driving performance in HIV infection. *Neurology* 2004; **26** : 1417–22.

Marra C, *et al.* ACTG 736:CSF HIV-1 and cognitive function in individuals receiving potent ART. *13th CROI*, session **70**, abstract no. 361; 2006.

Martin C, *et al.* Indinavir-based treatment of HIV-1 infected patients: Efficacy in the central nervous system. *AIDS* 1999; **13**: 1227–32.

Masliah E, *et al.* Spectrum of human immunodeficiency virus-associated neocortical damage. *Ann Neurol* 1992; **32**: 321–9.

Mayeux R, *et al.* Mortality risks in gay men with human immunodeficiency virus infection and cognitive impairment. *Neurology* 1993; **43**: 176–82.

McArthur JC, *et al.* The diagnostic utility of elevation in cerebrospinal fluid beta 2-microglobulin in HIV-1 dementia. Multicenter AIDS Cohort Study. *Neurology* 1992; **42**: 1707–12.

McArthur JC, *et al.* Dementia in AIDS patients: Incidence and risk factors. *Neurology* 1993; **43**: 2245–52.

McArthur JC, *et al.* Human immunodeficiency virus-associated dementia: An evolving disease. *J NeuroVirol* 2003; **9**: 205–21.

McArthur JC, *et al.* Attenuated central nervous system infection in advanced HIV/AIDS with combination antiretroviral therapy. *Arch Neurol* 2004; **61**: 1687–96.

McArthur JC, *et al.* Neurological complications of HIV infection. *Lancet Neurol* 2005; **4**: 543–55.

Merrill J, *et al.* Induction of interleukin-1 and tumor necrosis factor alpha in brain cultures by human immunodeficiency virus type 1. *J Virol* 1992; **66**: 2217–25.

Miller EN, *et al.* Neuropsychological performance in HIV-1-infected homosexual men: MACS. *Neurology* 1990; **40**: 197–203.

Miller RF, et al. Detection of 14–3–3 brain protein in cerebrospinal fluid of HIV infected patients. Sex Transm Infect 2000; 76: 408.

Mintz M, et al. Neurology 1996; 47: 1583–5.

Monteiro de Almeida S, et al. Dynamics of monocyte chemoattractant protein type one (MCP-1) and HIV viral load in human cerebrospinal fluid and plasma. J Neuroimmunol 2005; 169: 144–52.

Moore DJ, et al. Cortical and subcortical neurodegeneration is associated with HIV neurocognitive impairment. AIDS 2006; 20: 879–87.

Morgello S, et al. Effects of hepatic function and hepatitis C virus on the nervous system assessment of advanced-stage HIV-infected individuals. AIDS 2005; 19(Suppl 3): S116–22.

Nath A, et al. Synergistic neurotoxicity by human immunodeficiency virus proteins Tat and gp120: Protection by memantine. Ann Neurol 2000; 47: 186–94.

Nath A, et al. Molecular basis for interactions of HIV and drugs of abuse. J AIDS 2002; 31: S62–9.

Navia BA, Price RW. The acquired immunodeficiency syndrome dementia complex as the presenting or sole manifestation of human immunodeficiency virus infection. Arch Neurol 1987; 44: 65–9.

Navia BA, et al. The AIDS dementia complex: Clinical features. Ann Neurol 1986; 19: 517–24.

Navia BA, et al. A phase I/II trial of nimodipine for HIV-related neurologic complications. Neurology 1998; 51: 221–8.

Neuenburg JK, et al. HIV-related neuropathology, 1985 to 1999: Rising prevalence of HIV encephalopathy in the era of highly active antiretroviral therapy. J Acquir Immune Defic Syndr 2002; 31: 171–7.

Oshiro Y, et al. Novel cerebroprotective agents with central nervous system stimulating activity. 2. Synthesis and pharmacology of the 1-(acylamino)-7-hydroxyindan derivatives. J Med Chem 1991; 34: 2014–23.

Pascal S, et al. Metabolic asymmetries in asymptomatic HIV-1 seropositive subjects: Relationship to disease onset and MRI findings. J Nucl Med 1991; 32: 1725–9.

Patton HK, et al. Gp120-induced alterations of human astrocyte function: Na+/H+ exchange, K+ conductance and glutamate flux. Am J Physiol Cell Physiol 2000; 279: C700–08.

Pemberton LA, Brew BJ. Cerebrospinal fluid S-100beta and its relationship with AIDS dementia complex. J Clin Virol 2001; 22: 249–53.

Pert CB, et al. Octapeptides deduced from the neuropeptide receptor-like pattern of antigen T4 in brain potently inhibit human immunodeficiency virus receptor binding and T-cell infectivity. Proc Nat Acad Sci 1986; 83: 9254–8.

Price RW, et al. Neurological outcomes in late HIV infection: Adverse impact of neurological impairment on survival and protective effect of antiviral therapy. AIDS 1999; 13: 1677–85.

Quasney MW, et al. Increased frequency of the tumor necrosis factor-alpha-308 A allele in adults with human immunodeficiency virus dementia. Ann Neurol 2001; 50: 157–62.

Ragin AB, et al. Disease burden in HIV-associated cognitive impairment: A study of whole-brain imaging measures. Neurology 2004; 63: 2293–7.

Ragin AB, et al. Diffusion tensor imaging of subcortical brain injury in patients infected with human immunodeficiency virus. J Neurovirol 2005; 11: 292–8.

Ranki A, et al. Abundant expression of HIV Nef and Rev proteins in brain astrocytes in vivo is associated with dementia. AIDS 1995; 9: 1001–8.

Rapp SR, et al. Effect of estrogen plus progestin on global cognitive function in postmenopausal women: the Women's Health Initiative Memory Study: A randomized controlled trial. J Am Med Assoc 2003; 289: 2663–72.

Resnick L, et al. Early penetration of the blood-brain-barrier by HIV. Neurology 1988; 38: 9–14.

Reynolds IJ, Aizeman E. Pentamidine is an N-methyl-D-aspartate receptor antagonist and is neuroprotective in vitro. J Neurosci 1992; 12: 970–5.

Richard A, et al. Interference of HIV-1 Nef in the sphingomyelin transduction pathway activated by tumour necrosis factor-alpha in human glial cells. AIDS 1997; 11: F1–7.

Riedel DJ, et al. Therapy insight: CNS manifestations of HIV-associated immune reconstitution inflammatory syndrome. Nat Clin Pract Neurol 2006; 2: 557–65.

Rippeth JD, et al. Methamphetamine dependence increases risk of neuropsychological impairment in HIV infected persons. JINS 2004; 10: 1–14.

Robert-Guroff M, et al. Stucture and expression of tat-, rev- and nef-specific transcripts of human immunodeficiency virus type 1 in infected lymphocytes and macrophages. J Virol 1990; 64: 3391–8.

Robinson B, et al. Modulation of human immunodeficiency virus infection by anticonvulsant drugs. J Neurovirol 2006; 12: 1–4.

Rosen CA, et al. Intragenic cis-acting art gene-responsive sequences of the human immunodeficiency virus. Proc Natl Acad Sci 1988; 85: 2071–5.

Rosenberg GA, Navratil M. Metalloproteinase inhibition blocks edema in intracerebral hemorrhage in the rat. Neurology 1997; 48: 921–6.

Ruben S, et al. Structural and functional characterization of human immunodeficiency virus tat protein. J Virol 1989; 63: 1–8.

Rumbaugh JA, Nath A. Developments in HIV neuropathogenesis. Curr Pharm Des 2006; 12: 1023–44.

Sacktor N. The epidemiology of human immunodeficiency virus-associated neurological disease in the era of highly active antiretroviral therapy. J Neurovirol 2002; 8: 115–21.

Sacktor N, et al. A comparison of cerebral SPECT abnormalities in

HIV-positive homosexual men with and without cognitive impairment. *Arch Neurol* 1995a; **52**: 1170–3.

Sacktor N, *et al.* Cerebral single-photon emission computed tomography abnormalities in human immunodeficiency virus type 1-infected gay men without cognitive impairment. *Arch Neurol* 1995b; **52**: 607–11.

Sacktor N, *et al.* Transdermal selegiline in HIV-associated cognitive impairment: pilot, placebo-controlled study. *Neurology* 2000; **54**: 233–5.

Sacktor N, *et al.* HIV-associated neurologic disease incidence changes: Multicenter Aids Cohort Study, 1990–1998. *Neurology* 2001; **56**: 257–60.

Sacktor N, *et al.* Response to systemic HIV viral load suppression correlates with psychomotor speed performance. *Neurology* 2003; **61**: 567–9.

Sacktor NC, *et al.* The International HIV Dementia Scale: A new rapid screening test for HIV dementia. *AIDS* 2005a; **19**: 1367–74.

Sacktor N, *et al.* A multicenter study of two magnetic resonance spectroscopy techniques in individuals with HIV dementia. *J Magn Reson Imaging* 2005b; **21**: 325–33.

Sacktor N, *et al.* Antiretroviral therapy improves cognitive impairment in HIV+ individuals in sub-Saharan Africa. *Neurology* 2006; **67**: 311–14.

Sadek JR, *et al.* Retrograde amnesia in dementia: Comparison of HIV-associated dementia, Alzheimer's disease, and Huntington's disease. *Neuropsychology* 2004; **18**: 692–9.

Saito Y, *et al.* Overexpression of nef as a marker for restricted HIV-1 infection of astrocytes in postmortem pediatric central nervous tissues. *Neurology* 1994; **44**: 474–81.

Sardar AM, *et al.* Dopamine deficits in the brain: The neurochemical basis of parkinsonian symptoms in AIDS. *Neuroreport* 1996; **7**: 910–12.

Schifitto G, *et al.* Randomized trial of the platelet-activating factor antagonist lexipafant in HIV-associated cognitive impairment. *Neurology* 1999; **53**: 391–6.

Schifitto G, *et al.* Clinical trials in HIV-associated cognitive impairment: Cognitive and functional outcomes. *Neurology* 2001; **56**: 415–8.

Schifitto G, *et al.* Valproic acid adjunctive therapy for HIV-associated cognitive impairment: A first report. *Neurology* 2006; **66**: 919–21.

Selnes OA, *et al.* HIV-1 infection: No evidence of cognitive decline during the asymptomatic stages. The Multicenter AIDS Cohort Study. *Neurology* 1990; **40**: 204–8.

Sevigny JJ, *et al.* Evaluation of HIV RNA and markers of immune activation as predictors of HIV-associated dementia. *Neurology* 2004; **63**: 2084–90.

Shelburne SA, *et al.* Immune reconstitution inflammatory syndrome. *Medicine* 2002; **81**: 213–27.

Shelburne SA, *et al.* Immune reconstitution inflammatory syndrome: More answers, more questions. *J Antimicrob Chemother* 2006; **57**: 167–70.

Sidtis JJ, *et al.* Zidovudine treatment of the AIDS dementia complex: Results of a placebo-controlled trial. *Ann Neurol* 1993; **33**: 343–9.

Stauber RH, Pavlakis GN. Intracellular trafficking and interactions of the HIV-1 Tat protein. *Virology* 1998; **252**: 126–36.

Stephans SE, Yamamoto BK. Methamphetamine-induced neurotoxicity: Roles for glutamate and dopamine efflux. *Synapse* 1994; **17**: 203–9.

Stout JC, *et al.* Progressive cerebral volume loss in human immunodeficiency virus infection: A longitudinal volumetric magnetic resonance imaging study. HIV neurobehavioral Research Center Group. *Arch Neurol* 1998; **55**: 161–8.

Su ZZ, *et al.* Identification of gene products suppressed by human immunodeficiency virus type 1 infection or gp120 exposure of primary human astrocytes by rapid subtraction hybridization. *J NeuroVirol* 2003; **9**: 372–89.

Sulkowski MS, *et al.* Hepatotoxicity associated with antiretroviral therapy in adults infected with human immunodeficiency virus and the role of hepatitis C or B virus infection. *J Am Med Assoc* 2000; **283**: 74–80.

Sung JH, *et al.* Protective effect of glutathione in HIV-1 lytic peptide 1-induced cell death in human neuronal cells. *J Neurovirol* 2001; **7**: 454–65.

Tarasow E, *et al.* Cerebral MR spectroscopy in neurologically asymptomatic HIV-infected patients. *Acta Radiol* 2003; **44**: 206–12.

Tarasow E, *et al.* Antiretroviral therapy and its influence on the stage of brain damage in patients with HIV-1H MRS evaluation. *Med Sci Monit* 2004; **10**(Suppl 3): 101–6.

Tardieu M, *et al.* Human immunodeficiency virus type 1-infected monocytic cells can destroy human neuronal cells after cell-to-cell adhesion. *Ann Neurol* 1992; **32**: 11–7.

Tatsch K, *et al.* Functional and morphological findings in early and advanced stages of HIV infection: A comparison of 99mTc-HMPAO SPECT with CT and MRI studies. *Nuklearmedizin* 1990; **29**: 252–8.

Taylor MJ, *et al.* MR spectroscopy in HIV and stimulant dependence. *J Int Neuropsychol Soc* 2000; **6**: 83–5.

Thompson PM, *et al.* Thinning of the cerebral cortex visualized in HIV/AIDS reflects CD4+ T lymphocyte decline. *Proc Natl Acad Sci USA* 2005; **102**: 15647–52.

Tomlinson GS, *et al.* Upregulation of microglia in drug users with and without pre-symptomatic HIV infection. *Neuropathol Appl Neurobiol* 1999; **25**: 369–79.

Tornatore C, *et al.* HIV-1 infection of subcortical astrocytes in the pediatric central nervous system. *Neurology* 1994; **44**: 481–7.

Tracey I, *et al.* Increased cerebral blood volume in HIV-positive patients detected by functional MRI. *Neurology* 1998; **50**(6): 1821–6.

Tucker KA, *et al.* Neuroimaging in human immunodeficiency virus infection. *J Neuroimmunol* 2004; **157**: 153–62.

Turchan J, *et al.* Neuroprotective therapy for HIV dementia. *Cur HIV Res* 2003; **1**: 373–83.

Valle LD, *et al.* Detection of HIV-1 Tat and JCV capsid protein, VP1, in AIDS brain with progressive multifocal leukoencephalopathy. *J Neurovirol* 2000; **6**: 221–8.

Venkataramana A, *et al.* Immune reconstitution inflammatory syndrome in the CNS of HIV-infected patients. *Neurology* 2006; **67**: 383–8.

Vignoli AL, *et al.* Neuronal glycolytic pathway impairment induced by HIV envelope glycoprotein gp120. *Mol Cell Biochem* 2000; **215**: 73–80.

Wachtmann LM, *et al.* Platelet decline: An early predictive hematologic marker of simian immunodeficiency virus central nervous system disease. *J Neurovirol* 2006; **12**: 25–33.

Wendel KA, McArthur JC. Acute meningoencephalitis in chronic human immunodeficiency virus (HIV) infection: Putative central nervous system escape of HIV replication. *Clin Infect Dis* 2003; **37**: 1107–11.

Wesselingh SL, *et al.* Intracerebral cytokine messenger RNA expression in acquired immunodeficiency syndrome dementia. *Ann Neurol* 1993; **33**: 576–82.

Wiley CA, *et al.* Cellular localization of human immunodeficiency virus infection within the brains of acquired immune deficiency syndrome patients. *Proc Natl Acad Sci* 1986; **83**: 7089–93.

Wilkie FL, *et al.* Mild cognitive impairment and risk of mortality in HIV-1 infection. *J Neuropsychiatry Clin Neurosci* 1998; **10**: 125–32.

Wilson ME, *et al.* Immune modulation by estrogens: role in CNS HIV-1 infection. *Endocrine* 2006; **29**: 289–97.

Wilt SG, *et al.* In vitro evidence for a dual role of tumor necrosis factor-alpha in human immunodeficiency virus type 1 encephalopathy. *Ann Neurol* 1995; **37**: 381–94.

Wojna V, *et al.* Prevalence of human immunodeficiency virus-associated cognitive impairment in a group of Hispanic women at risk for neurological impairment. *J Neurovirol* 2006; **12**: 356–64.

Wojna V, Nath A. Challenges to the diagnosis and management of HIV dementia. *AIDS Read* 2007; **16**: 615–16, 621–4, 629–32.

Wojtowicz-Praga S. Clinical potential of matrix metalloprotease inhibitors. *Drugs R D* 1999; **1**: 117–29.

Wong MH, *et al.* Frequency of and risk factors for HIV dementia in an HIV clinic in sub-Saharan Africa. *Neurology* 2007; **68**: 350–5.

Woody GE, *et al.* Non-injection substance use correlates with risky sex among men having sex with men: Data from HIVNET. *Drug Alcohol Depend* 1999; **53**: 197–205.

Wright E, *et al.* Neurologic disorders are prevalent in HIV-positive outpatients in the Asia–Pacific region. 2008; **71**: 50–6.

Wu YC, *et al.* AIDS dementia complex in China. *J Clin Neurosci* 2007; **14**: 8–11.

Yi Y, *et al.* Chemokine receptor utilization and macrophage signaling by human immunodeficiency virus type 1 gp120: Implications for neuropathogenesis. *J Neurovirol* 2004; **10**(Suppl 1): 91–6.

Yuen AW. Lamotrigine: A review of antiepileptic efficacy. *Epilepsia* 1994; **35**(Suppl 5): S33–6.

Zink MC, *et al.* Neuroprotective and anti-human immunodeficiency virus activity of minocycline. *J Am Med Assoc* 2005; **293**: 2003–11.

Chapter 16

Role of immunomodulation in management of infections of the CNS

Miles H. Beaman

Introduction

Central nervous system (CNS) infections are difficult to treat for many reasons, including the fact that many pathogens are insensitive to standard anti-microbial treatments, and also because of inadequate penetration of many anti-microbials across the blood–brain barrier (BBB). The fact that many CNS pathogens are intracellular makes anti-microbial penetration even more problematic. In addition, many of the adverse outcomes of CNS infections are due to immunologically mediated damage of the CNS, arising from immune activation triggered by the infection. For these reasons, immunomodulatory therapies are of interest either as a means to treat previously refractory infections or as a way to enhance existing treatments. This chapter provides a broad perspective of the spectrum of immunomodulatory therapies that are either currently available or in the process of being developed.

At the outset, it is necessary to understand the underlying immunopathogenesis of CNS infections (which varies widely according to the specific pathogen involved) and to use this knowledge to develop cogent treatment protocols relevant to each clinical scenario (initially tested in animal models and subsequently evaluated in clinical trials). Because many CNS infections commence outside of the CNS prior to dissemination (e.g. tuberculosis, cryptococcosis, and toxoplasmosis), therapies with only systemic effects can often exert a useful role in the treatment of these infections and they will be briefly discussed. On the other hand, regimens that induce local CNS immune responses are required for treatment of infections that are already established in the CNS and will also be discussed, but this therapeutic approach is in its infancy compared to that of immunomodulatory therapy for either autoimmunity or cancer (some of which will also be illustrated here, but which are discussed in greater detail in other chapters).

Immunological responses to pathogens are essential for successful host defense and commence with a phase of immune activation directed against the foreign organism. Excessive immune activation (either in magnitude or duration) can, however, exert potentially deleterious bystander effects such that, at an appropriate time, the immune response needs to be deactivated in order to prevent unintended host damage (Grau and Modlin, 1991; Griffin, 2003). All components and steps along these activation and inhibitory pathways are subject to regulation, including by antigen (Tischner et al., 2006), immune complexes, B and T cell networks, cytokines, and the endocrine system. In general, protective responses to CNS infection include homing of T lymphocytes (T cells) to the CNS from the periphery and the activation of resident CNS macrophages/antigen presenting cells (predominantly microglia) (Aloisi et al., 2000) to produce activating cytokines (Wu et al., 2000).

This chapter will focus predominantly on therapeutic immunomodulation with cytokines, as these are currently the most promising agents for this mode of treatment, although there are several potential barriers to their successful application. The cytokine network provides a redundant, overlapping series of positive and negative regulatory signals to modulate host responses to infection. This redundancy has often been the cause of failure of experimental therapies when the approach has been to target a single component of a cytokine cascade. Design of trials involving the use of either cytokines or their inhibitors must also take into account the specific immunopathogenesis of the particular infection that is being studied, including the fact that cytokines can function in either an autocrine, paracrine, or endocrine manner (Beaman, 1994). Failure of anti-cytokine therapies in sepsis stem, in part, from the heterogeneous nature of the infections

Inflammatory Diseases of the Central Nervous System, ed. T. Kilpatrick, R. M. Ransohoff and S. Wesselingh. Published by Cambridge University Press. © Cambridge University Press 2010

(with many differing pathogeneses) that are being treated. Another important factor to be considered in trial design is that differing doses and timing of the delivery of a given cytokine can produce significantly different effects. More than one receptor is often activated by a given cytokine, and these can act in either synergistic or antagonistic ways: such receptors can be either membrane-bound or circulate in the blood or lymphatics (Fernandez-Botran, 1991). It is also now apparent that at the individual patient level, some cytokines can be overproduced, whereas others are relatively underproduced and in some instances inherited mutations of cytokine receptors can prevent adequate cytokine-induced signaling: all of these factors could result in severe infection-related disease. Where cytokine deficiency is posited, it is possible to administer either the cytokine directly or a DNA construct containing the relevant gene (Rodriguez et al., 2000). On the other hand, where overproduction is operative, inhibition of activity can be achieved by either specific blocking antibodies or by the administration of a soluble receptor that prevents the cytokine from binding to its membrane-bound receptor (Fernandez-Botran, 1991). The degree of penetration of therapeutic agents into the CNS and to the site of disease also must be taken into account: unfortunately, such data are not available currently for many therapeutic candidates. Non-cytokine therapies can also affect cytokine expression, and will be briefly mentioned.

Immunization

Human studies

The ultimate form of preventative immunomodulation is by immunization. Effective vaccines are widely used to prevent many infections that can affect the CNS, including both bacteria (e.g. *Streptococcus pneumoniae*, *Haemophilus influenzae*, *Neisseria meningiditis*, *Mycobacterium tuberculosis*, *Bordetella pertussis*, *Corynebacterium diptheriae*, *Clostridium tetani*, *Salmonella typhi*) and viruses (e.g. measles, mumps, rubella, varicella, rabies, polio, influenza, Japanese B Encephalitis Virus [JEV], yellow fever virus [YFV], and tick-borne encephalitis [TBE]).

Other vaccines that are available but are only used for specific patient groups include those for *Bacillus anthracis* and *Coxiella burnetti*. A dengue fever vaccine is in clinical trial at present. An apparently effective Lyme disease vaccine has been withdrawn from the market for commercial reasons. An HSV-2 vaccine is currently available to prevent genital herpes, but it is unknown whether this will also reduce CNS complications, including Mollaret's meningitis.

Passive immunization with specific immunoglobulin is also available to prevent or treat tetanus, rabies, botulism, and vaccinia. On the other hand, pooled immunoglobulin has been used in hypogammaglobulinemic patients with chronic enterovirus meningitis.

Animal studies

An insight into how vaccines can induce immunomodulatory effects locally within the CNS comes from a murine model of rabies. In this instance, an attenuated rabies vaccine strain activated many innate immune pathways, including those initiated by interferon-α and β (IFN-α and β), whereas wild-type rabies failed to activate such pathways (Wang et al., 2005). Interestingly, a rabies vaccine over-expressing tumor necrosis factor-α (TNF-α) reduced neuronal replication of wild-type virus more effectively than a vaccine strain without the TNF construct, underscoring the importance of inducing an inflammatory response (Faber et al., 2005).

Pharmacological agents

Corticosteroids (CS)

The first agents used for immunomodulation of infection in humans, including of the CNS, were corticosteroids. Clinical studies of these agents predated an understanding of the pathogenesis of infections, especially the role of pro-inflammatory cytokines in bacterial infections such as meningitis (Saez-Llorens et al., 1990a). The major effect of corticosteroids in vitro is a broad spectrum reduction in pro-inflammatory cytokine release, in part by suppression of nuclear factor-kappa beta (NF-κβ) transcription pathways. The uncontrolled use of corticosteroids as adjunctive therapy in severe CNS infections has confounded analysis of studies focusing on other immunomodulatory therapies. Corticosteroids may also be indicated for non-immunomodulatory reasons in CNS infection, especially if either cerebral edema or mass effect with hydrocephalus is present. Corticosteroids have been used in the management of brain abscess and cryptococcosis for these indications.

Cytokines and growth factors

There are numerous cytokines that can influence the host response to infection. This section discusses some of the principal players, many of which have been modulated in experimental contexts to assess their potential role as therapeutic candidates/targets. Interferon-α (IFN-α) is a key representative of a family of type 1 interferons that are produced by leukocytes (especially monocytes) and which induce many intracellular proteins that are protective against viral infection. Therapeutic human use was initially for treatment of malignancy, where many of the dose-limiting toxicities (neutropenia, influenza-like symptoms, and hepatotoxicity) of peripheral administration were characterized (Krown, 1986). Significant side effects have been noted with intrathecal administration of IFN-α, including neurotoxicity (Cianchetti et al., 1994; Finsterer et al., 2005) and generalized seizures (Caksen et al., 2003). A novel way of increasing the half-life of IFN-α has been found by generating a fusion protein with human albumin, and this product has shown good effect in a phase II study of hepatitis C virus (HCV) infection (Balan et al., 2006).

There has been some evidence that IFN-α may be overproduced in HIV infection with detrimental effects, so the effects of IFN-α blockade by immunization-induced antibodies were studied and found to be beneficial (Gringeri et al., 1999).

Interferon-β (IFN-β) is a type 1 interferon that is produced by fibroblasts, which binds to the same receptor as IFN-α and also induces the production of proteins with antiviral effect. The IFN-β has been shown in vitro to inhibit the ability of glial cells to activate T cells (Teige et al., 2006). Peripheral delivery of IFN-β gene is efficacious in reducing allergic encephalomyelitis in a murine model (Schaefer et al., 2006) and is well established to be effective in reducing disease activity in multiple sclerosis (Wingerchuk, 2008).

Interferon-γ (IFN-γ) is mainly produced by T lymphocytes (especially T-helper 1 [TH-1]) and natural killer (NK) cells and activates macrophages to kill intracellular pathogens (such as *Toxoplasma, Listeria, Leishmania, Mycobacteria,* and *Trypanosoma*) (Murray, 1988; Flesch et al., 1997). It can induce oxidative and non-oxidative mediated cytotoxicity in macrophages, but also stimulates activation pathways via STAT-1, IFN-γ receptor 1, interleukin [IL]-12 and IL-23 to induce protective immunity (Novelli and Casanova, 2004). Deficiency of this cytokine is notable in chronic granulomatous disease and replacement therapy reduces the risk of infective complications (Todd and Goa, 1992; Gallin, et al., 1995).

Interferon-omega is a newly developed IFN that is now in clinical trial for the treatment of HCV, where it has good antiviral effects (Buckwold et al., 2006).

Granulocyte-colony stimulating factor (G-CSF) is produced by monocytes and endothelial cells and stimulates the proliferation, differentiation, and activation of neutrophils. It has been used extensively for chemotherapy-induced neutropenia, especially for febrile neutropenia. The commonest side effect is bone pain.

Granulocyte-macrophage colony-stimulating factor (GM-CSF) is produced by many sources, including T cells and monocytes, and stimulates both the production and activity of neutrophils, monocytes, and eosinophils. It was initially used in the treatment of chemotherapy-induced neutropenia, but has been predominantly supplanted by G-CSF for this indication, partly because of its higher incidence of side effects including fever, myalgia, and dyspnea.

Epidermal growth factor (EGF) has been delivered by genetic means in a Sindbis encephalitis model and resulted in reduced viral levels and inflammation (van Marle et al., 2003).

Interleukin-1 (IL-1) levels have been manipulated by delivery of an IL-1 receptor antagonist but this strategy was not shown to be beneficial in the management of sepsis in humans (Opal et al., 1997). In addition, an IL-1 receptor antagonist did not provide demonstrable efficiency in animal models of bacterial meningitis (Paris et al., 1995).

Interleukin-2 (IL-2) is an important cytokine that is predominantly produced by TH-1 cells and which activates T and NK cells, resulting in IFN-γ and TNF-α release (with subsequent macrophage activation). Interleukin-2 has been used in human therapy for malignancy (Lotze et al., 1986) and in HIV infection for over 20 years, although its precise role in the latter condition is still awaiting the outcome of two long-term controlled trials (Vento et al., 2006). The production of pegylated (PEG)-IL-2 has increased the half-life of the agent and simplified administration schedules (Teppler et al., 1993). Construction of an IL-2/Ig fusion protein has also resulted in an increase in the therapeutic half-life (Craiu et al., 2001). In addition, a novel way of delivering IL-2 has been described using a vaccinia virus construct (Mukherjee et al., 2003). Each of these approaches could be explored in the future for management of CNS pathogens. Potentially serious complications of IL-2 therapy in humans have been described, including gut perforation (Heimann and Schwartentruber, 2004) and Graves Disease (Jimenez et al., 2004).

Interleukin-4 (IL-4) is a pleiotropic cytokine that is produced by T cells and which deactivates macrophages and enhances antibody production. It shares some common effects with the related cytokine IL-13. It binds to two different receptors, namely the class I IL-4R (comprising IL-4Ralpha/IL-2Rgamma chains) on T cells and the class II IL-4R (comprising IL-4Ralpha/IL-13Ralpha chains) on endothelial cells, which also binds IL-13. Binding of the receptor activates STAT-6 and deletions of STAT-6 and IL-4 have been shown to have similar effects. An IL-13 antagonist has been described which also inhibits IL-4 activity (Kioi et al., 2004). It has been shown that a soluble IL-4 receptor administered by inhalation acts as a cytokine antagonist and this agent has been reported to have benefit in the treatment of asthma (Borish et al., 2001). One mechanism by which IL-4 could influence infective processes is via the inhibition of expression of important inflammatory cytokines such as TNF-α, IL-1 and IFN-γ (Lee et al., 1995). Hence, several strategies are now available to either enhance or ablate the physiological effects of IL-4 in infections whose pathogenesis is potentially significantly affected by this cytokine. For example, many infections appear to be aggravated by IL-4 (e.g leishmaniasis, schistosomiasis: Donnelly et al., 2008; listeria: Szalay et al., 1996; paracoccidioides: Coltri et al., 2008; echinococcus: Al-Qaoud and Abdul-Hafez, 2008; and possibly tuberculosis: Roy et al., 2008). On the other hand, the course of legionella (Newton et al., 2000), toxoplasma (Suzuki et al., 1996), trichinella (Urban et al., 2000), Borrelia burgodorfori (Moro et al., 2001), and coxsackievirus (Jiang et al., 2008) infections is less severe in the presence of IL-4.

Interleukin-6 (IL-6) is a pleiotropic cytokine, but appears to be predominantly pro-inflammatory and causes deleterious effects in several animal models of CNS infection (Suzuki et al., 1997). A primate model of Lyme borreliosis demonstrated high IL-6 expression in the brain during infection (Pachner et al., 1997). A humanized anti-IL6 receptor antibody (tocluzimab) has now been introduced for clinical use in rheumatology (Smolen and Maini, 2006) and could have application in the treatment of infectious diseases in which IL-6 activity is thought to be deleterious.

Interleukin-7 (IL-7) is produced by endothelial cells, as well as other sources, and plays a role in T cell regulation, including selectively increasing CD8+ cells. The IL-7 has now been administered, and is well tolerated, in humans with malignancy (Rosenberg et al., 2006), so its potential role in the treatment of CNS infections could be pursued.

Interleukin-10 (IL-10) is a negative regulatory cytokine predominantly produced by TH-2 lymphocytes and which suppresses macrophage function. It is produced by glial cells in CNS infections such as N. meningitidis and Borrellia burgdorferi (Rasley et al., 2006). As IL-10 has now been safely administered to humans (Angel, et al., 2000), it may be time to study its role in those CNS infections where immune responses appear to have adverse effects.

Interleukin-12 (IL-12) is an important pro-inflammatory cytokine shown to have protective effects in many intracellular infections that can cause CNS disease, such as TB and toxoplasmosis (Gazzinelli et al., 1993). It is a heterodimeric protein comprising unrelated p40 and p35 subunits. The p40 subunit is generally secreted in excess and homodimers act as an IL-12 antagonist. When p40 binds a different subunit (p19) it forms the related cytokine IL-23. The IL-12 is produced by microglia and astrocytes (Constantinescu et al., 2005), dendritic cells, macrophages, and B-cells, and stimulates T cells and NK cells to produce IFN-γ. Production of IL-12 has been noted to be deficient in HIV patients (Gately, 1996).

Recombinant IL-12 has been safely administered to humans with HIV infection and Kaposi's sarcoma (Little et al., 2006), as well as to patients with HCV infection (albeit without significant benefit) (Zeuzem et al., 1999). Deficiency of the IL-12 receptor β1, which predisposes to mycobacterial infection (Filipe-Santos et al., 2006), has been rectified in vitro by retroviral-mediated gene transfer of the receptor (which is utilized by both IL-12 and IL-23 pathways) into human T cells obtained from IL-12 receptor-deficient patients (Bosticardo et al., 2004). Whether this is a viable therapy for in-vivo use remains uncertain.

Sequential therapy with exogenous IL-12 followed by IFN-alpha-2β has been administered without toxicity to patients with advanced cancer with measurable effects upon peripheral blood mononuclear cells (PBMC) (Eisenbeis et al., 2005). Gene therapy in humans using the IL-12 gene has been trialed in cancer patients, but unfortunately no major benefits were identified (Sangro et al., 2005). The IL-12 gene has been successfully delivered to mice using a Semliki virus vector for treatment in a brain tumor model (Yamanaka et al., 2002), and has also been administered nasally to mice to augment the effects of cytotoxic agents in a tumor model (Duan et al., 2006). Another method of safely delivering the IL-12 gene to healthy human controls has been described using CMV Towne strain vaccine (Jacobson et al., 2006). Such approaches could also ultimately have implications for the treatment of human CNS infections.

An anti-IL12 antibody has been developed for the treatment of Crohn's disease (Mannon *et al.*, 2004), a strategy that has been shown to block antigen presentation by microglia and astrocytes (Constantinescu *et al.*, 2005). Study of patients with Crohn's disease using this antibody suggests that IL-12 is an important protective cytokine in the defense against tuberculosis, as use of the antibody appeared to increase the risk of infection (Fieschi *et al.*, 2005). On the other hand, anti-IL-12 therapy has had beneficial effect in a murine model of Lyme arthritis (Anguita *et al.*, 1996). An anti-IL-12 p40 autovaccine has been studied in mice and protects against autoimmune inflammation as well as *Leishmania* infection (Uyttenhove *et al.*, 2004). Other strategies to inhibit interleukin-12 activity have also been tested in man including use of the antifungal itraconazole (Inoue *et al.*, 2004) and ginseng (Larsen *et al.*, 2004).

Interleukin-13 (IL-13) is a cytokine produced by TH-2 lymphocytes that has a prominent role in allergic diseases and responses to parasitic infection. It has also been reported to be relevant in *Listeria* infection (Flesch *et al.*, 1997).

Interleukin-15 (IL-15) is an important mediator of antiviral immunity (Aurelius *et al.*, 1994) and is produced in the CNS by microglia (Hanisch *et al.*, 1997). It is important in both the differentiation of NK cells and expansion of CD8+ T cells and shares a receptor (IL-2R) with IL-2.

Interleukin-16 (IL-16) is produced by many cells and has chemoattractant properties for lymphocytes and monocytes (Archin *et al.*, 2003). A potential role for IL-16 in the immune reconstitution of HIV-infected patients has been proposed (Cruikshank *et al.*, 2000)

Interleukin-17 (IL-17) is a pro-inflammatory cytokine produced by several cell types, including a subset of T-helper cells (Th-17 cells). Its induction occurs as a result of IL-23 and TGF-β activity via toll-like receptor 4 (TLR-4) (Happel *et al.*, 2003). An anti-IL-17A autovaccine has been studied in mice and protects against autoimmune inflammation (Uyttenhove and Van Snick, 2006).

Interleukin-18 (IL-18) has been demonstrated to play an important role in neuro-inflammation (Felderhoff-Mueser *et al.*, 2005). It is produced by many cell types, including microglia and astrocytes (Okamura *et al.*, 1998). This cytokine is secreted as a pro-cytokine and is processed by IL-1B-converting enzyme (ICE). Interleukin-18 binds its own receptor (homology has been reported with IL-1 receptor-related protein) and it signals via mechanisms similar to those induced by IL-1 (e.g. via MyD88 and IRAK) (Akira, 2000). The effects of receptor binding include NK cell activation, IFN-γ induction and activation of naive T cells to secrete IFN-γ. Many of the actions of IL-18 are exerted synergistically with IL-12 (via induction of IL-18 receptors). Levels of IL-18 in the CSF but not the serum have been shown to be elevated in HIV patients with cerebral opportunistic infections (von Giesen *et al.*, 2004). A novel method of delivering IL-18 to the brain using a Sindbis virus construct containing DNA encoding the cytokine has been described in a mouse brain tumor model (Yamanaka and Xanthopoulos, 2005), a strategy that could ultimately have relevance for the treatment of human cerebral infections.

Interleukin-23 (IL-23), as discussed above, shares a common structural subunit (p40) with IL-12 but also has its own unique subunit (p19), which is expressed by both microglia and astrocytes (Constantinescu *et al.*, 2005). Previous studies of p40 blockade in models of infection inferred only a role for IL-12 in these effects, but it is now appreciated that these protocols appear to have also inhibited IL-23 activity (Kreymborg *et al.*, 2005). In contrast to IL-12, IL-23 appears to exert most of its pro-inflammatory effect via IL-17 and IL-6 induction. The IL-23 has already been delivered to murine lung via an adenovirus vector (Happel *et al.*, 2005), and mechanisms to deliver it to the brain should also be pursued.

Interleukin-27 (IL-27) appears to be an important negative regulator of the immune activation mediated by T cells via IL-17. It is therefore likely to be an important immune modulator in both CNS infections and autoimmune disorders.

Tumor necrosis factor-α (TNF-α) is a pro-inflammatory cytokine that is well recognized to mediate adverse effects on the host, particularly in septicemia (Dinarello, 2000) and experimental meningitis (Mustafa *et al.*, 1989). It also mediates protective responses in some infections (Chang *et al.*, 1992). A TNF mimetic, TNF 70–80, has been shown to provide protection in a murine model of BCG infection (Briscoe *et al.*, 2000). In addition, TNF antagonism induced by the agents infliximab or etanercept has been shown to be useful in the treatment of autoimmune disease such as rheumatoid arthritis, but increases the risk of mycobacterial reactivation (Wallis et al., 2004) particularly with etanercept. The TNF-related apoptosis-inducing ligand (TRAIL) induces death of neurones, an effect that has been suppressed by flupirtine maleate in in-vitro studies (Dorr et al., 2005). The effects of TNF-α are often mediated via NF-κβ and subsequent iNOS induction, a pathway that can be antagonized by a variety of NF-κβ inhibitors (e.g. BAY-11–7082, MG-132, and helenalin) in vitro (Davis et al., 2005).

(CD 40)-ligand engages CD40 expressed on microglia, CD4+ T cells, B cells, and monocytes resulting in the production of IFN-γ (Subauste et al., 1999), IL-12 (Pietrella et al., 2004), and TNF-α (Tan et al., 1999). The CD40 has also been shown to be up-regulated by microglia in HIV infection (D'Aversa et al., 2002).

Erythropoietin (EPO) is a growth factor for red blood cells that has receptors in neuronal tissue and which has recently been recognized as an important modulator of neuroprotection (Hasselblatt et al., 2006), as well as a promoter of neuronal stem cell differentiation into astrocytes (Park et al., 2006).

Non-cytokine therapies

Cimetidine is a histamine-2 receptor antagonist that has been used extensively for the treatment of peptic ulceration. Its immunomodulatory effects have been useful for allergy management. It inhibits histamine-induced activation of suppressor T cells in vitro, and has been shown to significantly reduce healing time in herpes zoster infection (Miller et al., 1989). A small randomized study showed that cimetidine resulted in improvement in clinical disability scores in patients with subacute sclerosing panencephalitis (SSPE) (Anlar et al., 1993).

Nitric oxide (NO) is produced via inducible NO synthase (iNOS) and initiates one of the important non-oxidative killing pathways for macrophages infected with intracellular pathogens, as well as being a regulator of the blood–brain barrier (Komatsu et al., 1999a, 1999b). Interestingly, neuro-inflammation induced by the feline immunodeficiency virus (FIV) has been shown to be mediated by STAT-1 and NO pathways, which can be specifically inhibited by the inhibitor aminoguanidine (Zhu et al., 2005).

Peroxisome proliferator-activated receptor-gamma (PPAR-γ) is a nuclear receptor that, after activation, acts as a transcription factor to regulate gene expression and thereby modulate the immune response. Natural and synthetic PPAR-γ (Xue et al., 2002) agonists are now recognized, which inhibit microglial activation and cytokine production (Bernardo and Minghetti, 2006). Interestingly, PPAR-γ agonists have been used for some years in the treatment of arthritis (i.e. non-steroidal anti-inflammatories [NSAIDS]) and in the treatment of metabolic side effects of diabetes (glitazones). Recently, both ibuprofen and pioglitazone have been shown to reduce glial inflammation in a murine model of Alzheimer's disease (Heneka et al., 2005). These agents should therefore be further evaluated in models of CNS infection.

Statins act as inhibitors of HMG Co-A and have been extensively used clinically as cholesterol-lowering agents, but they also have potent anti-inflammatory properties. Simvastatin has been shown to reduce both MHC class II expression by astrocytes (Zeinstra et al., 2006) and the motility of microglia (Kuipers et al., 2006). Simvastatin also reduces human BBB permeability (Ifergan et al., 2006), and it exhibits an antiviral effect in HCV infection, particularly in combination with IFN-α (Ikeda et al., 2006). Statins could also have useful effects in other infections and deserve further study in this context.

Toll-like receptors (TLR) are important mediators of the innate immune system (Aderem and Ulevitch, 2000) that are present on the surface of dendritic cells, macrophages, and granulocytes and which bind molecular motifs on many pathogens, leading to the activation of immune cells (Ozato et al., 2002). The TLR 7/8 activate NK cells to produce IFN-γ (Hart et al., 2005), whereas TLR-2 pathways appear to be particularly important in mediating inflammatory cytokine production by microglia in HSV encephalitis (Aravalli et al., 2005). The TLR-3 is expressed in response to rabies and HSV infections (Jackson et al., 2006).

Intercellular adhesion molecules (ICAMS) are, in part, responsible for mediating leukocyte homing, which is an important step in the induction of neuroprotective responses to CNS infection. An important aspect of this process is the induction of expression of ICAM1 by IFN-α (Dietrich et al., 2002; Greenwood et al., 2002). Interference with ICAM-1 signaling has been shown to reduce neural inflammation (Turowski et al., 2005).

Artemisinins are potent anti-malarial agents that have been extensively used in the treatment of cerebral malaria. Although their effect was assumed to be solely due to parasite killing, they have now been shown to inhibit NF-κβ and prostaglandin production and they could therefore exert some of their effects through immunomodulation (Reddy et al., 2006).

Cannabinoids (CB) have been known to affect CNS function for millennia. More recently, cannabinoid receptors have been identified on microglia and have been shown to affect local immune function by enhancing microglial migration and proliferation but also by reducing their activation. Cannaboids thus have a potentially important role in the regulation of cerebral inflammation (Carrier et al., 2005). The CB2 receptor is up-regulated in simian immunodeficiency virus-induced encephalitis (Benito et al., 2005). An oral cannabinoid preparation (Dronabinol) has been available for use by HIV patients for some years and could have useful immunomodulatory effects.

Estrogens have been known to be immunomodulatory for some time (Maret et al., 2003), and have been shown to inhibit CNS cytokine production (Matejuk et al., 2001). The 17-beta estradiol inhibits microglial function during brain injury, partly by reducing the expression of inflammatory mediators such as TNF-α (Elisabetta et al., 2006). Estrogens have proven beneficial in MS models, with both 17-beta estradiol (Polanczyk et al., 2003) and a highly selective estrogen receptor ligand, namely propyl pyrazole triol (PPT), having been shown to reduce CNS inflammation (Morales et al., 2006).

Androstenedione and other androgenic steroids (Padgett and Sheridan, 1999) are known immunomodulators and widespread experience exists in their clinical use in endocrinology and sports medicine.

Vitamin D has been in clinical use for many years for endocrinological disease and is known to have potent peripheral immunological actions (Tsoukas et al., 1984). The 1,25 dihydroxy vitamin D3 has been described as inducing useful reduction in inflammatory cytokine production during murine Pseudomonas ocular infection (Xue et al., 2002).

Vitamin E has been known to be important in immunomodulation and dietary supplementation enhances immune responses (Meydani et al., 1997). A novel dual vitamin E-like antioxidant, IRFI 042, inhibits NF-κβ and has been shown to have anti-inflammatory action in an animal model of myocarditis (Altavilla et al., 2000).

Immunomodulation in specific infections

Bacterial meningitis

Bacterial meningitis (BM) has a high incidence of serious sequelae despite adequate antibiotic therapy,

and much of this is mediated by immune processes (van Deuren et al., 1994; Mustafa et al., 1989). In response to this revelation, several immunomodulatory strategies have been both tested and validated as having therapeutic utility in experimental models of bacterial meningitis. Administration of IL-10 in a murine model of pneumococcal meningitis successfully modulated meningeal inflammation (Paris et al., 1997). Pneumococcal meningitis has also been shown to induce local production of IL-18, and ablation of this cytokine reduces deleterious inflammation (Zwijnenburg et al., 2003). Blocking IL-18 with either specific antibody or an IL-18 receptor antagonist could therefore be a useful therapeutic strategy. The TNF-α inhibitor thalidomide reduces the CSF pleocytosis and also intrathecal levels of this cytokine in rabbit models of Haemophilus and pneumococcal meningitis (Burroughs et al., 1995; Paris et al., 1997). Another TNF-α inhibitor, pentoxyfylline, also reduced meningeal inflammation in a rabbit model of meningitis (Saez-Llorens et al., 1990b). Inhibition of TNF activity can also be mediated by blocking the activity of TNF-α converting enzyme which is necessary for the conversion of pro- to mature TNF. Such an effect has been achieved using the broad-spectrum metalloproteinase inhibitor BB-1101, which not only reduces CSF TNF-α levels in an animal model of pneumococcal meningitis, but which has also been reported to reduce neuronal injury and mortality (Leib et al., 2000). Finally, inhibition of NF-κβ by the inhibitors ALLN and BAY 11–7085 has been reported to significantly reduce meningeal inflammation (Koedel et al., 2000).

Randomized controlled trials have established the beneficial effects of corticosteroids in bacterial meningitis (in doses equivalent to dexamethasone 0.15 mg/kg qid for 2–4 days), predominantly in H. influenzae meningitis of infancy and childhood, with improvement in the profiles of key biomarkers such as CSF levels of IL-1β and TNF-α, as well as a reduction in sensorineural deafness and improved prognostic scores having been observed (Lebel et al., 1988; Odio et al., 1991; Schaad et al., 1993). Since H. influenzae B vaccination has almost eliminated this pathogen from the developed world, the role of routine corticosteroid use in meningitis in this setting is now unclear, especially given that studies which included children with S. pneumoniae meningitis have not shown such impressive benefits (Kanra et al., 1995; Wald et al., 1995; Molyneux et al., 2002). One controlled study of adult meningitis did not show any beneficial effect of dexamethasone (Thomas et al., 1999). More recent controlled data have, however, suggested that adults with meningitis could derive benefit from dexamethasone, especially when the cause is *S. pneumoniae*, with reduced mortality having being observed (de Gans *et al.*, 2002). Successful dexamethasone therapy in BM is correlated with a reduction in CSF TNF-α levels (Ohga *et al.*, 1999). Alternative therapeutic approaches have also been assessed, for example an uncontrolled trial of G-CSF has shown an apparent reduction in the complication rate amongst 22 patients with *Streptococcus pneumoniae* meningitis (de Lalla *et al.*, 2000).

Tuberculosis (TB) is a ubiquitous infection that appears to be increasing in prevalence, and multi-drug resistance (MDR) results in impaired responses to existing anti-microbials. Immunomodulation could, therefore, provide an important therapeutic option in this increasingly difficult to treat infection. Initial TB infection occurs through the pulmonary portal, with disease of the CNS occurring early in children but later (due to reactivation of tuberculomata) in adults.

Interferon-γ is critical in host defense against mycobacterial infection, including tuberculosis (Kamijo *et al.*, 1993). Pro-inflammatory cytokines, especially TNF-α and IL-1, are important in mediating tissue inflammation in humans with pulmonary TB (Flesch and Kaufmann, 1993; Tsao *et al.*, 2000) with TNF-α reported to be critical in the formation of the granulomata (Kindler *et al.*, 1989). On the other hand, numbers of IL-2-responsive cells have been reported to be reduced in patients with TB (Schauf *et al.*, 1993). Concordant with this observation, it is now recognized that deficiencies in activation pathways dependent on IFN-γ and IL-12 can predispose to mycobacterial disease, including disseminated disease and disease due to normally minimally pathogenic species such as BCG (Holland *et al.*, 2000). Low CSF IFN-γ levels are associated with poor outcome in TB meningitis (Simmons *et al.*, 2006). Replacement therapy has been of value in some patients, but those who have IL-12 receptor deficiencies may not show a good response to IFN-γ therapy (Ulrichs *et al.*, 2005). Studies in which patients with pulmonary tuberculosis have been administered subcutaneous (Palmero *et al.*, 1999) and aerosolized (Giosue *et al.*, 1998, 2000) IFN-α, aerosolized IFN-γ (Condos *et al.*, 1997; Giosue *et al.*, 2000; Koh *et al.*, 2004), IL-2 (Johnson *et al.*, 1995, 1997, 2003; Holland *et al.*, 2000) and IL-12 (Johnson *et al.*, 1997) have yielded variable results.

Tumor necrosis factor-α has also been reported to be an important mediator of adverse effects of tuberculosis meningitis (TBM) both in animal models (Tsenova *et al.*, 1999) and in humans (Tsai *et al.*, 1996). Inhibition of TNF-α by thalidomide enhanced survival and reduced brain pathology in an animal model of TBM (Tsenova *et al.*, 1998). Unfortunately, despite these promising animal model data, a randomized controlled trial of thalidomide in the treatment of childhood TBM showed no useful clinical responses (Schoeman *et al.*, 2004). The same authors, however, reported a small cohort of patients with intractable intracranial tuberculosis infection who appeared to benefit from thalidomide (Schoeman *et al.*, 2006).

Beneficial effects of corticosteroids have been noted in TBM, and their use has been recommended in patients with a depressed conscious state at presentation (Molavi and Le Frock, 1985). Although dexamethasone has been shown to suppress the production of inflammatory cytokines in response to *M. tuberculosis* by human microglia and astrocytes (Rock *et al.*, 2005), clinical studies do not reveal a reduction in CSF pro-inflammatory cytokines in patients with TB meningitis treated with this agent (Simmons *et al.*, 2005). A meta-analysis did not find evidence of benefit in adults, although a recent controlled trial revealed prolongation of survival but without beneficial effect upon the chronic sequelae of TBM (Thwaites *et al.*, 2004).

Listeria monocytogenes is an intracellular pathogen that is an important cause of meningoencephalitis and current anti-microbial therapy has suboptimal response rates. Animal models have identified a prominent role for pro-inflammatory cytokines (including IFN-γ, IL-12 and IL-18) in the protective response against this organism (Sugawara, 2000). Rising levels of IL-6 and falling levels of IFN-γ are a particularly poor prognostic sign (Kim *et al.*, 2001). In a murine model of listeriosis, administration of recombinant IL-12 enhanced resistance to infection (Wagner *et al.*, 1994). The administration of both recombinant IL-13 (possibly via induction of IL-12) and recombinant IL-1 have also been reported to significantly reduce the organism load in murine models (Flesch *et al.*, 1997; Czuprynski *et al.*, 1994). The G-CSF also appears to be important in protection against murine listeriosis, as G-CSF knockouts have adverse outcome in comparison with wild-type mice (Lieschke *et al.*, 1994): studies of G-CSF supplementation in human listeriosis would therefore be of great interest. Mice deficient in IL-10 have been observed to display a severe hyperinflammatory response to *Listeria* meningoencephalitis (Deckert *et al.*, 2001), suggesting that judicious supplementation of IL-10 could be a cogent therapeutic strategy. Blockade of TNF-α in the treatment of rheumatoid arthritis appears to increase the risk of listeriosis (Aparicio et al., 2003): it is therefore paradoxical that neutralization of TNF-α in a murine model of listeriosis appeared to be protective (Nakane et al., 1999). Finally, dexamethasone completely protected mice from death in a model of listeriosis but the mechanism of action is uncertain as suppression of multiple inflammatory cytokines was noted (Nakane et al., 1994).

Viral infections

Herpesviridae

Herpes simplex type 1 (HSV-1) causes a potentially devastating encephalitis, which does not always respond well to specific antiviral therapy. Recovery from herpes simplex viral encephalitis (HSVE) has been associated with the appearance of TNF-α in the CSF (Aurelius et al., 1994). Animal studies suggest a useful role for T-1 cytokines (Osorio et al., 2002) and IL-15 in the response to HSV-1 infections (Gosselin et al., 1999). A common model for studying defenses against HSV-1 involves a corneal infection protocol that results in spread of the virus to the optic nerve and, subsequently, the brain and trigeminal ganglion. In this model, although successful defense is correlated with a T-1 cytokine response (Osorio et al., 2002), IL-4 (a Th-2 cytokine) provided better protection than either IFN-γ or IL-2 (Osorio and Ghiasi, 2003). The model has also enabled a number of strategies designed to deliver genes encoding IFN-β (using a plasmid construct) (Cui and Carr, 2000), IFN-α (using a CMV vector) (Noisakran et al., 2000), IL-2 (Ghiasi et al., 2002), IL-4 (Osorio and Ghiasi, 2003), IL-12 p35 (Osorio and Ghiasi, 2005), and IL-16 (Archin et al., 2003) to be tested, but further work is required to identify the best cytokine/supplementation protocol for therapeutic trial in humans. In other studies, treatment of mice with recombinant CD40L protected marrow transplant recipients from mortality after HSV-1 infection (Beland et al., 1998). Androstenedione has also been shown to be protective in a murine model of HSV encephalitis by increasing levels of IFN-γ in the trigeminal ganglion (Carr, 1998). A retrospective study of 45 patients with HSV encephalitis who were treated with acyclovir has concluded that corticosteroid use (equivalent to a median dose of 64 mg of prednisolone daily for a median of 6 days) was an independent predictor of improved outcome (Kamei

et al., 2005). In-vitro studies using human neural cell lines demonstrate synergistic activity of acyclovir and IFN-α (Hanada et al., 1989).

Focal viral encephalitis of children is a clinical entity that has overlap with HSVE with a retrospective case series reporting successful use (with a decrease in both mortality and adverse sequelae) of a combination of acyclovir and IFN-β (5 mU/kg/d) (Wintergerst and Behloradsky, 1992). A recently conducted small controlled trial did not, however, find any superiority of combination therapy (Wintergerst et al., 2005), but in this study only 14 of 59 enrolled patients had proven encephalitis, such that conclusions were drawn from a very small data set and indicating that the role of IFN-β in the context is not, as yet, definitely clarified.

Varicella zoster virus (VZV) infection, in particular its dissemination, has been reported to be inhibited by the administration of IFN-α (Merigan et al., 1978; Winston et al., 1988). A case report has also suggested that IFN-α was useful in the treatment of zoster myelitis that was unresponsive to acyclovir (Nakano et al., 1992).

Cytomegalovirus (CMV) is an important opportunistic pathogen, especially in AIDS patients in whom it can cause retinitis, polyradiculoneuritis, and encephalitis. A retroviral murine model of CMV retinitis has revealed beneficial effects of exogenous IL-2 (Dix and Cousins, 2003) but not IL-12 (Dix et al., 1997).

Epstein–Barr virus (EBV), in particular its viral load, has been reported to be diminished in HIV patients receiving IL-2 treatment (Burighel et al., 2006), raising the possibility that this cytokine could be used for serious complications of this common infection. A case report described a beneficial response to IFN-γ therapy in the context of cerebral EBV (Andersson et al., 1999).

Papovaviridae

Progressive multifocal leukoencephalopathy (PML) occurs in immunocompromised patients and is caused by the JC virus. The pharmaceutical agent cytarabine has been used but with variable results in this condition. A case report documented successful treatment of PML with cytarabine combined with IFN-α (Steiger et al., 1993), but similar regimens have also been reported to be inefficacious (Heide et al., 1995). Case reports of progression of PML despite IFN-β monotherapy have also been described (Nath et al., 2006). A case report of sustained response to IL-2 has recently been published (Kunschner and Scott, 2005). The use of highly active antiretroviral therapy (HAART) in patients with underlying HIV has also resulted in improvement in PML (Albrecht *et al.*, 1998). The HAART regimen has, itself, been shown to result in significant restoration of normal cytokine secretion in HIV patients (Amirayan-Chevillard *et al.*, 2000). An uncontrolled study of HIV patients with PML who received HAART compared treatment with IFN-α (3 mU daily) to 32 untreated historical controls (Huang *et al.*, 1998) and reported delayed clinical progression in the IFN-α treated group. However, subsequent retrospective studies (Geschwind *et al.*, 2001) have cast doubt on whether IFN-α adds anything to the beneficial effects of HAART (Albrecht *et al.*, 1998).

Togaviridae

Alphaviruses comprise a group that includes important causes of human encephalitis, for example western equine encephalitis, eastern equine encephalitis, and Venezuelan equine encephalitis. The group also includes Sindbis virus which causes encephalitis in animals but polyarthritis in humans and which is a common model for studying the pathogenesis of encephalitis. Interferon-α and β have been shown to protect mice infected with Sindbis virus (Ryman *et al.*, 2000). However, other investigators have found IFN-γ to be a more important protective factor against this infection (Binder and Griffin, 2001). On the other hand, inhibition of iNOS (by *N*ω-nitro-L-arginine methyl ester [L-NAME]) in mice increases mortality in Sindbis encephalitis, probably by inhibiting neuroprotective mechanisms rather than by modulating immunopathogenesis (Tucker *et al.*, 1996).

Flaviviridae

Japanese B encephalitis (JEV) is a cause of severe encephalitis which has recently spread from continental Asia, westwards to India and southwards to Papua New Guinea and northern Australia. A role for IFN-α in JEV has been investigated in a randomized double-blind placebo-controlled trial of 112 infected Vietnamese children (Solomon *et al.*, 2003), but when the agent was administered at 10 mU/m^2 for 7 days it did not have any demonstrable beneficial effects. On the other hand, IL-12 has been shown to suppress protective immune responses in JEV infection when administered with a vaccine (Orange *et al.*, 1995).

St Louis encephalitis (SLEV) has been shown to be amenable to treatment with IFN-α in a murine model (Brooks and Philpotts, 1999). In an uncontrolled

series, 15 patients with SLEV infection were reported to exhibit superior clinical improvement after the administration of IFN-α 2b (3 mU daily) compared to 17 untreated patients (Rahal *et al.*, 2004).

West Nile virus (WNV) causes a potentially fatal encephalitis, and recently its distribution has extended into the Western Hemisphere with very rapid establishment in northern America. The virus has been shown to be sensitive to ribavirin and IFN-α in vitro (Anderson and Rahal, 2002). Individual cases of WNV encephalitis have appeared to improve with IFN-α monotherapy (Sayao *et al.*, 2004; Kalil *et al.*, 2005). However, failures have also been reported with this treatment (Chan-Tack and Forrest, 2005).

Paramyxoviridae

Measles can be complicated by encephalitis and can induce a severe depression of immune responses, predisposing to secondary infection (Griffin, 1995). Vitamin A has been shown in a controlled trial to improve outcome in children with acute measles infection (Hussey and Klein, 1990). Interferon-β has also been shown via neutralization studies to be critical in antiviral defense in a murine model of acute measles encephalitis (Finke *et al.*, 1995).

Subacute sclerosing panencephalitis (SSPE) is a devastating late complication of measles virus infection due to viral persistence in the CNS (Garg, 2002). Patients with SSPE have shown impaired plasma interferon activity (Gadoth *et al.*, 1989), and when SSPE patients were treated with an interferon-inducer (isoprinosine), their mononuclear cells demonstrated restored interferon production. Early studies of IFN-α monotherapy by intraventricular (IV) (Panitch *et al.*, 1986) and various other routes as treatment of SSPE suggested useful clinical effects in some patients (Yoshioka *et al.*, 1989).

A large non-randomized study of 98 patients with SSPE demonstrated significant survival advantage using monotherapy with isoprinosine (Jones *et al.*, 1982). A small study of patients with SSPE also showed stabilization in 3 of 7 patients treated with a combination of oral isoprinosine and IFN-β (Anlar *et al.*, 1998). An uncontrolled study comparing the efficacy of two therapeutic regimens of IFN-β delivery (60 μg IM weekly vs. 22 μg alternate daily) concluded that the latter regimen had better efficacy (Anlar *et al.*, 2004). An uncontrolled comparison of isoprinosine versus combined therapy with isoprinosine and IFN-α suggested superior activity of combination therapy

(Gokcil et al., 1999) in adult-onset SSPE, but another study concluded that isoprinosine provided no additional benefit (Anlar et al., 1997). A further uncontrolled study in SSPE found improved remission rates and longer survival periods amongst 13 patients receiving combined cytokine and antiviral therapy comprising subcutaneous (SC) IFN-α, isoprinosine and lamivudine, compared to 13 who did not receive any treatment (Aydin et al., 2003). Case reports have also suggested useful activity of high-dose intravenous ribavirin when used alone in SSPE (Hosoya et al., 2001). An uncontrolled case series studied combination therapy using intraventricular ribavirin and IFN-α in 10 cases of SSPE, most of whom had failed IFN-α monotherapy. Both a clinical response and a reduction in CSF measles antibody titers were documented (Hara et al., 2003).

A number of controlled trials have also been conducted. In one such trial, isoprinosine did not exert any identifiable activity when used as monotherapy (Haddad and Risk, 1980). On the other hand, a randomized, controlled trial of 121 patients with SSPE showed that combination therapy comprising IFN-α (1 mU/m^2 twice weekly) and isoprinosine (100 mg/kg/d) had similar response rates to isoprinosine therapy alone (Gascon et al., 2003). This study had a large drop out rate, however, and an intention to treat analysis was not reported. A small, randomized study showed improvement in clinical disability scores using cimetidine as an immunomodulator in SSPE (Anlar et al., 1993).

In conclusion, although some uncontrolled studies have reported beneficial effects of IV IFN-α used either with or without isoprinosine or ribavirin in patients with SSPE, it is clear that more rigorous controlled trials are required to confirm efficacy and to establish the optimal therapeutic regimen. One possibility that also needs to be explored is whether IFN-β could provide a viable alternative to IFN-α. Such studies also need to control for the adjunctive use of corticosteroids, which has confounded prior studies. Late relapses in some patients who initially responded to immunotherapy (Anlar et al., 1997), including one relapse that occurred 18 years after an apparent response (Miyazaki et al., 2005) suggest that very prolonged courses of therapy (some authors suggest life-long) could be required.

Rhabdoviridae

Rabies is currently a uniformly fatal infective disease of the brain. In an open study of four rabid patients evaluated combination therapy with intravenous and intraventricular IFN-α and tribavirin, but no clinical effect was observed (Warrell et al., 1989).

Orthomyxoviridae

Influenza A is an important cause of viral encephalitis, and the 1919 pandemic caused millions of cases of encephalitis lethargica, which is characterized by parkinsonian features. Human influenza encephalitis induces high levels of pro-inflammatory cytokines in the CSF, including IL-6 (Aiba et al., 2001), as well as by systemic immune activation (Kawada et al., 2003).

A DNA vaccine containing the IL-12 and GM-CSF genes had useful protective effects in a murine model of influenza A infection (Operschall et al., 1999). Ablation of IL-18 appears to have deleterious effects, with reduced microglial activation and reduced local IFN-γ production in a murine model of influenza A encephalitis (Mori et al., 2001). The effect of supplementation with IL-18 should therefore be studied in influenza infections. A TLR-7/8 agonist has been developed and had potent antiviral activity against influenza A in rats (Hammerbeck et al., 2006) and therefore also warrants further study.

Arenaviridae

Lymphocytic choriomeningitis virus (LCMV) is a zoonotic infection that is usually transmitted to humans from rats. Some inflammatory cytokines have been shown to be important mediators of deleterious inflammation in LCMV infection (Asensio et al., 1999). Gene therapy-based delivery of IFN-α appears to exacerbate LCMV encephalitis, with induction of both inflammation and neurodegeneration (Akwa et al., 1998). On the other hand, the IL-12 has been shown to suppress protective immune responses in LCMV infection when administered with a vaccine (Orange et al., 1995). Exogenous pathogen-specific memory T cells delivered to a murine model of LCMV infection have been shown to induce protective immunological responses, including CNS dendritic cell recruitment, TNF-α production, and microglial activation (Lauterbach et al., 2006).

Retroviridae

Infection can cause a myelopathy that, in a case report, has been suggested to respond clinically to corticosteroids (McArthur et al., 1990). In addition, systemic IFN-α (6 mU/alt d) has resulted in improvement of motor function and reduction in proviral DNA levels in 5 of a case series of 7 patients with HTLV-1-associated myelopathy (HAM) (Yamasaki et al., 1997).

Picornaviridae

In a single case study of chronic echovirus meningoencephalitis, a child with underlying agammaglobulinemia has been reported to have responded to therapy with intrathecal IFN-β (von der Wense et al., 1998).

Parasites

A number of immunomodulatory therapies have been considered for the treatment of toxoplasmic encephalitis (TE). On the one hand, corticosteroids did not provide additional benefit over anti-microbials alone in humans with TE (Luft et al., 1993). On the other hand, IFN-γ was shown to be critical in modulating murine TE (Suzuki et al., 1989) and treatment with this cytokine significantly improved outcome (Suzuki et al., 1990). Similar treatments in immunodeficient rats infected with toxoplasmosis have also been effective (Benedetto et al., 1991). Animal models of TE have also revealed a useful synergistic effect of adjunctive IFN-γ, supplementing standard anti-parasitic therapies (Araujo and Remington, 1991; Khan et al., 2001). Importantly, patients with AIDS do not produce IFN-γ in response to opportunistic infections, including toxoplasmosis (Murray et al., 1984). Exogenous IFN-γ has been shown to enhance killing of *Toxoplasma* by monocytes obtained from both immune-competent and immunosuppressed patients (Murray et al., 1987) in vitro. The IFN-γ, along with TNF-α and IL-6, also enhanced *T. gondii* killing by fetal microglia in vitro (Chao et al., 1994). A human trial of IFN-γ therapy of TE was planned, but never reported due to inadequate case recruitment (Remington, personal communication, 2006).

A beneficial effect of IL-2 therapy in murine toxoplasmosis has been reported (Sharma et al., 1985). The main role of IL-2 in murine models appears to be in inducing IFN-γ production (Villegas et al., 2002). Somewhat surprisingly, IL-4, a down-regulator of IFN-γ, is protective against the development of TE in mice (Suzuki and Yang, 1996). The protective effects do, however, appear to be time-dependent, with long-term detrimental effects subsequently becoming apparent (Roberts et al., 1996). On the other hand, IL-6 causes deleterious effects in vitro (Beaman, 1994), but is protective in animal models of toxoplasma infection (Suzuki et al., 1997). The IL-7 has been shown to have important protective effects in murine toxoplasmosis (Kasper et al., 1995) and ablation of IL-10 worsens murine toxoplasmosis, indicating that supplementation with IL-10 could have a therapeutic role (Gazzinelli et al., 1996; Neyer et al., 1997). Similarly, IL-12 has been shown to exert a protective effect in murine models of toxoplasmosis (Gazzinelli et al., 1993; Scharton-Kersten et al., 1995). Interleukin-15 plays a prominent role in defense during toxoplasmic encephalitis (Schluter et al., 2001). One important mechanism of action of IL-15 appears to be mediated via priming of the anti-toxoplasma CD4+ response in the periphery (Khan and Kasper, 1996; Combe et al., 2006). In combination, these data suggest that therapeutic immunomodulation with IL-15 should be studied further in the management of toxoplasmosis, in general, and specifically in patients with complicating CNS infection. Interleukin-23 has been shown to provide partial protection in murine toxoplasmosis if IL-12 is deficient (Lieberman et al., 2004). Interleukin-27 receptor-deficient mice develop severe *T. gondii* neuro-inflammation associated with a prominent IL-17 response (Stumhofer et al., 2006). The in-vitro administration of IL-27 to naive primary T cells suppressed the development of Th-17 cells (IL-17-producing T cells) by IL-6 and TGF-β, raising the possibility of a therapeutic role for exogenous IL-27 in toxoplasmic encephalitis.

Malaria is complex condition whose immunopathogenesis is heavily influenced by cytokine production (Medana et al., 2001; Angulo and Fresno, 2002; Aubouy et al., 2002). Cytokine dysregulation, including high levels of IL-10 and IFN-γ, are a feature of severe falciparum malaria in humans (Wenisch et al., 1995). Unfortunately, corticosteroids appear to worsen outcome when used in cerebral malaria (Prasad and Rahal, 2000). In-vitro studies performed on PBMC isolated from patients with severe falciparum malaria suggest that IL-10 is important in suppressing the production of pro-inflammatory cytokines (such as IL-6) which have detrimental effects (Ho et al., 1998). Supplementation with IL-10 should therefore be evaluated in malaria models. Pentoxifylline is a TNF-α inhibitor with demonstrated benefit in a murine model of malaria, but it has proved ineffective in human falciparum malaria in a placebo-controlled trial of 45 patients (Looareesuwan et al., 1998). This negative result occurred independent of successful suppression of TNF-α levels in the pentoxyfylline-treated group (Wenisch et al., 1998). A recent study of murine cerebral malaria showed that human EPO prevented death from this disease (Kaiser et al., 2006).

Table 16.1 Immunomodulators with effects in human CNS infection

Agent	Indication	Level of evidence	References
Corticosteroids	*H. influenzae* meningitis in children	1b	Lebel *et al.*, 1988; Odio *et al.*, 1991; Schaad *et al.*, 1993
	Adult bacterial meningitis	2b	de Gans *et al.*, 2002
	Tuberculous meningitis	3b	Thwaites *et al.*, 2004
	HSVE	3b	Kamei *et al.*, 2005
	Cysticercosis	5	Nash *et al.*, 2003
IFN-α	SSPE	3b	Anlar *et al.*, 1997
	HAM	4	Yamasaki *et al.*, 1997
	SLEV	4	Rahal *et al.*, 2004
IFN-β	SSPE	3b	Anlar *et al.*, 2004
	Focal viral encephalitis of children	4	Wintergerst and Behlohradsky, 1992
Inosiplex	SSPE	3b	Gascon *et al.*, 2003
IFN-α; inosiplex	SSPE	3b	Gascon *et al.*, 2003
IFN-α; inosiplex+ lamivudine	SSPE	4	Aydin *et al.*, 2003
IFN-β	HSVE	4	Wintergerst and Behlohradsky, 1992
G-CSF	Pneumococcal meningitis	4	de Lalla *et al.*, 2000

HAM = HTLV-1 associated myelopathy

Cysticercosis is caused by the larval form of the pork tapeworm, *Taenia solium*. It is an important cause of CNS disease in the developing world and the commonest cause of epilepsy in those regions. Type 2 cytokines are prominent in the CSF of patients with active neurocysticercosis (Rodrigues *et al.*, 2000; Aguilar-Rebolledo *et al.*, 2001). Corticosteroids have not been studied in well conducted, controlled trials for management of cysticercosis, but are often used when initiating anti-parasitic therapy (Nash, 2003). Anecdotal experience indicates that corticosteroids do not always prevent serious complications such as cerebral infarction or raised intracranial pressure (Takayanagui and Jardim, 1992).

Fungi

Cryptococcus neoformans is an important opportunistic CNS pathogen that causes cryptococcal meningitis, particularly in AIDS patients who appear to have impaired production of pro-inflammatory cytokines (Lortholary *et al.*, 2001). Interleukin-4 has been shown to impair defense against cerebral *C. neoformans* infection, and ablation of this cytokine with specific antibody reduces cerebral fungal burden, whereas supplementation with IL-4 increased the burden in a murine model (Kawakami *et al.*, 1999). Some of these latter effects appear to be mediated by reduced IL-12- and IL-18-mediated induction of IFN-γ. Interleukin-12 is important in early defense against pulmonary cryptococcal infection, and neutralization of IL-12 inhibits the induction of Th responses that prevent cerebral dissemination in a murine model (Pietrella *et al.*, 2004). Interleukin-18, when administered alone, has also been shown to prevent cerebral dissemination in a murine model of cryptococcus infection (Kawakami *et al.*, 1997) and appears to exert beneficial effects independent of IL-12 and via systemic induction of IFN-γ (Kawakami *et al.*, 2000). The combined administration of IL-12 and IL-18 had beneficial, synergistic effects in this model, partly mediated by suppression of IL-4-induced effects and partly by enhancement of IFN-γ induction (Kawakami *et al.*,

233

Table 16.2 Immunomodulators that have been administered to humans and which could have effect in CNS infections

Agent	Indication	References
IFN-α	HSVE, VZE, PML, HTLV1, SLEV, WNV	Balan *et al.*, 2006
IFN-γ	Toxoplasmosis, TBM, Listeriosis, HSVE, Cryptococcosis, EBV	Gallin *et al.*, 1995
IL-2	HSVE, Toxoplasmosis, PML, CMV, EBV	Teppler *et al.*, 1993
IL-7	Toxoplasmosis	Rosenberg *et al.*, 2006
IL-10	Malaria, Toxoplasmosis	Angel *et al.*, 2000
IL-12	Cryptococcosis, TBM, Toxoplasmosis, HSVE, JEV, Influenza	Little *et al.*, 2006
IL-16	HSVE	Cruikshank *et al.*, 2000
EPO	Malaria	Hasselblatt *et al.*, 2006
Anti-IFN-α	LCMV	Gringeri *et al.*, 1999
Anti-IL-6	Lyme Disease	Smolen and Maini, 2006
Anti-IL-12	Lyme Disease	Mannon *et al.*, 2004
Dexamethasone	Listeriosis	Nakane *et al.*, 1999
G-CSF	Listeriosis	Lieschke *et al.*, 1994
Thalidomide	BM, Malaria	Paris *et al.*, 1997
Androgens	HSVE	Carr, 1998

SLEV = St. Louis Encephalitis Virus

1999). Mice with IL-23 deficiency have also been reported to exhibit impaired recruitment and activation of mononuclear cells, including microglia, in response to cryptococcal infection (Kleinschek *et al.*, 2006). Signaling via CD40 induces B cell maturation and is important in inducing IL-12 production, which, as indicated above, is critical in successful defense against *Cryptococcus* (Pietrella *et al.*, 2004). Ablation of this signaling pathway results in an increase in the cerebral fungal burden in *C. neoformans* infection.

Conclusion

Currently, few immunomodulatory agents have been shown to have beneficial effects in human CNS infections (Table 16.1). This chapter has outlined the plethora of immunomodulators that could influence human infections. Perhaps the best way forward is to focus on agents that have already been administered to humans, but which have yet to be studied for efficacy in clinical infections (Table 16.2). Clearly, significant therapeutic benefits could be defined.

References

Aderem A, Ulevitch R. Toll-like receptors in the induction of the innate immune response. *Nature* 2000; **406**: 782–7.

Aguilar-Rebolledo F, *et al.* Interleukin levels in cerebrospinal fluid from children with neurocysticercosis. *Am J Trop Med Hyg* 2001; **64**: 35–40.

Aiba H, *et al.* Predictive value of serum interleukin-6 level in influenza virus-associated encephalopathy. *Neurology* 2001; **57**: 295–9.

Akira S. The role of IL-18 in innate immunity. *Curr Opin Immunol* 2000; **12**: 59–63.

Akwa Y, *et al.* Transgenic expression of IFN-alpha in the central nervous system of mice protects against lethal neurotropic viral infection but induces inflammation and neurodegeneration. *J Immunol* 1998; **161**: 5016–26.

Albrecht H, *et al.* Highly active antiretroviral therapy significantly improves the prognosis of patients with HIV-associated progressive multifocal leukoencephalopathy. *AIDS* 1998; **12**: 1149–54.

Aloisi F, *et al.* Glia-T cell dialogue. *J Neuroimmunol* 2000; **107**: 111–7.

Al-Qaoud KM, Abdul-Hafez SK. The induction of T helper type 1 response by cytokine gene transfection protects mice against secondary hydatidosis. *Parasitol Res* 2008; **102**: 1151–5.

Altavilla D, *et al.* IRFI 042, a novel dual vitamin E-like antioxidant, inhibits activation of nuclear factor-kappa B and reduces the inflammatory response in myocardial ischaemia-reperfusion injury. *Cardiovasc Res* 2000; **47**: 515–28.

Amirayan-Chevillard N, *et al.* Impact of highly active anti-retroviral therapy (HAART) on cytokine production and monocyte subsets in HIV-infected patients. *Clin Exper Immunol* 2000; **120**: 107–12.

Anderson JF, Rahal J. Efficacy of interferon alpha-2b and ribavirin against West Nile virus in vitro. *Emerg Infect Dis* 2002; **8**: 107–8.

Andersson J, *et al.* Interferon gamma (IFN-gamma) deficiency in generalized Epstein–Barr virus infection with interstitial lymphoid and granulomatous pneumonia, focal cerebral lesions, and genital ulcers: Remission following IFN-gamma substitution therapy. *Clin Infect Dis* 1999; **28**: 1036–42.

Angel JB, *et al.* A multicenter, randomized, double-blind, placebo-controlled trial of recombinant human interleukin-10 in HIV-infected subjects. *Aids* 2000; **14**: 2503–8.

Anguita J, *et al.* Effect of anti-interleukin 12 treatment on murine Lyme borreliosis. *J Clin Invest* 1996; **97**: 1028–34.

Angulo I, Fresno M. Cytokines in the pathogenesis of and protection against malaria. *Clin Diagnost Lab Immunol* 1145; **9**: 1145–52.

Anlar B, *et al.* Cimetidine as an immunomodulator in subacute sclerosing panencephalitis: A double blind, placebo-controlled study. *Pediatr Infect Dis J* 1993; **12**: 578–81.

Anlar B, *et al.* Long-term follow-up of patients with subacute sclerosing panencephalitis treated with intraventricular alpha-interferon. *Neurology* 1997; **48**: 526–8.

Anlar B, *et al.* Beta-interferon plus inosiplex in the treatment of subacute sclerosing panencephalitis. *J Child Neurol* 1998; **13**: 557–9.

Anlar B, *et al.* Retrospective evaluation of interferon-beta treatment in subacute sclerosing panencephalitis. *Clin Ther* 2004; **26**: 1890–4.

Aparicio AG, *et al.* Report of an additional case of anti-tumor necrosis factor therapy and Listeria monocytogenes infection: comment on the letter by Gluck *et al. Arthrit Rheumat* 2003; **48**: 1764–5.

Araujo FG, Remington JS. Synergistic activity of azithromycin and gamma interferon in murine toxoplasmosis. *Antimicrob Agents Chemother* 1991; **35**: 1672–3.

Araujo FG, *et al.* Treatment with interleukin 12 in combination with Atovaquone or Clindamycin significantly increases survival of mice with acute toxoplasmosis. *Antimicrob Agents Chemother* 1997; **41**: 188–90.

Aravalli RN, *et al.* Cutting edge: TLR2-mediated pro-inflammatory cytokine and chemokine production by microglial cells in response to herpes simplex virus. *J Immunol* 2005; **175**: 4189–93.

Archin NM, *et al.* Delayed spread and reduction in virus titer after anterior chamber inoculation of a recombinant of HSV-1 expressing IL-16. *Invest Ophthalmol Vis Sci* 2003; **44**: 3066–76.

Asensio VC, *et al.* Chemokines and the inflammatory response to viral infection in the central nervous system with a focus on lymphocytic choriomeningitis virus. *J Neurovirol* 1999; **5**: 65–75.

Aubouy A, *et al.* Plasma and in vitro levels of cytokines during and after a *Plasmodium falciparum* malaria attack in Gabon. *Acta Tropica* 2002; **83**: 195–203.

Aurelius E, *et al.* Cytokines and other markers of intrathecal immune response in patients with herpes simplex encephalitis. *J Infect Dis* 1994; **170**: 678–81.

Aydin OF, *et al.* Combined treatment with subcutaneous interferon-alpha, oral isoprinosine, and lamivudine for subacute sclerosing panencephalitis. *J Child Neurol* 2003; **18**: 104–8.

Balan V, *et al.* A Phase I/II study evaluating escalating doses of recombinant human albumin-interferon-alpha fusion protein in chronic hepatitis C patients who have failed previous interferon-alpha-based therapy. *Antivir Ther* 2006; **11**: 35–45.

Beaman M. Cytokine therapy of infectious diseases. In: Schwartz M, Remington J (Eds.). *Current Topics in Infectious Diseases.* Cambridge, MA: Blackwell Scientific Publications, 1994; **14**: 228–51.

Beaman MH, *et al.* Enhancement of intracellular replication of *Toxoplasma gondii* by interleukin-6: Interactions with interferon-γ and tumor necrosis factor-α. *J Immunol* 1994; **153**: 4583–7.

Beland JL, *et al.* Recombinant CD40L treatment protects allogeneic murine bone marrow transplant recipients from death caused by herpes simplex virus-1 infection. *Blood* 1998; **92**: 4472–8.

Benedetto N, *et al.* Effect of rIFN-gamma and IL-2 treatments in mouse and nude rat infections with *Toxoplasma gondii*. *Eur Cytokine Netw* 1991; **2**: 107–14.

Benito C, *et al.* A glial endogenous cannabinoid system is upregulated in the brains of macaques with simian immunodeficiency virus-induced encephalitis. *J Neurosci* 2005; **25**: 2530–6.

Bernardo A, Minghetti L. PPAR-gamma agonists as regulators of microglial activation and brain inflammation. *Curr Pharm Des* 2006; **12**: 93–109.

Binder GK, Griffin DE. Interferon-gamma-mediated site-specific clearance of alphavirus from CNS neurons. *Science* 2001; **293**: 303–6.

Borish LC, *et al.* Efficacy of soluble IL-4 receptor for the treatment of adults with asthma. *J Allergy Clin Immunol* 2001; **107**: 963–70.

Bosticardo M, *et al.* Retroviral-mediated gene transfer restores IL-12 and IL-23 signaling pathways in T cells from IL-12 receptor beta1-deficient patients. *Mol Ther* 2004; **9**: 895–901.

Briscoe H, *et al.* A novel tumor necrosis factor (TNF) mimetic peptide prevents recrudescence of *Mycobacterium bovis* bacillus Calmette–Guerin (BCG) infection in CD4(+) T cell-depleted mice. *J Leukocyte Biol* 2000; **68**: 538–44.

Brooks TJ, Philpotts R. Interferon-alpha protects mice against lethal infection with St Louis encephalitis virus delivered by the aerosol and subcutaneous routes. *Antiviral Res* 1999; **41**: 57–64.

Buckwold VE, *et al.* Antiviral activity of CHO-SS cell-derived human omega interferon and other human interferons against HCV RNA replicons and related viruses. *Antiviral Res* 2007; **73**: 118–25.

Burighel N, *et al.* Differential dynamics of Epstein–Barr virus in individuals infected with human immunodeficiency virus-1 receiving intermittent interleukin-2 and antiretroviral therapy. *Haematologica* 2006; **91**: 244–7.

Burroughs MH, *et al.* Effect of thalidomide on the inflammatory response in cerebrospinal fluid in experimental bacterial meningitis. *Microb Pathogen* 1995; **19**: 245–55.

Caksen H, *et al.* Onset of generalized seizures after intrathecal interferon therapy of SSPE. *Pediatr Neurol* 2003; **29**: 78–9.

Carr DJ. Increased levels of IFN-gamma in the trigeminal ganglion correlate with protection against HSV-1-induced encephalitis following subcutaneous administration with androstenediol. *J Neuroimmunol* 1998; **89**: 160–7.

Carrier EJ, *et al.* Endocannabinoids in neuroimmunology and stress. *Curr Drug Targets CNS Neurol Disord* 2005; **4**: 657–65.

Chang H, *et al.* Role of tumour necrosis factor in chronic murine *Toxoplasma gondii* encephalitis. *Immun Infect Dis* 1992; **2**: 61–8.

Chan-Tack KM, Forrest G. Failure of interferon alpha-2b in a patient with West Nile virus meningoencephalitis and acute flaccid paralysis. *Scand J Infect Dis* 2005; **37**: 944–6.

Chao CC, *et al.* Human microglial cell defense against *Toxoplasma gondii*. The role of cytokines. *J Immunol* 1994; **152**: 1246–52.

Cianchetti C, *et al.* Toxic effect of intraventricular interferon-alpha in subacute sclerosing panencephalitis. *Ital J Neurol Sci* 1994; **15**: 153–5.

Coltri C, *et al.* Therapeutic administration of KM+ lectin protects mice against *Paracoccidioides brasiliensis* infection via interleukin-12 production in a toll-like receptor 2-dependant mechanism. *Am J Pathol* 2008; **173**: 423–32.

Combe CL, *et al.* Lack of IL-15 results in the suboptimal priming of CD4+ T cell response against an intracellular parasite. *Proc Natl Acad Sci* 2006; **103**: 6635–40.

Condos R, *et al.* Treatment of multidrug-resistant pulmonary tuberculosis with interferon-gamma via aerosol. *Lancet* 1997; **349**: 1513–15.

Constantinescu CS, *et al.* Astrocytes as antigen-presenting cells: Expression of IL-12/IL-23. *J Neurochem* 2005; **95**: 331–40.

Craiu A, *et al.* An IL-2/Ig fusion protein influences CD4(+) T lymphocytes in naive and simian immunodeficiency virus-infected rhesus monkeys. *AIDS Res Human Retrovir* 2001; **17**: 873–86.

Croce M, *et al.* Sequential immunogene therapy with interleukin-12- and interleukin-15-engineered neuroblastoma cells cures metastatic disease in syngeneic mice. *Clin Cancer Res* 2005; **11**: 735–42.

Cruikshank WW, *et al.* Interleukin-16 [Review]. *J Leukocyte Biol* 2000; **67**: 757–66.

Cui B, Carr DJ. A plasmid construct encoding murine interferon beta antagonizes the replication of herpes simplex virus type I in vitro and in vivo. *J Neuroimmunol* 2000; **108**: 92–102.

Czuprynski CJ, *et al.* Effects of murine recombinant interleukin 1 alpha on the host response to bacterial infection. *J Immunol* 1994; **140**: 962–8.

D'Aversa TG, *et al.* CD40–CD40L interactions induce chemokine expression by human microglia: Implications for human immunodeficiency virus encephalitis and multiple sclerosis. *Am J Pathol* 2002; **160**: 559–67.

Davis RL, *et al.* Effects of mechanistically distinct NF-kappaB inhibitors on glial inducible nitric-oxide synthase expression. *Nitric Oxide* 2005; **12**: 200–9.

de Gans J, *et al.* Dexamethasone in adults with bacterial meningitis. *N Engl J Med* 2002; **347**: 1549–56.

de Lalla F, *et al.* Safety and efficacy of recombinant granulocyte colony-stimulating factor as an adjunctive therapy for *Streptococcus pneumoniae* meningitis in non-neutropenic adult patients: A pilot study. *J Antimicrob Chemother* 2000; **46**: 843–6.

Deckert M, *et al*. Endogenous interleukin-10 is required for prevention of a hyperinflammatory intracerebral immune response in *Listeria monocytogenes* meningoencephalitis. *Infect Immun* 2001; **69**: 4561–71.

Dietrich JB. The adhesion molecule ICAM-1 and its regulation in relation with the blood–brain barrier. *J Neuroimmunol* 2002; **128**: 58–68.

Dinarello CA. Proinflammatory cytokines. *Chest* 2000; **118**: 503–8.

Dix RD, Cousins SW. Interleukin-2 immunotherapy of murine cytomegalovirus retinitis during MAIDS correlates with increased Intraocular CD8+ T-cell infiltration. *Ophthalm Res* 2003; **35**: 154–9.

Dix RD, *et al*. Systemic cytokine immunotherapy for experimental cytomegalovirus retinitis in mice with retrovirus-induced immunodeficiency. *Invest Ophthalmol Vis Sci* 1997; **38**: 1411–17.

Donnely S, *et al*. Helminth 2-Cys peroxiredoxin drives Th2 responses through a mechansim involving alternatively activated macrophages. *FASEB J* 2008; **22** : 4022–32.

Dorr J, *et al*. Tumor-necrosis-factor-related apoptosis-inducing-ligand (TRAIL)-mediated death of neurons in living human brain tissue is inhibited by flupirtine-maleate. *J Neuroimmunol* 2005; **167**: 204–9.

Duan X, *et al*. Intranasal interleukin-12 gene therapy enhanced the activity of ifosfamide against osteosarcoma lung metastases. *Cancer* 2006; **106**: 1382–8.

Eisenbeis CF, *et al*. Phase I study of the sequential combination of interleukin-12 and interferon alfa-2b in advanced cancer: Evidence for modulation of interferon signalling pathways by interleukin-12. *J Clin Oncol* 2005; **23**: 8835–44.

Elisabetta V, *et al*. The endogenous estrogen status regulates microglia reactivity in animal models of neuroinflammation. *Endocrinology* 2006; **147**: 2263–72.

Faber M, *et al*. Overexpression of tumor necrosis factor alpha by a recombinant rabies virus attenuates replication in neurons and prevents lethal infection in mice. *J Virol* 2005; **79**: 15405–16.

Felderhoff-Mueser U, *et al*. IL-18: A key player in neuroinflammation and neurodegeneration? *Trends Neurosci* 2005; **28**: 487–93.

Fernandez-Botran R. Soluble cytokine receptors: Their role in immunoregulation. *FASEB J* 1991; **5**: 2567–74.

Fieschi C, *et al*. High risk of infectious disease caused by salmonellae and mycobacteria infections in patients with Crohn disease treated with anti-interleukin-12 antibody. *Clin Infect Dis* 2005; **40**: 1381.

Filipe-Santos O, *et al*. Inborn errors of IL-12/23- and IFN-gamma-mediated immunity: molecular, cellular, and clinical features. *Semin Immunol* 2006; **18**: 347–61.

Finke D, *et al*. Gamma interferon is a major mediator of antiviral defense in experimental measles virus-induced encephalitis. *J Virol* 1995; **69**: 5469–74.

Finsterer J, *et al*. Multifocal leukoencephalopathy and polyneuropathy after 18 years on interferon alpha. *Leuk Lymphoma* 2005; **46**: 277–80.

Flesch IE, Kaufmann SH. Role of cytokines in tuberculosis [Review]. *Immunobiology* 1993; **189**: 316–39.

Flesch IE, *et al*. Effects of IL-13 on murine listeriosis. *Int Immunol* 1997; **9**(4): 467–74.

Fukuda T, *et al*. Treatment with Y-40138, a multiple cytokine production modulator, inhibits lipopolysaccharide- or tumour necrosis factor-alpha-induced production of pro-inflammatory cytokines and augments interleukin-10. *J Pharm Pharmacol* 2005; **57**: 1461–6.

Gadoth N, *et al*. The interferon system in subacute sclerosing panencephalitis and its response to isoprinosine. *Brain Dev* 1989; **11**: 308–12.

Gallin JI, *et al*. Interferon-gamma in the management of infectious diseases. *Ann Intern Med* 1995; **124**: 216–24.

Garg R. Subacute sclerosing panencephalitis. *Postgrad Med J* 2002; **78**: 63–70.

Gascon G, *et al*. Randomized treatment study of inosiplex versus combined inosiplex and intraventricular interferon-alpha in subacute sclerosing panencephalitis (SSPE): International multicenter study. *J Child Neurol* 2003; **18**: 819–27.

Gately MK, Mulqueen MJ. Interleukin-12 – Potential clinical applications in the treatment and prevention of infectious diseases. *Drugs* 1996; **52** (Suppl 2): 18–25.

Gazzinelli R, *et al*. Interleukin-12 is required for the T-lymphocyte-independent induction of interferon-g by an intracellular parasite and induces resistance in T-cell-deficient hosts. *Proc Natl Acad Sci* 1993; **90**: 6115–19.

Gazzinelli RT, *et al*. In the absence of endogenous IL-LO, mice acutely infected with *Toxoplasma gondii* succumb to a lethal immune response dependent on CD4(+) T cells and accompanied by overproduction of IL-12, IFN-gamma, and TNF-alpha. *J Immunol* 1996; **157**(2): 798–805.

Geschwind MD, *et al*. The relative contributions of HAART and alpha-interferon for therapy of progressive multifocal leukoencephalopathy in AIDS. *J Neurovirol* 2001; **7**: 353–7.

Ghiasi H, *et al*. Overexpression of interleukin-2 by a recombinant herpes simplex virus type 1 attenuates pathogenicity and enhances antiviral immunity. *J Virol* 2002; **76**: 9069–78.

Giosue S, *et al*. Effects of aerosolized interferon-alpha in patients with pulmonary tuberculosis. *Am J Respir Crit Care Med* 1998; **158**: 1156–62.

Giosue S, *et al*. Aerosolized interferon-alpha treatment in patients with multi-drug-resistant pulmonary tuberculosis. *Eur Cytok Network* 2000; **11**: 99–104.

Gokcil Z, *et al*. Alpha-interferon and isoprinosine in adult-onset

237

subacute sclerosing panencephalitis. *J Neurol Sci* 1999; **162**: 62–4.

Gosselin J, *et al.* Interleukin-15 as an activator of natural killer cell-mediated antiviral response. *Blood* 1999; **94**: 4210–19.

Grau G, Modlin R. Immune mechanisms in bacterial and parasitic diseases: Protective immunity versus pathology. *Curr Opin Immunol* 1991; **3**: 480–5.

Greenwood J, *et al.* Lymphocyte migration into the central nervous system: Implication of ICAM-1 signalling at the blood–brain barrier. *Vascul Pharmacol* 2002; **38**: 315–22.

Griffin D. Immune responses during measles virus infection. *Curr Top Microbiol Immunol* 1995; **191**: 117–34.

Griffin DE. Immune responses to RNA-virus infections of the CNS [Review]. *Nature Rev Immunol* 2003; **3**: 493–502.

Gringeri A, *et al.* Active anti-interferon-alpha immunization: A European–Israeli, randomized, double-blind, placebo-controlled clinical trial in 242 HIV-1-infected patients (the EURIS study). *J AIDS Human Retrovirol* 1999; **20**: 358–70.

Haddad FS, Risk W. Isoprinosine treatment in 18 patients with subacute sclerosing panencephalitis: A controlled study. *Ann Neurol* 1980; **7**: 185–8.

Hammerbeck DM, *et al.* Administration of a dual toll-like receptor 7 and toll-like receptor 8 agonist protects against influenza in rats. *Antiviral Res* 2006; **73**: 1–11.

Hanada N, *et al.* Combined effects of acyclovir and human interferon-alpha on herpes simplex virus replication in cultured neural cells. *J Med Virol* 1989; **29**: 7–12.

Hanisch UK, *et al.* Mouse brain microglia express interleukin-15 and its multimeric receptor complex functionally coupled to Janus kinase activity. *J Biol Chem* 1997; **272**: 288853–60.

Happel KI, *et al.* Pulmonary interleukin-23 gene delivery increases local T-cell immunity and controls growth of *Mycobacterium tuberculosis* in the lungs. *Infect Immun* 2005; **73**: 5782–8.

Happel KI, *et al.* Cutting edge: Roles of toll-like receptor 4 and IL-23 in IL-17 expression in response to *Klebsiella pneumoniae* infection. *J Immunol* 2003; **170**: 4432–6.

Hara S, *et al.* Combination therapy with intraventricular interferon-alpha and ribavirin for subacute sclerosing panencephalitis and monitoring measles virus RNA by quantitative PCR assay. *Brain Dev* 2003; **25**: 367–9.

Hart OM, *et al.* TLR7/8-mediated activation of human NK cells results in accessory cell-dependent IFN-gamma production. *J Immunol* 2005; **175**: 1636–42.

Hasselblatt M, *et al.* The brain erythropoietin system and its potential for therapeutic exploitation in brain disease. *J Neurosurg Anesthesiol* 2006; **18**: 132–8.

Heide W, *et al.* Failure of cytarabine/interferon therapy in progressive multifocal leukoencephalopathy. *Ann Neurol* 1995; **37**: 412–13.

Heimann DM, Schwarzentruber D. Gastrointestinal perforations associated with interleukin-2 administration. *J Immunother* 2004; **27**: 254–8.

Heneka MT, *et al.* Acute treatment with the PPARgamma agonist pioglitazone and ibuprofen reduces glial inflammation and Abeta1–42 levels in APPV717I transgenic mice. *Brain* 2005; **128**: 1442–53.

Ho M, *et al.* Endogenous interleukin-10 modulates proinflammatory response in *Plasmodium falciparum* malaria. *J Infect Dis* 1998; **178**: 520–4.

Holland SM. Cytokine therapy of mycobacterial infections. *Adv Intern Med* 2000a; **45**: 431–52.

Holland SM. Treatment of infections in the patient with Mendelian susceptibility to mycobacterial infection. *Microbes Infect* 2000b; **2**: 1579–90.

Hosoya M, *et al.* High-dose intravenous ribavirin therapy for subacute sclerosing panencephalitis.

Antimicrob Agents Chemother 2001; **45**: 943–5.

Huang SS, *et al.* Survival prolongation in HIV-associated progressive multifocal leukoencephalopathy treated with alpha-interferon: An observational study. *J Neurovirol* 1998; **4**: 324–32.

Hussey GD, Klein M. A randomized, controlled trial of vitamin A in children with severe measles. *N Engl J Med* 1990; **323**: 160–4.

Ifergan I, *et al.* Statins reduce human blood–brain barrier permeability and restrict leukocyte migration: Relevance to multiple sclerosis. *Ann Neurol* 2006; **60**: 45–55.

Ikeda M, *et al.* Different anti-HCV profiles of statins and their potential for combination therapy with interferon. *Hepatology* 2006; **44**: 117–25.

Inoue H, *et al.* Modulation of the human interleukin-12p40 response by a triazole antifungal derivative, itraconazole. *Scand J Infect Dis* 2004; **36**: 607–9.

Jackson AC, *et al.* Expression of Toll-like receptor 3 in the human cerebellar cortex in rabies, herpes simplex encephalitis, and other neurological diseases. *J Neurovirol* 2006; **12**: 229–34.

Jacobson MA, *et al.* Safety and immunogenicity of Towne cytomegalovirus vaccine with or without adjuvant recombinant interleukin-12. *Vaccine* 2006; **24**(25): 5311–9.

Jiang Z, *et al.* Remission of CVB3-induced viral myocarditis by in vivo Th2 polarization via hydrodynamics-based interleukin-4 gene transfer. *J Gene Med* 2008; **10**: 918–29.

Jimenez C, *et al.* Graves' disease after interleukin-2 therapy in a patient with human immunodeficiency virus infection. *Thyroid* 2004; **14**: 1097–102.

Johnson BJ, *et al.* rhuIL-2 adjunctive therapy in multidrug resistant tuberculosis: A comparison of two treatment regimens and placebo. *Tuberc Lung Dis* 1997; **78**: 195–203.

Johnson BJ, *et al.* Clinical and immune responses of tuberculosis patients treated with low-dose IL-2 and multidrug therapy. *Cytokin Molec Ther* 1995; **1**: 185–96.

Johnson JL, *et al.* Randomized trial of adjunctive interleukin-2 in adults with pulmonary tuberculosis [Comment]. *Am J Respir Crit Care Med* 2003; **168**: 185–91.

Jones CE, *et al.* Inosiplex therapy in subacute sclerosing panencephalitis. A multicentre, non-randomised study in 98 patients. *Lancet* 1982; **1**: 1034–7.

Kaiser K, *et al.* Recombinant human erythropoietin prevents the death of mice during cerebral malaria. *J Infect Dis* 2006; **193**: 987–95.

Kalil AC, *et al.* Use of interferon-alpha in patients with West Nile encephalitis: Report of 2 cases. *Clin Infect Dis* 2005; **40**: 764–6.

Kamei S, *et al.* Evaluation of combination therapy using aciclovir and corticosteroid in adult patients with herpes simplex virus encephalitis. *J Neurol Neurosurg Psychiatry* 2005; **76**: 1544–9.

Kamijo R, *et al.* Mice that lack the interferon-gamma receptor have profoundly altered responses to infection with bacillus Calmette–Guerin and subsequent challenge with lipopolysaccharide. *J Exp Med* 1993; **178**: 1435–40.

Kanra GY, *et al.* Beneficial effects of dexamethasone in children with pneumococcal meningitis. *Pediatr Infect Dis J* 1995; **14**: 490–4.

Kasper LH, *et al.* IL-7 stimulates protective immunity in mice against the intracellular pathogen, *Toxoplasma gondii. J Immunol* 1995; **155**: 4798–804.

Kawada J, *et al.* Systemic cytokine responses in patients with influenza-associated encephalopathy. *J Infect Dis* 2003; **188**: 690–8.

Kawakami K, *et al.* Il-18 protects mice against pulmonary and disseminated infection with *Cryptococcus neoformans* by inducing IFN-gamma production. *J Immunol* 1997; **159**: 5528–34.

Kawakami K, *et al.* Interleukin-4 weakens host resistance to pulmonary and disseminated cryptococcal infection caused by combined treatment with interferon-gamma-inducing cytokines. *Cell Immunol* 1999; **197**: 55–61.

Kawakami K, *et al.* Reduced host resistance and Th1 response to *Cryptococcus neoformans* in interleukin-18 deficient mice. *FEMS Microbiol Lett* 2000; **186**: 121–6.

Khan AA, *et al.* Activity of gatifloxacin alone or in combination with pyrimethamine or gamma interferon against *Toxoplasma gondii. Antimicrob Agents Chemother* 2001; **45**: 48–51.

Khan IA, Kasper L. IL-15 augments CD8+ T cell-mediated immunity against *Toxoplasma gondii* infection in mice. *J Immunol* 1996; **157**: 2103–8.

Kim D, *et al.* Relationships between IFNgamma, IL-6, corticosterone, and *Listeria monocytogenes* pathogenesis in BALB/c mice. *Cell Immunol* 2001; **207**: 13–18.

Kindler V, *et al.* The inducing role of tumor necrosis factor in the development of bactericidal granulomas during BCG infection. *Cell* 1989; **56**: 731–40.

Kioi M, *et al.* Mechanism of action of interleukin-13 antagonist (IL-13E13K) in cells expressing various types of IL-4R. *Cell Immunol* 2004; **229**: 41–51.

Kleinschek MA, *et al.* IL-23 enhances the inflammatory cell response in *Cryptococcus neoformans* infection and induces a cytokine pattern distinct from IL-12. *J Immunol* 2006; **176**: 1098–106.

Koedel U, *et al.* Pharmacologic interference with NF-kappaB activation attenuates central nervous system complications in experimental pneumococcal meningitis. *J Infect Dis* 2000; **182**: 1437–45.

Koh WJ, *et al.* Six-month therapy with aerosolized interferon-gamma for refractory multidrug-resistant pulmonary tuberculosis. *J Korean Med Sci* 2004; **19**: 167–71.

Komatsu T, *et al.* Neuronal expression of NOS-1 is required for host recovery from viral encephalitis. *Virology* 1999a; **258**: 389–95.

Komatsu T, *et al.* Regulation of the BBB during viral encephalitis: Roles of IL-12 and NOS. *Nitric Oxide* 1999b; **3**: 327–39.

Kreymborg K, *et al.* IL-23: changing the verdict on IL-12 function in inflammation and autoimmunity. *Expert Opin Ther Targets* 2005; **9**: 1123–36.

Krown S. Interferons and interferon inducers in cancer treatment. *Semin Oncol* 1986; **13**: 207–17.

Kuipers HF, *et al.* Simvastatin affects cell motility and actin cytoskeleton distribution of microglia. *Glia* 2006; **53**: 115–23.

Kunschner L, Scott. T. Sustained recovery of progressive multifocal leukoencephalopathy after treatment with IL-2. *Neurology* 2005; **65**: 1510.

Larsen MW, *et al.* Ginseng modulates the immune response by induction of interleukin-12 production. *APMIS* 2004; **112**: 369–73.

Lauterbach H, *et al.* Adoptive immunotherapy induces CNS dendritic cell recruitment and antigen presentation during clearance of a persistent viral infection. *J Exp Med* 2006; **203**: 1963–75.

Lebel MH, *et al.* Dexamethasone therapy for bacterial meningitis. Results of two double-blind, placebo-controlled trials. *N Engl J Med* 1988; **319**: 964–71.

Lee JD, *et al.* Interleukin-4 inhibits the expression of tumour necrosis factors α and β, interleukins-1β and -6 and interferon-γ. *Immunol Cell Biol* 1995; **73**: 57–61.

Leib SL, *et al.* Matrix metalloproteinases contribute to brain damage in experimental pneumococcal meningitis. *Infect Immun* 2000; **68**: 615–20.

Lieberman LA, *et al.* IL-23 provides a limited mechanism of resistance to acute toxoplasmosis in the absence of IL-12. *J Immunol* 2004; **173**: 1887–93.

Lieschke GJ, *et al.* Mice lacking granulocyte colony-stimulating factor have chronic neutropenia, granulocyte and macrophage progenitor cell deficiency, and impaired neutrophil mobilization. *Blood* 1994; **84**: 1737–46.

Little RF, *et al*. Activity of subcutaneous interleukin-12 in AIDS-related Kaposi sarcoma. *Blood* 2006; **107**: 4650–7.

Long MT, Baszler TV. Neutralization of maternal IL-4 modulates congenital protozoal transmission: Comparison of innate versus acquired immune responses. *J Immunol* 2000; **164**: 4768–74.

Looareesuwan S, *et al*. Pentoxifylline as an ancillary treatment for severe falciparum malaria in Thailand. *Am J Trop Med Hyg* 1998; **58**: 348–53.

Lortholary O, *et al*. Immune mediators in cerebrospinal fluid during cryptococcosis are influenced by meningeal involvement and human immunodeficiency virus serostatus. *J Infect Dis* 2001; **183**: 294–302.

Lotze M, *et al*. Clinical effects and toxicity of interleukin-2 in patients with cancer. *Cancer* 1986; **58**: 2764–72.

Luft BJ, *et al*. Toxoplasmic encephalitis in patients with the acquired immunodeficiency syndrome. *N Engl J Med* 1993; **329**: 995–1000.

Mannon PJ, *et al*. Anti-interleukin-12 antibody for active Crohn's disease. *N Engl J Med* 2004; **351**: 2069–79.

Maret A, *et al*. Estradiol enhances primary antigen-specific CD4 T cell responses and Th1 development in vivo. Essential role of estrogen receptor alpha expression in hematopoietic cells. *Eur J Immunol* 2003; **33**: 512–21.

Matejuk A, *et al*. 17 beta-estradiol inhibits cytokine, chemokine, and chemokine receptor mRNA expression in the central nervous system of female mice with experimental autoimmune encephalomyelitis. *J Neurosci Res* 2001; **65**: 529–42.

McArthur JC, *et al*. Steroid-responsive myeloneuropathy in a man dually infected with HIV-1 and HTLV-I. *Neurology* 1990; **40**: 938–44.

Medana IM, *et al*. Central nervous system in cerebral malaria: "Innocent bystander" or active participant in the induction of immunopathology? [Review].

Immunol Cell Biol 2001; **79**: 101–20.

Merigan T, *et al*. Human leukocyte interferon for the treatment of Herpes Zoster in patients with cancer. *N Engl J Med* 1978; **298**: 981–7.

Meydani SN, *et al*. Vitamin E supplementation and in vivo immune response in healthy elderly subjects. A randomized controlled trial. *J Am Med Assoc* 1997; **277**: 1380–6.

Miller A, *et al*. Cimetidine as an immunomodulator in the treatment of herpes zoster. *J Neuroimmunol* 1989; **22**: 69–76.

Miyazaki M, *et al*. Long-term follow-up of a patient with subacute sclerosing panencephalitis successfully treated with intrathecal interferon alpha. *Brain Dev* 2005; **27**: 301–3.

Molavi A, Le Frock J. Tuberculous meningitis. *Med Clin North Am* 1985; **69**: 315–31.

Molyneux EM, *et al*. Dexamethasone treatment in childhood bacterial meningitis in Malawi: A randomised controlled trial. *Lancet* 2002; **360**: 211–18.

Morales LB, *et al*. Treatment with an estrogen receptor alpha ligand is neuroprotective in experimental autoimmune encephalomyelitis. *J Neurosci* 2006; **26**: 6823–33.

Mori I, *et al*. Impaired microglial activation in the brain of IL-18-gene-disrupted mice after neurovirulent influenza A virus infection. *Virology* 2001; **287**: 163–70.

Moro MH, *et al*. Gestational attenuation of Lyme arthritis is mediated by progesterone and IL-4. *J Immunol* 2001; **166**: 7404–9.

Mukherjee S, *et al*. Dendritic cells infected with a vaccinia virus interleukin-2 vector secrete high levels of IL-2 and can become efficient antigen presenting cells that secrete high levels of the immunostimulatory cytokine IL-12. *Cancer Gene Therapy* 2003; **10**(8): 591–602.

Murray H. Interferon-gamma, the activated macrophage and host defence against microbial

challenge. *Ann Intern Med* 1988; **108**: 595–608.

Murray H, *et al*. Impaired production of lymphokines and immune (gamma) interferon in the acquired immunodeficiency syndrome. *N Engl J Med* 1984; **310**: 883.

Murray HW, *et al*. In vitro and in vivo activation of human mononuclear phagocytes by interferon-gamma. Studies with normal and AIDS monocytes. *J Immunol* 1987; **138**: 2457–62.

Mustafa M, *et al*. Role of tumor necrosis factor alpha (cachectin) in experimental and clinical bacterial meningitis. *Pediatr Infect Dis J* 1989; **8**: 907–8.

Nakane A, *et al*. Protection by dexamethasone from a lethal infection with *Listeria monocytogenes* in mice. *FEMS Immunol Med Microbiol* 1994; **9**: 163–70.

Nakane A, *et al*. Endogenous cytokines during a lethal infection with *Listeria monocytogenes* in mice. *FEMS Microbiol Lett* 1999; **175**: 133–42.

Nakano T, *et al*. Recurrent herpes zoster myelitis treated with human interferon alpha: A case report. *Acta Neurol Scand* 1992; **85**: 372–5.

Nash TE. Human case management and treatment of cysticercosis. *Acta Trop* 2003; **87**: 61–9.

Nath A, *et al*. Progression of progressive multifocal leukoencephalopathy despite treatment with beta-interferon. *Neurology* 2006; **66**: 149–50.

Newton C, *et al*. Induction of interleukin-4 (IL-4) by *Legionella pneumophila* infection in BALB/c mice and regulation of tumor necrosis factor alpha, IL-6, and IL-1 beta. *Infect Immun* 2000; **68**: 5234–40.

Neyer LE, *et al*. Role of interleukin-10 in regulation of T-cell-dependent and T-cell-independent mechanisms of resistance to *Toxoplasma gondii*. *Infect Immun* 1997; **65**: 1675–82.

Noisakran S, *et al*. IFN-alpha 1 plasmid construct affords protection against HSV-1 infection in transfected

L929 fibroblasts. *J Interfer Cytokin Res* 2000; **20**: 107–15.

Novelli F, Casanova J. The role of IL-12, IL-23 and IFN-gamma in immunity to viruses. *Cytokine Growth Factor Rev* 2004; **15**: 367–77.

Odio CM, *et al.* The beneficial effects of early dexamethasone administration in infants and children with bacterial meningitis. *N Engl J Med* 1991; **324**: 1525–31.

Ohga S, *et al.* Cerebrospinal fluid cytokine levels and dexamethasone therapy in bacterial meningitis. *J Infect* 1999; **39**: 55–60.

Okamura H, *et al.* Interleukin-18: A novel cytokine that augments both innate and acquired immunity. *Adv Immunol* 1998; **70**: 281–312.

Opal SM, *et al.* Confirmatory interleukin-1 receptor antagonist trial in severe sepsis: A phase III, randomized, double-blind, placebo-controlled, multicenter trial. The Interleukin-1 Receptor Antagonist Sepsis Investigator Group. *Crit Care Med* 1997; **25**: 1115–24.

Operschall E, *et al.* Enhanced protection against viral infection by co-administration of plasmid DNA coding for viral antigen and cytokines in mice. *J Clin Virol* 1999; **13**: 17–27.

Orange JS, *et al.* Mechanism of interleukin 12-mediated toxicities during experimental viral infections: Role of tumor necrosis factor and glucocorticoids. *J Exp Med* 1995; **181**: 901–14.

Osorio Y, Ghiasi H. Comparison of adjuvant efficacy of herpes simplex virus type 1 recombinant viruses expressing TH1 and TH2 cytokine genes. *J Virol* 2003; **77**: 5774–83.

Osorio Y, Ghiasi H. Recombinant herpes simplex virus type 1 (HSV-1) codelivering interleukin-12p35 as a molecular adjuvant enhances the protective immune response against ocularHSV-1 challenge. *J Virol* 2005; **79**: 3297–308.

Osorio Y, *et al.* The role of T(H)1 and T(H)2 cytokines in HSV-1-induced corneal scarring. *Ocul Immunol Inflamm* 2002; **10**: 105–16.

Ozato K, *et al.* Toll-like receptor signaling and regulation of cytokine gene expression in the immune system [Review]. *Biotechniques* 2002; Suppl S: 66.

Pachner AR, *et al.* Interleukin-6 is expressed at high levels in the CNS in Lyme neuroborreliosis. *Neurology* 1997; **49**: 147–52.

Padgett DA, Sheridan JF. Androstenediol (AED) prevents neuroendocrine-mediated suppression of the immune response to an influenza viral infection. *J Neuroimmunol* 1999; **98**: 121–9.

Palmero D, *et al.* Phase II trial of recombinant interferon-alpha2b in patients with advanced intractable multidrug-resistant pulmonary tuberculosis: Long-term follow-up. *Int J Tuberc Lung Dis* 1999; **3**: 214–18.

Panitch HS, *et al.* Subacute sclerosing panencephalitis: Remission after treatment with intraventricular interferon. *Neurology* 1986; **36**: 562–6.

Paris MM, *et al.* Effect of interleukin-1 receptor antagonist and soluble tumor necrosis factor receptor in animal models of infection. *J Infect Dis* 1995; **171**: 161–9.

Paris MM, *et al.* The effect of interleukin-10 on meningeal inflammation in experimental bacterial meningitis. *J Infect Dis* 1997; **176**: 1239–46.

Park MH, *et al.* ERK-mediated production of neurotrophic factors by astrocytes promotes neuronal stem cell differentiation by erythropoietin. *Biochem Biophys Res Commun* 2006; **339**: 1021–8.

Pietrella D, *et al.* Disruption of CD40/CD40L interaction influences the course of *Cryptococcus neoformans* infection. *FEMS Immunol Med Microbiol* 2004; **40**: 63–70.

Polanczyk M, *et al.* The protective effect of 17beta-estradiol on experimental autoimmune encephalomyelitis is mediated through estrogen receptor-alpha. *Am J Pathol* 2003; **163**: 1599–605.

Prasad K, Garner P. Steroids for treating cerebral malaria. *Cochrane Database Syst Rev* 2000; **2**: CD000972.

Rahal JJ, *et al.* Effect of interferon-alpha2b therapy on St. Louis viral meningoencephalitis: Clinical and laboratory results of a pilot study. *J Infect Dis* 2004; **190**: 1084–7.

Rasley A, *et al.* Murine glia express the immunosuppressive cytokine, interleukin-10, following exposure to *Borrelia burgdorferi* or *Neisseria meningitidis*. *Glia* 2006; **53**: 583–92.

Reddy AM, *et al.* Artemisolide from *Artemisia asiatica*: Nuclear factor-kappaB (NF-kappaB) inhibitor suppressing prostaglandin E2 and nitric oxide production in macrophages. *Arch Pharm Res* 2006; **29**: 591–7.

Roberts CW, *et al.* Different roles for interleukin-4 during the course of *Toxoplasma gondii* infection. *Infect Immun* 1996; **64**: 897–904.

Rock RB, *et al.* *Mycobacterium tuberculosis*-induced cytokine and chemokine expression by human microglia and astrocytes: Effects of dexamethasone. *J Infect Dis* 2005; **192**: 2054–8.

Rodrigues V, *et al.* Interleukin-5 and interleukin-10 are major cytokines in cerebrospinal fluid from patients with active neurocysticercosis. *Brazil J Med Biolog Res* 2000; **33**: 1059–63.

Rodriguez FH, *et al.* Cytokine therapeutics for infectious diseases [Review]. *Curr Pharmaceut Des* 2000; **6**: 665–80.

Rosenberg SA, *et al.* IL-7 administration to humans leads to expansion of CD8+ and CD4+ cells but a relative decrease of CD4+ T-regulatory cells. *J Immunother* 2006; **29**: 313–19.

Roy E, *et al.* Beneficial effect of anti-interleukin-4 antibody when administered in a murine model of tuberculosis infection. *Tuberculosis* 2008; **88**: 197–202.

Ryman KD, *et al.* Alpha/beta interferon protects adult mice from fatal Sindbis virus infection and is an important determinant of cell and tissue tropism. *J Virol* 2000; **74**: 3366–78.

Saez-Llorens X, *et al.* Molecular pathophysiology of bacterial

241

meningitis: current concepts and therapeutic implications. *J Pediatr* 1990a; **116**: 671–84.

Saez-Llorens X, *et al*. Pentoxifylline modulates meningeal inflammation in experimental bacterial meningitis. *Antimicrob Agents Chemother* 1990b; **34**: 837–43.

Sangro B, *et al*. Gene therapy of cancer based on interleukin 12. *Curr Gene Ther* 2005; **5**: 573–81.

Sayao AL, *et al*. Calgary experience with West Nile virus neurological syndrome during the late summer of 2003. *Can J Neurol Sci* 2004; **31**: 194–203.

Schaad UB, *et al*. Dexamethasone therapy for bacterial meningitis in children. Swiss Meningitis Study Group. *Lancet* 1993; **342**: 457–61.

Schaefer C, *et al*. Gene-based delivery of IFN-beta is efficacious in a murine model of experimental allergic encephalomyelitis. *J Interferon Cytokine Res* 2006; **26**: 449–54.

Scharton-Kersten T, *et al*. Role of IL12 in induction of cell-mediated immunity to *Toxoplasma gondii Res Immunol* 1995; **146**: 539–45. [Erratum appears in *Res Immunol* 1996; **147**(2): 121.]

Schauf V, *et al*. Cytokine gene activation and modified responsiveness to interleukin-2 in the blood of tuberculosis patients. *J Infect Dis* 1993; **168**: 1056–9.

Schluter D, *et al*. Regulation of microglia by CD4+ and CD8+ T cells: Selective analysis in CD45-congenic normal and *Toxoplasma gondii*-infected bone marrow chimeras. *Brain Pathol* 2001; **11**: 44–55.

Schoeman JF, *et al*. Intractable intracranial tuberculous infection responsive to thalidomide: Report of four cases. *J Child Neurol* 2006; **21**: 301–8.

Schoeman JF, *et al*. Adjunctive thalidomide therapy for childhood tuberculous meningitis: Results of a randomized study. *J Child Neurol* 2004; **19**: 250–7.

Sharma SD, *et al*. In vivo recombinant interleukin 2 administration enhances survival against a lethal

challenge with *Toxoplasma gondii*. *J Immunol* 1985; **135**: 4160–3.

Simmons CP, *et al*. The clinical benefit of adjunctive dexamethasone in tuberculous meningitis is not associated with measurable attenuation of peripheral or local immune responses. *J Immunol* 2005; **175**: 579–90.

Simmons CP, *et al*. Pretreatment intracerebral and peripheral blood immune responses in Vietnamese adults with tuberculous meningitis: Diagnostic value and relationship to disease severity and outcome. *J Immunol* 2006; **176**: 2007–14.

Smolen JS, Maini. R. Interleukin-6: A new therapeutic target. *Arthritis Res Ther* 2006; **8**(S2): S5.

Solomon T, *et al*. Interferon alfa-2a in Japanese encephalitis: A randomised double-blind placebo-controlled trial. *Lancet* 2003; **361**: 821–6.

Steiger MJ, *et al*. Successful outcome of progressive multifocal leukoencephalopathy with cytarabine and interferon. *Ann Neurol* 1993; **33**: 407–11.

Stumhofer JS, *et al*. Interleukin 27 negatively regulates the development of interleukin 17-producing T helper cells during chronic inflammation of the central nervous system. *Nat Immunol* 2006; **7**: 937–45.

Subauste CS, *et al*. CD40–CD40 ligand interaction is central to cell-mediated immunity against *Toxoplasma gondii*: Patients with hyper IgM syndrome have a defective type 1 immune response that can be restored by soluble CP40 ligand trimer. *J Immunol* 1999; **162**: 6690–700.

Sugawara I. Interleukin-18 (IL-18) and infectious diseases, with special emphasis on diseases induced by intracellular pathogens [Review]. *Microb Infect* 2000; **2**: 1257–63.

Sugawara I, *et al*. IL-4 is required for defense against mycobacterial infection. *Microbiol Immunol* 2000; **44**: 971–9.

Suzuki Y, *et al*. Importance of endogenous IFN-γ for prevention of toxoplasmic encephalitis in

mice. *J Immunol* 1989; **143**: 2045–50.

Suzuki Y, *et al*. Treatment of toxoplasmic encephalitis in mice with recombinant gamma interferon. *Infect Immun* 1990; **58**: 3050–5.

Suzuki Y, Yang Q. IL-4 is protective against development of toxoplasmic encephalitis. *J Immunol* 1996; **157**: 2564–9.

Suzuki Y, *et al*. Impaired resistance to the development of toxoplasmic encephalitis in interleukin-6-deficient mice. *Infect Immun* 1997; **65**: 2339–45.

Szalay G, *et al*. IL-4 neutralization or TNF-alpha treatment ameliorate disease by an intracellular pathogen in IFN-gamma receptor-deficient mice. *J Immunol* 1996; **157**: 4746–50.

Takayanagui OM, Jardim E. Therapy for neurocysticercosis. Comparison between albendazole and praziquantel. *Arch Neurol* 1992; **49**: 290–4.

Tan J, *et al*. Activation of microglial cells by the CD40 pathway: relevance to multiple sclerosis. *J Neuroimmunol* 1999; **97**: 77–85.

Teige I, *et al*. IFN-beta inhibits T cell activation capacity of central nervous system APCs. *J Immunol* 2006; **177**: 3542–53.

Teppler H, *et al*. Efficacy of low doses of the polyethylene glycol derivative of interleukin-2 in modulating the immune response of patients with human immunodeficiency virus type 1 infection. *J Infect Dis* 1993; **167**: 291–8.

Thomas R, *et al*. Trial of dexamethasone treatment for severe bacterial meningitis in adults. *Intens Care Med* 1999; **25**: 475–80.

Thwaites GE, *et al*. Dexamethasone for the treatment of tuberculous meningitis in adolescents and adults. *N Engl J Med* 2004; **351**: 1741–51.

Tischner D, *et al*. Antigen therapy of experimental autoimmune encephalomyelitis selectively induces apoptosis of pathogenic T cells. *J Neuroimmunol* 2006; **183**: 146–50.

Todd P, Goa K. Interferon gamma-1b. A review of its pharmacology and therapeutic potential in chronic granulomatous disease. *Drugs* 1992; **43**: 111–22.

Tsai ML, *et al.* Cerebrospinal fluid interleukin-6, interleukin-8, and tumor necrosis factor-alpha in children with central nervous system infections. *Acta Paediatr Sin* 1996; **37**: 16–21.

Tsao TC, *et al.* Imbalances between tumor necrosis factor-alpha and its soluble receptor forms, and interleukin-1 beta and interleukin-1 receptor antagonist in BAL fluid of cavitary pulmonary tuberculosis. *Chest* 2000; **117**: 103–9.

Tsenova L, *et al.* Tumor necrosis factor alpha is a determinant of pathogenesis and disease progression in mycobacterial infection in the central nervous system. *Proc Natl Acad Sci* 1999; **96**: 5657–62.

Tsenova L, *et al.* A combination of thalidomide plus antibiotics protects rabbits from mycobacterial meningitis-associated death. *J Infect Dis* 1998; **177**: 1563–72.

Tsoukas CD, *et al.* 1,25-dihydroxyvitamin D3: A novel immunoregulatory hormone. *Science* 1984; **224**: 1438–40.

Tucker PC, *et al.* Inhibition of nitric oxide synthesis increases mortality in Sindbis virus encephalitis. *J Virol* 1996; **70**: 3972–7.

Turowski P, *et al.* Pharmacological targeting of ICAM-1 signaling in brain endothelial cells: Potential for treating neuroinflammation. *Cell Mol Neurobiol* 2005; **25**: 153–70.

Ulrichs T, *et al.* Variable outcome of experimental interferon-gamma therapy of disseminated Bacillus Calmette–Guerin infection in two unrelated interleukin-12Rbeta1-deficient Slovakian children. *Eur J Pediatr* 2005; **164**: 166–72.

Urban JF, *et al.* Stat6 signaling promotes protective immunity against *Trichinella spiralis* through a mast cell- and T cell-dependent mechanism. *J Immunol* 2000; **164**: 2046–52.

Uyttenhove C, Van Snick J. Development of an anti-IL-17A auto-vaccine that prevents experimental auto-immune encephalomyelitis. *Eur J Immunol* 2006; **36**: 2868–74.

Uyttenhove C, *et al.* Development of an anti-IL-12 p40 auto-vaccine: Protection in experimental autoimmune encephalomyelitis at the expense of increased sensitivity to infection. *Eur J Immunol* 2004; **34**: 3572–81.

van Deuren M, *et al.* Differential expression of proinflammatory cytokines and their inhibitors during the course of meningococcal infections. *J Infect Dis* 1994; **169**: 157–61.

van Marle G, *et al.* Human immunodeficiency virus type 1 envelope-mediated neuropathogenesis: Targeted gene delivery by a Sindbis virus expression vector. *Virology* 2003; **309**(1): 61–74.

Vento S, *et al.* Interleukin-2 therapy and CD4+ T cells in HIV-1 infection. *Lancet* 2006; **367**: 93–5.

Villegas EN, *et al.* Susceptibility of interleukin-2-deficient mice to *Toxoplasma gondii* is associated with a defect in the production of gamma interferon. *Infect Immun* 2002; **70**: 4757–61.

von der Wense A, *et al.* Intrathecal interferon therapy in chronic echovirus meningoencephalitis in Bruton type agammaglobulinemia. *Klin Padiatr* 1998; **210**: 51–5 [in German].

von Giesen HJ, *et al.* Serum and cerebrospinal fluid levels of interleukin-18 in human immunodeficiency virus type 1-associated central nervous system disease. *J Neurovirol* 2004; **10**: 383–6.

Wagner RD, *et al.* Recombinant interleukin-12 enhances resistance of mice to *Listeria monocytogenes* infection. *Microb Pathog* 1994; **17**: 175–86.

Wald ER, *et al.* Dexamethasone therapy for children with bacterial meningitis. Meningitis Study Group. *Pediatrics* 1995; **95**: 21–8.

Wallis RS, *et al.* Granulomatous infectious diseases associated with tumor necrosis factor antagonists. *Clin Infect Dis* 2004; **38**: 1261–5.

Wang ZW, *et al.* Attenuated rabies virus activates, while pathogenic rabies virus evades, the host innate immune responses in the central nervous system. *J Virol* 2005; **79**: 12554–65.

Warrell MJ, *et al.* Failure of interferon alfa and tribavirin in rabies encephalitis. *Br Med J* 1989; **299**: 830–3.

Wassie L, *et al.* Ex vivo cytokine mRNA levels correlate with changing clinical status of Ethiopian TB patients and their contacts over time. *PLoS ONE* 2008; **3**: e1522.

Wenisch C, *et al.* Elevated serum levels of IL-10 and IFN-gamma in patients with acute *Plasmodium falciparum* malaria. *Clin Immunol Immunopathol* 1995; **74**: 115–7.

Wenisch C, *et al.* Effect of pentoxifylline on cytokine patterns in the therapy of complicated *Plasmodium falciparum* malaria. *Am J Trop Med Hyg* 1998; **58**: 343–7.

Wingerchuk D. Current evidence and therapeutic strategies for multiple sclerosis. *Semin Neurol* 2008; **28**: 56–68.

Winston D, *et al.* Recombinant interferon-alpha-2a for treatment of Herpes Zoster in immunocompromised patients with cancer. *Am J Med* 1988; **85**: 147–51.

Wintergerst U, Behlohradsky B. Acyclovir versus acyclovir plus beta-interferon in focal viral encephalitis in children. *Infection* 1992; **20**: 207–12.

Wintergerst U, *et al.* Therapy of focal viral encephalitis in children with aciclovir and recombinant beta-interferon – results of a placebo-controlled multicenter study. *Eur J Med Res* 2005; **10**: 527–31.

Wu DT, *et al.* Mechanisms of leukocyte trafficking into the CNS. *J Neurovirol* 2000; **6**(Suppl 1): S82–5.

Xue ML, *et al.* 1 Alpha,25-Dihydroxyvitamin D-3 inhibits pro-inflammatory cytokine and chemokine expression in human corneal epithelial cells colonized with *Pseudomonas aeruginosa*. *Immunol Cell Biol* 2002; **80**: 340–5.

Yamanaka R, Xanthopoulos K. Induction of antigen-specific immune responses against malignant brain tumors by intramuscular injection of sindbis DNA encoding gp100 and IL-18. *DNA Cell Biol* 2005; **24**: 317–24.

Yamanaka R, *et al*. Marked enhancement of antitumor immune responses in mouse brain tumor models by genetically modified dendritic cells producing Semliki Forest virus-mediated interleukin-12. *J Neurosurg* 2002; **97**: 611–18.

Yamasaki K, *et al*. Long-term, high dose interferon-alpha treatment in HTLV-I-associated myelopathy/tropical spastic paraparesis: A combined clinical, virological and immunological study. *J Neurol Sci* 1997; **147**: 135–44.

Yoshioka H, *et al*. Administration of human leukocyte interferon to patients with subacute sclerosing panencephalitis. *Brain Dev* 1989; **11**: 302–7.

Zeinstra E, *et al*. Simvastatin inhibits interferon-gamma-induced MHC class II up-regulation in cultured astrocytes. *J Neuroinflam* 2006; **3**: 16.

Zeuzem S, *et al*. A phase I/II study of recombinant human interleukin-12 in patients with chronic hepatitis C. *Hepatology* 1999; **29**: 1280–7.

Zhu Y, *et al*. Lentivirus infection causes neuroinflammation and neuronal injury in dorsal root ganglia: Pathogenic effects of STAT-1 and inducible nitric oxide synthase. *J Immunol* 2005; **175**: 1118–26.

Zwijnenburg PJG, *et al*. Interleukin-18 gene-deficient mice show enhanced defense and reduced inflammation during pneumococcal meningitis. *J Neuroimmunol* 2003; **138**: 31–7.

Neuro-inflammation: an emerging therapeutic target in neurological disease

Joseph M. Antony and Christopher Power

Introduction

The design of therapeutics for neurological diseases represents one of the greatest challenges in medicine today, in large part because of the complexities underlying the pathogenesis of neurological diseases, the difficulties in delivering drugs to the nervous system, and the burgeoning costs of drug development. The impact of neurological disease burden is immense as the number of people with age-related nervous system diseases is on the rise, which is compounded by the increasing numbers of patients afflicted with drug- and infectious disease-related nervous system pathologies (Lucas *et al.*, 2006). Many neurological diseases are characterized by varying degrees of inflammation within the nervous system. Indeed, all of the major nervous system diseases identified worldwide by the WHO including stroke, dementia, head injury, Parkinson's disease, multiple sclerosis, epilepsy, and neurological infections are associated with some degree of inflammation within the nervous system as a response to the underlying disease process (Rogers *et al.*, 2007). For the most part, inflammation is a beneficial response to injury, which enhances recovery of affected tissues. However, when inflammation extends beyond its reparative limits in terms of duration and magnitude, the potential for tissue damage is high, leading to increased neurological disability including blindness, weakness, ataxia, and pain. In this regard, multiple sclerosis (MS) has generated substantial interest in terms of the science underlying neuro-inflammation, which is defined by coordinated interactions between the environment, genes, and infectious agents. Multiple sclerosis represents the prototypic neuro-inflammatory disease characterized by both adaptive and innate immune responses within the nervous system manifested as localized inflammation and demyelination with ensuing axon damage. This conceptualization of MS has also spawned a considerable spectrum of therapeutic options, each of which has been shown to have impressive results in animal models, but with modestly beneficial effects in human subjects. Similarly, other neurodegenerative diseases including Alzheimer's disease (AD), stroke, and amyotrophic lateral sclerosis (ALS) have been modeled in murine models but thus far, all efforts to prevent or treat these diseases have progressed minimally beyond experimental models. Nevertheless, due to the complex nature of the human genome and its interaction with a diverse ecological and socio-cultural niche, diverse treatment strategies designed on the basis of their efficacy in experimental models have been translated into human therapies. Moreover, optimism remains high, given the number of therapeutics designed for neurological disorders that are in various clinical phases. Indeed, this is ample proof that the pharmaceutical industry will continue to invest in the design and development of neurological therapies. However, as with most drugs, caution must be exercised when drugs to combat neuro-inflammatory or -degenerative disorders are prescribed, as the risk of off-target (side) effects remains. Hence, it is necessary to understand the mechanisms of action of these drugs: this chapter therefore attempts to summarize the actions of some of the commonly used immunotherapeutics. The discussion will concentrate on the central nervous system (CNS), focusing on MS and other diseases in which inflammation and neurodegeneration appear to be linked, including HIV-associated dementia (HAD), Alzheimer dementia (AD), Parkinson's disease (PD), stroke, and amyotrophic lateral sclerosis (ALS).

Inflammatory Diseases of the Central Nervous System, ed. T. Kilpatrick, R. M. Ransohoff and S. Wesselingh. Published by Cambridge University Press. © Cambridge University Press 2010.

Neuro-inflammation

The CNS consists of several groups of highly differentiated and complex cells (neurons, astrocytes, monocytoid cells, oligodendrocytes, ependymal and endothelial cells) that are functionally integrated by cell-to-cell contacts and/or synapses, but are phenotypically diverse depending on their location and function in the CNS. The healthy brain enjoys a relatively immune privileged status in that it lacks resident natural killer (NK) cells, T and B lymphocytes, a lymphatic system and has limited ability for capillary endothelium to bind leukocytes. Expression of major histocompatibility complex (MHC) class I and II molecules is low on neuroectodermal cells but monocytoid cells including resident microglia and perivascular macrophages (Kaur *et al.*, 2001), which originate from mesenchymal macrophages and monocytes during development and are the professional antigen-presenting cells of the CNS, readily express detectable MHC class I and II molecules (Neumann, 2001). Neurons can also express high levels of MHC class I after axotomy (Maehlen *et al.*, 1988) and cytokine treatment (Neumann *et al.*, 1997). The blood–brain barrier (BBB) is a tight anatomic barrier that excludes proteins and cells in the blood from entering the CNS under normal conditions (Johnson, 1998). It consists of tight junctions between mitochondria-rich endothelial cells in CNS vessels, basal lamina, and a continuous covering provided by extended foot processes derived from astrocytes and microglia. The BBB has evolved to maintain homeostatic differences in the constituents of the blood and CSF, and acts as a selective barrier to maintain ionic concentrations of the internal environment within a narrow physiological range (Lowenstein, 2002). Although the BBB separates the CNS from circulating leukocytes and antibodies, the circumventricular organs allow free interaction between blood components and the CNS (Steinman, 2004). The choroid plexus is a highly vascularized area containing fenestrated endothelial cells unlike the brain parenchymal endothelial cells associated with a tight BBB (Kosugi *et al.*, 2002). The intrinsic cells of the nervous system including neurons and glia (astrocytes, oligodendrocytes, and microglia) can be also regarded as two distinct populations including "target" cells that are susceptible to pathogenic injury and death (neurons and oligodendrocytes) and effector cells (microglia and astrocytes), which, together with circulatory leukocytes, mediate the fate of target cells during neuro-inflammation.

Cellular components of neuro-inflammation

Neuro-inflammation represents the activation of immune cells within the nervous system, involving multiple cell types with a broad range of possible outcomes depending on the individual cells and their products. The generation and selection of a diverse population of immunocompetent but naive lymphocytes from a large number of precursor cells in the primary lymphoid organs (PLO) and the efficient initiation of an immune response by immunocompetent cells on antigen capture in the secondary lymphoid organs (SLO) lead to antigen recognition and response while maintaining tolerance to self-antigens. Lymphocyte homing and trafficking link the PLO and SLO with each other and with the extralymphoid sites of the body (Brocke *et al.*, 1999). It is now increasingly appreciated that the CNS is not immunologically isolated from the rest of the body, although there are fundamental differences in the nature of the induced innate and adaptive immune responses generated within the CNS.

In the event of an immune response to an antigen in the CNS, immunological cues are sent from the CNS to the periphery for recruitment of leukocytes to eliminate the antigen, remove debris, and promote repair. However, eradication of the antigen from the CNS can lead to immunological damage in part due to bystander effects, which can be beyond the prescribed protective or reparative effects. Infiltration of effector leukocytes through the BBB and its interaction with the CNS components contribute to the pathogenesis of several CNS diseases. The entry of leukocytes into the CNS is generally restricted by the tight junctions and by the lack of adhesion molecules on cerebral capillary endothelial cells (Griffin, 2003). However, studies have also shown that activated T cells regularly transmigrate across the BBB as part of the normal immunological surveillance of all tissues. Transendothelial migration of activated $CD4^+$ T cells takes place due to interaction of P-selectin glycoprotein ligands expressed by activated T cells with P-selectin, which is expressed at low levels by normal cerebrovascular endothelial cells, but levels of both these molecules increase during an inflammatory response, increasing surveillance and migration of activated T cells (Ransohoff *et al.*, 2003; Callahan and Ransohoff, 2004).

Activated T cells can cross antigen- or cytokine-stimulated endothelial cells of the BBB, independent of antigen specificity. The general mechanism consists of:

1. Tethering and rolling: circulating leukocytes first tether to and then roll on endothelial cells expressing adhesion molecules. The tethering and rolling steps are mediated by the selectins, as well as α_4 integrins. Selectins on the endothelium interact with carbohydrate-counter receptors on the leukocyte surface, tethering leukocytes that slow down and roll along the endothelium even in the presence of shear forces that guide movement of leukocytes through the bloodstream.

2. Integrin activation: signaling through $G_{\alpha i}$ proteins activates integrins expressed on leukocytes.

3. Leukocyte arrest: firm adhesion occurs when integrins bind to their endothelial ligands with high affinity.

4. Diapedesis: chemokines, acting through G-protein-coupled receptors (GPCRs), mediate leukocyte transmigration into tissue (Ransohoff et al., 2003). While this process is well-defined for T cells in the CNS, it is widely assumed that a similar mechanism also contributes to the entry of other leukocytes such as neutrophils (Kelly et al., 2007). However, monocyte/macrophage infiltration of the CNS is less clearly understood, particularly in the context of viral infections such as HIV or tuberculosis.

In addition to activation, proliferation, and eventual entry into the CNS by T cells, neutrophils, and monocytoid cells, there is also a robust innate immune system within the CNS. Innate immunity within the CNS is mediated chiefly by resident microglia and perivascular macrophages, together with a subset of astrocytes. Although there is widely recognized phenotypic diversity within these cell types, they act both in concert and independently to protect the CNS from injury as a first line of defense. At the same time, the potential for these effector cell types to be dysregulated is substantial, resulting in the release of neurotoxic factors including cytokines, chemokines, reactive oxygen species, and proteases together with aberrant neurotrophin expression. The ensuing outcome is damage to target cells including neurons and oligodendrocytes, causing injury to target cell processes (myelination for oligodendrocytes or synapses for neurons) or cell death. It is also worth bearing in mind that neurons are also capable of modulating innate immune responses through expression of MHC class I molecules and other cell surface molecules (i.e. CD200), together with the expression of cytokines, chemokines, free radicals, and proteases, but the roles of these neuronal events in innate immunity remain incompletely understood. None the less, nitric oxide produced by neurons exerts both pro-apoptotic and anti-apoptotic effects and induces soluble guanylyl cyclase, elevating cyclic GMP in the brain and it also displays cGMP-independent activity. It is notable that β-amyloid down-regulates the NO/cGMP/CREB signaling in AD, which suggests that multiple biochemical signaling pathways can be activated to promote neuronal survival (Thatcher et al., 2006). Activation of innate immunity has the capacity to cause ongoing target cell injury and death through the direct cytotoxic actions of secreted molecules or indirectly by disruption of the BBB with ensuing edema and entry of cytotoxic agents present in the adjacent circulation. Thus, neuro-inflammation is closely coupled with neurodegeneration and many of the molecules released by effector cells result in the activation of specific signaling pathways in target cells with specific outcomes including necrosis or programmed cell death defined by apoptosis, caspase-independent cell death, or autophagy, which has multiple potential outcomes (Bredesen et al., 2006).

Immunotherapy

Immunotherapy has become an important option for the treatment of several neurological disorders and a range of drugs with different modes of action have been approved with varying degrees of efficacy. A time-honoured means of controlling neuro-inflammation has been global immunosuppression, which has significant side-effects including the potential to interfere with protective immunity. Inflammation and the events surrounding it are a key component of various neurodegenerative disorders including MS, HIV-associated neurological disorders, ALS, and AD, and can be viewed as attempts by the immune system to protect neural tissue. The immune system is therefore truly Janus-faced, with protective as well as destructive components and future rational drug design therefore requires a targeted approach. Immunotherapy is most feasible if the underlying condition, as well as the signaling that drives both pathogenesis and treatment are understood. Unfortunately, for many chronic inflammatory neurological disorders the disease processes are uncertain.

Owing to the complex immunological network underlying most neuro-inflammatory diseases, combination therapies are likely to be more beneficial in the long term. However, whether combination therapies might lead to synergism or antagonism is often hard to predict. Efforts to predict and verify drug interactions via interrogation of cell signaling pathways remain comparatively primitive, but the advent of new technologies and experimental tools including systems biology approaches, together with multiplatform "Omics" technologies, are likely to open new avenues for the analysis and development of combination therapies. It is also important to note that most immunotherapies require long-term administration to achieve a desirable theraupeutic effect and in this context cumulative side-effects can necessitate drug withdrawal.

The issues facing immunotherapy development have been further complicated by extrapolating findings from rodent models to human patients, as recently observed in the case of AD patients vaccinated with β-amyloid, of whom several went on to develop post-vaccination meningoencephalomyelitis despite previously successful results in APP transgenic mice (Orgogozo et al., 2003).

In the following sections, we will review clinically-approved and experimental immunotherapies.

Immunomodulatory agents

Glucocorticosteroids (GCs)

Glucocorticoids remain the first line of treatment for acute relapses in MS and the treatment of vasogenic edema associated with other neurological infections including brain abscesses and bacterial meningitis. This family of drugs includes both natural and synthetic corticosteroids and their releasing factors such as ACTH. The GCs represent a class of immunomodulatory agents whose actions are mediated through intracellular steroid receptors. The glucocorticosteroid–receptor complex binds glucocorticosteroid-responsive motifs in DNA, resulting in transcriptional modulation of a variety of genes, particularly affecting NFκB and as a consequence, down-regulating several cytokines including interferon-γ (IFN-γ) and tumor necrosis factor-α (TNF-α). Other inflammatory mediators including arachidonic acid metabolites such as prostaglandins and leukotrienes are also suppressed by GCs. Since many inflammatory mediators are largely chemotactic, GCs also influence the distribution and trafficking of leukocytes (Teixeira et al., 1998). In fact, GCs are likely to exert effects on both adaptive and innate immune pathways. Unfortunately, the side-effects associated with long-term GC therapy usually preclude protracted use but the recognition of steroids synthesized within the nervous system, termed neurosteroids, holds promise for this group of molecules in the treatment of neuro-inflammation (Reddy, 2004).

Interferon (IFN)-β

The different IFN-β subtypes represent the first established biologic therapies for MS, which have been termed disease-modifying therapies. The IFN-β is a type-1 interferon as it shares the same receptor as IFN-α. Type 1 interferons are produced upon stimulation by viruses or other agents. Along with IFN-γ, a type-II interferon, type-1 interferons increase expression of MHC class I, which enhances recognition of an infected cell by CD8[+] T lymphocytes. The IFN-γ enhances MHC class II, whereas the expression of this antigen-presenting molecule is inhibited by IFN-α and -β. Of interest, the use of IFN-γ as a therapeutic agent in MS patients resulted in a worsened clinical outcome (Johnson and Panitch, 1988). The interferons induce expression of chemokines and the adhesion molecule, soluble vascular cell adhesion molecule 1, while down-regulating another, namely Very late antigen- (VLA-)4, on peripheral blood lymphocytes. In addition, IFN-β induces expression of the anti-inflammatory cytokine interleukin-10 (IL-10), and decreases leukocyte transmigration (Alder et al., 2006). The IFN-β is a standard therapy used in MS and it could theoretically act through its anti-viral and anti-inflammatory effects although the mechanism of actions remains unclear (Yong, 2002). Until recently, it has been widely assumed that immunotherapeutic actions of IFN-β are chiefly exerted on lymphocytes outside the CNS, perhaps preventing their eventual entry into the CNS or diminishing their levels of activation. However, recent work has suggested the beneficial effects of endogenous type-1 interferons to limit the severity of experimental autoimmune encephalomyelitis, an animal model of MS, are due principally to their actions upon the innate immune system (Prinz et al., 2008). While the IFN-β derivatives reduce the relapse frequency and improve the neuroradiological outcome and quality of life in MS patients, their impact on long-term neurological disability remains uncertain.

Glatiramer acetate (GA)

Like IFN-β, GA is a putative disease-modifying therapy which is approved for MS treatment, but there is wide interest in its use for neurodegenerative diseases because of its capability to modify both adaptive and innate immune responses. Glatiramer acetate is a synthetic basic random co-polymer of the four amino acids, L-glutamic acid, L-lysine, L-alanine, and L-tyrosine in a molar residue ratio of 0.14:0.34:0.43:0.1 with an average molecular mass of 4700–11000 kDa. This mixture resembles myelin basic protein (MBP) and can suppress experimental autoimmune encephalomyelitis (EAE), the mouse model of MS. Since the D-amino acids also bind to MHC class II molecules as effectively as the L-isomer, competition with myelin antigens for binding to the MHC class II molecules might not be the only mechanism by which GA acts to suppress EAE in mice. Upon recognition of cross-reactive MBP in the CNS, the GA-reactive suppressor T cells could exert down-regulatory functions. Glatiramer acetate might also act as a regulatory altered peptide ligand or T cell receptor antagonist on MBP-specific T cells; hence, circulating MBP-specific T cells might be tolerized or exhibit a shifted cytokine profile. In addition, GA has also recently been posited to exert its beneficial effects via the innate immune system (Weber et al., 2007), possibly through polarization of monocytoid cells and presumed protective effects directly on neurons (Yong et al., 2007).

Intravenous immunoglobulin (IVIg)

Intravenous immunoglobulin is widely used for different neuroimmune disorders including acute demyelinating encephalomyelitis (ADEM), Guillain–Barré Syndrome (GBS) and myasthenia gravis (MG) (Matney and Huff, 2007). Although the exact mode of action of IVIg is incompletely understood, several mechanisms such as blockade of Fc receptors, neutralization of circulating antibodies, or increased clearance of immune complexes might be responsible. It might also interfere with the α4 integrin-dependent leukocyte recruitment (Lapointe et al., 2004). Because of its relatively easy use and safety, it has remained a mainstay of immunotherapy in neuroimmune disorders. A more complete understanding of its mechanism(s) of action might provide important additional insights into disease processes and their treatment.

Plasmapheresis and thymectomy

Plasmapheresis is used for CNS and peripheral nervous system (PNS) neuroimmune disorders including ADEM, GBS, and MG. Plasmapheresis presumably involves removal of circulating antibodies and inflammatory molecules and improvement is due to its tacit removal of antigen-specific pathogenic antibodies or complement-fixing antibodies.

Thymectomy is often performed for MG in order to avoid the development of a thymoma, but potential consequences include the absence of negative selection of high affinity T cells in the thymus via which autoimmune diseases might arise. However, many patients have undergone thymectomy without significant short- or long-term adverse immunological outcomes. Nevertheless, thymectomy is an invasive procedure that might eventually become obsolete due to further advances in immunotherapy.

Antibody therapies

During an inflammatory response, leukocyte recruitment to the site of inflammation is mediated by complement, leukotrienes, prostaglandin, neuropeptides, chemokines, and cytokines which can be selectively targeted with specific therapeutic antibodies (Chavarria and Alcocer-Varela, 2004). Likewise, the importance of selectins and integrins in leukocyte trafficking through the CNS vasculature is best elucidated in EAE. Although myelin oligodendrocyte glycoprotein (MOG)-induced mice express limited levels of P-selectin in the CNS vasculature, leukocyte rolling is inhibited by blocking this selectin, suggesting its requirement for initial recruitment of encephalitogenic T cells. Therapeutically, dual inhibition of α_4-integrin and P-selectin could have synergistic effects and provide optimal benefit in the treatment of human disease (Kerfoot and Kubes, 2002). In fact, blocking $\alpha_4\beta_1$ integrin leads to reduced infiltration of leukocytes into the CNS, perhaps by affecting fibronectin-mediated leukocyte migration (Yednock et al., 1992). Commercially available and therapeutically viable antibody antagonists have been produced against the $\alpha_4\beta_1$ integrin for treatment of MS with high therapeutic efficiency (Ropper, 2006), as recently shown for natalizumab, a recombinant humanized antibody of the IgG4 isotype (which does not fix complement) directed to the α_4 integrins ($\alpha_4\beta_1$ and $\alpha_4\beta_7$) (Langer-Gould et al., 2005). One month after an infusion of 300 mg of natalizumab, there was binding and greater than 80% saturation of α4-integrin on peripheral blood leukocytes despite the elimination half-life of 6–9 days. However, a potential setback to this treatment protocol was the unexpected development of progressive multifocal leukoencephalopathy (PML). A demyelinating disease, PML is caused by the human polyomavirus JC virus, which is activated in the periphery and succeeds in CNS infection (Bartt, 2006). This infection in humans was diagnosed in at least five patients who were treated with natalizumab. An extensive study revealed risk of PML in approximately 1 in 1000 patients treated with natalizumab for 18 months, although the risk of longer-term therapy remains unknown (Yousry et al., 2006). Another potential drawback of anti-VLA4 therapy is that it might also reduce the protective role(s) of neuro-inflammation (Schwartz and Kipnis, 2005).

Other potential selective antibodies that could be used in the future include rituximab, which binds to CD20 on B lymphocytes, daclizimab, which targets the IL-2 receptor on lymphocytes and alemtuzumab which targets CD52 on lymphocytes and monocytes. Each of these antibodies has been shown to be beneficial in the treatment of MS in either uncontrolled or phase II trials of MS patients (Bielekova et al., 2004; Cross et al., 2006; Coles et al., 2008; Hauser et al., 2008). However, it is important to recall that rational antibody therapies can have adverse outcomes. Tumor necrosis factor (TNF-α) is highly expressed in the CNS during MS with presumed adverse effects, yet parenterally administered anti-TNF-receptor antibodies exacerbated the disease course (Nash and Florin, 2005). In addition, the administration of alemtuzumab was associated with the development of immune thrombocytopenic purpura and thyroid disease (Coles et al., 2008). Independent of these caveats, the delivery of specific antibodies holds immense promise for the treatment of MS and other diseases involving leukocyte activation and entry into the nervous system.

In ex-vivo assays and mouse models of AD, passive immunization with antibodies to β-amyloid revealed that when bound to plaques, the N-terminus of the antibodies facilitate Fc receptor-mediated microglial phagocytosis of the plaques. Since peripheral administration of this antibody could also decrease plaque load, a peripheral sink model was proposed whereby a net increase in blood β-amyloid levels is consequent to an increase in the β-amyloid efflux from the brain. Thus, passive immunization has been suggested to be a suitable alternative to active immunization as the adverse side effects that occur with the latter might

be avoided (Brendza and Holtzman, 2006). Additionally, off-label uses for therapeutic antibodies could grow with time given recent successes in the application of anti-TNF-α receptor antibodies to uncommon diseases such as neurosarcoidosis (Salama et al., 2006).

Peptides and ligands

Recombinant T cell receptor (TCR) ligands that contain soluble MHC domains linked to specific antigenic peptides were able to reverse demyelination and axonal loss in an EAE model of MS and appear to function by switching the inflammatory cells from a TH1 profile (producing IFN-γ, TNF-α and IL-12) to that of a TH2 profile (producing IL-4, IL-5 and IL-13), which might promote neuronal protection and survival in the CNS (Wang et al., 2006). However, a recent clinical trial in MS patients using an altered peptide ligand failed to show benefit in MS (Bielekova et al., 2000). Another trial using an MBP-derived peptide in the treatment of secondary progression MS is currently in progress (Warren et al., 2006).

Unlike cytokines, which have pleiotrophic effects, chemokines target specific leukocyte subsets. Expression of chemokine receptors such as CXCR3, CXCR4, CCR5, and others either on leukocytes or endothelial cells can lead to infiltration by neutrophils and macrophages through chemotaxis, followed by chemokine-receptor-expressing lymphocytes. Thus, blocking chemokine receptors might be a rational therapeutic strategy. Furthermore, several chemokine receptors are expressed on neurons and might mediate neurotoxic effects, which could also be abrogated by selective receptor antagonists (Woodruff et al., 2006). A recent study describes the use of vasoactive intestinal peptide (VIP) in an EAE model which revealed that VIP induces a major population of T regulatory lymphocytes in vivo which is CD4[+]CD25[+]Foxp3[+]neuropilin[hi] and inhibits effector T cell proliferation through direct cellular contact (Fernandez-Martin et al., 2006).

Immunosuppressive agents

Mycophenolate motefil and azathioprine

Azathioprine (AZA) and mycophenolate motefil are immunosuppressive agents, which have been proposed as treatments for MS and other neuroinflammatory disorders (Confavreux and Moreau, 1996). Mycophenolate motefil inhibits DNA synthesis, while AZA is converted into its metabolite

6-mercaptopurine, which, in turn, competes with its analog, hypoxanthine, thus affecting DNA, RNA, and protein synthesis. Azathioprine induces B and T cell lymphopenia by acting on proliferating lymphocytes, thus inhibiting mitogen-driven and antibody responses. Azathioprine also exerts mild anti-inflammatory properties by inhibiting pro-monocyte cell division (Sugiyama et al., 2003). To date, the use of these drugs in MS is not supported by appropriately powered randomized controlled trials, but perhaps they might prove to be useful in the future as adjunct therapies.

Immunophilin-binding agents

Inhibition of calcineurin is achieved by the immunophilin-binding agents including cyclosporin, rapamycin, and FK506. These drugs block transcription of pro-inflammatory genes including IL-2 and chiefly target T lymphocytes (Creput et al., 2007). While these drugs are used widely in transplantation, their use in neuro-inflammatory disorders has not been supported by clinical trials for neurological diseases to date. However, given their potential neuro-protective effects, as demonstrated in experimental models (Medyouf et al., 2007), they could yet prove to be useful in the future.

Cyclophosphamide

Cyclophosphamide has been used for many years in the treatment of MS patients, as well as in other neuro-inflammatory disorders. Cyclophosphamide is an alkylating agent of the nitrogen mustard type. Its activated form, phosphoramide mustard, alkylates or binds intracellular molecular structures including nucleic acids, where cross-linking can cause either cytotoxicity or inhibition of protein synthesis. The numbers and function of T and B lymphocytes are effectively suppressed by cyclophosphamide (Stepkowski et al., 2000). More recently, there has been an interest in using very high dose cyclophosphamide in efforts to suppress disease progression in patients with advanced MS (Scott and Figgitt, 2004).

Mitoxantrone

Mitoxantrone is a member of the anthracendione family that is chemically similar to anthracyclins such as doxorubicin and daunorubicin and has both immunosuppressive and immunomodulatory effects. It mediates its effects by intercalating with DNA and inducing single-and double-strand breaks as well as inhibiting DNA repair by inhibition of topoisomerase II. Several inflammatory cells including macrophages, T, and B cells are suppressed, while the secretion of inflammatory mediators, including cytokines is modulated by mitoxantrone (Morrissey et al., 2005). This drug has been recommended as a first-line treatment for patients with MS who have an aggressive clinical course and as a second-line drug in those with relapsing remitting and secondary progressive disease who are unresponsive to interferon-β derivatives or GA. The drug should be directed to patients who demonstrate active inflammatory disease either clinically or neuroradiologically. There are ongoing concerns regarding the capacity of mitoxantrone to induce acute myeloid leukemia and to cause cardiotoxicity (Fox, 2006).

Cladribine (2-chlorodeoxyadenosine)

Cladribine (2-chlorodeoxyadenosine) is a relatively selective lymphocytotoxic drug, which has been shown to cause a significant reduction in MRI inflammatory lesions, but variable clinical results in terms of an influence upon either relapse rate or disability progression have been reported (Martinez-Rodriguez et al., 2007). Cladribine is used effectively as an oral therapy in neoplastic diseases to preferentially deplete lymphocytes and has a well-established safety profile. Though information on its long-term use and safety profile in MS is lacking, preliminary data indicate its effectiveness in the treatment of MS (Leist and Vermersch, 2007).

Teriflunomide

Teriflunomide is a dihydro-orotate dehydrogenase inhibitor that induces apoptosis of cells arrested in the G1 phase and blocks cellular proliferation (Ringshausen et al., 2008) of B cell chronic lymphoid leukemia (B-CLL). In the context of MS, oral delivery of teriflunomide resulted in a reduction in the annual relapse rate amongst patients, as well as reduced MRI lesions (O'Connor et al., 2006).

Laquinimod

Laquinimod is a small molecule with high oral bioavailability with favorable pharmacokinetics and which has been shown to exert significant effects upon inflammatory cells by shifting the profile of cytokine production from pro-inflammatory to an anti-inflammatory repertoire, without causing general immunosuppression in mouse models of MS (Yang et al., 2004). Interestingly, laquinimod has been shown to act synergistically with interferons to reduce disease progression in EAE (Runstrom et al., 2006). In MS patients, oral laquinimod was well tolerated and was effective in suppressing the development of active lesions visible on MRI in relapsing forms of MS (Polman et al., 2005).

Fingolimod

Fingolimod or FTY720 is an oral sphingosine 1-phosphate receptor modulator, which in EAE was shown to effectively preserve the integrity of the BBB and to reduce inflammation, reverse paralysis, normalize electrophysiological responses, and to decrease demyelination (Balatoni et al., 2007). It is currently in Phase III trials, but clinical data from Phase II trials have shown promising results with a relapse reduction of over 50% compared to placebo controls and with an acceptable safety profile.

Fumaric acid esters (FAE)

Fumaric acid esters (FAE) include diethyl fumarate and ethylhydrogen fumarate with the former being rapidly hydrolyzed to methyl hydrogen fumarate, which might be the active metabolite. In a chronic mouse model of MS, FAE given preventatively can effectively reduce clinical disease severity, as well as reduce inflammatory cell infiltrates. The FAE appear to exert their action predominantly on CD4$^+$ T cells by polarizing these to a Th2 profile, as well as inducing apoptosis of lymphocytes and dendritic cells by preventing nuclear entry of NFκB (Loewe et al., 2002; Treumer et al., 2003). In a clinical trial, FAE was well tolerated, with a reduction in disease activity, as measured by significant improvements in MRI lesions, though patients in this prospective, open-label, baseline-controlled exploratory study were few in number. Nevertheless, the results obtained were intriguing and thus warrant further study (Schimrigk et al., 2006).

Methotrexate

Methotrexate is a potent immunosuppressive drug that might act through inhibition of dyhydrofolate reductase as well as via its anti-inflammatory and immunoregulatory activities, which has been used in open label studies in patients with MS (Calabresi et al., 2002). However, long-term administration of oral methotrexate is not without undesirable side effects, and there have been reports of hepatic fibrosis. Recently, it has been suggested that oral methotrexate should not be used in either relapsing remitting or progressive MS due to lack of supportive evidence of efficacy (Gray et al., 2006).

Small molecule neuroimmune modulators

Neurotransmission modulators

Glutamate is the most abundant neurotransmitter in the CNS and is released as well as taken up by neurons and glia. It has the capacity to exert neuropathogenic effects through Ca$^+$-dependent excitotoxicity, mediated through the NMDA and AMPA receptors. Memantine has been used as an antagonist of the NMDA-R, but also reduces β-amyloid-induced apoptosis and neurotoxicity in the hippocampus.

Inhibition of acetylcholinesterase by donepezil and galantamine increases the availability of neuronal acetylcholine. Upon release from pre-synaptic vesicles following depolarization, acetylcholine interacts with muscarinic and nicotinic cholinergic receptors. While the effects of acetylcholine are assumed to be largely on neurons, it has become evident that there are acetylcholine receptors on microglia (Shytle et al., 2004) and astrocytes (Xiu et al., 2005), which might influence the extent and effects of neuro-inflammation.

Antioxidants

β-Amyloid induces the enzymes cyclooxygenase (COX)-1 and -2, which results in increased production of prostaglandins and reactive oxygen species. The levels of vitamin E in AD patients are low and supplementation with vitamin E has been found to induce cholinergic signaling, which is attenuated by β-amyloid in animal models (Huang et al., 2000). While some antioxidants such as acetyl-L-carnitine, normally produced by mitochondria, can facilitate uptake of acetyl CoA during fatty acid oxidation and can enhance acetylcholine production, others, such as aged garlic, scavenge reactive oxygen species and induce cellular antioxidant enzymes (Frank and Gupta, 2005).

Non-steroidal anti-inflammatory drugs (NSAIDS)

The NSAIDS reduce neurotoxic inflammatory responses in the brain and some including ibuprofen, indomethacin, and sulindac also reduce β-amyloid in culture systems, which might be due to non-selective inhibition of COX-1 (Aisen et al., 2003). While clinical trials of NSAIDS in AD have failed to show any benefits, their chronic use is closely associated with a lower risk of developing AD.

Signaling inhibitors

The blood–brain barrier comprises endothelial cells forming a tight junction and is compromised during neuro-inflammation, allowing for inflammatory cells in the blood to infiltrate the CNS. Tight junction proteins including occludins are lost due to proteolytic actions of matrix metalloproteinases (MMPs). Transmigration of monocytes that otherwise invade the barrier and cause neuro-inflammation in the brain can be effectively blocked by the MMP inhibitor, BB-3103 (Reijerkerk *et al.*, 2006). Moreover, studies using the MMP inhibitor, prinomastat, have demonstrated marked neuroprotection via the prevention of proteolytic cleavage of a chemokine in models of HIV-associated dementia (Johnston *et al.*, 2001).

One of the downstream effectors of the small GTP-binding protein of the Rho GTPase subfamily is Rho-coiled-coil-containing protein kinase (ROCK). Rho-GTPases function by switching between a biologically inactive state (GDP-bound) and an active state (GTP-bound). Activation of ROCK leads to phosphorylation of various substrates including the myosin light chain (MLC). In regions of neuronal injury, the Rho-ROCK pathway is stimulated when neurite growth inhibitors released in the microenvironment bind to specific receptors, which impedes neurite outgrowth. Accumulation of β-amyloid or neurofibrillary tangles containing phosphorylated tau protein are a feature of Alzheimer's disease and the tau protein is a substrate for ROCK. The amount of β-amyloid aggregates was found to be lowered by incorporating NSAIDS in animal models of the disease, which, in turn, impede the ROCK pathway. Inhibitors of ROCK also interfere with the gamma secretase pathway thus reducing the amyloid burden. Drugs such as lovastatin, the flavenoid luteolin, and phenyltransferase inhibitors, which are effective in MS, likely act by inhibiting the Rho-ROCK pathway. Further, the infiltration of inflammatory cells into the CNS is prevented by blocking ROCK since leukocytes require RhoA and ROCK for diapedesis across the endothelium. Inhibitors of ROCK can contribute to remyelination in vitro and thus hold promise for inducing functional recovery in autoimmune-damaged CNS tissue (Mueller *et al.*, 2005).

The glycogen synthase kinase-3 (GSK3) family is highly conserved throughout evolution and regulates the cell cycle, stem cell differentiation and renewal, apoptosis, the circadian rhythm, transcription, and insulin action, making it a target of choice for neurodegenerative diseases. Indeed, amyloid precursor protein (APP) is a GSK3β substrate and GSK3β is also involved in Wnt and sonic hedgehog signaling. There are over 30 GSK3 inhibitors available, most of which bind to the ATP binding pocket and which therefore compete with ATP at this site within GSK. These inhibitors are, in general, low molecular weight (<600 Da) species with flat hydrophobic heterocycles comprising part of their structures. However, the inhibitors often exhibit an affinity for other kinases resulting in undesirable side effects (Gerdes and Katsanis, 2005).

Natural product inhibitors

Bilobalide is a terpene trilactone, a component of *Ginkgo biloba* leaves, and was shown to have neuroprotective effects in models of cerebral ischemia and edema by preventing the uncoupling of mitochondrial oxidative phosphorylation and maintaining the respiratory activity under ischemic conditions. It also induces antioxidant enzymes such as superoxide dismutase and catalase but prevents induction of iNOS, protecting neuronal cells from NO-induced damage (Defeudis, 2002). Likewise, crocin, a derivative of saffron, appears to prevent neuronal injury, possibly through the regulation of free radicals (Zheng *et al.*, 2007).

Antibiotics

The tetracyclines, minocycline and doxycycline, have been shown to be neuroprotective and to suppress neuro-inflammation in models of stroke, MS, ALS, and AD, usually at doses far exceeding those that can be tolerated by humans. Nonetheless, these tetracyclines seem to suppress cytokine and protease expression while also inhibiting cell death in certain target cells (Lee *et al.*, 2004). The β-lactam antibiotics such as ceftriaxone are highly effective in a mouse model of ALS and induced the expression of the glutamate transporter, EAAT2, which is suppressed in ALS. However, short-term clinical trials in humans that tested this drug were negative (Carri *et al.*, 2006).

Endocrine therapy

Since the brain is a target for gonadal steroids, estrogens could have the potential to affect the incidence of AD. Estrogen receptors act as ligand-activated transcription factors, which translocate to the nucleus after binding and initiate transcription of target genes (Pozzi *et al.*, 2006). Estrogens have also been found to be neuroprotective in a variety of contexts including oxidative stress, excitotoxicity, and ischemia, while also helping to modulate the plasticity of neurons, to enhance glucose transport, and to increase cerebral blood flow. However, estrogens could also exert negative effects within the CNS (Henderson, 2006). Other potentially neuroprotective compounds that might exert regulatory actions on neuro-inflammation include growth hormone, insulin-like growth factor-1, erythropoietin, and the neurotrophins including nerve growth factor, brain derived neurotrophic factor, and neurotrophin-3. Clinical trials with these agents have yielded mixed results, depending on the disease and the individual compound.

Antiepileptic drugs (AEDs)

The mechanisms of action of many AEDs has come under renewed scrutiny over the past 5 years, fuelled by a better understanding of the roles of different ion channels. Axonal degeneration caused by experimental anoxia within the white matter of the CNS is a Ca^{2+}-dependent process. This can be triggered by a sustained sodium influx that reverses the Na^+–Ca^{2+} exchanger, resulting in an import of Ca^{2+} that can damage axons within the anoxic white matter. The energy failure in MS is due to ATP depletion, which leads to inhibition of Na^+–K-ATPase and the persistently activated Na^+ channels allow Na^+ ions to enter the axoplasm. Consistent with these observations, phenytoin and flecainide, both Na^+ channel blockers, have been shown to promote axon survival. The expression of $Na_v1.6$ channels has also been detected in microglia and macrophages in MS lesions, suggesting their importance in neuropathogenesis (Waxman, 2006). Indeed, several studies now indicate that AEDs which block sodium channels including phenytoin, carbamazepine, and limotrigine, could exert their beneficial effects in EAE through inhibition of $Na_v1.6$ expressed on macrophages and microglia (Bechtold et al., 2006; Black et al., 2007). This same channel is also expressed on T cells, raising the possibility of using AEDs in the treatment of MS and other neuroimmune diseases. Clinical trials of AEDs in the treatment of MS are in progress. Recent studies suggest that valproic acid might exert neuroprotective effects among patients with HIV-associated dementia (Schiffito et al., 2006), possibly through reduced neuronal phosphorylated beta-catenin and tau (Dou et al., 2003), although these results remain controversial (Cysique et al., 2006).

Future perspectives

Inflammation provides a setting for the formation of several bioactive compounds that have widely differing roles, depending on the tissue affected and on the timing and duration of exposure. Increasingly sophisticated approaches to the treatment of inflammatory disorders could allow selective modulation of these processes for maximal therapeutic benefit.

New therapeutic candidates

The catecholamines including dopamine, norepinephrine, and epinephrine appear to modulate the immune response by acting as transmitters between the nervous and the innate immune systems and also as autocrine/paracrine mediators in the immune cells. Endogenous catecholamines might have a role in the pathogenesis of MS, since activation-induced production of dopamine was found to be impaired in leukocytes from MS patients, which might be due to interferon-γ. Of interest, interferon-β therapy, by virtue of its immunomodulatory role, was found to induce the release of catecholamines, to support normal T cell function (Cosentino et al., 2005).

Other compounds that are being investigated for use in MS therapy include the statins, which are cholesterol-lowering drugs and which act as inhibitors of 3-hydroxy-3-methylglutaryl coenzyme A (HMG CoA) reductase, a key intermediate in cholesterol synthesis. Statins have been shown to have both anti-inflammatory and neuroprotective properties (Stuve et al., 2004). They prevent and reverse chronic and relapsing EAE (Paintlia et al., 2006) and are thus being tested in clinical trials of MS patients.

Cytokine secretion and proliferation and activation of T cells are dependent on the intracellular levels of cAMP. The level of cAMP is controlled by adenylate cyclase which is involved in its synthesis and its degradation is regulated by phosphodiesterases. The type IV phosphodiesterase is expressed in cells of the immune system and the CNS and its inhibition will raise intracellular cAMP levels, thus reducing cytokine production and T cell proliferation, thereby potentially reducing the severity of diseases such as MS. Inhibition of type IV phosphodiesterase using the agent mesopram has been shown to reduce disease severity in animals with EAE. However, in clinical trials side effects seem to restrict the therapeutic utility of mesopram. Newer versions of phosphodiesterase inhibitors are currently being tested (Dyke and Montana, 2002).

Several small molecule inhibitors have been designed as therapeutics for rational therapy of MS. Of these, one inhibitor designed against α4-integrin was found to reverse the clinical course of disease in a guinea pig model of MS. Interestingly, the molecule also induced closure of the BBB, thereby reducing edema and inflammation in the CNS and preventing accumulation of inflammatory-mediated damage (Piraino *et al.*, 2005). As an alternative approach, using a computer-aided screening approach, an organic molecule TJU103 was identified to specifically inhibit autoreactive CD4 T cells by disrupting the function of CD4 during activation. Administration of this inhibitor either shortly before or after the onset of clinical symptoms reduced the severity in mouse models of EAE (Edling *et al.*, 2002).

Gene therapy

In EAE mice, small interfering RNAs against T-bet, a transcription factor that regulates the release of gamma interferon in CD4 T cells, were used to transduce myelin-specific T cells. These cells were then adoptively transferred into mice, which subsequently did not develop signs of EAE (Lovett-Racke *et al.*, 2004). Another therapeutic approach to MS might incorporate restriction of axonal damage as well as regeneration including the potentiation of oligodendrocyte differentiation: indeed, the use of viral vectors such as HSV1 to deliver fibroblast growth factor-2 intrathecally resulted in the amelioration of the disease course and neuropathology of EAE. In addition, the numbers of oligodendrocyte precursors and myelin-forming oligodendrocytes were both increased in areas of demyelination and axonal loss upon delivery of the gene therapy (Ruffini *et al.*, 2001). Similarly, delivery of either insulin-like growth factor 1 or vascular endothelial growth factor using viral vectors ameliorated disease in mouse models of ALS (Carri *et al.*, 2006).

Vaccination

In mouse models of virus-induced demyelinating disease, vaccination by oral administration of live virus induced protection against the disease, mediated by the early infiltration of antibody-producing B cells into the CNS, together with virus-specific CD4 and CD8 T cells (Kang *et al.*, 2007).Vaccination against IL-17, a molecule that is implicated in the pathogenesis of MS and several other autoimmune diseases, was also successful in ameliorating disease in mouse models of MS

(Uyttenhove and Van Snick, 2006). Vaccination with DNA is also a novel approach to target the inflammatory cells that contribute to disease pathogenesis. In this approach, DNA sequences encoding for the alpha and beta chains of the T cell receptor were incorporated into an expression vector that was capable of inducing a protective immune response in mice with EAE (Buch and Waisman, 2006).

Drug delivery

Since the HIV-1 Tat protein was shown to cross cell membranes when tagged to larger peptides, this system has been used to create Tat fusion proteins incorporating glia-derived neurotrophic factor (GDNF). Such a fusion protein has been shown to transduce mouse neurons and to protect cells from caspase-3-mediated death by elevating Bcl-xL proteins, following optic nerve transection (Killie *et al.*, 2005). Due to the impermeability of the BBB, other methods employed to deliver neurotrophic factors include implanting cells that produce ciliary neurotrophic factor (CNTF) directly to injury sites within the CNS. These cells are immunoisolated by encapsulations, which allow transfer of nutrients and oxygen but prevent host rejection (Emerich and Thanos, 2006).

Nanoparticles also hold promise for the optimization of the delivery of drugs to the CNS. For example, the quinoline derivative, clioquinol (CQ), which is a Cu/Zn chelator known to solubilize β-amyloid plaques, has been shown to cross the BBB when delivered intravenously as polymeric nanoparticles. Similarly, D-penicillamine can be delivered through nanoparticles and functions to chelate copper to reverse the metal-induced precipitation of amyloid beta. In addition, thioflavine when incorporated into polymeric nanoparticles has been used as a probe for the detection of amyloid beta in plaques (Roney *et al.*, 2005).

Bone marrow transplantation

Severe cases of MS that are resistant to various treatment options are potential candidates for bone marrow transplant (BMT) or autologous hematopoietic stem cell transplantation (HSCT). On the completion of various clinical trials, it was reported that high-dose immunosuppression followed by HSCT was effective as it reduced disease progression in several patients, although unavoidable side-effects due to marked immunosuppression and a significant mortality have also been noted (Cavaletti, 2006).

Conclusion

Multiple immunotherapies targeting neuro-inflammation and associated neural cell injury or death are in clinical use, while many experimental therapies show promise. It is likely that a combined approach, targeting both neuro-inflammation and the various mechanisms that underpin neural cell damage are most likely to yield the best outcomes.

Nonetheless, the limited efficacy of the existing immunotherapies, which are apparently relatively specific in their actions, underscores the remarkable redundancy and plasticity of neuro-inflammation and the need for ongoing investigation into its fundamental mechanisms and consequences, as a preamble to the design of more potent treatment options.

References

Aisen PS, *et al*. Effects of rofecoxib or naproxen vs placebo on Alzheimer disease progression: a randomized controlled trial. *J Am Med Assoc* 2003; **289**: 2819–26.

Alder J, *et al*. Interferon-gamma dose-dependently inhibits prostaglandin E2-mediated dendritic-cell-migration towards secondary lymphoid organ chemokines. *Vaccine* 2006; **24**: 7087–94.

Balatoni B, *et al*. FTY720 sustains and restores neuronal function in the DA rat model of MOG-induced experimental autoimmune encephalomyelitis. *Brain Res Bull* 2007; **74**: 307–16.

Bartt RE. Multiple sclerosis, natalizumab therapy, and progressive multifocal leukoencephalopathy. *Curr Opin Neurol* 2006; **19**: 341–9.

Bechtold DA, *et al*. Axonal protection achieved in a model of multiple sclerosis using lamotrigine. *J Neurol* 2006; 253:1542–51.

Bielekova B, *et al*. Encephalitogenic potential of the myelin basic protein peptide (amino acids 83–99) in multiple sclerosis: Results of a phase II clinical trial with an altered peptide ligand. *Nat Med* 2000; **6**: 1167–75.

Bielekova B, *et al*. Humanized anti-CD25 (daclizumab) inhibits disease activity in multiple sclerosis patients failing to respond to interferon beta. *Proc Natl Acad Sci USA* 2004; **101**: 8705–8.

Black JA, *et al*. Exacerbation of experimental autoimmune encephalomyelitis after withdrawal of phenytoin and carbamazepine. *Ann Neurol* 2007; **62**: 21–33.

Bredesen DE, *et al*. Cell death in the nervous system. *Nature* 2006; **443**: 796–802.

Brendza RP, Holtzman DM. Amyloid-beta immunotherapies in mice and men. *Alzheimer Dis Assoc Disord* 2006; **20**: 118–23.

Brocke S, *et al*. Antibodies to CD44 and integrin alpha4, but not L-selectin, prevent central nervous system inflammation and experimental encephalomyelitis by blocking secondary leukocyte recruitment. *Proc Natl Acad Sci USA* 1999; **96**: 6896–901.

Buch T, Waisman A. Protection from autoimmunity by DNA vaccination against T-cell receptor. *Meth Mol Med* 2006; **127**: 269–80.

Calabresi PA, *et al*. An open-label trial of combination therapy with interferon beta-1a and oral methotrexate in MS. *Neurology* 2002; **58**: 314–17.

Callahan MK, Ransohoff RM. Analysis of leukocyte extravasation across the blood–brain barrier: Conceptual and technical aspects. *Curr Allergy Asthma Rep* 2004; **4**: 65–73.

Carri MT, *et al*. Targets in ALS: designing multidrug therapies. *Trends Pharmacol Sci* 2006; **27**: 267–73.

Cavaletti G. Current status and future prospective of immunointervention in multiple sclerosis. *Curr Med Chem* 2006;**13**: 2329–43.

Chavarria A, Alcocer-Varela J. Is damage in central nervous system due to inflammation? *Autoimmun Rev* 2004; **3**: 251–60.

Coles AJ, *et al*. Alemtuzumab vs. Interferon Beta-1a in early multiple sclerosis. *N Engl J Med* 2008; **359**: 1786–801.

Confavreux C, Moreau T. Emerging treatments in multiple sclerosis: Azathioprine and mofetil. *Mult Scler* 1996; **1**: 379–84.

Cosentino M, *et al*. Interferon-gamma and interferon-beta affect endogenous catecholamines in human peripheral blood mononuclear cells: Implications for multiple sclerosis. *J Neuroimmunol* 2005; **162**: 112–21.

Creput C, *et al*. New therapeutic targets for antibodies and recombinant proteins in organ transplantation. *Curr Opin Mol Ther* 2007; **9**: 153–9.

Cross AH, *et al*. Rituximab reduces B cells and T cells in cerebrospinal fluid of multiple sclerosis patients. *J Neuroimmunol* 2006; **180**: 63–70.

Cysique LA, *et al*. Valproic acid is associated with cognitive decline in HIV-infected individuals: A clinical observational study. *BMC Neurol* 2006; **6**: 42.

Defeudis FV. Bilobalide and neuroprotection. *Pharmacol Res* 2002; **46**: 565–8.

Dou H, *et al*. Neuroprotective activities of sodium valproate in a murine model of human immunodeficiency virus-1 encephalitis. *J Neurosci* 2003; **23**: 9162–70.

Dyke HJ, Montana JG. Update on the therapeutic potential of PDE4 inhibitors. *Expert Opin Investig Drugs* 2002; **11**: 1–13.

Edling AE, *et al*. An organic CD4 inhibitor reduces the clinical and pathological symptoms of acute experimental allergic encephalomyelitis. *J Autoimmun* 2002; **18**: 169–79.

Emerich DF, Thanos CG. Intracompartmental delivery of CNTF as therapy for Huntington's disease and retinitis pigmentosa. *Curr Gene Ther* 2006; **6**: 147–59.

Fernandez-Martin A, *et al*. VIP prevents experimental multiple sclerosis by downregulating both inflammatory and autoimmune components of the disease. *Ann NY Acad Sci* 2006; **1070**: 276–81.

Fox EJ. Management of worsening multiple sclerosis with mitoxantrone: A review. *Clin Ther* 2006; **28**: 461–74.

Frank B, Gupta S. A review of antioxidants and Alzheimer's disease. *Ann Clin Psychiatry* 2005; **17**: 269–86.

Gerdes JM, Katsanis N. Small molecule intervention in microtubule-associated human disease. *Hum Mol Genet* 2005; **14** Spec No. 2: R291–300.

Gray OM, *et al*. A systematic review of oral methotrexate for multiple sclerosis. *Mult Scler* 2006; **12**: 507–10.

Griffin DE. Immune responses to RNA-virus infections of the CNS. *Nat Rev Immunol* 2003; **3**: 493–502.

Hauser SL, *et al*. B-cell depletion with rituximab in relapsing-remitting multiple sclerosis. *N Engl J Med* 2008; **358**: 676–88.

Henderson VW. Estrogen-containing hormone therapy and Alzheimer's disease risk: understanding discrepant inferences from observational and experimental research. *Neuroscience* 2006; **138**: 1031–9.

Huang HM, *et al.* Amyloid beta peptide impaired carbachol but not glutamate-mediated phosphoinositide pathways in cultured rat cortical neurons. *Neurochem Res* 2000; **25**: 303–12.

Johnson KP, Panitch HS. Effects of experimental recombinant interferons on multiple sclerosis. *Trans Am Clin Climatol Assoc* 1988; **100**: 171–6.

Johnson RT. *Viral Infections of the Nervous System.* 2nd edn (ed. Mark Placito EH). Philadelphia: Lippincott-Raven Publishers, 1998; 265–314.

Johnston JB, *et al.* HIV-1 Tat neurotoxicity is prevented by matrix metalloproteinase inhibitors. *Ann Neurol* 2001; **49**: 230–41.

Kang BS, *et al.* Oral administration of live virus protects susceptible mice from developing Theiler's virus-induced demyelinating disease. *Virology* 2007; **366**: 185–96.

Kaur C, *et al.* Origin of microglia. *Microsc Res Tech* 2001; **54**: 2–9.

Kelly M, *et al.* Modulating leukocyte recruitment in inflammation. *J Allergy Clin Immunol* 2007; **120**: 3–10.

Kerfoot SM, Kubes P. Overlapping roles of P-selectin and alpha 4 integrin to recruit leukocytes to the central nervous system in experimental autoimmune encephalomyelitis. *J Immunol* 2002; **169**: 1000–6.

Kilic E, *et al.* TAT-GDNF in neurodegeneration and ischemic stroke. *CNS Drug Rev* 2005; **11**: 369–78.

Kosugi I, *et al.* Innate immune responses to cytomegalovirus infection in the developing mouse brain and their evasion by virus-infected neurons. *Am J Pathol* 2002; **161**: 919–28.

Langer-Gould A, *et al.* Progressive multifocal leukoencephalopathy in a patient treated with natalizumab. *N Engl J Med* 2005; **353**: 375–81.

Lapointe BM, *et al.* IVIg therapy in brain inflammation: etiology-dependent differential effects on leucocyte recruitment. *Brain* 2004; **127**: 2649–56.

Lee CZ, *et al.* Doxycycline suppresses cerebral matrix metalloproteinase-9 and angiogenesis induced by focal hyperstimulation of vascular endothelial growth factor in a mouse model. *Stroke* 2004; **35**: 1715–9.

Leist TP, Vermersch P. The potential role for cladribine in the treatment of multiple sclerosis: clinical experience and development of an oral tablet formulation. *Curr Med Res Opin* 2007; **23**: 2667–76.

Loewe R, *et al.* Dimethylfumarate inhibits TNF-induced nuclear entry of NF-kappa B/p65 in human endothelial cells. *J Immunol* 2002; **168**: 4781–7.

Lovett-Racke AE, *et al.* Silencing T-bet defines a critical role in the differentiation of autoreactive T lymphocytes. *Immunity* 2004; **21**: 719–31.

Lowenstein PR. Immunology of viral-vector-mediated gene transfer into the brain: An evolutionary and developmental perspective. *Trends Immunol* 2002; **23**: 23–30.

Lucas SM, *et al.* The role of inflammation in CNS injury and disease. *Br J Pharmacol* 2006; **147** (Suppl 1): S232–40.

Maehlen J, *et al.* Axotomy induces MHC class I antigen expression on rat nerve cells. *Neurosci Lett* 1988; **92**: 8–13.

Martinez-Rodriguez JE, *et al.* Cladribine in aggressive forms of multiple sclerosis. *Eur J Neurol* 2007; **14**(6): 686–9.

Matney SE, Huff DR. Diagnosis and treatment of myasthenia gravis. *Consult Pharm* 2007; **22**: 239–48.

Medyouf H, *et al.* Targeting calcineurin activation as a therapeutic strategy for T-cell acute lymphoblastic leukemia. *Nat Med* 2007; **13**: 736–41.

Morrissey SP, *et al.* Mitoxantrone in the treatment of multiple sclerosis. *Int MS J* 2005; **12**(3): 74–87.

Mueller BK, *et al.* Rho kinase, a promising drug target for neurological disorders. *Nat Rev Drug Discov* 2005; **4**: 387–98.

Nash PT, Florin TH. Tumour necrosis factor inhibitors. *Med J Aust* 2005; **183**: 205–8.

Neumann H. Control of glial immune function by neurons. *Glia* 2001; **36**: 191–9.

Neumann H, *et al.* Major histocompatibility complex (MHC) class I gene expression in single neurons of the central nervous system: differential regulation by interferon (IFN)-gamma and tumor necrosis factor (TNF)-alpha. *J Exp Med* 1997; **185**: 305–16.

O'Connor PW, *et al.* A Phase II study of the safety and efficacy of teriflunomide in multiple sclerosis with relapses. *Neurology* 2006; **66**: 894–900.

Orgogozo JM, *et al.* Subacute meningoencephalitis in a subset of patients with AD after Abeta42 immunization. *Neurology* 2003; **61**: 46–54.

Paintlia AS, *et al.* Immunomodulatory effect of combination therapy with lovastatin and 5-aminoimidazole-4-carboxamide-1-beta-D-ribofuranoside alleviates neurodegeneration in experimental autoimmune encephalomyelitis. *Am J Pathol* 2006; **169**: 1012–25.

Piraino PS, *et al.* Suppression of acute experimental allergic encephalomyelitis with a small molecule inhibitor of alpha4 integrin. *Mult Scler* 2005; **11**: 683–90.

Polman C, *et al.* Treatment with laquinimod reduces development of active MRI lesions in relapsing MS. *Neurology* 2005; **64**: 987–91.

Pozzi S, *et al.* Estrogen action in neuroprotection and brain inflammation. *Ann NY Acad Sci* 2006; **1089**: 302–23.

Prinz M, *et al.* Distinct and nonredundant in vivo functions of IFNAR on myeloid cells limit autoimmunity in the central nervous system. *Immunity* 2008; **28**: 675–86.

Ransohoff RM, *et al.* Three or more routes for leukocyte migration into the central nervous system. *Nat Rev Immunol* 2003; **3**: 569–81.

Reddy DS. Role of neurosteroids in catamenial epilepsy. *Epilepsy Res* 2004; **62**: 99–118.

Reijerkerk A, et al. Diapedesis of monocytes is associated with MMP-mediated occludin disappearance in brain endothelial cells. *FASEB J* 2006; **20**: 2550–2.

Ringshausen I, et al. The immunomodulatory drug Leflunomide inhibits cell cycle progression of B-CLL cells. *Leukemia* 2008; **22**: 635–8.

Rogers J, et al. Neuroinflammation in Alzheimer's disease and Parkinson's disease: Are microglia pathogenic in either disorder? *Int Rev Neurobiol* 2007; **82**: 235–46.

Roney C, et al. Targeted nanoparticles for drug delivery through the blood–brain barrier for Alzheimer's disease. *J Control Release* 2005; **108**: 193–214.

Ropper AH. Selective treatment of multiple sclerosis. *N Engl J Med* 2006; **354**: 965–7.

Ruffini F, et al. Fibroblast growth factor-II gene therapy reverts the clinical course and the pathological signs of chronic experimental autoimmune encephalomyelitis in C57BL/6 mice. *Gene Ther* 2001; **8**: 1207–13.

Runstrom A, et al. Inhibition of the development of chronic experimental autoimmune encephalomyelitis by laquinimod (ABR-215062) in IFN-beta k.o. and wild type mice. *J Neuroimmunol* 2006; **173**: 69–78.

Salama B, et al. Optic neuropathy in refractory neurosarcoidosis treated with TNF-alpha antagonist. *Can J Ophthalmol* 2006; **41**: 766–8.

Schifitto G, et al. Valproic acid adjunctive therapy for HIV-associated cognitive impairment: A first report. *Neurology* 2006; **66**: 919–21.

Schimrigk S, et al. Oral fumaric acid esters for the treatment of active multiple sclerosis: an open-label, baseline-controlled pilot study. *Eur J Neurol* 2006; **13**: 604–10.

Schwartz M, Kipnis J. Protective autoimmunity and neuroprotection in inflammatory and noninflammatory neurodegenerative diseases. *J Neurol Sci* 2005; **233**: 163–6.

Scott LJ, Figgitt DP. Mitoxantrone: A review of its use in multiple sclerosis. *CNS Drugs* 2004; **18**: 379–96.

Shytle RD, et al. Cholinergic modulation of microglial activation by alpha 7 nicotinic receptors. *J Neurochem* 2004; **89**: 337–43.

Steinman L. Elaborate interactions between the immune and nervous systems. *Nature Immunol* 2004; **5**: 575–81.

Stepkowski SM. Molecular targets for existing and novel immunosuppressive drugs. *Expert Rev Mol Med* 2000; **2**: 1–23.

Stuve O, et al. Statins as potential therapeutic agents in multiple sclerosis. *Curr Neurol Neurosci Rep* 2004; **4**: 237–44.

Sugiyama K, et al. Comparison of suppressive potency between azathioprine and 6-mercaptopurine against mitogen-induced blastogenesis of human peripheral blood mononuclear cells in-vitro. *J Pharm Pharmacol* 2003; **55**: 393–8.

Teixeira MM, et al. The role of lipocortin-1 in the inhibitory action of dexamethasone on eosinophil trafficking in cutaneous inflammatory reactions in the mouse. *Br J Pharmacol* 1998; **123**: 538–44.

Thatcher GR, et al. NO chimeras as therapeutic agents in Alzheimer's disease. *Curr Alzheimer Res* 2006; **3**: 237–45.

Treumer F, et al. Dimethylfumarate is a potent inducer of apoptosis in human T cells. *J Invest Dermatol* 2003; **121**: 1383–8.

Uyttenhove C, Van Snick J. Development of an anti-IL-17A auto-vaccine that prevents experimental auto-immune encephalomyelitis. *Eur J Immunol* 2006; **36**: 2868–74.

Wang C, et al. Antigen-specific therapy promotes repair of myelin and axonal damage in established EAE. *J Neurochem* 2006; **98**: 1817–27.

Warren KG, et al. Intravenous synthetic peptide MBP8298 delayed disease progression in an HLA Class II-defined cohort of patients with progressive multiple sclerosis: Results of a 24-month double-blind placebo-controlled clinical trial and 5 years of follow-up treatment. *Eur J Neurol* 2006; **13**: 887–95.

Waxman SG. Ions, energy and axonal injury: Towards a molecular neurology of multiple sclerosis. *Trends Mol Med* 2006; **12**: 192–5.

Weber MS, et al. Type II monocytes modulate T cell-mediated central nervous system autoimmune disease. *Nature Med* 2007; **13**: 935–43.

Woodruff TM, et al. Therapeutic activity of C5a receptor antagonists in a rat model of neurodegeneration. *FASEB J* 2006; **20**: 1407–17.

Xiu J, et al. Expression of nicotinic receptors on primary cultures of rat astrocytes and up-regulation of the alpha7, alpha4 and beta2 subunits in response to nanomolar concentrations of the beta-amyloid peptide(1–42). *Neurochem Int* 2005; **47**: 281–90.

Yang JS, et al. Laquinimod (ABR-215062) suppresses the development of experimental autoimmune encephalomyelitis, modulates the Th1/Th2 balance and induces the Th3 cytokine TGF-beta in Lewis rats. *J Neuroimmunol* 2004; **156**: 3–9.

Yednock TA, et al. Prevention of experimental autoimmune encephalomyelitis by antibodies against alpha 4 beta 1 integrin. *Nature* 1992; **356**: 63–6.

Yong VW. Differential mechanisms of action of interferon-beta and glatiramer acetate in MS. *Neurology* 2002; **59**: 802–8.

Yong VW, et al. Experimental models of neuroprotection relevant to multiple sclerosis. *Neurology* 2007; **68**: pS32–7; discussion S43–54.

Yousry TA, et al. Evaluation of patients treated with natalizumab for progressive multifocal leukoencephalopathy. *N Engl J Med* 2006; **354**: 924–33.

Zheng YQ, et al. Effects of crocin on reperfusion-induced oxidative/nitrative injury to cerebral microvessels after global cerebral ischemia. *Brain Res* 2007; **1138**: 86.

Index

Note: page numbers in *italics* refer to figures and tables

abacavir 211
acetyl-L-carnitine 252
acrolein 23
acute disseminated encephalomyelitis
  (ADEM) 9, 97–106
  acute hemorrhagic leukoencephalitis
    105–6
  brainstem involvement 99–100
  classification 101
  clinical features 98–9
  cognitive impairment 102
  consensus definitions 103
  demyelination 98
    recurrence 103
  encephalopathy 104–5
  epidemiology 97
  gray matter lesions 100
  imaging 99–101, *100*
  immunoglobulin therapy
    102, 249
  investigations 99–101
    laboratory 99
  lesion resolution 101
  MS risk differentiation
    104–5, *104*
  neurophysiology 99
  outcome 102–3
  pathophysiology 97–8
  plasmapheresis 102, 249
  post-vaccination 97, 104
  prodromal illness 97, 104
  progression to MS 103–4
  recurrent 103–4
  spinal cord involvement 101
  steroid therapy 101–2
    recurrence after 103
  treatment 101–2
  white matter abnormalities
    99–100
acute hemorrhagic leukoencephalitis
  (AHLE) 105–6
adaptive immune reactivity 2, 4–5
  cellular components 5
  clonal diversity 4–5
adaptive immune response 1
  activation in viral infections 128–9
  detrimental 132–3
  cyclic adenosine monophosphate
    (cAMP) 254

adenosine triphosphate (ATP)
  microglia activation 18
  MS pathology 61–2
adhesion molecules
  acute disseminated
    encephalomyelitis 98
  HIV infection 142
  MS demyelination activity
    staging 54
  MS lesions 52–3
AIDS dementia complex *see* HIV-
  associated dementia (HAD)/
  HIV dementia (HIV-D)
alphavirus
  encephalomyelitis 132
  immunomodulation 230
Alzheimer's disease, microglia role in
  neurodegeneration 17
Alzheimer's pathology, HIV-associated
  dementia 148
aminoguanidine 23, 226
amyloid precursor protein
  deposition in traumatic brain injury
    185–6
  HIV-associated dementia 148
amyloidosis of CNS 116
amyotrophic lateral sclerosis
  30, 31
androstenedione 227
angioimmunolymphoproliferative
  lesions (AIL) 119
animal models
  acute viral encephalitis 126, *127*
  dendritic cells 28–9
  HIV dementia 145
  malaria 177–8
  MS 56
  TNF-alpha 190–1
  see also experimental autoimmune
    encephalomyelitis (EAE)
antibiotics 253
antibody therapies 249–50
antiepileptic drugs 254
antigen(s)
  immune response 246
  in-situ presentation 90–1
antigen presentation
  cross-presentation 87, 92
  dendritic cells 90–1

immune reactivity 6–7
  viral encephalitis 129
antigen-presenting cells
  activation via innate immune
    receptors 4
  cross-presentation 87
  dendritic cells 5
  macrophages in MS 49
  microglia in MS 49
  professional 6–7
  T cell priming 91–2
anti-glutaminergic agents 213–214
anti-inflammatory adjunctive
  treatment, bacterial meningitis
  166–8
antioxidants 252
antiphospholipid syndrome 120
antiretroviral agents
  HIV dementia 210–11
  see also highly active antiretroviral
    therapy (HAART)
apoptosis, Purkinje cells 17
aquaporin 4 (AQP-4), neuromyelitis
  optica 58–9
Arenaviridae immunomodulation 231
artemisinins 226
asthma, IL-4 immunomodulation
  223–4
astrocytes
  activation *187*
  antigen presentation 6
  B cell activating factor 7
  HIV infection 140
  HIV-associated dementia 145
  inflammation in traumatic brain
    injury 188
  innate immunity 247
  macrophage regulation 145
  malaria 179
  microglia regulation 145
  neuro-inflammation regulation 3
  neurotrophin production 192
astrogliosis, traumatic brain
  injury 192
autoimmunity
  B cells 10
  infection association 3–4
  promotion by innate immune
    activity 3–4

axons
  diffuse injury 185–6
    TNF-alpha 190
  MS pathology 61–3, *62*
    cortical demyelination
      63–4
    immune-mediated damage *80*
  remodeling of connections *81*
azathioprine 250–1

B cell activating factor 7
B cell chronic lymphoid leukemia
  (B-CLL) 251
B cell lymphoma, intravascular 119
B lymphocytes
  adaptive immune reactivity 5
  autoimmunity role 10
  CNS 7
  CNS immune reactivity 10
  CNS milieu 7–8
  experimental autoimmune
    encephalomyelitis 7
  immunoglobulin rearrangement in
    CNS 9–10
  lymphoid tissues 8
  MS lesions 48–9
  viral encephalitis 128–9
bacteria/bacterial infections
  entry into CNS 161–2
  immunomodulation 227–9
  mucosal colonization/invasion/
    spread 161–2
  survival in subarachnoid space 162
BAFF (B cell activating factor of the
  tumor necrosis family) 77
Balo's concentric sclerosis
  hypoxia 52
  lesions *59*
  pathological heterogeneity 59
Behçet's syndrome, CNS vasculitis
  119–20
benign angiitis of the central nervous
  system (BACNS) 109
  see also reversible vasoconstrictive
    disease states (RVDS)
bilobalide 253
biphasic disseminated encephalitis
  103–4
blood–brain barrier (BBB) 35, 246
  bacterial docking structures 42
  bacterial invasion 162
  cerebral malaria 177
  damage in MS 50
  endothelial cells 5–6, 35,
    37–41
    tight junctions 35–6
  HIV infection crossing 139, 140
  immune cells crossing 35–7, *36*

immune privilege 87
  leukocyte routes across 40–1
  matrix metalloproteinases 214
  pathogens crossing 35–7, *36*
  post-capillary venules 36
  regional differences 36
  T cell migration 5–6, 38–9, 247
  tight junctions 50
  Trojan horse mechanism for
    crossing 41, 42
blood–CSF barrier *see* epithelial
  blood–cerebrospinal fluid
  barrier
bone marrow transplantation 255
Borrelia burgdorferi 112
brain gangliosides 129
brain injury *see* traumatic brain
  injury (TBI)
brain-derived neurotrophic factor
  (BDNF) 22, 23
  HIV-associated dementia 144
  MS lesion repair 60
  neuro-immune cross-talk in
    MS 75–6

calcineurin inhibition 251
calcium ion-dependent protein
  kinases 18
cannabinoids 22, 227
catecholamines 254
CCL2
  bacterial meningitis 165
  HIV-associated dementia
    143–4
CCL3 165
CCL4 165
CCL5 143–4
CCR1 49
CCR2 177–8
CCR5
  MS 49
  T cell migration in malaria
    177–8
CCR7 31
CD4+ T cells
  CD8+ T cell-mediated
    disease 92–3
  EAE 38, 89
  HIV dementia 202
  HIV infection 139, 140
  malaria 178–9
  migration 246
  MS 89
  viral clearance
    from glial cells 131
    from neurons 130–1
CD8+ T cell-mediated autoimmune
  disease 87–93

CD8+ T cells 87
  EAE 89
  HIV infection 139, 140
  malaria 178–9
  MS 48, 89
    dendritic cell role 89–90
    lesions 51
    neuro-immune cross-talk
      79–80
  paraneoplastic neurologic
    degeneration 88
  priming of CNS antigen-specific
    91–2
  viral clearance
    from glial cells 131
    from neurons 130–1
CD36 sequestration in malaria 176
CD40 ligand immunomodulation 226
central nervous system (CNS)
  amyloidosis 116
  immune privilege 87
  immunological quiescence 127
  sarcoid vasculitis 115–16
cerebral angiography, primary
    angiitis of the central nervous
    system 121
cerebral atherosclerosis 120
cerebral malaria *see* malaria; cerebral
cerebral edema
  TNF-alpha 190
  traumatic brain injury 186
cerebrospinal fluid (CSF)
  changes in HIV dementia 206
  oligoclonal bands in MS 105
chemokine(s) 20
  bacterial meningitis inflammatory
    response 165
  CXCLs in B cell infiltration of CNS 7
  HIV infection 143–4
  immunomodulation 250
  innate immunity 247
  leukocyte transmigration 247
  microglia 21
  MS 49
    neuro-immune cross-talk 77
  T cells
    migration in malaria 177–8
    recruitment across BBB 39
  traumatic brain injury 193–4
  viral infections 128
chemokine receptors
  T cell migration in malaria 177–8
  see also CCRs
children
  chronic infantile neurological
    cutaneous and articular
    syndrome 2
  focal viral encephalitis 229

2-chlorodeoxyadenosine 251
choroid plexus 37
    leukocyte migration into CSF 41
chronic granulomatous disease, β
        immunomodulation 223
chronic infantile neurological
        cutaneous and articular
        syndrome 2
cimetidine immunomodulation 226
circumventricular organs 37, 41
cladribine 251
cognitive impairment, acute
        disseminated
        encephalomyelitis 102
complement
    bacterial meningitis inflammatory
        response 165
    HIV infection 142
    microglia activation 19
complement cascade
    HIV-associated dementia 142
    MS cortical lesions 64
corticosteroids see glucocorticosteroids
CPI-1189 213
Crohn's disease, IL-12
        immunomodulation 224–5
cross-presentation 87, 92
Cryptococcus neoformans
        immunomodulation 233–4
CX3CL1 21, 23
    HIV-associated dementia
        143–4
    neuro-immune cross-talk in
        MS 77
    viral infections 128
CXC3R1 77, 128
CXCL1 165
CXCL8 165
CXCL12 143–4
cyclo-oxygenase (COX) 252
    inhibition 252
cyclophosphamide 251
cysticercosis, immunomodulation 233
cytokines
    bacterial meningitis inflammatory
        response 164–5
    HIV infection 142–3
    immunomodulation 221–6
        bacterial meningitis 227
    innate immunity 247
    malaria 178
    microdialysis use in detection 194
    microglia 21
    MS
        demyelination activity staging 54
        neuro-immune cross-talk 76–7
    pro-inflammatory 20
        leukocyte migration 52

traumatic brain injury
        188–93
    detection 194
    viral infections 128
cytomegalovirus (CMV)
        immunomodulation 229
cytotoxicity, MS lesions 51

DAPTA 212
dementia see HIV-associated dementia
        (HAD)/HIV dementia
        (HIV-D)
demyelinating disease 120
dendritic cells 27–32
    adaptive immune reactivity 5
    animal models 28–9
    antigen presentation 90–1
    CCR7 expression 31
    CD8+ T cell activation 89–90
    CNS inflammation induction/
        remission 31
    constitutive 28
    derivation 27–8
    inflammatory 28
    inflammatory disorders 28–9
    lineage differentiation 30–1
    localization in human brain/spinal
        cord 29–30
    lymphoid 27–8
    maturation 27
    migration 27
        to lymphoid organs 7
    MS 29–30
        CD8+ T cell activation 89–90
    myeloid 27–8, 30–1
    peripheral 28
    plasmacytoid 30
    precursors 30–1
    professional antigen-presenting
        cells 6–7
    recruitment from blood 30
    subtypes 27–8, 29
    T cell interactions 31
    viral clearance 31
diapedesis 247
diffuse axonal injury 185–6
    TNF-alpha 190
disseminated encephalitis
    biphasic/multiphasic 103–4
    see also acute disseminated
        encephalomyelitis (ADEM)
DNA viruses, acute viral
        encephalitis 125
donepezil 252
doxycycline 253
drug use/abuse
    CNS vasculitis 119
    HIV dementia association 205–6

drugs, pharmaceutical see
        pharmacological agents
dysferlin, MS 50

echovirus meningoencephalitis 232
edavarone, minocycline
        effects 22
encephalitis
    biphasic disseminated 103–4
    CMV 229
    disseminated 103–4
    echovirus meningoencephalitis 232
    equine encephalitis viruses 230
    focal viral of children 229
    herpes simplex viral 229
    HIV 137–8
    influenza virus 231
    Japanese B encephalitis 230
    lymphocytic choriomeningitis 231
    measles 230
    multiphasic disseminated
        103–4
    Sindbis virus 230
    St Louis encephalitis 230
    toxoplasmic 232
    West Nile virus 230
    see also subacute sclerosing
        panencephalitis (SSPE)
        immunomodulation; viral
        encephalitis, acute
encephalomyelitis see acute
        disseminated encephalomyelitis
        (ADEM)
encephalopathy, acute disseminated
        encephalomyelitis 104–5
endocannabinoids 22
endocrine therapy 253–4
endothelial cells
    changes in cerebral
        malaria 177
    see also blood–brain barrier (BBB);
        endothelial cells
epidermal growth factor
        (EGF) 223
epithelial blood–cerebrospinal fluid
        barrier 37
    bacterial invasion 162
    immune cell crossing 41
Epstein–Barr virus (EBV)
        immunomodulation 229
equine encephalitis viruses 230
erythropoietin 226
Escherichia coli 161
estradiol, 17-beta 227
estrogens 253–4
    HIV dementia therapy 214
    immunomodulation 227
excitotoxicity, MS lesions 52

263

experimental autoimmune
    encephalomyelitis (EAE)
  acute disseminated
    encephalomyelitis similarities
    97–8
  B lymphocytes 7
  CD4$^+$ T cells 89
  CD8$^+$ T cells 89
  dendritic cells 28–9, 31
    myeloid 31
  endothelial blood–brain barrier 38
  gene therapy 255
  α immunomodulation 223
extracellular signal-related kinase
    (ERK) 19

familial cold autoinflammatory
    syndrome 2
fingolimod 252
Flaviviridae immunomodulation 230
flavonoids, HIV dementia therapy 214
FMS-like tyrosine kinase ligand
    (FLT3L) 31
focal viral encephalitis of
    children 229
fraktalkine see CX3CL1
fumaric acid esters 252
fungal infections, immunomodulation
    233–4

galantamine 252
GAP-43, MS lesions 64
gene therapy 255
germinal center-like formations 8
giant cell arteritis, CNS vasculitis 120
Ginkgo biloba 253
Glasgow Coma Scale, traumatic brain
    injury 185
glatiramer acetate
  immunomodulation 249
  MS treatment 81–2, 249
glial cells
  acute viral encephalitis 127
  viral clearance 131
glial-derived neurotrophic factor
    (GDNF) 255
  neuro-immune cross-talk in
    MS 75
glucocorticosteroids
  acute disseminated
    encephalomyelitis 101–2
    recurrence after 103
  immunomodulation 222, 233, 248
  mechanism of action 167
  meningitis
    administration 168
    anti-inflammatory adjunctive
      treatment 167–8

complications impact 167–8
  immunomodulation 227–8
  mortality effects 167
reversible vasoconstrictive disease
    states 118
side effects 168
glutamate 252
  MS lesions 52
  multiple sclerosis 62
L-glutamate 20
  microglia activation 18
glutamate excitotoxicity 20
glutamic acid decarboxylase
    (GAD) 133
glutathione therapy 213
glycogen synthase kinase 3
    (GSK3) 253
glycolipids, immunological
    effects 129
gp120, HIV dementia 209–10
GPI glycan, cerebral malaria 176–7
granulocyte colony-stimulating factor
    (G-CSF) immunomodulation
    223, 233
  Listeria monocytogenes 228–9
granulocyte–macrophage colony-
    stimulating factor
    (GM-CSF) 223
granulomatous angiitis of the central
    nervous system (GACNS) 109,
    110–13
  clinical signs 110–11
  CNS amyloidosis 116
  CNS biopsy 111–12
  CNS sarcoid vasculitis 115–16
  diagnosis 111–13
  differential diagnosis 112
  disease activity monitoring 122
  etiology 111
  infections 111
  lumbar puncture 111
  management 112–13
  neuro-imaging 111
  treatment 112–13
  see also primary angiitis of the
    central nervous system
    (PACNS)
Guillain–Barré syndrome 249
  plasmapheresis 249

head injury see traumatic brain
    injury (TBI)
hemozoin, cerebral malaria 176–7
hepatitis C
  CNS vasculitis 118–19
  HIV dementia association 205
  ω immunomodulation 223
herpes simplex viral encephalitis 229

herpes simplex virus (HSV)
    immunomodulation 229
  TLR 226
highly active antiretroviral therapy
    (HAART)
  cognitive disorders 201
  HIV dementia 147–8, 202,
    202, 203, 208, 210–11, 212
  progressive multifocal
    leukoencephalopathy
    immunomodulation
    229–30
HIV encephalitis 137–8
HIV infection
  adhesion molecules 142
  astrocytes 140, 145
  blood–brain barrier crossing 42,
    139, 140
  bystander hypothesis 141
  cannabinoid immunomodulation
    227
  CD4$^+$ T cells 139, 140
  CD8$^+$ T cells 139, 140
  chemokines 143–4
  chronic 137–49
  CNS vasculitis 118–19
  complement 142
  cytokines 142–3
  dendritic cells 30
  direct injury hypothesis 141
  epidemiology 137
  gp120 209–10
  granulomatous angiitis of the central
    nervous system differential
    diagnosis 112
  IL-2 immunomodulation 223
  IL-12 immunomodulation 224–5
  immune response 138–9
  indirect hypothesis 141
  matrix metalloproteinases 142
  minor cognitive motor
    disorder 201
  molecular response 142–5
  natural history 139–40
  neurocognitive disorders 201–14
  neurons 140–1
    loss 137–8, 208
  neurotrophins 144
  perivascular macrophages 138–9,
    208
  progressive multifocal
    leukoencephalopathy
    immunomodulation 229–30
  synaptodendritic injury 209
  tat 209
  tropism 138
  viral replication control 139–40
  viral spread to CNS 131, 132

HIV-associated dementia (HAD)/HIV
    dementia (HIV-D) 137, 201–14
  adjunctive therapies 211–14
  Alzheimer's pathology 148
  amyloid precursor protein 148
  animal models 145
  antiretroviral agents 210–11
  astrocytes 145
  CD4$^+$ T cells 202
  clinical features 202–3
  CNS escape 205
  complement cascade 142
  confounding illnesses 203–6, *204*
  CSF changes 206
  disease cofactors 205–6
  drug use/abuse association 205–6
  epidemiology 137
  gp120 209–10
  HAART 147–8, 202, *202, 203, 208,*
    210–11, 212
  hepatitis C association 205
  immune tolerance 146–7
  kynurenine pathway 146–7
  late development 145–6
  macrophages 141
  molecular response 142–5
  monocytes 146
  neurotrophins 144
  onset 201–2
  pathogenesis 141, 146
  pathology 137–8, 208–10
  pre-HAART 202–3
  quinolinic acid 146–7
  radiological features 206–8, *207*
  risk factors 202
  tat 209
  viral evolution 146
HIV-associated neurocognitive
    disorders (HAND) 201–14
  adjunctive therapies 211–14
  antiretroviral agents 210–11
  clinical features 202–3
  confounding illnesses 203–6, *204*
  CSF changes 206
  disease cofactors 205–6
  evolution 201–2
  genetic susceptibility 205
  HAART *202, 203, 208,* 210–11, *212*
  hepatitis C association 205
  pathology 208–10
  prevalence 201–2
  radiological features 206–8, *207*
Hodgkin's lymphoma, CNS vasculitis 119
host defense 221
host response, acute viral encephalitis
    129–5
human T cell lymphotropic virus 1
    (HTLV-1) 231

humoral immune response, antigen-
    specific 133
hypoxia
  Balo's concentric sclerosis 52
  MS lesions 51–2
  traumatic brain injury 186
hypoxia-inducible factors (HIF),
    MS 51–2

immune activation 221
immune cells
  access to CNS 35–42
  migration across brain barriers
    35–41
immune privilege 87, 90–1
immune reactivity
  antigen presentation 6–7
  see also adaptive immune reactivity
immune reconstitution inflammatory
    illness (IRIS) 203–4
immune response
  to antigen 246
  antigen-specific 128
    humoral 133
  HIV infection 138–9
  induction in viral infections 127–8
  neuropathology generation 131–3
  regulation of local 129–30
  see also adaptive immune response;
    innate immune response
immunization 222
immunoglobulin therapy
  acute disseminated
    encephalomyelitis 102
  intravenous 249
immunoglobulins
  brain tissue in multiple sclerosis 9
  intrathecal production 8–9
  oligoclonal bands in CSF 7,
    8–9, 105
  polyspecific intrathecal response 9
  rearrangement in CNS 9–10
immunomodulation 221–34
  bacterial infections 227–9
  bacterial meningitis 227–8
  corticosteroids 222
  cytokines 221–6
  fungal infections 233–4
  immunization 222
  parasitic infections 232–3
  tuberculosis 228
  viral infections 229–32
immunomodulators 222–7, *233, 234,*
    248–50
  small molecule neuro-immune
    modulators 252–4
immunophilin-binding agents 251
immunosuppressive agents 250–2

immunotherapy
  combination 248
  neuro-inflammation 247–8
  see also immunoglobulin therapy;
    immunomodulation;
    immunomodulators
indoleamine 2,3-dioxygenase (IDO)
    pathway 179
infections
  acute disseminated
    encephalomyelitis prodromal
    illness 97, 104
  autoimmunity association 3–4
  CNS vasculitis 118–19, *119*
  fungal 233–4
  granulomatous angiitis of the central
    nervous system 111
  immune response induction
    127–8
  immunomodulation 221–34
  interferon response induction
    127–8
  viral 229–32
  see also bacteria/bacterial infections;
    parasitic infections
inflammation
  development 128–9
  lipopolysaccharide model 187
  macrophages 187
  traumatic brain injury 187–8
  see also neuro-inflammation
inflammatory mediators,
    malaria 178
influenza virus immunomodulation 231
innate immune response 1, *2*
  activation in bacterial meningitis
    163–4
  brain pathology modulation 4
  CNS autoimmunity
    promotion 3–4
  CNS resident cells 3
  injurious 131–2
  neuro-inflammation 247
α_4-integrin 38, 249–50
  leukocyte migration across
    BBB 39
integrins 249–50
  activation 165, 247
intercellular adhesion molecule 1
    (ICAM-1)
  acute disseminated
    encephalomyelitis 98
  choroid plexus epithelium 41
  HIV infection 142
  immunomodulation 226
  inflammatory cell recruitment across
    BBB 39–40
  T cell interaction with BBB 39

intercellular adhesion molecule 2
(ICAM-2)
inflammatory cell recruitment across
BBB 39–40
T cell interaction with BBB 39
interferon
MS therapy 81–2, 248, 254
response induction in viral infections
127–8
interferon alpha (α)
immunomodulation 223,
233, 248
herpes simplex virus 229
Listeria monocytogenes 228–9
toxoplasmic encephalitis 232
tuberculosis 228
varicella zoster virus 229
malaria 178, 179
viral clearance from neurons
130–1
interferon beta (β) 223
immunomodulation 233
interferon omega (ω) 223
interleukin 1 (IL-1)
bacterial meningitis inflammatory
response 164–5
immunomodulation 223
microglia 21
traumatic brain injury 189–90
interleukin 1 type 1 receptor antagonist
(IL-1ra) 21
interleukin 2 (IL-2)
immunomodulation 223
cytomegalovirus 229
Epstein–Barr virus 229
toxoplasmic encephalitis 232
interleukin 4 (IL-4)
immunomodulation 223–4
herpes simplex virus 229
microglia 21
interleukin 6 (IL-6)
bacterial meningitis inflammatory
response 164–5
immunomodulation 224
traumatic brain injury 191–2
interleukin 6 receptor
(IL-6-R) 192
interleukin 7 (IL-7)
immunomodulation 224
toxoplasmic encephalitis 232
interleukin 8 (IL-8) 193–4
interleukin 10 (IL-10)
immunomodulation 224
bacterial meningitis 227
malaria 232
malaria 178, 232
traumatic brain injury
189–90, 193

interleukin 12 (IL-12)
immunomodulation 224–5
influenza virus 231
Listeria monocytogenes 228–9
toxoplasmic encephalitis 232
malaria 178
interleukin 13 (IL-13)
immunomodulation 225
Listeria monocytogenes 228–9
interleukin 15 (IL-15)
immunomodulation 225
toxoplasmic encephalitis 232
interleukin 16 (IL-16)
immunomodulation 225
interleukin 17 (IL-17) 31
immunomodulation 225
interleukin 18 (IL-18)
immunomodulation 225
bacterial meningitis 227
influenza virus 231
Listeria monocytogenes 228–9
interleukin 23 (IL-23)
immunomodulation 225
interleukin 27 (IL-27)
immunomodulation 225
toxoplasmic encephalitis 232
intravenous immunoglobulin
(IVIG) 249
ischemia, traumatic brain
injury 186
isoprinosine 230–1

Japanese B encephalitis 230
junction adhesion molecules (JAMs) 40

Kaposi's sarcoma, IL-12
immunomodulation 224–5
kynurenine pathway, HIV-associated
dementia 146–7

laquinimod 251–2
leukocytes
arrest 247
HIV infection 139
immune response role 246
migration 52, 247
recruitment in bacterial meningitis
165–6
rolling/tethering 247
ligands, immunomodulation 250
lipo-oligosaccharide 164
lipopolysaccharide (LPS),
inflammation model 187
lipoteichoic acid 163–4
Listeria monocytogenes 161
immunomodulation 228–9
lymphocyte function-associated
antigen (LFA-1) 39–40

lymphocytes
MS demyelination activity staging 54
see also B lymphocytes;
T lymphocytes
lymphocytic choriomeningitis
detrimental adaptive immunity 132
immunomodulation 231
lymphoid organs, primary/secondary
246
lymphoid tissues
B cell containing 8
tertiary 91
lymphoma, intravascular B-cell 119
lymphotoxin-alpha (LT-alpha) 8
malaria 178

macrophages
BBB damage 50
foamy 49–50, 53
HIV-associated dementia 141
inflammation 187
matrix metalloproteinase
expression 53
MS lesions 49–50
demyelination activity staging 54
neuro-immune cross-talk 79–80
perivascular 15
HIV infection 138–9, 208
innate immunity 247
phenotypes 49–50
regulation by astrocytes 145
traumatic brain injury 187
major histocompatibility complex
(MHC) class I 246
expression by microglia 6
inducibility in neurons 6
MS 48
major histocompatibility complex
(MHC) class II 246
glatiramer acetate
immunomodulation 249
MS demyelination activity
staging 54
malaria, cerebral 173–9
animal models 177–8
artemisinin immunomodulation 226
astrocytes 179
bioactive parasite products 176–7
blood–brain barrier changes 177
burden 173
cellular involvement 178–9
clinical features 173
complications 173
cytokines 178
development mechanisms 175
endothelial cell changes 177
epidemiology 173
IL-10 178

IL-12 178
immunity 173
immunomodulation 232
indoleamine 2,3-dioxygenase
    pathway 179
inducible NOS 178
inflammatory mediators 178
lymphotoxin-alpha 178
microvascular obstruction 177
mortality 173
neuropathology 174–5
    CNS role in induction 179
NK cells 178
retina 175
ROS 178
sequestration 174–6, *175*
    receptors *176*
T cells 178–9
TNF-alpha 178
malignancy
    IL-2 immunomodulation 223
    IL-7 immunomodulation 224
    IL-12 immunomodulation 224–5
malignancy-associated CNS
    vasculitis 119
mannose-binding lectin pathway 165
matrix metalloproteinase(s) (MMPs)
    bacterial meningitis 166
    blood–brain barrier function 214
    HIV dementia 214
    HIV infection 142
    MS lesions 53
matrix metalloproteinase (MMP)
    inhibitors 253
    HIV dementia therapy 214
measles 230
memantine 212, 252
meningitis, bacterial 161–8
    anti-inflammatory adjunctive
        treatment 166–8
    brain damage mediators 166
    chemokines in inflammatory
        response 165
    complement in inflammatory
        response 165
    cytokines in inflammatory response
        164–5
    entry into CNS 161–2
    glucocorticoid therapy 167–8
        administration 168
        anti-inflammatory adjunctive
            treatment 167–8
        complications impact 167–8
        immunomodulation 227–8
    immunomodulation 227–8
        IL-1 223
    inflammatory response 164–6

innate immune response activation
    163–4
    invasion through BBB 162
    leukocyte recruitment 165–6
    matrix metalloproteinases 166
    neuropathology 166
    NOD proteins 164
    peroxynitrite 166
    reactive oxygen species 166
    toll-like receptors 163–4
    transcellular passage across brain
        barriers 42
    tuberculosis 228
meningitis, cryptococcal 233–4
meningitis, viral
    echovirus meningoencephalitis 232
    see also lymphocytic
        choriomeningitis
methamphetamine abuse, HIV
    dementia association 205–6
methotrexate 252
microbial infections, immunoglobulin
    oligoclonal bands in CSF 7
microdialysis, cytokine detection 194
microglia 15–23
    activation 15, 17–18, *187*
    antigen presentation 6
    ATP receptors 18
    biochemical activators 18–19
    calcium ion-dependent protein
        kinases 18
    chemotactic response 16, 23
    drug actions 22–3
    EGFP expression
    HIV infection 137–9
    immunoregulatory effects 129–30
    innate immunity 247
    ion channel changes 18
    MS lesions 49–50
    neurodegeneration 17
    origins 15–16
    parenchymal 91
    pathogenic mediators 19–21
    pathophysiological functions 17
    perivascular 91
    physiological function 16–17
    post-mitotic neuron death 17
    progenitors 16
    proliferation 16–17
    protective mediators 21–2
    PRRs 3
    regulation by astrocytes 145
    toxin actions 22–3
minocycline 253
    HIV dementia therapy 214
    microglia effects 22
minor cognitive motor disorder
    (MCMD) 201

clinical features 202–3
CNS escape 205
confounding illnesses 203–6
disease cofactors 205–6
onset 201–2
pre-HAART 202–3
mitochondria, dysfunction in MS 61–2
mitogen-activated protein kinases
    (MAPKs) 19
mitoxantrone 251
    MS treatment 81–2
monocyte chemoattractant protein 1
    (MCP-1) 194
monocytes, HIV-associated dementia
    146
mononuclear inflammatory cells, viral
    encephalitis 128–9
Muckle-Wells syndrome 2
multiphasic disseminated encephalitis
    103–4
multiple sclerosis (MS) 47–57
    acute disseminated
        encephalomyelitis
        differentiation 104–5, *104*
    adhesion molecules 52–3
    animal models 56
    antigen cross-presentation 87, 92
    antigen-presenting cells 49
    ATP dysfunction 61–2
    axonal connection remodeling *81*
    axonal pathology 61–3, *62*
        cortical demyelination 63–4
        immune-mediated damage *80*
    B lymphocytes 48–9
    blood–brain barrier
        damage 50
        tight junctions abnormalities 50
    CD4$^+$ T cells 89
    CD8$^+$ T cells 48, 51, 89
        demyelination 89
        neuro-immune cross-talk 79–80
    chemokines 49
    chronic lesion remyelination 60
    cladribine therapy 251
    complement cascade in cortical
        lesions 64
    cortical lesions 63–4
        gray matter/white matter 64
    cytotoxicity 51
    demyelination
        axons 61–2
        CD8$^+$ T cells 89
        cortical lesions 63–4
        ion channels 62–3
        oligodendrocyte destruction
            59–60
    dendritic cells 29–30
    dysferlin 50

multiple sclerosis (MS) (cont.)
early disease remyelination 59–60
estrogen immunomodulation 227
excitotoxicity 52
GAP-43 64
germinal center-like formations 8
glucocorticoid immunomodulation 248
glutamate 52, 62
heterogeneity 53–7
clinical implications 57
pathological 56–7
therapeutic implications 57
hypoxia 51–2
hypoxia-inducible factors 51–2
immunoglobulin oligoclonal bands in CSF 7, 8–9, 105
immunoglobulins in brain tissue 9
immunologic classification 54–6
immunomodulation 248, 249
estrogen 227
glucocorticoids 248
inflammation
remyelination promotion 60
smoldering 80–1
inflammatory infiltrates 5
interferon therapy 81–2, 248, 254
laquinimod therapy 251–2
lesion pattern types 54–6, 54, 55
animal models 56
clinical course 57
macrophages 49–50
neuro-immune cross-talk 79–80
matrix metalloproteinases 53
MHC class I expression 48
microglia 49–50
mitochondrial dysfunction 61–2
mitoxantrone treatment 251
myelin oligodendrocyte glycoprotein 48
myelin phagocytosing cells 49
natalizumab 6, 52–3, 81–2, 249–50
neuro-immune balance 79
neuro-immune cross-talk 75–82
CD8+ T cells 79–80
functional evidence 78–82
macrophages 79–80
molecular mediators 75–8
neurodegeneration 80–1
neurotrophic factors 75–6
neuromyelitis optica pathogenic relationship 58
neuroprotective therapies 81–2
nitric oxide 50–1
demyelinated axons 61–2
oligodendrocytes
apoptosis 56–7
demyelinated plaques 60–1

pathological pattern similarity to animal models 56
progression from acute disseminated encephalomyelitis 103–4
reactive oxygen species 51
remyelination 59–61, 60
chronic lesions 60
early disease 59–60
heterogeneity 61
promotion by inflammation 60
risk 104–5, 104
small molecule inhibitors 255
smoldering inflammation 80–1
statins 254
synaptophysin 63–4
T lymphocytes in lesions 47–8
teriflunomide therapy 251
tissue damage effector mechanisms 50–3
tissue inhibitors of metalloproteinase 53
tissue plasminogen activator 53
treatment 64–6, 65
vascular endothelial growth factor 50
VCAM-1 52–3
myasthenia gravis 249
plasmapheresis 249
Mycobacterium tuberculosis
CNS vasculitis 118–19
see also tuberculosis
mycophenolate mofetil 250–1
myelin-associated glycoprotein (MAG) 54
myelin basic protein (MBP) 54, 249
myelin oligodendrocyte glycoprotein (MOG) 48, 54
myelin-phagocytosing cells 49
myelin-related protein (MRP) 54

NADPH oxidase (NOX) 19–20
NALP3 2
nanoparticles 255
natalizumab, MS treatment 6, 52–3, 81–2, 249–50
natural killer (NK) cells 178
natural product inhibitors 253
Neisseria meningitidis 161
TLR activation 163–4
transcellular passage across brain barriers 42
nerve growth factor (NGF) 22
HIV-associated dementia 144
neuro-immune cross-talk in MS 76
neuro-immune balance, multiple sclerosis 79

neuro-immune cross-talk in MS 75–82
molecular mediators 75–8
neurodegeneration 80–1
neurotrophic factors 75–6
neuro-inflammation
cellular components 246–7
immunosuppressive agents 250–2
immunotherapy 247–8
innate immune response 247
new therapies 254–5
pathology 246
small molecule neuro-immune modulators 252–4
therapeutic target 245–56
neuromyelitis optica
aquaporin 4 58–9
lesions 58
MS pathogenic relationship 58
pathological heterogeneity 57–9
neurons
acute viral encephalitis 126
cell death in traumatic brain injury 185–6
HIV infection 140–1
innate immune reactions 3
loss in HIV infection 137–8, 208
MHC class I inducibility 6
neuro-inflammation 247
viral clearance 130–1
neurotransmission modulators 252
neurotrophic factors, neuro-immune cross-talk in MS 75–6
neurotrophin(s)
astrocyte production 192
HIV infection 144
innate immunity 247
microglia 22
neurotrophin 3 (NT-3) 22
neurotrophin 4/5 (NT-4/5) 76
neutropenia
G-CSF immunomodulation 223
GM-CSF immunomodulation 223
neutrophils, traumatic brain injury 188
nimodipine 211
nitric oxide 20
immunomodulation 226
MS tissue damage 50–1
nitric oxide synthase, inducible (iNOS)
astrocytes 21
malaria 178
microglia 19, 20
minocycline actions 22
MS lesions 50–1
NOD proteins 164
NOD-like receptors (NLRs) 2
bacterial meningitis 164

non-Hodgkin's lymphoma 119
non-steroidal anti-inflammatory drugs
(NSAIDs) 252
nuclear factor-κB (NFκB) 3

occludin 50
oligodendrocyte progenitor cells
(OPCs) 60
oligodendrocytes
acute viral encephalitis 127
apoptosis in MS 56–7
destruction in demyelination in MS
59–60
MS demyelinated plaques 60–1
neuro-inflammation 247
OPC-14117 212
opiates, minocycline effects 23
Orthomyxoviridae
immunomodulation 231

Papoviridae immunomodulation
229–30
Paramyxoviridae immunomodulation
230–1
paraneoplastic cerebellar
degeneration 88
paraneoplastic neurologic
degeneration 88
CD8+ T cells 88
neuronal degeneration 90
Purkinje cells 88
parasitic infections 173–9
immunomodulation 232–3
neuro-inflammatory injury 174
parasitized red blood cells (PRBC)
capillary obstruction 177
sequestration 173, 175–6
Parkinson's disease,
neurodegeneration 17
pathogen-associated molecular
patterns (PAMPs) 1–2
cerebral malaria 176–7
pathogens
access to CNS 35–42
BBB crossing 35–7
entry across brain barriers 41–2
immunological response 221
paracellular crossing of BBB 42
pattern-recognition receptors (PRRs) 1
CNS cells 3
innate immune response activation
in bacterial meningitis 163–4
recognition of self 2–3
types 1–2
PECAM-1, leukocyte migration across
BBB 40
peptide immunomodulation 250
peptide T 212

peptidoglycans 163–4
peripheral immune system, CNS
communication 7
peroxisome proliferator activator
receptor-gamma (PPAR-
gamma) 226
peroxynitrite 19–20
bacterial meningitis 166
pharmacological agents
delivery 255
immunomodulation 222–7
see also immunomodulators;
immunosuppressive agents;
named drugs
phosphodiesterase inhibitors 254
Picornaviridae immunomodulation
232
plasmapheresis 249
acute disseminated
encephalomyelitis 102
Plasmodium 173
Plasmodium berghei ANKA (PbA)
177–8
Plasmodium falciparum erythrocyte
membrane protein 1
(PfEMP1) 176
platelet-activating factor (PAF)
antagonists 212–13
polyarteritis nodosa, CNS vasculitis
119–20
potassium channel K$_v$1.3 18
potassium channels, MS
demyelination 62–3
primary angiitis of the central
nervous system (PACNS)
109–16
associated with VZV infection
114–15
atypical 113–14
brain biopsy 114, 121–2
cerebral angiography 121
cerebral vasoconstriction 113
clinical subsets 110–16
conditions mimicking 110,
116–22
diagnosis 120–2
diagnostic criteria 109–10
disease activity monitoring 122
infections 118–19
mass lesions 113–14
neuro-imaging 120–1
reversible vasoconstrictive disease
states 116–18
differential diagnosis 118
spinal cord involvement 113
see also granulomatous angiitis of the
central nervous system
(GACNS)

prinomastat 253
progressive multifocal
leukoencephalopathy
immunomodulation 229–30
natalizumab-induced
249–50
proteolipid protein (PLP) 54
P-selectin 249–50
CD4+ T cell migration 246
P-selectin glycoprotein ligand
(PSGL-1) 38
Purkinje cells
apoptosis 17
paraneoplastic neurologic
degeneration 88

quinolinic acid, HIV-associated
dementia 146–7

rabies
immunomodulation 231
murine model 222
TLR immunomodulation 226
reactive oxygen species (ROS)
innate immunity 247
malaria 178
meningitis 166
MS 51
NOX 19–20
traumatic brain injury 186
retina, cerebral malaria 175
Retroviridae immunomodulation
231
reversible vasoconstrictive disease
states (RVDS) 116–18
angiography 116
clinical features 117–18
diagnosis 118
disease activity monitoring 122
laboratory tests 117
neuro-imaging 117
primary angiitis of the central
nervous system differential
diagnosis 118
treatment 118
Rhabdoviridae immunomodulation
231
rheumatoid arthritis, TNF-alpha
immunomodulation
225–6
Rho-coiled-coil-containing
protein kinase (ROCK)
253
Rho-GTPases 253
RIG-I-like receptors (RLRs) 2
rituximab 250
RNA viruses, acute viral
encephalitis 125

sarcoid vasculitis of CNS
115–16
selectins
acute disseminated
encephalomyelitis 98
CD4$^+$ T cell migration 246
experimental autoimmune
encephalomyelitis 38
see also P-selectin
selegiline 211–12
selenium 213
sepsis, IL-1 immunomodulation 223
septicemia, TNF-alpha
immunomodulation 225–6
sequestration in malaria 174–6, 175
parasitized red blood cells 173, 175–6
receptors 176
signaling inhibitors 253
Sindbis virus 230
SIV infection, viral spread to CNS
131, 132
small molecule inhibitors 255
small molecule neuro-immune
modulators 252–4
sodium channel Na$_v$1.6 18
sodium channels, MS demyelination 62–3
spermine 23
St Louis encephalitis 230
statins 226
MS therapy 254
steroids see glucocorticosteroids
stiff man syndrome 133
Streptococcus pneumoniae 161
crossing BBB 42
invasion through BBB 162
NOD proteins 164
TLR activation 163–4
subacute sclerosing panencephalitis
(SSPE) immunomodulation
230–1
cimetidine 226
subarachnoid space, bacterial
survival 162
synaptophysin, MS cortical
lesions 63–4
systemic vasculitides 119–20

T cell receptor (TCR) ligands 250
T lymphocytes
adaptive immune reactivity 5
in CNS 5
dendritic cells 31
HIV infection 139
malaria 177–9
migration through BBB 5–6,
38–9, 247
cerebral malaria 177–8
MS lesions 47–8

survival in CNS 130
viral encephalitis 128–9
see also T-helper (Th) cells
tat fusion proteins 255
HIV infection 209
teriflunomide 251
tetracycline 253
T-helper (Th) cells 47
immunoglobulin rearrangement in
CNS 9–10
thrombin, microglia activation 18–19
thymectomy 249
tight junctions, BBB endothelial cells
35–6
tissue inhibitors of metalloproteinase
(TIMP) 53
tissue plasminogen activator
(t-PA) 53
TMEV murine infection, detrimental
adaptive immunity 132–3
tocluzimab 224
Togaviridae immunomodulation 230
tolerance
HIV-associated dementia 146–7
TLRs 3
toll-like receptors (TLRs) 2
bacterial meningitis 163–4
brain pathology modulation 4
cerebral malaria 176–7
immunomodulation 226
microglia 3
recognition of self 2
tolerance role 3
Toxoplasma gondii (toxoplasmosis)
crossing BBB 42
IL-12 immunomodulation 224–5
toxoplasmic encephalitis 232
transforming growth factor beta (TGF-
beta) 193
traumatic brain injury (TBI) 185–95
amyloid precursor protein
deposition 185–6
astrocytes 188
astrogliosis 192
biochemistry 186
cerebral edema 186
chemokines 193–4
classification 185–6
cytokines 188–93
detection 194
hypoxia 186
IL-1 189–90
IL-6 191–2
IL-8 193–4
IL-10 193
inflammation 187–8
ischemia 186
macrophages 187

MCP-1 194
neuronal cell death 185–6
neutrophils 188
reactive oxygen species 186
secondary damage 186
TGF-beta 193
TNF-alpha 190–1
Trojan horse mechanism, BBB crossing
41, 42
tropomyosin receptor kinase (Trk)
family 22
tuberculosis
CNS vasculitis 118–19
immunomodulation 228
IL-12 224–5
meningitis 228
tumor necrosis factor alpha (TNF-
alpha) 20–1
animal models of inflammation
190–1
bacterial meningitis
immunomodulation 227, 228
inflammatory response 164–5
cerebral edema 190
diffuse axonal injury 190
immunomodulation 225–6
malaria 232
meningitis 227, 228
malaria 178
immunomodulation 232
rabies vaccine 222
receptors 191
traumatic brain injury 190–1
tumor necrosis factor alpha (TNF-
alpha) inhibitor 213
tumor necrosis factor (TNF) gene
family 8
tumor necrosis factor receptors
(TNFRs) 20–1

vaccines 222, 255
valproic acid 213
varicella zoster virus 229
CNS vasculitis 118–19
granulomatous angiitis of the central
nervous system differential
diagnosis 112
neurovascular syndrome 114–15
primary angiitis of the central
nervous system association
114–15
vascular cell adhesion molecule 1
(VCAM-1)
choroid plexus epithelium 41
HIV infection 142
MS lesions 52–3
vascular endothelial growth factor
(VEGF), MS lesions 50

vasculitis, CNS
  granulomatous *112*
  infections 118–19, *119*
  lymphocytic *114*
  malignancy-associated 119
  mononuclear inflammatory
    infiltrate *115*
  sarcoid 115–16
vasculitis, systemic 119–20
vasoactive intestinal peptide
    (VIP) 250
verapamil, reversible
    vasoconstrictive disease
    states 118
viral clearance
  acute viral encephalitis
    129–5
  dendritic cells 31

viral encephalitis, acute 125–34
  adaptive immune response
    activation 128–9
    detrimental 132–3
  animal models 126, *127*
  antigen presentation 129
  apoptosis 130
  B lymphocytes 128–9
  causes *126*
  cellular targets 126–7
  immune response
    antigen-specific humoral 133
    induction 127–8
    injurious innate 131–2
    local 129–30
    neuropathology generation 131–3
  immune-mediated clearance
    mechanisms 130–1

  interferon response induction 127–8
  microglial cell immunoregulatory
    effects 129–30
  mononuclear inflammatory cells
    128–9
  T cell survival in CNS 130
  T lymphocytes 128–9
  viruses causing 125–6
viral infections, immunomodulation
    229–32
vitamin D immunomodulation 227
vitamin E immunomodulation 227, 252

West Nile virus 230
  stiff man syndrome 133

zidovudine 210–11
zonula occludens (ZO1) 50